Infectious Lesions of the Central Nervous System

Vsevolod Zinserling

Infectious Lesions of the Central Nervous System

Springer

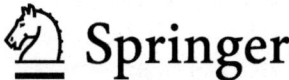

Vsevolod Zinserling
Institute of Experimental Medicine
Almazov National Medical Research Center
Saint Petersburg, Russia

ISBN 978-3-030-96262-3 ISBN 978-3-030-96260-9 (eBook)
https://doi.org/10.1007/978-3-030-96260-9

This Springer imprint is published by the registered company Springer Nature Switzerland AG
The registered company address is: Gewerbestrasse 11, 6330 Cham, Switzerland

Introduction

According to WHO, every year 2 million people suffer from infectious diseases, while 17 million of them die. Currently, infectious diseases are spreading across the planet much faster than before. In addition, since 1970, at least one new infectious disease has been reported every year. A new coronavirus infection turned out to be very significant for the whole world. Among the various clinical, epidemiological, pharmacological, and molecular biological approaches, morphological methods are in the shadow. In the manual "Infectious Pathology of the Respiratory Tract," we were able to fill partially this gap, including, along with numerous practical materials, general approaches to the study of infectious pathology that have developed in the Russian scientific school. This book continues the planned series of publications.

The history of the study of neuroinfections can be traced back to the drawings of changes characteristic of polio in ancient Egyptian papyri. However, there are very few modern summarizing works devoted to these issues in the world literature. Especially noticeable is the lack of research on morphological aspects. Studies concerning the morphology of neuroinfections are very sparsely presented in the periodical literature, Internet resources, and materials of international congresses on pathology, neuropathology, neurology, and infectology.

Many of the current infections can cause brain damage: meningococcal, pneumococcal, Mycobacteria tuberculosis, syphilis, herpes, HIV, covid-19, tick-borne encephalitis, poliomyelitis, and some other diseases with well-studied etiology and clinical and morphological changes. Nevertheless, complete statistical data related to morbidity, mortality, and lethality due to brain lesions in them is absent and many important issues still remain unclear.

At the same time, there are many pathogens, about the diseases by which we do not have any statistical data, nor accurate information about the pathogenesis and structural changes: influenza, intrauterine encephalitis, chlamydiosis, mycoplasmosis, etc. Data on mixed etiology of brain lesions is extremely scarce.

Data on the possible role of biological pathogens for the development of many noninfectious processes have been obtained: schizophrenia, Alzheimer and Parkinson diseases, ischemic insults, autism, migraine, and disorder of consciousness, but the views of the investigators are controversial. We present our own and literary data that infectious factor cannot be ignored.

The fact that the brain is an immunoprivileged site of the body is widely known, but there is evident lack of important details concerning its defense mechanisms, especially of their structural equivalent. Many aspects of relations between pathogen and brain matter, including its maturation, stay undescribed especially in chronic process.

This manual summarizes the long-term clinical, pathological, and experimental observations of the author and his staff, carried out over several decades in Leningrad/Saint-Petersburg, Russia, in the V.A. Almazov Research Center, the S. P. Botkin Clinical Infectious Hospital, Medical Faculty of St. Petersburg University Pediatric Medical Institute/Academy/University at the Department of Pathological Anatomy, Research Institute of Children's Infections, the Research Institute of Medical Mycology, the Research Institute of Phthisiopulmonology, together with many specialists of various profiles. As coauthors of individual chapters, some specialists who study in-depth certain issues are involved. Thus, Y.R. Zyuzya made an essential contribution in the chapter devoted to tuberculosis and syphilis (Chaps. 13 and 14) and provided numerous excellent illustrations for other diseases. YI Vainshenker made an outstanding contribution in Chap. 17 presenting “hidden” encephalitis in prolonged disorders of consciences basing on her long-term special studies. Chapter 20 (Some Noncommunicable Diseases of the Central Nervous System with a Possible Infectious Etiology) was written with efficient collaboration of V.A. Orlova, I.I. Mikhailova, A.A. Garbuzov, D.A. Khavkina, P.V. Chukhliaev, T.A. Ruzhentsova I. L. Naidenova, A. B. Danilov, A.V. Simonova, E. G. Filatova, I. A. Pavlovsky, O. V. Bystrova, A.M. Zatevalov, S.L. Bezrodny, and T.Sh. Sadekov.

The author is also grateful to his colleagues (N.A. Lugovskaya, A.N. Isakov, and V.E. Karev) who provided a number of illustrations from their observations. We also set ourselves the task of providing fairly complete information on the issues under consideration from the modern literature.

Clinical experience confirms the old aphorism "Qui bene diagnoscit, bene curat" (who diagnoses well, treats well); we considered it right to dwell in detail on the issues of etiology, pathogenesis, and clinical, laboratory, and morphological diagnostics.

We hope that the data provided in the manual will be of interest to doctors of various specialties: neurologists, neuropathologists, infectious diseases specialists, internists, pediatricians, psychiatrists, radiologists, pathologists, and forensic medical experts, including those working in nonspecialized institutions. We look forward to all constructive suggestions and critical comments.

Contents

1 Microbiology and Molecular Biology in Diagnostics

The importance of an accurate laboratory verification of the etiology of infectious lesions on both clinical and morphological materials is difficult to overestimate, especially in connection with the emergence of modern possibilities of dexiotropic therapy [1–4]. Our general views on infectious disease pathology have been formulated previously [5]. It is obvious that, taking into account the peculiarities of the tissues located behind the blood-brain barrier (BBB), virological, bacteriological, and molecular biological research should primarily be carried out on materials obtained from the area of the assumed infectious process. At the same time, a number of objective and subjective circumstances lead to the fact that, in practice, this rather elementary principle is often violated. The most accessible and quite informative object of research is cerebrospinal fluid (CSF) obtained in patients with lumbar puncture and in infants with fontanelle puncture. The contraindication for their implementation is pronounced brain edema with a threat of dislocation or the beginning of its implementation. At a clinical autopsy, it is also strongly recommended to take cerebrospinal fluid for laboratory tests. Technically, it is most convenient to do this with a pipette from a large tank at the time of the extraction of the brain, trying as much as possible to ensure possible sterility and at the same time to prevent the mixing of the liquor with blood. Theoretically, CSF fluid can be subjected to all currently known laboratory tests. In this chapter, we give a brief overview of those in which we have our own many years of positive experience.

- Isolation of viruses according to classical virological methods, including developing chicken embryos and a variety of cell cultures. The effectiveness of this method against many viruses is quite low, which can be explained by both objective (a relatively small number of viral particles, the possibility of the presence of various inhibitors) and subjective (insufficient use of cell culture sets and insufficient number of passages) reasons. It should be noted that the isolation of viruses from CSF, as well as from other materials, is currently rare for a variety of reasons.
- Determination of interferon and its individual subpopulations (viral, immune).
- Determination of antiviral antibodies in the complement-binding reaction. It is necessary to note our long-term positive experience of such diagnostics on autopsy material; it is obvious that the detection of antibodies in the titer of 1:20 can be considered diagnostic. Titers above 1:80 in the study of this material are extremely rare.
- Bacteriological cultures using a wide range of nutrient media. In the study of CSF, the cultures on blood, chocolate, and whey agar are regulated. It should be noted that despite the sterility of the CSF in the norm, the seeding of

V. Zinserling, *Infectious Lesions of the Central Nervous System*,
https://doi.org/10.1007/978-3-030-96260-9_1

any microorganism in it does not yet clearly indicate that it is the causative agent of the disease. It is a well-known phenomenon that a number of microbes under the influence of therapy and/or the protective mechanisms of the central nervous system begin to seed with difficulty while maintaining their etiological role. This applies primarily to *Neisseria meningitidis*. In the terminal period, there is a significant increase in the permeability of the blood-brain barrier, leading to the fact that postmortem CSF is relatively rarely sterile. As a result, in practice, we had to deal with observations when, in the clinical picture of meningococcemia, pneumococcus was isolated from the CSF during postmortem bacteriological examination. The presumed diagnosis of pneumococcemia was abandoned only after an in-depth study of the biological properties of this strain, which turned out to be apathogenic:

- The bacterioscopy of the liquor sediment (and in the case of the examination of the sectional material and smears from the soft meninges) can be quite informative. At the same time, it should be remembered that the morphology of almost all microorganisms in the conditions of the infectious process and treatment is quite variable, and they can only vaguely resemble classical drawings in atlases and smears of pure cultures. As the most striking example, we should mention the *Hemophilus influenzae* bacillus, which in clinical practice often bacterioscopically looks quite like large gram-negative polymorphic cocci. Gram staining also does not always give the expected clear, unambiguous results. The clearest results can be obtained by applying a methylene blue stain. For direct microscopy, the smears are filled with 1–2 drops of ink, against which encapsulated yeast cells are detected. The capsule does not miss the carcass particles and forms characteristic rims. The sensitivity of CSF microscopy with ink staining is 40–70%. The spectrum of nosological forms under consideration is limited to meningococcal and pneumococcal purulent meningitis, viral and mycotic meningoencephalitis, rabies, toxoplasmosis, and amebiasis.
- There is a small positive experience of immunofluorescence diagnostics of a number of microorganisms (pneumococci, meningococci) in the sediment of the cerebrospinal fluid, including in those observations in which they were no longer seeded. The widespread adoption of this method in practice is limited by both the lack of commercial sera and the possibility of frequent intersections between pathogens. In addition, it should be remembered the exceptional ability of staphylococci to nonspecifically adsorb all known diagnostic sera, which in conditions of frequent neglect of controls is fraught with the danger of erroneous conclusions.
- Cytological studies of stained CSF smears are also very promising, especially in clinical practice [6]. For their preparation at low cytosis, ultracentrifugation is the most optimal. Unfortunately, currently this method is rarely used, almost exclusively for the diagnosis of tumors.
- The cerebrospinal fluid can also be a substrate for other additional methods of bacteriological diagnostics, including the so-called rapid diagnostic methods: RAL (latex agglutination reaction) for detecting the antigens of a number of bacterial agents.
- Modern molecular biological methods, primarily polymerase chain reaction (PCR), can also be successfully used to detect a number of viral, bacterial, mycoplasma, and fungal pathogens in the CSF. Currently, several companies commercially produce kits for the diagnosis of many infectious antigens. Systems for dot hybridization are now much less common.
- Recently, there have been very encouraging data on the possibility of using mass spectrometry based on the determination of the unique protein spectrum of different pathogens for the detection and identification of various microorganisms. At the same time,

high specificity and speed and economy are achieved. Existing methods and devices are aimed at working with pure cultures of bacterial and mycotic pathogens, but there are prospects for their detection directly in tissues.

A more limited number of methods can be used for the laboratory study of materials from the brain, which can be obtained both by autopsy and by taking a biopsy. Among them, we should mention (a) virus isolation, (b) determination of interferon, and (c) bacteriological studies. The bacterioscopic and IF examination of smears is possible. In our experience, smears are most informative only in cases when they are taken at the autopsy by the pathologist himself, smears prints are made from an unidentified surface of a piece of brain tissue by a laboratory virologist, or the bacteriologist does not carry positive information. It is always most advisable to examine smears prints from various areas of the soft meninges. In clinical practice, the diagnostic value is also traditionally attached to the determination of glucose and electrolytes. A laboratory examination of the CSF and brain is preferably carried out in conjunction with the study of blood and other available objects by similar methods, which allows for a deep analysis of each observation. The final etiological diagnosis is established only on the basis of a comprehensive analysis of all laboratory, clinical, and, in some cases, morphological data. It is not excluded that the final judgment about the cause of brain damage will be different from the result of any laboratory study. Therefore, in our practice, there was a case when the diagnosis of herpetic meningoencephalitis (with complete noncharacteristic structural changes) was not made despite the isolation of the herpes simplex virus from the brain tissue. It should also be borne in mind that, in some cases, with purulent neuroinfections, it is possible to form a "block" in the upper part of the spinal canal, which leads to a sad fact for the clinical diagnosis that the indicators obtained during puncture do not correspond to the true state of the soft membranes of the brain and the hypodiagnosis of purulent meningitis.

In the modern literature [7] are presented different molecular assays such as polymerase chain reaction (PCR), including multiplex, isothermal amplification, deoxyribonucleic acid (DNA) microarrays, in situ hybridization, and next-generation sequencing. Among the mentioned methods revealing host response are antigenic enzyme-linked immunosorbent assays (ELISA) and luciferase immunoprecipitation system (LIPS). The most common approaches are bead-based assays for the detection of cytokines and chemokines, which indicate immune activation consistent with infection, which can be used for insights into pathogenesis and prognosis, for indications of genetic differences underlying innate and adaptive immunity, and as biomarkers for viral reactivation. It was also elaborated the biomarker discovery platforms that quantitate levels of specific host ribonucleic acid (RNA) populations in tissues and body fluids through the use of microarrays or RNA sequencing (transcriptomics), host proteins (proteomics), or products of metabolic processes (metabolomics) through mass spectroscopy. These methods should allow the integration of large data sets to gain insights into the impact of environmental perturbations on function at the level of individual cells, organs, or entire organisms. These insights have the potential to lead to new treatment strategies in the future.

It should also be noted that without the joint work and participation of virologists, bacteriologists, and molecular biologists, who have the ability to use modern adequate methods, progress in solving many fundamental questions about the pathogenesis of infectious brain lesions that remain mysterious to this day would be impossible.

References

1. Kradin RL, editor. Diagnostic pathology of infectious diseases. Elsevier; 2018. p. 698.
2. Procop GW, Pritt BS, editors. Pathology of infectious diseases. Elsevier; 2015. p. 706.

3. Hofman P. Infectious disease and parasites. Springer Reference; 2016. p. 343.
4. Schmitt BH. Atlas of infectious disease pathology. Springer; 2017. 255
5. Zinserling VA. Infectious pathology of the respiratory tract. Springer; 2021. ISBN 978-3-030-66324-7
6. Torzewski M, Lackner KJ, Bohl J, Sommer C. Integrated cytology of cerebrospinal fluid. Berlin-Heidelberg: Springer Verlag; 2008. p. 93S.
7. Lipkin WI, Hornig M. Diagnostics and discovery in viral central nervous infections. Brain Pathol. 2015;2s5:600–4.

2 Defense Mechanisms and Local Immunity of the Brain

2.1 Blood-Brain Barrier: Structural and Functional Features

Ideas about the blood-brain barrier (BBB) began to form in the early twentieth century, and the term itself was first proposed by L.S. Stern and R. Gauthier in 1921. Since then, a number of both physiological and morphological works have been devoted to this issue. It should be emphasized, however, that the vast majority of researchers have studied its permeability to dyes, various biochemical substances, and drugs in normal conditions in various animals and humans. There is practically no work devoted to BBB in conditions of infectious pathology. The issues of BBB formation in ontogenesis are also poorly studied. The most complete summary of modern ideas about the BBB is given by S.A. Dando et al. [1].

It is customary to distinguish three major divisions of the BBB: hemato-cerebral (hemato-neuronal), hematoliquor, and cerebrospinal fluid-encephalic. In addition, the arachnoid and soft meninges also participate in the formation of the BBB.

The blood-brain barrier is also heterogeneous in different parts of the brain. It includes the capillary endothelium, the basal lamina, and the underlying glial cells. It is distinguished by its special structure in the area of the area postrema, the hillock of the hypothalamus, the epiphysis, and the pituitary gland (Fig. 2.1).

In most parts of the brain, the main barrier function is attributed to the capillary endothelium, which is characterized by the absence of both external and intracellular fenestrations and perforations. In the area of intercellular junctions, dense contacts are determined, although the possibility of their structural lability is noted. The state of brain capillaries and their polarized microvascular endothelial cells are responsible for BBB structure and functional integrity because of their tight junctions (Tjs). Some substances, in particular leukotrienes (LT), C4, D4, E4, can lead to the weakening of tight contacts, causing the contraction of individual endothelial cells. Under the endothelium is a solid three-layer basal plate of considerable thickness (up to 40–80 nm). In its dublicature may be located processes of the pericytes. The basal plate varies in thickness and is not always homogeneous. In its composition, at least five main components are determined: type IV collagen, laminin (which includes type 1 and type 2), proteoglycan, entactin, and fibronectin. It is interesting to note that the chains of $\alpha 2$ laminin 2 (merosin) are present only in the basement membrane of the central nervous system (CNS) but not in the peripheral nervous system. The bodies or, more often, the processes of astrocytic glial cells are attached to the basement membrane. The processes of astrocytes are separated by intercellular slits, forming an extracellular space (in the old literature called the Virchow-Robin space). The reality of the

V. Zinserling, *Infectious Lesions of the Central Nervous System*,
https://doi.org/10.1007/978-3-030-96260-9_2

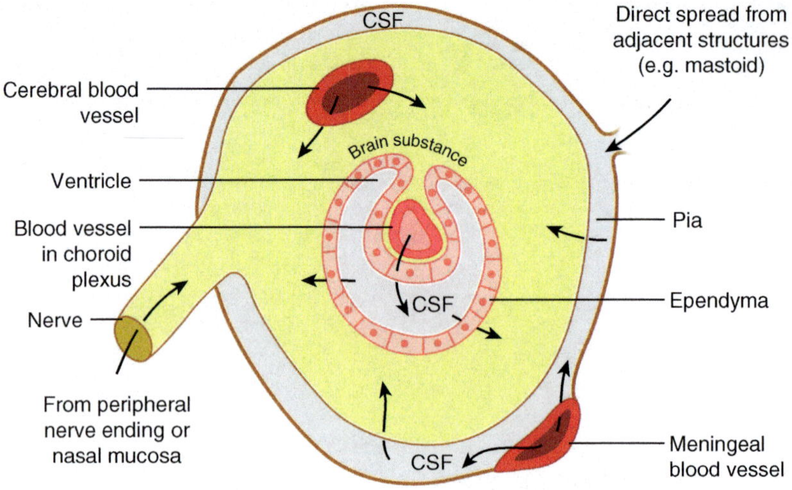

Fig. 2.1 Schematic overview of blood-brain barrier and possible ways of pathogen entry

existence of this space has been debated in the morphological literature for decades; some authors considered it as an artifact, and now it is recognized by almost all researchers. According to various estimates, the extracellular space accounts for 5–20% of the brain mass. Between the legs of astrocytes, as a rule, in the distal parts, there are also tight contacts, which allow us to speak of a perivascular glial coupling. The role of perivascular gliocytes is considered insufficiently studied.

In the areas of the area postrema, hypothalamus, epiphysis, and neurohypophysis, the fenestrated endothelium of the capillaries is described. The fenestras are closed by a very thin diaphragm with a hole in the center. Between the endothelial cells and the perivascular space lies the basal plate. The second basal plate separates the perivascular space from the processes of astrocytes. In the perivascular space, collagen fibers and fibroblasts are detected. It is believed that the described fenestras are necessary either for neurosecretion or chemoreceptor function (area postrema).

The BBB in the area of the vascular plexus is represented by cells of a specialized epithelium, on the surface of which microvilli and rare cilia are determined. Dense contacts are determined between the cells, mainly near the apical ends. Intercellular slits in the epithelium of the vascular plexus are closed by dense connections at the apical end of the cells and open toward the capillaries. The main function of these cells is the secretion of cerebrospinal fluid (CSF). In humans, about 500 ml of fluid is secreted in 24 h. The total surface area of the choroidal epithelium is 200 cm^2. Epithelial cells lie on a fairly thick basal plate, below which is the pericapillary space, which contains the collagen protofibrils. Endothelial cells are fenestrated.

The wall of the cerebral ventricles is lined with flattened ependymal cells, which also have microvilli and a few cilia on their surface. Below are the basal plate and the processes of the glial cells.

At present, new data on the molecular biology of the blood-brain barrier have been obtained. The main attention of researchers is drawn to the tight and adherent junctions between endothelial cells in the brain substance. Proteins that characterize their state were studied: claudin-5, occludin, JAM (junctional adhesion molecule, contact adhesion molecule), cytoplasmic accessory protein, cathedrin (cadhedrin). There is interesting evidence that their expression, determined by immunohistochemistry (IHC), allows us to judge the permeability of the BBB, especially in experimental studies. However, it should be noted that there is no information in the available literature about the use of this approach in clinical infectious neuropathology.

The biological barrier surrounding the peripheral nerves is also important (Fig. 2.2). The axial cylinders are surrounded by a basal plate. Around

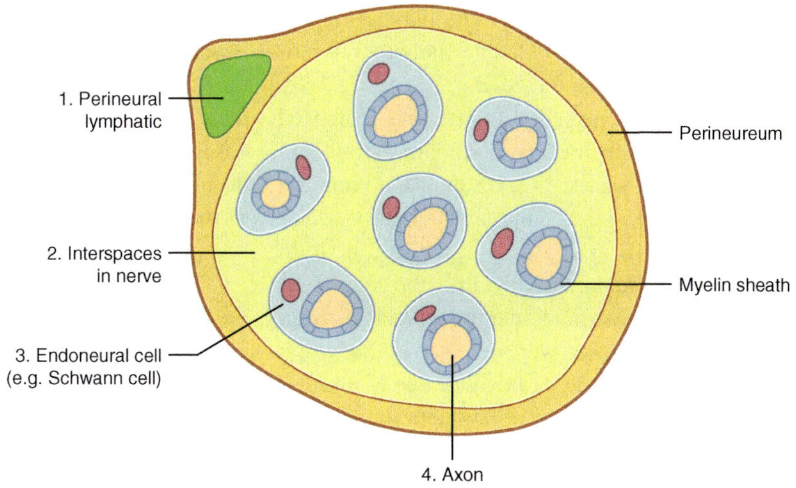

Fig. 2.2 Schema of biological barrier around peripheral nerves

them is the endoneurium, which contains collagen fibers and capillaries. The endothelial cells of the capillaries lie on the basal plates. On the outside of the nerve bundle is located three to five layers of the perineural epithelium.

Violation of BBB permeability often occurs in those places (area postrema, hypothalamus, choroidal plexus) where, due to functional necessity, there is a violation of the endothelial lining [2]. The main "barrier" load is carried by the endotheliocytes of the brain capillaries and astrocytes, which, surrounding the capillaries with processes, regulate various types of exchange between the blood and the cerebrospinal fluid. Violations of the BBB significantly increase the likelihood of (1) the penetration of infectious agents into the brain tissue and (2) the development of autoimmune processes. Many factors that damage the BBB are described. The key factors for the adhesion of white blood cells to endothelial cells (with the participation of special endotheliocyte molecules) with subsequent migration through the BBB are the proteins alpha and beta integrins. The results of a number of studies indicate that BBB dysfunction is associated with the effect of inflammatory mediators and cytokines. In particular, in Alzheimer's disease, due to certain mediators, high-molecular proteins and various components of the immune system enter the brain. Cytokines (interleukins (ILs)-1, -2, and -6 and tumor necrosis factor alpha (TNFa)) are transported to the central nervous system, produced by glial elements, and then positively affect this production (cascade), which violate the BBB. Interferon-gamma and -alpha and TNFa, by increasing the induction of adhesion molecules on endotheliocytes, play a major role in the migration of T lymphocytes to the central nervous system. Microbial antigens and their complexes with immunoglobulins (Igs), interleukin-1, leukotriene B4, and the cytokines macrophage inflammatory protein-1 alpha (MIP-1α) and macrophage inflammatory protein-1 beta (MIP-1β), produced by microglia, can serve as chemoattractants, which stimulate the migration of white blood cells through the blood-brain barrier. The role of cytokines in this respect may also be indirect: the combination of signals from different cytokines included the "migration" phenotype of lymphocytes, which under this condition significantly more actively penetrated the BBB.

Immunostimulated monocytes in the BBB model stimulated the formation of free gaps between endotheliocytes, resulting in a 20-fold increase in the number of migrating lymphocytes. Some authors note the influence of a number of other substances on the functioning of the BBB. For example, the state of laminin α-2, a protein that is part of the basement membrane of endotheliocytes and Schwann cells; the gradient of sodium bicarbonate concentrations; and the level of biosynthesis in endotheliocytes affect the transport of glucose through the BBB, and the monocarboxylate transporter can play an important role in the passage of lactate and other monocarboxylates through the BBB.

It has been repeatedly shown that increased BBB permeability occurs in inflammatory and autoimmune diseases. As a result of the violation of the integrity of the components of the vascular wall of the BBB in scrapie encephalitis, albumin penetrated more intensively into the cerebellar tissue. In experimental meningoencephalitis in mice, myelin antigens were detected in the lymph nodes. It is assumed that this was due to a violation of the BBB. Foci of inflammation and damage to the brain tissues of various etiologies can be zones of BBB violation, while the local immune system of the brain may lose its natural immunological tolerance. One of the important reasons that violate the state of the BBB is active neuroimmunization; against its background, the passage of labeled antibodies (AT) to neuroantigens in various parts of the brain sharply increases, which contributes to the emergence of a vicious circle of mutually reinforcing immunopathological processes. In addition, hypoxia, electrolyte imbalance, intoxication, microtrauma, metalloproteinases synthesized by capillary endothelial cells, astroglia, and microglia are considered as factors contributing to the violation of BBB permeability.

Currently, the factors of individual microbes that allow them to overcome the BBB are also being studied quite intensively. At the same time, the study is mainly carried out using in vitro models, which are represented by one- or two-layer cell cultures (endothelial cells with tight contacts and underlying epithelial cells). The most complete data in this regard are given in the review [2]. Thus, among the invasive proteins should be noted those of *Escherichia coli* IbeA, IbeB, AslA, YijP, and OmpA; *Neisseria meningitidis* Opc, Opa, and PilC; *Listeria monocytogenes*, InlB; *Streptococcus pneumoniae* CbpA; HIV-gp120; and Sindbis virus E2 glycoprotein.

The study of cellular receptors that bind pathogens in the structures of the BBB has also begun. For *E. coli*, this is IbeA, and for pneumococcus, it is a receptor for PAF (platelet-activating factor). For the human immunodeficiency virus (HIV), the main receptor is CD4, and additional heparin-sulfate-containing chemokine receptors CCR5 and CXCR4. It should be noted that the data obtained in model experiments can, in most cases, be considered only as preliminary, and we do not have evidence of the complete adequacy of the cell model in vitro to the real, much more complex BBB in humans.

Thus, the problem of BBB permeability is multifaceted. On the one hand, BBB dysfunction contributes to the progression (it is possible, and the occurrence) of autoimmune and chronic infectious diseases of the central nervous system; on the other hand, these diseases aggravate BBB disorders. Moreover, it is important to emphasize that the BBB is an actively functioning system, many of the capabilities of which are still unknown today.

Recently, significant clarifications have been made to the concepts of fluid circulation within the brain [3], according to which the concept of interstitial fluid (ISF) is introduced, flowing between the arteries and veins in the brain substance, actually performing the multifaceted functions of the lymphatic system absent in it (Figs. 2.3 and 2.4). The existence of the glymphatic system in the CNS is declared [4]. It should be noted that despite the obvious importance of this system both for the spread of various biological pathogens and protective facts, these aspects of the problem are not considered in these reviews.

2.2 Features of the Immune Response within the Central Nervous System

Immune response within the CNS is frequently characterized by such terms as "immunological privilege of the brain," "autonomy," and "compartmentalization of the immune response."

Nowadays, in reality, the interactions between the brain and the immune system are intensive and are based upon numerous mechanisms recently updated by R. Dantzer [4]. In this fundamental review based upon more than 250 publications, the questions related to the interaction

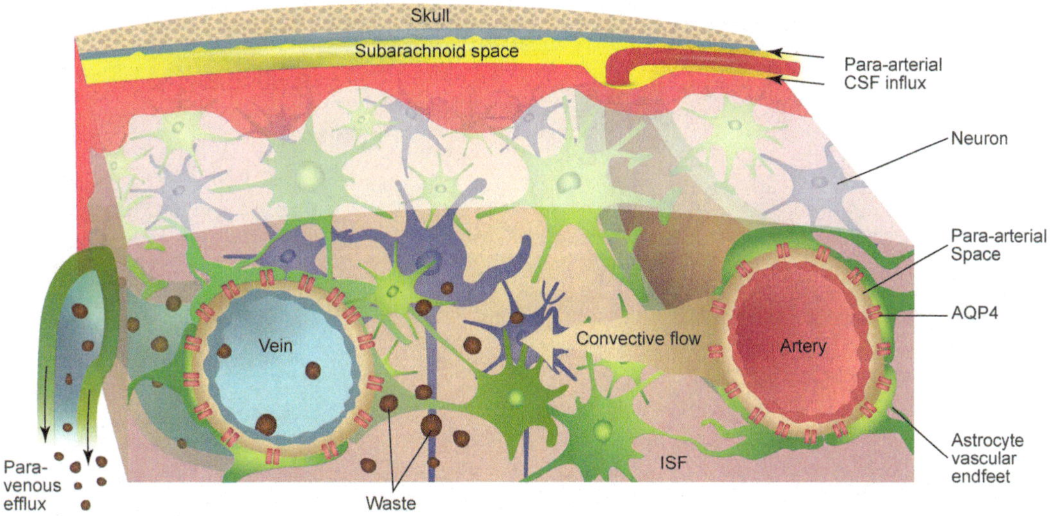

Fig. 2.3 Circulation of cerebrospinal fluid and interstitial fluid through the glymphatic pathway

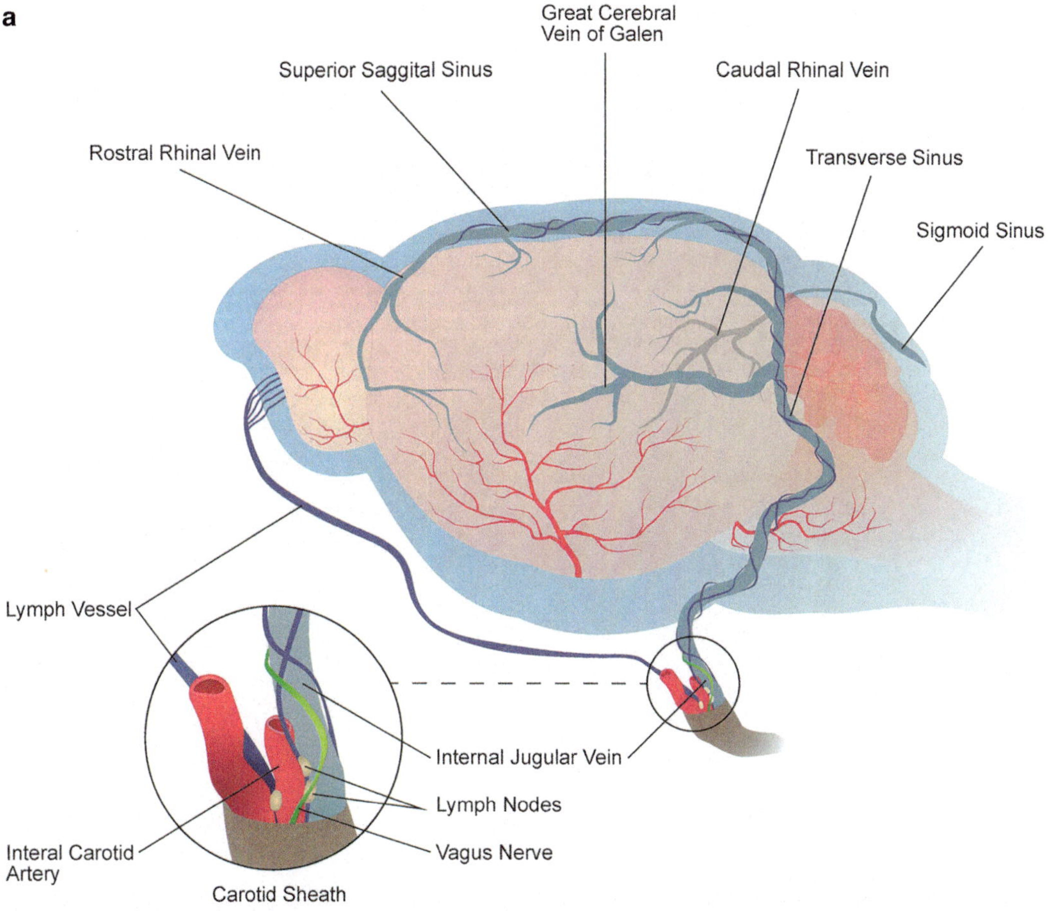

Fig. 2.4 Postglymphatic pathways. (**a**) Outflow of ISF and metabolites into the subarachnoid through the perineural spaces. (**b**) Circulation of CSF and metabolites into venous blood through arachnoid granulations protruding into the dural sinuses via lymphatic vessels and along the olfactory nerves (passing through the cribriform plate)

b

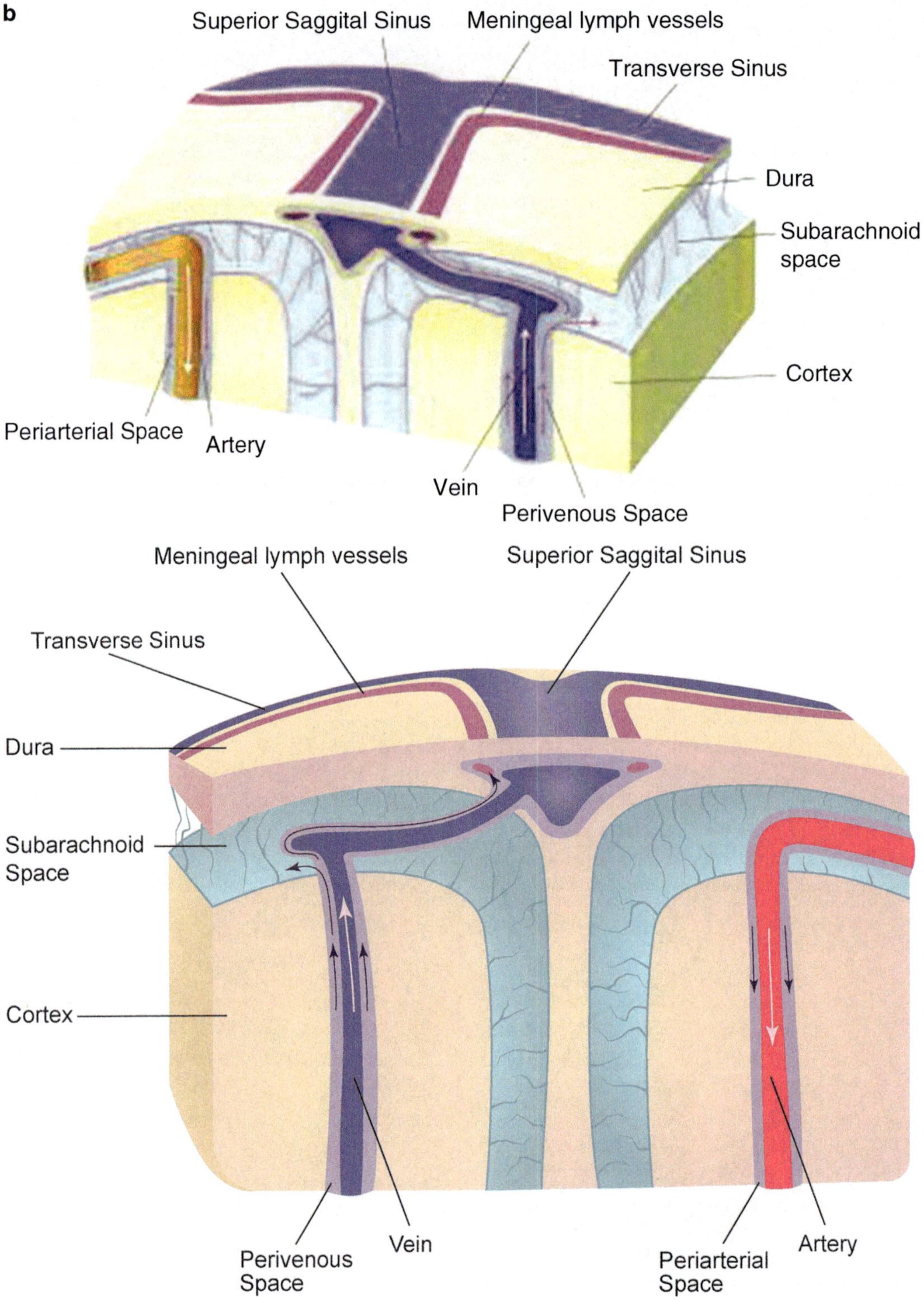

Fig. 2.4 (continued)

between the central nervous and immune systems in the course of infection are not highlighted. In Russian literature, neuroimmune interactions were, for a long time, have been successfully studied by E. Korneva and her collaborators [5].

A large number of studies are devoted to the determination of IgG and IgM in the CSF in various diseases, mainly in multiple sclerosis. Using the calculations of the ratio of the content of immunoglobulins in the blood and CSF, all authors who studied this question unanimously came to the conclusion that the local synthesis of immunoglobulins in CSF is predominant. These data were also confirmed when determining the oligoclonal origin of IgG in the central nervous system. Numerous studies of a number of neuroinfections have shown the diagnostic significance of the appearance in the CSF of specific antibodies to their pathogens in their absence or significantly lower content in the blood. Such data initially appeared in relation to herpes mumps and lymphocytic choriomeningitis.

Speaking about the antibodies contained in CSF, it should be borne in mind that the immune complexes formed by them together with the antigen do not attach any fractions of complement, as a result of which they do not have a cytolytic effect. In such conditions, there are prerequisites for the temporary inactivation of the pathogen, and the possibility, under certain conditions, of the collapse of the immune complex with the release of a viable pathogen creates, according to the same authors, conditions for the chronicity of viral brain lesions.

The exact location of the production of immunoglobulins and antibodies within the central nervous system remains unclear. In the literature, there are only isolated indications of the ability of CSF lymphocytes to produce antibodies in vitro and the presence of B lymphocytes in the CSF with ultrastructural signs of secretion. However, the correlation between the antibody content and the number of plasma cells in the CSF has not been studied by anyone. Of interest are the results of an experimental study [6], which showed on a model of meningoencephalitis caused by the Sindbis virus that T lymphocytes (mainly subpopulations of Lyt-2) appear in the soft meninges at the beginning (on the third day of infection), which are gradually replaced by macrophages and B lymphocytes by the 14th day.

There are quite numerous data on the appearance of both viral and immune interferons in the CSF during neuroinfections. The synthesis of both viral and immune interferons can also occur within the central nervous system.

In later studies, the pathogenesis of the immune response within the central nervous system was studied in more detail. A very interesting and in-depth study, which was awarded the R. Virchow Prize in 1998, was performed on a model of experimental mouse toxoplasmosis [7]. Using IHC, a fairly significant basal expression was shown in the normal brain of IL-10 and IL-1ß in the neurons of the choroidal plexus epithelial cells. Microglial cells expressed TNF-α, IL-1β, and IL-10. Under the conditions of the infectious process caused by toxoplasmas, intracerebral cytokine production increased significantly, and newly "recruited cells" also took part in it. TNF-α and IL-10 were the most widely synthesized, which were detected both in microglial cells and macrophages and in T lymphocytes carrying both CD4 and CD8 receptors. The production of IL-2 was limited to T-helpers. IL1β-a was produced by T-suppressors, microglial cells, and macrophages. Immunofluorescence (IF) was equally produced by both helper and suppressor populations of T lymphocytes. The ability of astrocytes to synthesize TNF-α under the conditions of this experiment was also shown. It was clearly shown that IF (carries the function of protection against protozoa (toxoplasmas)). TNF1 factor was also shown to be associated with a sharp decrease in the expression of INOS (inducible nitric oxide synthase) in lung and brain tissues, which in turn correlated with animal death. Under the conditions of the toxoplasma infection process, there was also a sharp activation of immunologically important cell surface molecules on the microglial and endothelial cells of blood vessel antigens of classes 1 and 2 of the large histocompatibility complex (MHC) and intercellular adhesion molecules ICAM-1, among the ligands of which can be called LFA-1 (leucocyte function-associated antigen), CD43, and LCA (leucocyte common antigen). With the help of these molecules, microglial cells can enter into direct intercellular interactions with other immunocompetent cells, primarily T lymphocytes. Interesting data were also obtained on the value of IL-10 in brain tissue, which has a pronounced immunosuppressive effect and is synthesized in nerve cells, epithelial cells of the choroidal plexus, and microglia. In conditions of inflammation, this cytokine also begins to be secreted by CD4, CD8, lymphocytes, and macrophages. The neutralization of IL-10 with a specific antiserum leads to the increased production of other protective cytokines (IL-2, IL4, IFNy, and TNF-α) and a significant decrease in the number of protozoa in the tissue. In connection with the obtained data, the author suggests that this cytokine is important for preventing damage to the central nervous system tissue due to the hyperproduction of cytokines, which stimulate the immune process, such as TNF-α, which also has a neurotoxic effect. It is obvious that these data, on the one hand, allow us to fairly accurately explain the severe course of toxoplasmosis in conditions of immunodeficiency (in particular, in HIV infection), and on the other hand, they reveal some mechanisms of intercellular interactions that provide an immune response within the central nervous system to various infectious processes.

An important role in the pathogenesis of CNS lesions in acute neuroinfections belongs to antibodies and sensitized T lymphocytes, which react with the antigenic complex formed by the interaction of the pathogen with the most important components of the nervous tissue, including peptides, myelin lipoproteins, and glycoproteins, which leads to the often observed processes of demyelination with the destruction of myelin.

There is evidence that immune complexes that have a damaging effect are deposited primarily in the choroidal plexuses, subependymal regions, and soft meninges.

In the modern immunologic literature is widely discussed the role of toll-like receptors (TLR), which are expressed in a variety of mammalian immune systems related cell types and initiate signals in response to diverse pathogen-associated molecular patterns (PAMPs). TLRs are also present in the brain, where their expression is detected in microglia, astrocytes, oligodendrocytes, and even neurons and neuronal progenitor cells [8]. It is postulated that nearby the role in the innate immune response [9] TLR are now being recognized as modulators of CNS plasticity. In the CNS, microglia express several different TLRs that, when activated by PAMPs, induce the production of pro-inflammatory cytokines, including IL-6 and TNFα. Microglia can be activated during systemic infections without BBB being compromised, suggesting that PAMPs can cross the BBB and/or activate macrophages and microglia in circumventricular organs. Alternatively, macrophages and/or circulating cytokines can pass BBB and intercept invading pathogens in the brain and/or activated microglial cells. Localized activation of TLR4 in BBB-associated macrophages/microglia can trigger a "wave" of microglial activation that spreads within the brain parenchyma; this transcellular wave of innate immune cell activation is believed to be propagated by TNFα. TLR activation can and does result in different outcomes in different types of CNS cells. When TLR3 is activated in human astrocytes, a neuroprotective is suggested. Many aspects of the problem still stay unclear.

2.3 Features of Inflammatory Reactions within the Central Nervous System

It is quite widely believed that meningitis is initially always serous with lymphomonocytic infiltration of the soft meninges, and only then, in some cases, the inflammation becomes purulent. This raises many questions already purely theoretically since the ability of neutrophilic leukocytes to respond most quickly to the appearance of pyogenic pathogens in the tissues is well known. In addition, this position is not supported by the results of many experimental studies, including our own [9]. It should be noted that in our material with meningococcal infection, it was often possible to detect changes in the soft meninges, which could formally be designated as serous meningitis. However, a comparison of the results of morphological and various virological data made it possible to link these changes to the generalization of acute respiratory viral infections (see Chap. 9).

In purulent inflammation, neutrophilic leukocytes, due to the absence of opsonins in the cerebrospinal fluid and an incomplete set of complement components, do not have bactericidal properties, starting from the second day after the onset of the disease, and when leukocytes are destroyed, their hydrolytic enzymes cause damage to brain tissue, which is associated with residual symptoms of the catamnesis. It should be noted that in the first day after infection, a large number of bacteria without neutrophil cytosis in the cerebrospinal fluid is an unfavorable prognostic sign. In the following days, an increase in the content of granulocytes in the cerebrospinal fluid correlates with damage to brain tissue.

For about 3 days, the infiltration of the meninges, venous walls, and perivenous spaces in the brain substance is predominantly neutrophilic, followed by a gradual increase in the number of monocytes, lymphocytes, and macrophages, as well as the appearance of fibrin filaments. Starting from days 5 to 7, the appearance of connective-woven fibers is also noted. It should be mentioned that, in some cases, especially in pneumococcal meningoencephalitis, along with severe sclerosis, there may be areas with delimited fresh neutrophil infiltration. The outcome of purulent meningoencephalitis is adhesive processes, fibrosis of the membranes, abscesses, and hydrocephalus.

Along with hematogenic macrophages, usually located perivascularly and referred to in the modern literature as "perivascular macrophages," related microgliocytes and "epiplex cells" lying above the choroidal plexus epithelial cells have the ability to phagocytosis.

It is obvious that cytological studies of CSF should play a leading role in the clinical characterization of inflammation within the central nervous system. However, there are very few such studies in the literature. A number of studies have shown that during serous meningitis, there is a regular change in the cellular composition of the cerebrospinal fluid. At the same time, depending on the predominant cells, the syndromes of lymphocytic, lymphoid, and mononuclear phagocytes are distinguished. The lymphocytic cell syndrome is the most favorable in prognostic terms, the mononuclear phagocyte syndrome indicates a prolonged course of the process, and the lymphoid one is accompanied by the greatest severity of general cerebral and meningeal syndromes. In relation to purulent meningitis, it was shown that after severe neutrophilosis, which is observed in all variants of the course of the disease for 2–3 days, there are some differences in the cellular composition in different courses of the disease. With a favorable course of the disease, by fifth to sixth day, there is a presence of a cross: the number of monocytes and macrophages begins to predominate over neutrophils (proliferative phase), and starting from days 9 to 10, lymphocytes become the predominant cells (reparative phase). With a prolonged course of the disease, the intersection between mononuclear cells and segmentonuclear leukocytes occurs only by days 9–10, and significant numbers of monocytes and macrophages remain predominant up to a month.

Relative to other factors involved in inflammatory reactions within the central nervous system, information is rather scarce. Thus, complement activation can occur quite quickly: for example, in mice with experimental listeriosis meningitis, the level of expression of C3 mRNA and factor B reaches a maximum within 12 h. This expression is detected in pyramidal neurons, Purkinje cells, and white blood cells that infiltrate the subarachnoid space; both tumor necrosis factor-α and other mediators can regulate this process.

Anaphylatoxin C5a may play a role in the pathogenesis of bacterial meningitis as a mediator of inflammation. Receptors for it are found in the cells of the infiltrate (in the soft meninges), some neurons. An important regulator of the expression of these receptors is tumor necrosis factor-α, in the presence of which their expression is significantly increased in both *Listeria*-infected mice and healthy mice. In addition, there are data on the role of such factors as IL-8, GROa, McP-1, MIP1a, MIP1β, and MIP-2 in the development of bacterial infection in the central nervous system. For the development of autoimmune reactions, importance is attached to such factors as MIP1a, MIP1β, NCA3, IP10, KC, VCH-3, MCP-1, and RANTES (regulated on activation, normal T-cell expressed and secreted). For the response to viral antigens, the values of IL-8, IP-10, MIP-1α, MIP1β, MCP-3, lymphotactin, C10, MIP-2, and MCP-1 are considered.

Interferons, as inflammatory mediators, play a protective role in infections. Mice deprived of the ability to synthesize interferon-γ showed severe herpetic encephalitis, both clinically and morphologically (apoptosis of neurons), while control animals in this situation suffered infection asymptomatically; a number of authors believe that interferon-γ, by inhibiting apoptosis, protects nerve tissue from viral destruction.

In viral infections within the central nervous system, IFNa, IFNß, TNFy, IL-1, IL-6, IL-15, IL-18, IP-10, McP-3, MAP-1, and fractalkin are considered inflammatory mediators; pgE2, LTB4, LTC4, and complement fractions C3a and C5a are considered proinflammatory eucosanoids. IFNß, IL-1Ra, IL-4, IL-10, LDTGF-β, eucosinoid- LXA4, and some gangliosides have anti-inflammatory effects.

It should also be noted that IL-6 and TNF have neurotrophic and neuroprotective effects.

Neuroinflammation can be studied on animal models as well. Recently, one of preferred is zebrafish (*Danio rerio*) [10].

2.4 Pathways of Pathogens Entering the Central Nervous System

Pathways of pathogens penetrating the central nervous system were recently reviewed by S.J. Dando et al. [1].

One of the most well- and early-studied pathways of pathogens (neurotropic viruses) is their penetration into nerve cells through their peripheral processes. There is evidence that infection can occur through the mechanism of retrograde axonal transport or through perineural spaces. This pathway of infection is most well studied for rabies, starting with the classic works of Louis Pasteur, which received full scientific confirmation with the help of modern methods in the second half of the twentieth century. The infected saliva of a sick animal (wolf, dog, fox), when it bites a person, promotes the entry of the rabies virus into the nerve endings, thereby creating the prerequisites for its transportation. This pathway of infection has also been studied in some detail in some variants of herpetic lesions. The place of primary replication of the virus in most cases is the skin or mucous membranes, from where the viruses neurogenically enter the peripheral ganglia, where they remain protected from the reactions of the immune system and subsequently can get through direct intercellular connections already within the central nervous system. The axonal transport ability of rabies and herpes viruses was also proven in tissue cultures of neurons, while it could be specifically inhibited both in vitro and in vivo. It is also necessary to note the unconditional ability of the herpes virus for hematogenic transport.

The possibility of neuronal transport as one of the possible ways for viruses to enter the central nervous system cannot be excluded in other encephalitis caused by neurotropic viruses and transmitted by the bite of infected arthropods. In countries with a temperate climate, this is primarily tick-borne and mosquito-borne (Japanese) encephalitis.

The hematogenic pathway of CNS infection is recognized by most authors as the leading one. The blood-brain barrier does not allow biological pathogens to enter the central nervous system directly. On the contrary, activated lymphocytes and macrophages can relatively easily pass by the BBB as, being infected with viruses (especially paramyxoviruses, lentiviruses), mycoplasmas, and chlamydia, they can act as a "Trojan horse." Other pathogens enter the central nervous system due to their ability to infect endothelial cells (transcellular penetration). In the literature, there are indications of such properties of poliovirus, Sindbis virus, Semliki forest virus, and mouse retroviruses. Another group of viruses, such as mumps and eastern and western equine encephalitis, enter the CNS due to the direct infection of the choroidal plexus stroma or by passive transport to the CSF, so that the ependymal cells of the lateral ventricles contribute to the further spread of the pathogen.

Unfortunately, for many viruses that are fundamentally able to enter the central nervous system by hematogenic means, we do not have accurate data that allow us to generalize them as "endotheliotropic and epitheliotropic." This pathway is almost the only way for pathogenic bacteria and fungi to enter the central nervous system. It should also be particularly noted that almost 100% of the pathogen enters the central nervous system during a transplacental hematogenic infection of the fetus with many viruses, mycoplasmas, and chlamydia. The exact mechanisms for overcoming the blood-brain barrier remain not fully understood.

It should be noted that one of the significant factors that increase the permeability of the BBB for bacteria is viral infections involving the central nervous system tissues, primarily the soft meninges and choroidal plexuses [2]. Damage to the BBB can occur already in the first days of inflammatory disease, for example, tick-borne meningoencephalitis, judging by the dynamics of the ratio of albumin concentrations in blood serum and CSF.

It should also be noted that primary lesions with hematogenic pathogens entering the brain may have different localizations. In the case of viruses, these may be the pia mater, choroidal plexuses, and vessels of the brain substance. With bacterial processes, the first two options have to be met. In the vast majority of cases, purulent neuroinfections begin as meningitis, although the possibility of the primary development of choroiditis, ependymatitis, and, later, meningitis should be remembered. The different sequence of involvement of brain structures in the process is of essential clinical significance since in the case of the primary development of choroiditis, there will be no meningeal symptoms in the presence of general infectious and general cerebral symptoms, which significantly complicates the diagnosis and can lead to incorrect management tactics of the patient.

A number of authors have suggested that various neurotropic viruses can enter the brain directly from the nasal mucosa through the branches of the olfactory nerve, which, as is known in its structure, is a process of the most ancient structure—the olfactory brain. This path seems quite likely when analyzing many medical histories of neuroinfections, when viral encephalitis/meningoencephalitis is actually the primary disease. Given the objective difficulties in testing this hypothesis, most authors limit themselves to theoretical reasoning. An attempt was made to study this issue in experimental intranasal infection of mice with a neurotropic strain of the influenza virus. Despite the logical structure of the work, it is not sufficiently justified to focus on the promotion of viral particles only on the basis of IF microscopy data. The trigeminal nerve can also be considered a possible portal to the brain, but no direct evidence has been published until now [1].

Another pathway of infection is occasionally mentioned in the literature to be hypothetically possible. From anatomical studies, there are contacts between CSF and lymph in the neck, which does not theoretically exclude the lymph liquor pathway of infection. However, as far as we know, there are no specific clinical, morphological, or experimental data in this regard in the literature.

Bacterial agents can enter the central nervous system in otitis media with bone destruction in the roof of the tympanic cavity through the water supply of the cochlea or the internal auditory canal, directly in traumatic brain injuries. Often, purulent inflammation of the paranasal sinuses (sphenoid, latticed) is important, followed by infection of blood clots in the sinuses of the dura mater and the transition of infection to the soft membranes and the substance of the brain.

It is obvious that in a number of exceptional situations, it is possible to get pathogens (more often we are talking about bacteria) by contact. It is possible to distinguish three groups of circumstances when there is a violation of the integrity of the cranium and the bone case of the spinal cord:

1. CNS injuries—combat injuries associated with various violent actions and accidents. The occurrence of purulent pachyleptomeningitis and/or myelitis is possible only if the patient experiences pain for several hours and there is no antibiotic prophylaxis. Infection, in principle, can also occur with a relatively small injury (crack) in the area of the base of the brain, accompanied by cerebrospinal fluid.

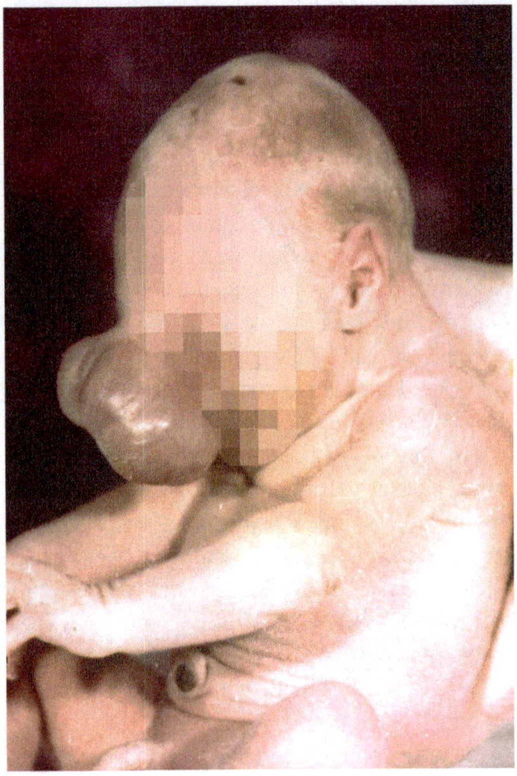

Fig. 2.5 Cerebral hernia in an infant

2. Congenital malformations, among which the most common are spina bifida, craniocerebral and spinal hernias (Fig. 2.5), and hydrocephalus—in many cases, purulent deposits, which are often the direct cause of death of children with such disorders, can be considered hospital infection, especially when trying to surgically correct the defects.
3. For neurosurgical operations.

2.5 Pathogenesis of Acute Inflammatory Reactions in the Brain

The nature of the course of acute neuroinfections is determined by various factors. First of all, it depends on the etiology as well as on the properties of a particular strain of a microorganism, the immunological reactivity of the host organism, its hereditary predisposition, its age, etc. The degree of cell damage may depend on factors such as the genetic properties of the pathogen, its virulence, and the number and functional state of CNS cells.

There are well-defined clinical and morphological criteria for distinguishing acute and chronic processes. Acute diseases include such neuroinfections that have the following characteristics:

- Acute, rapid onset.
- Distinct, including focal neurological symptoms that occur, as a rule, on the second to third day.
- Rapidly developing cerebral edema.
- Positive dynamics for an average of 1–2 months (if there is no fatal outcome).
- Certain morphological features: neuronal death, necrosis, neuronophagy, vasculitis, and a number of other changes, which will be discussed in more detail below.

In matters of pathogenesis, in particular the features of immunological reactions, the main damaging factors, the causes of tropism, and the persistence of pathogens, there are today many controversial and unclear points.

The acute course of NI is characteristic of most pathogens of a bacterial nature. However, meningoencephalitis caused by bacteria of the intestinal group, *Pseudomonas aeruginosa*, staphylococci, and pneumococci, due to various circumstances, often takes a prolonged course. Viral lesions of the central nervous system, in many cases, are also characterized by acute and chronic stages. Among them, the most important are the processes caused by herpes simplex virus, varicella zoster, measles, rubella, tick-borne encephalitis, polio, Coxsackie, and ECHO enteroviruses. For lesions caused by cytomegaloviruses, toxoplasmas, and *Candida albicans*, they are characterized by a subacute or chronic course, although in some cases it is very active. Viruses of the respiratory group (influenza, parainfluenza, and others), as a rule, cause an acute process in the brain, but a number of authors have demonstrated the possibility of their persistence in the central nervous system, and about 20% of patients after the acute phase have distinct neurological manifestations [11].

The course, nature, and topic of the lesion in acute neuroinfections largely depend on the tropism of pathogens. The clinical and morphological features of some diseases are largely due to rabies polio and tick-borne encephalitis. Most viruses are tropic to many tissues of the body, but it is believed that in the central nervous system, they specifically interact with cellular receptors, and this causes, unlike other cells, more pronounced changes [8]. The receptors identified so far relate to proteins, carbohydrate components of proteins, and lipids. Glycolipids containing sialic acid (gangliosides) are found in large quantities in the nervous tissue; they have a receptor function for rabies and influenza viruses, and the most active structures for binding viruses are gangliosides GT1b and GQ1b. For measles virus is known CD46 receptor (glycoprotein) in transgenic mice and in humans. Chemokine receptors, which are essential for the human immunodeficiency virus-1, on lymphocytes and macrophages, CCR3, CCR5, and CXCR4 can be expressed on neurons, astrocytes, and microgliocytes. A large cellular receptor for the Epstein-Barr virus, complement receptor type 2 (CR2, CD21), was found on various astrocyte cell lines. Enteroviruses can cause various forms and degrees of severity of damage to both internal organs and the central nervous system; this is due to the polymorphism of the clinical picture of enterovirus infection. The receptor for SARS CoVi2 is ACE2. Some pathogens have a tropism to the choroidal plexus, vascular walls, and meninges (respiratory viruses (RVs), rubella virus, and mycoplasma).

Pathogenetically, damage can occur, both directly related to the action of the microorganism and mediated. Damaging factors in bacteria are exotoxins and endotoxins. In particular, the enzymes that contribute to the invasion of meningococcus are hyaluronidase and neuraminidase, and the main pathogenic substance is a powerful endotoxin (lipopolysaccharide complex of the cell wall). The pathogenicity of pneumococcus is caused by cell-damaging hemolysins and leucocidin; the enzymes peptidase and hyaluronidase promote the spread of the microorganism; The M protein and capsule provide resistance to phagocytosis. The enzymes of streptococci are hyaluronidase and streptokinase (fibrinolysin), which contribute to the generalization of the process; the toxins are O-streptolysin, S-streptolysin, leucocidin, and cytotoxins. A large number of enzymes and toxins are produced by staphylococci; these enzymes include plasmocoagulase, hyaluronidase, lecithinase, and fibrinolysin, and the toxins are leucocidin, hemolysin (α, γ), and exfoliative toxins. The pathogenicity of *Hemophilus influezae* is associated with capsular polysaccharides (antiphagocytic properties) and endotoxin.

The cytopathic effect of viruses is carried out by the following mechanisms. As a result of the action of virus fusion proteins and the intense budding of viral particles, defects in the plasma membrane of the cell occur. During intracellular reproduction of virions, there occur virus-specific suppression of cell protein synthesis, destruction of lysosomes, release of enzymes and autolytic processes, as well as depletion of the cell's nutritional and energy resources. Accumulated viruses also have a mechanical effect on organelles. The spectrum of damage to brain cells after the virus has penetrated is very wide. In this case, biochemical and functional disorders are possible, as well as dystrophy, irreversible lysis, and cell death. The fact that some infected cells survive may indicate that sometimes the cell is able to suppress the transcription of the virus. Mycoplasmas, on the one hand, stimulate the synthesis of a number of cytokines (tumor necrosis factor, interleukin-6, nitric oxide) by macrophages and astrocytes in the brain of mice and, on the other hand, the formation of oxygen radicals by macrophages, which contribute to mycoplasma brain damage.

In response to infectious agents in the nervous system, immunological reactions occur, in which almost all parts of the immune system can participate: humoral and cellular immunity, interferon, and complement and macrophages.

For some acute viral encephalitis (measles, chickenpox), especially those that occur during the period of convalescence of infection, it is considered the main allergic mechanism of occurrence and progression. However, some studies have demonstrated the presence of viruses in the cells of the nervous system. It is possible that viral antigens may be a trigger in the development of immunopathological reactions. In this case, it is possible to assume the presence of a staged process: at the first stage, the action of the virus itself prevails, and then allergic mechanisms take effect. Numerous data strongly suggest the direct effect of the mumps virus on CNS tissues, which has a neurotropic effect, but most authors consider autoimmune processes to be important in the development of the disease. In this problem, it remains unclear why these viruses induce immunopathological reactions in the central nervous system, and in other organs, the outcome of infection is most often favorable. In such a situation, it is impossible to exclude the significance of a special form of persistence of agents in the cells of the nervous system and the immunological autonomy of the central nervous system violated by viruses. In acute mycoplasma encephalopathy, focal and multiple lesions of the cerebral hemispheres and cerebellum are regarded as manifestations of autoimmune reactions. After a study of patients with mycoplasma lesions of the central nervous system by nuclear magnetic resonance, it is believed that demyelination is a secondary process in relation to vascular damage. There is evidence that both processes are very significant in the pathogenesis of mycoplasmosis. The possibility of viral damage to oligodendrocytes with subsequent demyelination is also very likely, and autoantibodies play the role of "nurses."

The synthesis and activation of complements in the brain can not only play a protective role but also be important in a number of neurological diseases by damaging CNS tissues in the case of activation in an inappropriate place or appearance in increased amounts. Morphological manifestations of acute inflammatory diseases of the central nervous system are very diverse. They may depend on the etiology and underlying pathogenetic mechanisms. In some cases, all classic signs of inflammation can be found in the CNS tissues, including vasculitis, gliocyte's proliferation, in other cases the canges are limited to alterations in various cellular elements, hemodynamic disorders, and edema. Often there are changes specific to a particular pathogen.

2.6 Pathogenesis of Chronic Inflammatory Reactions in the Brain

In chronic infection, there is a persistence of a microorganism, more often a virus, with one or more symptoms of the disease, the development and maintenance of the pathological process with periods of exacerbation and remission. Latent infection is characterized by the preservation of the agent in the body with or without the production of infectious particles or by the reproduction and release of the pathogen into the external environment. A slow infection is characterised by persistence of the agent, its incubation period lasting for many months or even years, and after it slowly but steadily develops symptoms of the disease, always ending in death.

If for slow neuroinfections the etiological factors are mainly viruses and prions, for chronic and latent ones, they are almost all classes of microorganisms. At the same time, the vast majority of them can induce both acute and chronic courses. Rare exceptions are, perhaps, the human immunodeficiency virus and the cytomegaly virus in intrauterine infection; the acute period of infection caused by them is practically absent. In such a situation, it is reasonable to assume that the variant of the course depends both on the characteristics of the strain of a particular pathogen and on the reactivity of the macroorganism and its previous state.

The problem of chronic infectious lesions of the nervous system has a long history. In 1917, epidemic encephalitis (Economo) was described in 1934–1935. The scientific history of the study of slow neuroinfections began in the late forties and early fifties of the twentieth century after many years of research on mass diseases among sheep on farms in Iceland. To date, various forms of such lesions have been described in detail in both animals and humans. Neuroinfections, which can take a chronic course, are tick-borne (spring-summer) encephalitis, epidemic (Economy), Japanese (mosquito), encephalitis with HIV infection, measles, rubella, mumps, chickenpox, lymphocytic choriomeningitis, and Vilyuisk encephalomyelitis (attribution to neuroinfections is conditional). Slow neuroinfections include kuru, scrapie, Creutzfeldt-Jakob disease, amyotrophic leukospongiosis (caused by prions), multiple sclerosis, visna, subacute sclerosing panencephalitis, Aleutian mink disease, Born disease, and slow mouse influenza infection (caused by viruses or unspecified pathogens). The main areas of research of these diseases are the etiology of some clinical forms, the mechanisms of cytopathic action of microorganisms and the conditions for their implementation, the immunopathological mechanisms of pathogenesis (autoimmune, allergic), the effect of microorganisms on reactivity when they enter the host, and the causes of persistence in the central nervous system.

A chronic and slow course of neuroinfection can develop initially or after acute infection (and not necessarily with a lesion of the nervous system); in both cases, the main groups of causes of persistence are as follows:

- In the features of the central nervous system tissue, in particular, neurons with their lack of ability to divide.
- In the reactions of the immune system, a congenital or acquired immune disorder: it is appropriate to note that the interaction of micro- and macroorganisms in the form of chronic infection is not always due simply to a decrease in immunological reactivity, but it is often associated with the presence of immunopathological reactions in such diseases.
- Vital activity of the pathogens: there are many properties of microorganisms that prevent the immune system from fully performing its functions and often lead to the chronicity of the process or the development of slow NI.

In relation to the immune system, microorganisms, firstly, affect the induction of the immune response and, secondly, suppress its implementation, i.e., they evade the effectors of immunity.

Unfortunately, the details and subtle mechanisms of the development of a particular process in different people (when infected with a single agent) have not yet been largely revealed. At the same time, it should be noted that infectious diseases in the central nervous system acquire a chronic course more often than in other organs.

The features of the course of infections in the central nervous system are determined by the immunological "privilege" and anatomical isolation of the brain. This is manifested, in particular, in the possibility of local synthesis of specific immunoglobulins, cytokines, and complements; in the presence of specific receptors on brain cells in a number of microorganisms; in the great importance of autoimmune processes in the reactivity of the central nervous system; and in the tendency for persistence of pathogens of various classes (mainly viruses). Strong barriers to infection cause the relative rarity of CNS infection.

Infectious agents have a large number of components and properties that prevent them from being affected by the host's protective factors and sometimes damage these systems.

Immunodeficiency states are recognized by many authors as one of the important conditions for the persistence of pathogens in the central nervous system. It can be assumed that a variety of specific and severe immune deficits, including those that are not clinically manifested, may be important for the development of chronic and slow neuroinfections.

All known infectious agents have immunomodulatory activities to varying degrees.

Infection of immune cells with a large number of viruses able to penetrate and reproduce in them leading to the their destruction or disruption of their function. Thus, in T-lymphocytes loss of functional activity is of major importance. This situation very often leads to the establishment of persistent neuroinfections (Japanese encephalitis, herpes simplex virus (HSV), HIV). In addition, infected lymphoid cells can produce soluble immunosuppressive and immunomodulatory substances. Thus, in mice immunized with HSV, after stimulation by the same virus, a factor appears that suppresses the induction of specific T-killers, and as a result of the interaction of HSV with macrophages, factors that inhibit the production of interleukin (IL)-1 and other immune functions are secreted. A number of experimental models clearly show direct damage to the organs of the immune system (spleen, bone marrow) by HSV. The resulting immunosuppression can be specific and nonspecific, and the latter, if long-term, is accompanied by the development of a persistent infection. The suppression of the formation of virus-specific antibodies associated with damage to the function of B lymphocytes during their infection (Aleutian mink disease, visna, cytomegalovirus infection) is described.

Viruses, bacteria, and protozoa can cause a violation of numerous functions of macrophages, which often contributes to the progression and chronization of infection. In particular, there may be a violation of monocyte chemotaxis in influenza, HIV infection, and experiments on HSV I infection in animals (Immunology of the infectious process, 1993, Mims A. C. et al., 1995). In toxoplasmosis, the inhibition of attachment to macrophages and a decrease in lysosomal activity are described. The modulation of IL-I production by macrophages was observed under the influence of HIV type I and cytomegalovirus. There are many studies demonstrating ineffective phagocytosis, a toxic effect on phagocytes.

Some viruses negatively affect the immune system through mediators: either they destroy the immunocytes that produce them or inactivate the mediators after their production. This is of great importance for silt. In a number of viral infections (herpetic, influenza, rubella, HIV), in which the CNS is often involved in the process, a low level of IL is observed due to their weak synthesis or a decrease in the expression of receptors to these mediators. As a result of suppressing the secretion or blocking or weakening the sensitivity of infected cells to cytokines, the expression of human leukocyte antigen (HLA) and other immunosuppressive molecules on the surface of infected cells may decrease.

A number of viruses are able to block the action of interferon or elude it, and DNA-containing viruses are more resistant than RNA-containing ones. Blocking can be carried out by inactivating an interferon-induced virus.

2.7 Persistent Brain Lesions and their Pathogenesis

The possibility of persistent brain damage by various viruses has been known for a long time. In the literature, there is evidence of latent brain damage by herpes simplex virus, measles, rubella, and a number of other viruses. At the same time, an infectious virus (herpes for example), can be not isolated, but the viral genome detected as multiple extrachromosomal copies of DNA characterized by covalently closed rings associated with nucleosomes. The only viral RNA transcripts found in neurons during latency are latency-associated transcripts (LAT). Within the LAT sequences, open reading frames are present and proteins can be expressed. Further analysis showed that the ability to multiply in cell cultures and cause latent infections in vivo does not change in viruses with a mutation in the LAT gene. It should also be noted that most researchers have studied the reactivation of persistent viral infections in nerve cells.

Based on our material [11], 23 children were found to have an isolated brain lesion with RV or with its sharp predominance over changes in other organs (Table 2.1). These children had a coincidence of the results of an IF study of smears from meninges, serological of cerebrospinal fluid, and histological of brain, which allowed us to diagnose brain lesions caused by a certain respiratory viruses. The signs of damage due to the same virus in the lungs, as well as other internal organs, according to the results of the IF study of lung smears, serological of blood and histological either were absent (in 15 people), or were expressed to a much lesser extent (in 8 people). Among the children assigned to this group, girls predominated (16) as only seven were boys. At the age of 1–5 months, four children died; at 6–11 months, ten children; at 1–2 years, six children; at 3–6 years, two children; and at over 7 years, one child.

Most of the children (13) died from hypertoxic forms of meningococcal infection, accompanied

Table 2.1 Some results of laboratory studies of children with isolated brain lesions due to respiratory viruses

Name, initial, age	Underlying disease and its duration	IF results		Serological results		Results of histological examination[a]	
		Lungs	Meninges	Blood	CSF	Lungs	Brain
Julia S., 2 years and 10 months	Meningococcal infection, 1 day	Neg	PI3	Ad 1:80	PI3 160/80	Moderate serous desquamative pneumonia	Mononuclear infiltration, vasculitis, proliferation of ependymal cells of the lateral ventricles and choroid plexuses
Elena S., 1 year and 8 months	Encephalomyelopolyradiculoneuritis, 5 days	RS, PI, A2	B[b],	A1 80/40	B 1:80, A2 1:20	Moderate proliferation of bronchocytes	Cells with light nuclei in meninges
Elena M., 8 years	Abscess of the right hemisphere of the brain?	Neg	Ad	B40, PI 20/0	Ad 1:40	Residual changes in influenza, pillow-like proliferation of bronchocytes	Cells with enlarged hyperchromic nuclei near the abscess capsule
Ekaterina E., 10 months	Necrotic herpetic meningoencephalitis, 10 days	A3, PI	RS	A3 80/40, PI 320, HSV20	RS 80HSV 40	Residual changes in influenza, proliferation of bronchocytes	Papillary growths of bronchocytes of the cerebral ventricles
Dmitry B., 1.5 months	Toxoplasmic meningoencephalitis, 28 days	B	B, Ad	B40, A3 20/20	Ad1:40	Exfoliated alveolocytes with basophilic cytoplasm	In meninges, cells with enlarged hyperchromic nuclei

A3, B—influenza viruses A and B; Ad—adenovirus; PI—parainfluenza virus; RS—respiratory syncytial virus; HSV–herpes simplex virus

[a]Only changes associated with respiratory viruses

[b]By virological study was isolated influenza B virus from the brain. Laboratory results related to viruses causing isolated brain lesions are underlined

by Waterhouse-Friderichsen syndrome, during the first days after the onset of the disease. Purulent pneumococcal meningoencephalitis with a duration of several days to 1 month was detected in three children. Other diseases that appeared in the main diagnosis are purulent meningoencephalitis caused by group D streptococci, brain abscess, purulent meningoencephalitis with ventriculitis caused by *Escherichia*, toxoplasma meningoencephalitis, herpetic necrotic meningoencephalitis, and acute respiratory viral infection. The clinical manifestations of the disease in all deceased children were typical of the abovementioned main diagnoses, which fully fit the changes found during the clinical autopsy. As an example, we present the results of the laboratory and morphological studies of materials from five children, which allowed us to identify isolated lesions of the brain by respiratory viruses.

Most often, isolated brain lesions were associated with respiratory syncytial (RS) virus (seven cases) or adenoviruses (four cases), and one time the detected changes were caused by influenza A0 and B and parainfluenza type 3 viruses. When the brain was affected by all listed pathogens, structural changes characteristic of this etiology of the process were naturally determined (see Chap. 7). In electron microscopy (EM), the cytoplasm of the cells of the lining of the vascular plexus of one child naturally revealed single or lying in groups (2–4) rounded formations surrounded by a membrane, corresponding in structure to viral particles.

The clinical and morphological analysis revealed no significant differences during the main diseases in the children of the analyzed group compared to the course of similar diseases without isolated brain lesions of respiratory viruses. This made us analyze in detail the background states of the deceased children.

Three children were diagnosed with intrauterine generalized infections (mycoplasmosis, cytomegaly, and toxoplasmosis), and the last child was also diagnosed with severe combined primary immunodeficiency. Etiologically unencrypted perinatal encephalopathies were observed in four children. Their manifestations were delayed psychomotor development, moderate hydrocephalus, epileptiform seizures from 1.5 months, and periodic temperature rising to 39° without catarrhal phenomena (one child each). The pregnancy of the mothers of two children occurred with the threat of miscarriage—one child was born in a socially disadvantaged family. In the anamnesis of one of the children were noted repeated acute respiratory infections, including the phenomenon of false croup.

Special attention was paid to those structural changes within the brain that may be associated with the long course of the inflammatory process. Moderate meningeal sclerosis was detected in four cases, and sclerosis in the vascular plexus, partially with the appearance of psammoma bodies, was detected in four cases of varying severity. Small, mostly subependimar glial proliferation was detected in two cases. In the stroma of the choroidal plexus in one of the children with EM, viral particles were detected. Together, the above changes were completely absent in the three deceased children. An example of this group is the following observation.

Julia S., 2 years and 10 months old, became acutely ill with symptoms of acute respiratory infections. On the third day of the disease, there was a sharp deterioration in her condition. On the basis of a hemorrhagic rash, a meningococcal infection was diagnosed, and after 1 h and 45 min of hospitalization, the child died.

During the autopsy (pathology by V.A. Zinserling), the phenomena of laryngotracheobronchitis and focal bronchopneumonia were revealed. The brain weighs 1130 g. The soft medulla is edematous and cloudy. The convolutions are flattened, and the blood vessels are dilated. The lateral ventricles are slit shaped.

During the cytological examination, meningocytes and individual diplococci, similar to meningococci, predominate in the smear from the soft meninges. The smears from the lungs contain a moderate amount of neutrophils and intranuclear fuchsinophilic inclusions. IF examination of smears with MMO revealed a specific glow with serum for parainfluenza-3; serum for influenza A1, A3, and B; parainfluenza 1 and 2; adenovirus; and mycoplasma of pneumonia, and there was no lightening. In the IF study of lung smears, the results are negative.

Serological examination revealed antibodies to adenoviruses (1:80), RS virus (1:40), mycoplasma of pneumonia (1:20), and no antibodies to parainfluenza in the blood. In the serological study of CSF with serum for type 3 parainfluenza before treatment with cysteine, the antibody titer was 1:160, and after treatment, it was 1:80. No antibodies to other viruses were detected.

Histological examination revealed sharp edema of meninges; they contain a significant number of mononuclear lymphocytes with an enlarged cytoplasm. Focally lymphocytic infiltration is determined. In various parts of the brain, there are small areas of nerve cell loss and glial proliferation. The walls of almost all blood vessels are swollen, the nuclei of endotheliocytes are enlarged in size, some form small growths, and the walls and perivascular spaces are sometimes infiltrated by the cells of the lymphoid series. Vascular plexuses are sharply full blooded, and their cells are mostly dystrophic, changed, and separated from each other. Along with this, there are complexes of cells that are closely adjacent to each other and form structures that resemble "pillows." Their cytoplasm is enlarged in size and is colored basophilically. In the stroma of the choroidal plexus, there are sometimes growths of collagen fibers. Moderate pillow-like growths were also detected on the part of the ependymocytes of the lateral ventricles. Serous desquamative pneumonia was detected in the lungs, and leukocyte pneumonia was detected in some areas. The growth of alveolocytes and bronchocytes, in particular, typical for parainfluenza pincushion, could not be detected. In the parenchymal organs, there is a sharp fullness and dystrophic change.

2.8 Conclusion

The observation was generally regarded as a case of mixed infection. Meningococcal infection was the leading cause of death. Isolated changes caused by the type 3 parainfluenza virus were clearly identified among the brain lesions. Laboratory-morphological comparisons, primarily the results of the serological examination of CSF, allow us to talk about the duration of the process for at least 1 month.

In eight children who died from hypertoxic forms of meningococcal infection, the laboratory morphological analysis revealed, along with the most pronounced changes caused by RV within the brain, moderate signs of damage to the same pathogen and other organs. Among the children of this group, there were four boys and four girls. One child died at the age of 3 months, four at the age of 6–11 months, two at 1–3 years, and two at the age of 3–7 years.

The clinical course of meningococcal infection in all these children also had no significant features. Among the identified background conditions, attention was drawn to one of the children with intrauterine syphilis, another child with an unspecified perinatal infection accompanied by hypoxic encephalopathy and convulsive syndrome, and a third child who had splenectomy for nonspherocytic hemolytic anemia. Five children have a premorbid background without peculiarities.

According to the etiology, viral infections with predominant brain damage turned out to be influenza A1, influenza B, and adenovirus. In one observation, the etiology of the process, according to the conducted studies, was associated with influenza A2 and in another case mixed (adenovirus and influenza A0-swine virus). The nature of the changes caused by these viruses in the brain did not differ fundamentally from those described in the previous subgroup and later in Chap. 7.

References

1. Dando SA, Mackay-Sim A, Norton R, et al. Pathogens penetrating the central nervous system: infection pathways and the cellular and molecular mechanisms of invasion. Clin Microbiol Rev. 2014;27(4):691–726.
2. Jamil Al-Obaidi MM, Mohd Desa MN. Mechanisms of blood brain barrier disruption by different types of bacteria, and bacterial-host interactions facilitate the bacterial pathogen invading the brain. Cell Mol Neurobiol. 2018;38:1349–68.
3. Dantzer R. Neuroimmune interactions: from the brain to the immune system and vice versa. Physiol Rev. 2018;98:477–504.

4. Plog BA, Nedergaard M. The glymphatic system in central nervous system health and disease: past, present, and future. Annu Rev Pathol. 2018;13:379–94. https://doi.org/10.1146/annurev-pathol-051217-111018.
5. Korneva EA, Shanin SN, Novikova NS, Pugach VA. Cell molecular basis of neuroimmune interactions during stress. Ross Fiziol Zh Im I M Sechenova. 2017;103(3):217–29. (in Russian)
6. Griffin DE, Hess JL, Moench TR. Immune responses in the central nervous system. Toxicol Pathol. 1987;15(3):294–302. https://doi.org/10.1177/0191262338701500307.
7. Deckert- Schlüter M, Schlüter D, Theisen F, Wiestler OD, Hof H. Activation of innate immune system in murine congenital toxoplasma encephalitis. J Neuroimmunol. 1994;53(1):47–51. https://doi.org/10.1016/0165-5728(94)90063-9.
8. Okun E, Griffioen KJ, Mattson MP. Toll-like receptor signaling in neural plasticity and disease. Trends Neurosci. 2011;34(5):269–81.
9. Ransohoff RM, Brown MA. Innate immunity in the central nervous system. J Clin Invest. 2012;122(4):1164–71. https://j.c.i.me/58644/pdf
10. Ya BV, Belova AS, Bashirzade AA, et al. Models of traumatic brain injury in zebrafish (Danio rerio) Rus. Fisiol Zh im Sechenova. 2021;107(9):1059–76. (in Russian)
11. Zinserling VA, Chukhlovina ML (2011) Infectious Lesions of nervous system. Issues of etiology, pathogenesis and diagnostics. Saint-Petersburg, ElbiSPb. 583 p (In Russian).

3 Neuroplasticity and its Possible Role in Infectious Pathology

The wide prevalence of diseases that lead to disability due to brain damage makes it essential to study various mechanisms of neurorehabilitation, among which neurogenesis has recently become an important role. Neurogenesis is the process that leads to the formation of functioning neurons from neural stem cells. Over the past 20 years, a large amount of data on neurogenesis in the brain in adult animals have been obtained [1]. Despite the fact that the development of the human brain in the prenatal period has been studied quite well, the number of works devoted to the process of formation of new neurons in the adult brain is not so large. Among other things, this is due to the difficulty of obtaining brain tissue from a living person, including from patients whose disease has not ended in a fatal outcome. In addition, it is currently not sufficiently studied how functionally complete the newly formed neurons and their connections are. This chapter is devoted to the study of neurogenesis in the adult human brain. For brain development in embryos and fetuses, see Sect. 16.1.

Although in 1894S. Ramon-y-Cajal, describing the phenotype of central nervous system (CNS) cells, defined brain structures as static and unable to form new cells [2], already in 1912, proliferating cells were first demonstrated in the wall of the lateral ventricles of the brain in rats [3]. Since then, for almost 100 years, a lot of new data have been obtained. The subventricular zone and the subgranular zone of the dentate gyrus of the hippocampus are considered "traditional" neurogenic zones [4, 5]. However, most of the research has been done on animals. There are very few works performed on materials in humans today.

In 1996, the ability of adult sensorineural olfactory cells to proliferate and differentiate was first demonstrated in vitro. The olfactory epithelium was obtained from both autopsy (8–25 h after death) and biopsy materials (the maximum age of the patient is 72 years). Under the influence of neural recombinant (the main fibroblast growth factor), bipolar cells were differentiated, becoming immunopositive to some neuronal (but not glial) proteins. Using radioautography with 3H-thymidine, it was proved that these neurons appeared in vitro [6]. P. Eriksson et al. demonstrated that new neurons are formed from dividing progenitor cells in the dentate gyrus of an adult hippocampus. Division was documented using bromodeoxyuridine (BrdU), and their neuronal affiliation was documented by staining them with NeuN (nucleus neurons) and NCE (neuron-specific enolase), which were coexpressed with bromodeoxyuridine. At the same time, among BrdU+ cells, both HCE+ and NeuN+ (young neurons, about 22% of cells) and ORSM+ (glial fibrillar acid protein) cells (young astroglia, about 18% of cells) were found. No cross-reaction to neuronal and glial markers was observed; however, in all observations, there were BrdU+ cells that expressed neither glial nor

V. Zinserling, *Infectious Lesions of the Central Nervous System*,
https://doi.org/10.1007/978-3-030-96260-9_3

neuronal markers and were morphologically similar to undifferentiated cells. In addition to the dentate gyrus, the authors studied the subventricular zone near the caudate nucleus, in which BrdU+ cells were found that coexpressed neither ORSM nor NeuN, which suggested that low-differentiated progenitors were located in this zone. The study was conducted on autopsy materials from five patients suffering from squamous cell carcinoma of the root of the tongue, larynx, or pharynx without metastases to the brain. All patients received an intravenous injection of BrdU (the patients were not receiving antitumor therapy at that time) [7].

In a study by C.L. Spalding, the number of newly formed cells in the human hippocampus was estimated by measuring 14C in the deoxyribonucleic acid (DNA) of proliferating cells. Part of the hippocampal neurons appear postnatally, but 35% of the human hippocampal neurons are subject to "turnover," while in mice this figure is 10%. In the adult hippocampus, 700 new neurons are formed daily, resulting in the replacement of 1.75%. The number of newly formed neurons decreases slightly with age. The incorporation of 14C into the human body occurred through the consumption of plants containing 14C as a consequence of nuclear tests. The study was conducted on the autopsy material of patients from 19 to 92 years old. The hippocampal tissues of the nucleus cells were isolated, which were then incubated with antibodies against NeuN. Furthermore, the nuclei of neurons and cells that were not neurons were separated by flow cytometry [8].

Later, by a similar method, it was found that markers of the neuroblast site DCX (doublecortin) type and PSA-NCAM (polysialylated neural cell adhesion molecule) type are detected not only in the subventricular zone but also in the striatum. The study was conducted on autopsy material. Nuclei were isolated from the striatum by centrifugation then identified as neuronal and glial by means of antibodies to NeuN and SOX10 (HMG-box associated with SRY) and flow cytometry [9]. It should be noted that in animals, neurogenic processes in the striatum were observed relatively long ago [10].

Another neurogenic zone in animals is the olfactory bulb (as part of the rostral migration flow) [11]. In humans, proliferating progenitor cells or immature neurons have not yet been detected in this zone, but in 2014, functional genomics proved the possibility of neurogenesis in the olfactory bulb of an adult. A fifth of the genes expressed in the olfactory bulb serves for the functioning and development of the nervous system, half of which were associated with axonogenesis. Other genes that were expressed were associated with signal transmission or response to chemical stimuli. The study was conducted on two olfactory bulbs from one patient (surgical material) [12].

3.1 Neurogenesis and Age

In animal experiments, it was shown that proliferation in neurogenic zones decreases with age [13, 14]. There are very few works devoted to how the process of formation of new neurons in the human brain changes depending on age. Among them is a study by N.S. Roy et al., who in laboratory conditions studied neurogenesis from progenitor cells obtained from the dentate gyrus of an adult hippocampus (surgical material for temporal lobectomy). The isolated cells were transfected with plasmid DNA carrying the hGFP (humanized green fluorescent protein) gene. Plasmid DNA was placed in front of genes encoding nestin (a neuroepithelial protein) or T-α1-tubulin (an early neuronal protein). The fluorescent cells were sorted by flow cytometry. The fluorescent cells were sorted by flow cytometry, nestin + and T-α1 - tubulin+cells separately. The authors showed that both cells in the test tube were transformed into neurons (expression of βIII-tubulin or MAP-2 (MT-associated protein-2)), and many of them incorporated BrdU+, which indicates the appearance of these cells during cultivation in the laboratory. The study was conducted on eight male patients aged 5–63 years, while the authors do not indicate any differences depending on age [15].

R. Knoth et al. investigated changes in neurogenesis in humans and animals with age. It was found that the immunohistochemical (IHC) characteristics of neurogenesis in the adult hippocampus are similar to those in rodents. As a person ages, the total number of DCX+ cells in the hippocampus decreases exponentially. Unlike animals, humans have not been able to detect morphologically a clear subgranular zone, as in rodents. At the same time, in the early postnatal period, along with the transformation, 14 more markers were detected in the cells: proliferation markers – PCNA protein protein (nuclear antigen of proliferating cells), Ki67, mkm2 (yeast of the species Saccharomyces cereviseae minichromosome repair 2 homologues); progenitor cell markers – nestin and Sox2; maturation markers – PSA concern-NCAM, calretinin, Tuc4, BTIII-tubulin, NeuN, Carta2, GAD67; cell line markers – NeuroD1, Prox1. By the age of 40–50, Tuc4, MAP2, NeuroD1, and Ki67 are no longer coexpressed with DCX. In individuals over 75 years of age, only the proteins PCNA, Sox2, nestin, βIII-tubulin (aka Tuj1), calretinin, NeuN, GAD67, and Prox1 are found in the cells together with the body. The study was conducted on archived autopsy materials from patients of both sexes aged from 1 day to 100 years with positive and negative controls and with a study on hypoxia-induced proteins. Western blotting, IHC, and in situ hybridization were used for the study [16].

In the recent literature, data appeared concerning the role of Toll-like receptors (TLRs) in neural plasticity (E. Okun et al. 2009) [17]. TLRs influence the proliferation of neural progenitor cells, their differentiation, neurite outgrowth, and behavioral plasticity. Although the experimental studies strongly implicate these receptors in neuroplasticity, the distinction between the developmental and functional effects of a life-long deficiency of TLR as well as the specific roles for TLRs in neuroplasticity following infection and injury remain unclear. Little is known whether and how TLR signaling interacts with the signaling pathways involved in developmental and adult neuroplasticity. Probably complex TLR signaling network influences neural plasticity by both direct effects on neural progenitor cells and neurons and indirect glia-mediated processes.

Our limited experience of complex neuroplasticity studies [18] demonstrates that certain IHC staining (nestin, musashi, Tuc4, etc.) are informative and correlate with clinical and magnetic resonance imaging (MRI) data (Figs. 3.1 and 3.2).

There are only a few data about the influence of infectious pathogens on the development of the brain. In experiment on mice maternal inoculation with influenza the virus mimic polynosynic:polycytidylic acid resulting in abnormalities in social and locomotor behaviors

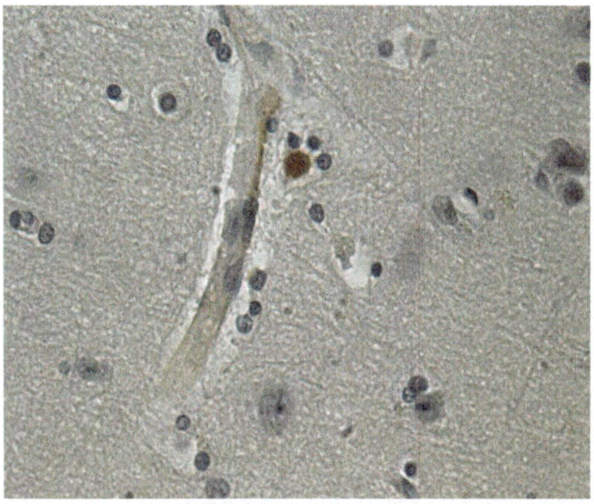

Fig. 3.1 Nestin+ cell in perivascular space in the left anterior cingulate cortex of 39y women recovering after posttraumatic vegetative state. X 320

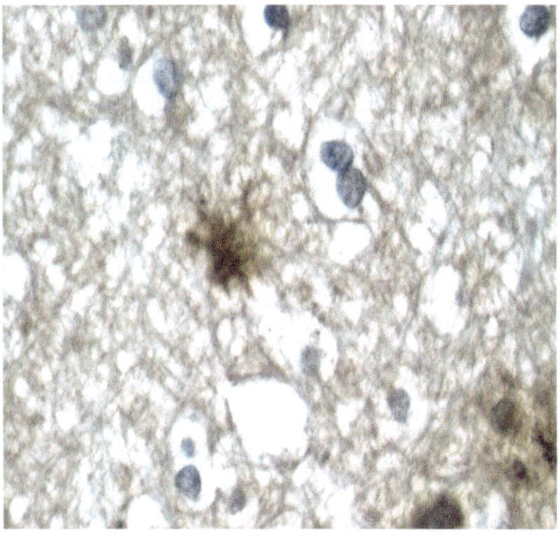

Fig. 3.2 TuC4+ cells with visible neurite outgrowths located in the right temporal lobe of the same women. X640

of the offspring [19]. These effects are associated with a reduction in neuronal stem cells. This model is considered relevant to human disease, primarily autism.

References

1. Belzung C, Wigmore P. Neurogenesis and neural plasticity. Springer; 2013. https://doi.org/10.1007/978-3-642-36232-3.
2. Cajal R. Les nouvelles idées sur la structure du système nerveux chez l'homme et chez vertebras. Paris: C. Reinwald; 1894.
3. Allen E. The cessation of mitosis in the central nervous system of the albino rat. Baltimore: Waverly Press; 1912.
4. Lois C, Alvarez-Buylla A. Proliferating subventricular zone cells in the adult mammalian forebrain can differentiate into neurons and glia. Proc Natl Acad Sci U S A. 1993;90(5):2074–7. https://doi.org/10.1073/pnas.90.52074.
5. Gould E, Reeves AJ, Fallah M, Tanapat P, Gross CG, Fuchs E. Hippocampal neurogenesis in adult Old World primates. Proc Natl Acad Sci U S A. 1999;96(9):5263–7. https://doi.org/10.1073/pnas.96.9.5263.
6. Murrel W, Bushell GR, Livesey J, McGrath J, et al. Neurogenesis in adult human. Neuroreport. 1998;7(6):1189–94. https://doi.org/10.1038/3305.
7. Eriksson PS, Perfilieva E, Bjork-Erikson T, et al. Neurogenesis in the adult human hippocampus. Nat Med. 1998;4(11):1313–7. https://doi.org/10.1038/3305.
8. Spalding KL, Bergmann O, Alkass K, et al. Dynamics of hippocampal neurogenesis in adult humans. Cell. 2013;153(6):1219–27. https://doi.org/10.1016/j.cell.2013.05.02.
9. Ernst A, Alkass K, Bernard S, et al. Neurogenesis in the striatum of the adult human brain. Cell. 2014;156(5):1072–83. https://doi.org/10.1016/j.cell.2014.01.044.
10. Reynolds BA, Weiss S. Generation of neurons and astrocytes from isolated cells of the adult mammalian central nervous system. Science. 1992;252(5052):1707–10. https://doi.org/10.1126/science.553558.
11. Altman J. Autoradiographic and histological studies of postnatal neurogenesis. IV Cell proliferation and migration in the anterior forebrain, with special reference to persisting neurogenesis in olfactory bulb. J Comp Neurol. 1969;137(4):433–57.
12. Lötsch J, Schaeffeler E, Mittelbronn M, et al. Functional genomics suggest neurogenesis in the adult human olfactory bulb. Brain Struct Funct. 2014;219(6):1991–2000. https://doi.org/10.1007/s00429-013-0618-3.
13. Seki T, Arai Y. Age-related production of new granule cells in the adult dentate gyrus. Neuroreport. 1995;6(18):2479–82. https://doi.org/10.1097/00001756-199512150-00010.
14. Kuhn HG, Dickinson-Anson H, Gage FH. Neurogenesis in the dentate gyrus of an adult rat: age related decrease of neuronal progenitor proliferation. J Neurosci. 1996;16(6):2027–33.
15. Roy NS, Wang S, Jiang L, et al. In vitro neurogenesis by progenitor cells isolated from the adult hippocampus. Nat Med. 2000;6(3):271–7. https://doi.org/10.1038/73119.
16. Knoth R, Singec I, Ditter M, et al. Murine features of neurogenesis in the human hippocampus across the lifespan from 0 to 100 years. PLoS One. 2010;5(1):e8809. https://doi.org/10.1371/j.pone.0008809.
17. Okun E, Griffioen KJ, Lathia JD, et al. Toll-like receptors in neurodegeneration. Brain Res Rev. 2009;59(2):278–92. https://doi.org/10.1016/j.brainresrev2008.09.001.
18. Vainshenker Y, Zinserling V, Korotkov A, Medvedev S. Noncanonical adult human neurogenesis and axonal growth as possible structural basis of recovery from traumatic vegetative state. Clin Med Insights Case Rep. 2017;10:1–10. https://doi.org/10.1177/1179954761773204O.
19. Malkova NV, Yu CZ, Hsiao EY, et al. Maternal immune activation yields offspring displaying mouse versions of the three core symptoms of autism. Brain Behav Immun. 2012;26:607–16.

4 General Principles of Morphological Diagnostics of Infectious Pathology in the Brain and Terminology

4.1 Principles of Postmortem Diagnosis

The recent years have been characterized by a significant increase in morbidity and mortality from the new coronavirus infection all over the world. Other infections remain important in many countries as well. In this regard, the pathological service is tasked with providing a reliable diagnosis of all infectious processes in the deceased, regardless of their significance for the onset of death, assessing the timeliness and effectiveness of the therapy and studying the morphological features of infections, depending on the patient population, environmental conditions, and the biological features of circulating pathogens [1]. A successful resolution of these issues is possible only if a qualified postmortem laboratory and morphological examination is carried out. General principles of infection diagnostics in pathology practice have been presented elsewhere [2, 3].

Best known and easy for diagnostics are the pathological processes caused by bacteria. Many experts have formed the opinion that for a successful diagnosis of bacterial infection, it is sufficient and necessary to have only a positive result of a postmortem bacteriological examination. At the same time, it should be remembered that often in practice, the range of isolated microorganisms is very much limited by the choice of nutrient media available in the laboratory, as well as the available opportunities for the accurate identification of isolated pathogens. Microorganisms such as anaerobic bacteria, L-forms, and mycoplasmas are not isolated in routine studies. At the same time, the bacteria often identified in postmortem cultures, especially those related to the so-called conditionally pathogenic ones, are not the pathogens of the studied process.

The long-term experience of the St. Petersburg/Leningrad school of pathologists specializing in infectious diseases suggests the need to determine the bacteriologically isolated pathogen in tissues during histobacterioscopic or cytological examination to verify its role in the etiology of the pathological process. The most important methods for histobacterioscopic examination are the azure-eosin staining (in any of its numerous modifications) or Gram staining to detect the vast majority of bacteria as well as periodic acid Schiff (PAS) reaction to detect fungi, pneumocysts, toxoplasmas, and mycoplasmas. Ziehl-Neelsen staining is also essential. It is most often used to detect mycobacteria (both tuberculosis and atypical) in smears and tissues. It should be noted, however, that in practice, false-negative staining by this method is often found. In addition, Ziehl-Neelsen staining can be very useful for detecting other pathogens, especially cryptosporidia. In our experience, it can also be very useful for detecting cryptococci; not only are the microbial cell and the lipopolysaccharide capsule

V. Zinserling, *Infectious Lesions of the Central Nervous System*,
https://doi.org/10.1007/978-3-030-96260-9_4

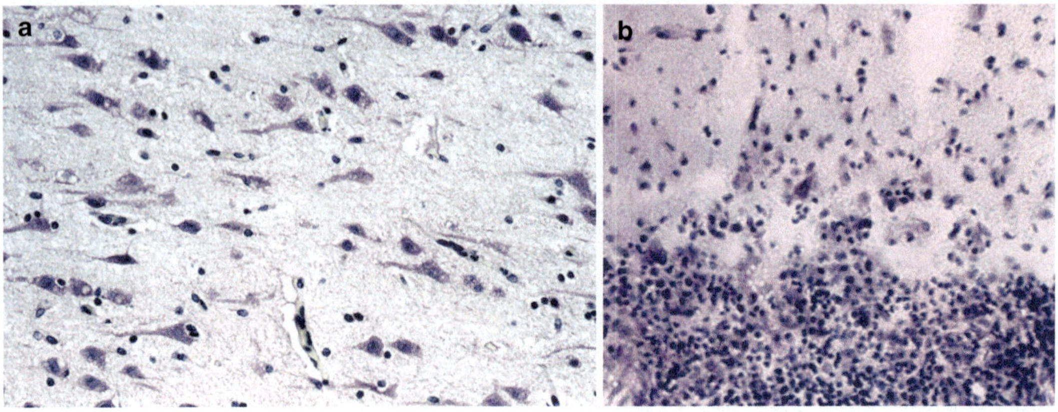

Fig. 4.1 Changes of neurons in staining by thionin according Nissl X600. (**a**) Heavy changes in brain neurons. (**b**) "Loss" of Purkinje cells in cerebellum

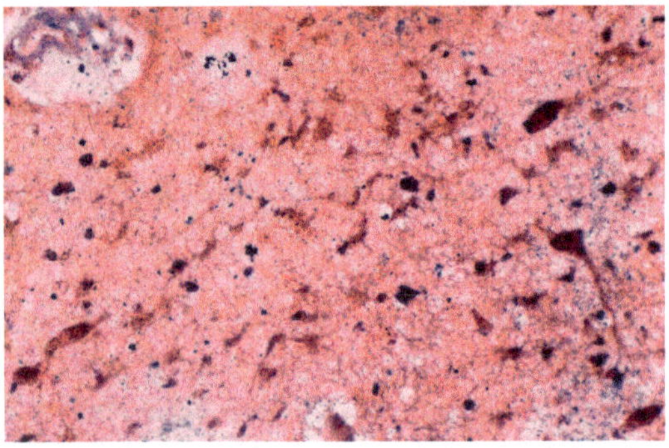

Fig. 4.2 Moderate activation of astroglia. Gold impregnation by Cajal in modification of Kitoh and Matsdushita X 200

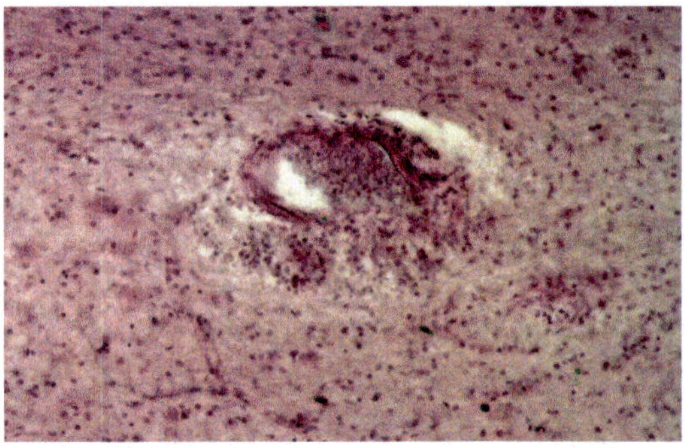

Fig. 4.3 Economo encephalitis. H-E after celloidin embedding. X 100

clearly stained, but also the structure of the microbial cells, in particular the nuclei, which are not detected with any other light-optical color, is traced. Lipopolysaccharide capsules, in particular cryptococci, are well colored with alcyan blue, in particular by Mowry. For better verification of mushrooms, impregnation with silver salts according to Grokkot is recommended.

An important task is also to distinguish cell populations in brain matter. In classical neuropathology, main attention has been drawn to Nissl staining, which allows judging better the state of neurons and glial populations (Fig. 4.1) and the different gold and silver impregnation methods (Cajal, Miagawa, etc.) (Fig. 4.2). Nowadays, the latter, due to inconstant results and high cost, are practically no longer used anywhere. Neuropathologists of previous generations preferred also embedding in celloidin (Fig. 4.3) due to numerous reasons, which are also not used anymore. Instead, in the market are presented numerous sera for immunohistochemical analysis, widely used in neurooncopathology and while studying neurodegenerative diseases. The most popular are NeuN- for neurons, glial fibrillary acidic protein (GFAP) for astrocytes, musashi 1 and nestin for progenitor neural cells, CD68 for macrophages and microglia, CD 31 and 34 for endothelium, etc. For the differentiation of macrophages and microglia, receptor p2Y12 was recently proposed [4]. We have to note that, in many cases, cell differentiation appears difficult. Detailed characteristics of cell reactions are unknown, even with the use of modern technologies in infectious pathology. In neu-

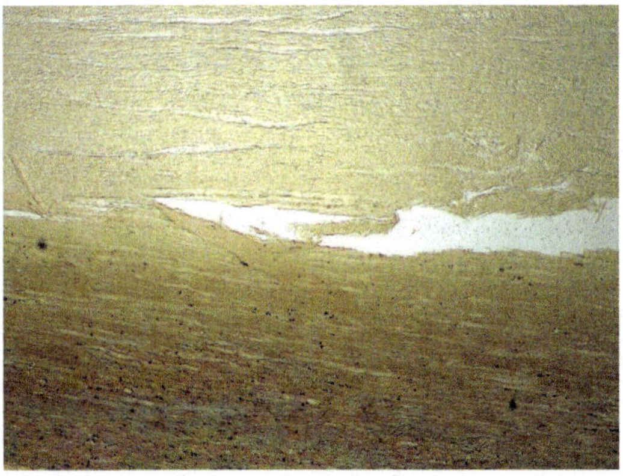

Fig. 4.4 Focal demyelinisation in rabbit nerve. Marchi method (staining with OsO4 in piece) X 50

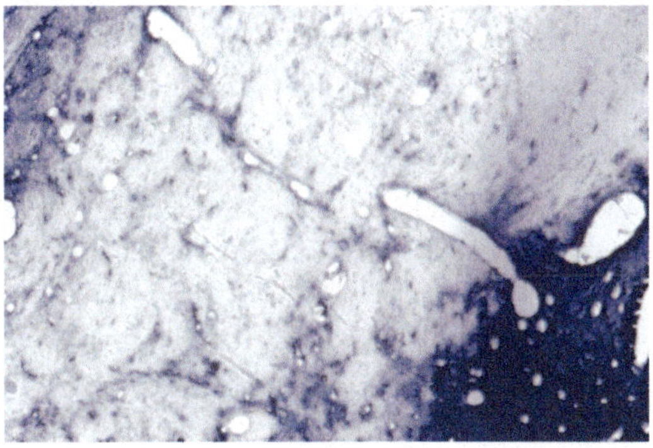

Fig. 4.5 Focal demyelinisation in brain matter. Luxol fast blue X 100

ropathology, it is extremely important to judge the preservation of myelin sheets. Among classical histological methods saining in piece with OsO4 was used (Fig. 4.4), nowadays totally replaced by other methods (Fig. 4.5).

Very valuable information can also be obtained by using an extremely simple and economical method of examination—postmortem smears (scraping or prints), stained using one of the simplest bacterioscopic methods.

The detection of structural changes characteristic of individual pathogens during macro- and microscopic examination is also of fundamental importance. To solve many pathogenetic problems, it is essential to compare the results of studies of the properties of microorganisms and the nature of the structural changes caused by them.

The widespread occurrence of immunodeficiency conditions of various origins contributes to a significant increase in the frequency of processes caused by pathogenic fungi. Only a few of them (*Candida*, *Aspergillus*, *Mucor*) can be isolated by routine bacteriological examination. The diagnosis of most mycotic processes requires the use of special studies in mycological laboratories, which exist only in a few large centers. The detection of typical fungal structures in the tissues, especially those with signs of a characteristic reaction, is of fundamental importance for the diagnosis.

Due to international contacts with countries with a tropical climate, the possibility of appearance of infectious diseases typical for them caused by a variety of protozoa is significantly increasing. In practice, it is impossible to conduct parasitological studies on clinical and sectional materials. Excluding the very limited possibilities of serological studies (in toxoplasmosis), the main diagnosis is also based on the determination of the characteristic structures of the pathogen in the tissues.

The tactics involved in pathological research fundamentally correspond to the general guidelines for a morphological study [1]. Before the autopsy, it is necessary to analyze the medical documentation in as much detail as possible, while planning the necessary additionary investigations during the autopsy. Because of the vast majority of infectious diseases, when conducting an autopsy of the deceased, it is a must to use protective clothing; even ordinary ones are enough: two dressing gowns, a rubberized apron, two pairs of protective gloves, and a cap. The gloves, apron tools, as well as dissection table should, after the autopsy, be treated with disinfection solution (3% chloramine). In the autopsy room, wet cleaning should be carried out daily with the use of disinfection solution, and the air should be neutralized with the help of ultraviolet lamps. The drains of the sectional table must pass through a sump tank with a disinfectant solution before entering the general sewer system. Compliance with the basic rules of personal hygiene, like a desirable shower after the autopsy, allows almost the elimination of the risk of infection of the staff participating in the autopsy.

Special rules are observed when opening the corpses of those who died from particularly dangerous infections or if they are suspected of such. When opening the corpse of a person who died of a plague or is suspected of it, a special protective suit has to be used [5, 6].

The most important feature of an autopsy in infectious diseases is the conduct of a wide range of laboratory and histological studies. To help the pathologist in collecting material for laboratory research and filling out directions, a laboratory assistant should be present in the autopsy. The material must be taken with a clean (if possible, sterile) instrument. It is advisable to take pieces of the tissue for sowing at the start of the autopsy; before placing them in a sterile dish, it is advisable to burn them over the flame of an alcohol lamp.

The most common bacterial lesions include purulent meningitis and meningoencephalitis. Their macroscopic diagnosis (opening the skull cavity is desirable in all cases) in most cases does not cause difficulties. In those who died at the earliest stages of the process, the most important differential diagnostic value for edema of the meninges and edema swelling of the brain (Fig. 4.6) is the cytological examination of smears prints. To assess the effectiveness of the therapy and complete the pathogenetic assessment of the observation, it is necessary to conduct a bacteriological study, for which it can be recommended to take a swab of pus from the surface of the meninges, cerebrospinal fluid (CSF), and choroidal plexuses. Plexus choriodeus is especially important, since in the part of the observations (clinically beginning with general cerebral symptoms in the absence of distinct meningeal signs), the initial reproduction of the pathogen occurs precisely in the choroidal plexuse, with the subsequent development of ventriculitis and only later meningitis.

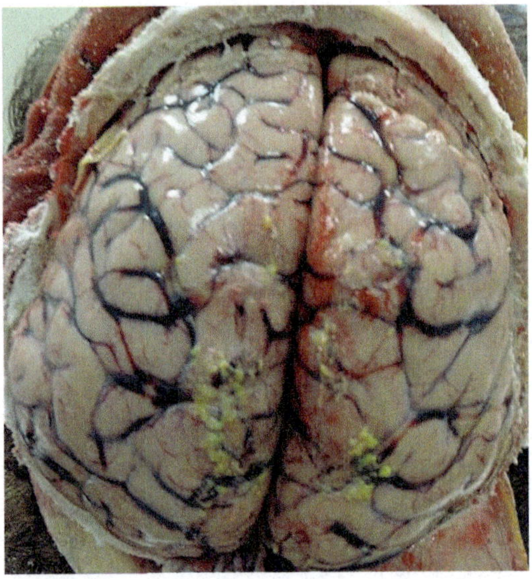

Fig. 4.6 Brain edema swelling. Unfixed macropreparation. Courtesy of N.A. Lugovsya

The most common bacterial pathogens of meningitis are meningococcus, pneumococcus, and *Hemophilus* rod. When evaluating the results of a bacteriological study, it should be remembered that all of them (especially hemophilic bacillus and, to a lesser extent, meningococcus) are very demanding on nutrient media, which very often leads to false-negative results in practical work. And for meningococcal, pneumococcal, and hemophilic infections, the use of test kits for determining antigens using the agglutination reaction in blood serum is of diagnostic importance.

It is also essential to determine the primary or secondary nature of the inflammatory process in the meninges, which necessitates a thorough morphological and bacteriological study of the tonsils, pharynx, lungs, ears, and paranasal sinuses. To make a reasonable thanatological conclusion, it is necessary to carefully assess the presence of at least minimal signs of all variants of dislocation (insertion) of the brain, changes in its mass, and consistency. It should be remembered that a significant part of bacterial processes develops in the background or together with viral ones.

4.2 Lifetime Clinical Diagnostics

The importance of reliable diagnosis and differential diagnosis of brain lesions in the practice of neurosurgeons, neurologists, and psychiatrists is obvious. Along with the clinical picture, which does not always allow an accurate diagnosis, a wide range of various radiological methods (MRI, PET-CT) and numerous laboratory methods are widely used. They are aimed to determin the characteristics of the spinal fluid, the presence of pathogens, cellular and humoral reactions. It should be emphasized that, in principle, it is possible to carry out all the most diverse reactions developed for blood serum in CSF.

Among the promising diagnostic methods for everyday medical practice is chromatography-mass spectrometry of microbial markers (MSMM), which is certified for clinical use and allows to simultaneously examine any biological material for 57 microorganisms. Unlike genetic methods, MSMM allows you to quickly determine the presence of herpesviruses (cytomegalovirus (CMV), herpes types 1 and 2, Epstein-Barr virus (EBV)), pathogenic and conditionally pathogenic microbes, aerobic and anaerobic bacteria, gram-negative "sticks," and actinomycetes, as soon as 3 h after the sample is received in the laboratory to assess the content of toxins, the total level of microorganisms, and the number of normoflora (bifidobacteria and lactobacilli).

A cytological study of CSF has been elaborated, first of all, for the detection of tumor cells and also, to a lesser extent, for the detection of bacterial, fungal, and protozoan pathogens [7].

At the same time, a cytological examination of the cell sediment with calculation of the cell formula is carried out, though extremely rarely and is almost not used in the diagnosis of infectious brain lesions, which is primarily associated with the need to increase the content of cell elements in a unit volume for counting, which can be achieved both by centrifugation and filtration. In principle, it is also possible to coagulate protein components in 70% ethyl alcohol, followed by the pouring of the resulting precipitate into the paraffin and then making histological preparations according to the standard method.

In our practice, CSF is periodically sent to the pathology department for cytological examination in order to detect some pathogens, primarily *Mycobacterium tuberculosis* and cryptococci. In addition to the hematoxylin-eosin review technique, it is possible to use the entire spectrum of bacterioscopic and immunocytochemical methods (see Sect. 5.2) (Figs. 4.7 and 4.8). In the study of V.E. Karev et al. was shown the diversity of CD3+ cells number in smears from CSF in course of purulent meningitis of different etiology [8]. Despite the availability of other methods, the complexity and some subjectivity in the interpretation of the results of cytological studies, the data obtained are of priority importance.

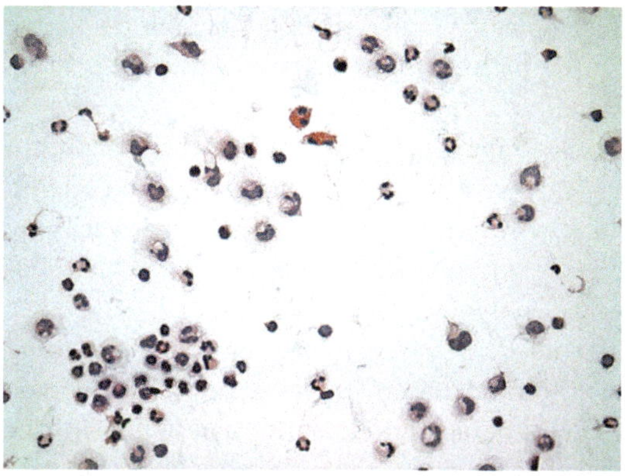

Fig. 4.7 Cytological picture of CSF H-E X600. Courtesy of V.E. Karev

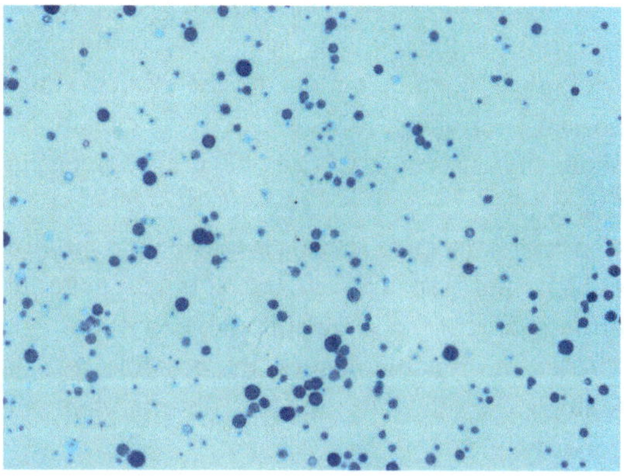

Fig. 4.8 Numerous cryptococci in smear from CSF. Staining by Ziehl-Neelsen X600. Courtesy of V.E. Karev

We have to state that in some clinical observations, there is a discrepancy between the results of the cytological examination of the "peripheral" CSF and the actual state of the soft meninges determined during a pathoanatomic autopsy. It can be assumed that there is a block in the cerebrospinal fluid pathways with the development of purulent inflammation. There are no alternative ways to verify the true state of the meninges.

In modern neurosurgical practice, morphological studies of biopsy and surgical material in the vast majority of cases are aimed at verifying tumors. In previous years (before the introduction of polymerase chain reaction (PCR) studies into practice), a brain biopsy aimed at identifying inclusions characteristic of herpes (Cowdry type 1 bodies) was considered the gold standard for diagnosing this infection. In principle, it is possible; although it is practiced extremely rarely, it is proposed to conduct a transfontanel biopsy in children in the first year of life.

There are no reliable data on the frequency of detection of inflammatory changes during morphological examination during the clinical diagnosis of a tumor; isolated cases occur in all neurosurgical centers. Our data are given in Chap. 19.

There is isolated evidence of the detection of inflammatory changes in the surgical material during the removal of an epileptogenic focus [9]. There is no reliable data on the possible role of biological pathogens in the development of epilepsy.

4.3 Conclusion

It should be noted that lifetime morphological studies play a relatively modest role in the clinical diagnosis of infectious brain lesions; they should be evaluated in comparison with data obtained using other methods. It seems that the wider use of CSF cytograms can be very useful for both predicting the course of various meningitis, primarily serous, and analyzing the mechanisms of the unfavorable course of the disease.

References

1. Alfsen C, Gulczyński J, Kholova I, et al. Code of practice for medical autopsies: a minimum standard position paper for pathology department performing medical (hospital) autopsies in adults. Virchows Arch. 2021:1–9. https://doi.org/10.1007/s00428-021-032242-y.
2. Kradin RL, editor. Diagnostic pathology of infectious diseases. Elsevier; 2018. p. 698.
3. Zinserling VA. Infectious pathology of the respiratory tract. Springer International Publishing. https://doi.org/10.1007/978-3-030-66325-4. ISBN 978-3—030-66324-7
4. Korzevskii DE, Tsyba DL, Kirik OV, Alekseeva OS. A comparison of microglia detection in mammals and humans using purinergic receptor P2Y12 labelling Zh. Evol Biokh Phisiol. 2021;57(5):363–72. (In Russian)
5. Wilson ML. Infectious diseases and the autopsy. Clin Infect Dis. 2006;43(5):602–3. https://doi.org/10.1086/506574.
6. Baj J, Ciesielka M, Buszewicz G, et al. COVID-19 in the autopsy room-requirements, safety, recommendations and pathological findings. Forensic Sci Med Pathol. 2021;17(1):101–13. https://doi.org/10.1007/s12024-020-00341-1.
7. Torzewski M, Lackner KJ, Bohl J, Sommer C. Integrated cytology of cerebrospinal fluid. Berlin-Heidelberg: Springer Verlag; 2008. p. 93S.
8. Karev VE, Skripchenko NV, Ivaschenko IA, et al. Possibilities of immunocytochemical phenotyping of cells in cerebrospinal fluid while children's bacterial meningitis Zh. Inf Dent. 2013;5(4):61–4. https://doi.org/10.22625/2072-6732-2013-5-4-61-64.
9. Sitovkaya DA, Zabrodskaya YM, Sokolova TV, et al. Structural heterogeneity of epileptic foci in local drug resistant epilepsy. Arkh Patol. 2020;82(6):5–15. https://doi.org/10.17116/patol2020820615.

5 Lesions of the Nervous System in Herpes

5.1 Introduction

Among infectious lesions of the nervous system, a special place is given to diseases associated with herpesviruses [1, 2]. The latter is due to both the wide prevalence of herpetic viruses and the severity of the damage to the nervous tissue caused by them. It is believed that for the first time, herpetic manifestations on the skin were described by the ancient Greek historian Herodotus, who lived in the fifth century BC, but even today issues on the etiology and pathogenesis of lesions in the nervous system with herpesvirus remain insufficiently studied.

5.2 Etiology and Epidemiology

Viruses from the *Herpesviridae* family (herpes simplex virus (HSV) types 1 and 2, chickenpox, shingles, cytomegaly, Epstein-Bar) and the lesions caused by them have attracted the attention of many researchers for many years [3]. The development of methods for culturing lymphoid cells and isolating the viruses that infect them led to the discovery in 1986 of herpesvirus type 6 and then types 7 and 8. Herpesviruses contain double-helix deoxyribonucleic acid (DNA); the virion consists of a lipoprotein envelope, a capsid, and a nucleoprotein. Known is high resistance of herpesviruses to freezing in the dried state, sensitivity to temperature effects - they die within 30 minutes at a temperature of 50 °C, are inactivated by phenol, formaldehyde, chloroform, alcohol. All herpesviruses are characterized by pantropism, the possibility to course the widest spectrum of pathological processes, survival in a latent state, and oncogenic properties. In spite of their intensive studies, which last for several decades, including decoding the genome, the diversity of their clinical impact remains partly unclear. All herpesviruses are neurotropic, and the data are summarized in Table 5.1.

Usually classified under herpesviruses are herpes simplex 1 and 2 serotypes (HSV-1 and HSV-2), which differ in antigenic determinants but also have common antigens, which makes it possible for them to develop cross-serological reactions. Cytomegaly will be discussed in Sect. 8.2 (brain complications of human immunodeficiency virus (HIV) infection) and Sect. 16.2, among other intrauterine encephalitides. Brain lesions in chickenpox/herpes zoster are presented in Sect. 7.6. For data related to the role of herpesviruses in noninfectious brain pathology, see Chaps. 17 and 20. Certain aspects of their evaluation in clinical pathology are summarized in Chap. 19. There are indications that HV6, 7, and 8 can be detected in nervous tissue, but their clinical relevance stays generally unclear and their histopathological features remain unknown [4].

Currently, it is established that herpesviruses have the following transmission routes: airborne, household contact, sexual, parenteral, and

V. Zinserling, *Infectious Lesions of the Central Nervous System*,
https://doi.org/10.1007/978-3-030-96260-9_5

Table 5.1 Clinical manifestations of infectious lesions caused by herpesviruses

Herpesviruses	Abbreviated Latin name	Systemic diseases or local lesions	Neurological diseases
1	2	3	4
Herpes simplex virus type 1 (HSV-1)	HSV-1	Stomatitis, gingivitis, keratitis, recurrent herpes simplex	Herpetic encephalitis
Herpes simplex type 2 (HSV-2)	HSV-2	Genital herpes, cervical cancer	Encephalitis of newborns, meningitis of adults, recurrent radiculitis
Varicella-zoster virus (VZV)	VZV	Varicella, herpes zoster	Neuropaths, neuralgia, meningitis, encephalitis, Guillain-Barre syndrome
Cytomegalovirus (CMV)	CMV	Generalized intrauterine infection, infectious mononucleosis, retinitis, pneumonitis	Encephalitis, Guillain-Barre syndrome
Epstein-Barr virus (EBV)	EBV	Infectious mononucleosis, Burkitt lymphoma, nasopharyngeal carcinoma	Encephalitis, meningitis, Guillain-Barre syndrome
Herpesvirus type 6 (HHV-6)	HHV-6	Exanthema in children, maculopapular rash in newborns	Encephalitis in children and adults
Herpesvirus type 7 (HHV-7)	HHV-7	Exanthema, cofactor for other infections, lymphadenopathy	Meningitis, encephalitis in children and adults, facial nerve neuropathy, vestibular neuronitis
Herpesvirus type 8 (HHV-8)	HHV-8	Kaposi sarcoma, Castleman disease, multiple myeloma	Primary lymphoma of the brain

vertical from mother to fetus. The first route of transmission occurs in cases where a herpetic infection proceeds in the form of acute respiratory disease; the second, most frequent, means is when the virus is contained in saliva or tear fluid, which can be transmitted when using common things like towels or plates, through kissing, or in case of noncompliance with sanitary standards in ophthalmological and dental offices. The sexual route of infection with herpes is associated with the fact that it is one of the most common infections transmitted in this way. The presence of viremia in generalized herpes explains an opportunity for a parenteral pathway. Such cases are described in people suffering from drug addiction.

Although HSV-1 and HSV-2 have a tropism to the skin, mucous membranes, and nervous system, they have different pathways of dissemination. HSV-1 is mainly spread by airborne droplets or by household contact with the lesion of the mucous membrane of the eyes, nose, and oral cavity. For HSV-2, the most characteristic is the sexual pathway of distribution with damage to the mucous membrane of the genitals, as well as transplacental transmission to the fetus. It is believed that in 95% of cases, herpetic encephalitis is caused by HSV-1. At the same time, in newborns and children of the first 6 months of life, the cause of encephalitis is more often HSV-2 (see also Sect. 16.2). In older individuals, HSV-2 mainly causes the development of serous meningitis, which can recur.

The source and reservoir of herpesviruses are men. At the same time, such laboratory animals as rabbits, guinea pigs, mice, rats, and hamsters are sensitive to them, so they are widely used in experimental studies. The infection of people with herpesvirus occurs at an early age, most often without clinical manifestations. At the same time, the herpesvirus has the ability to persist for many years in the sensitive ganglia, mainly of the trigeminal nerve, remaining in a latent form and causing exacerbations in the presence of various resolving factors. Currently, it is not possible to reduce its ability for latent existence even with the use of DNA vaccines, which, in the experiment, reduce the titer of the herpesvirus in the Gasser node by 100 times and induce a significant increase in the number of CD4 lymphocytes in it [5].

5.3 Pathology and Pathogenesis

The neurotropism of viruses belonging to the *Herpesviridae* family is well known. It is believed that the target of the herpesvirus is the structure of the nervous system [3]. After the virus is adsorbed on the surface of the epithelial cells of the skin or mucous membranes, after being released from the capsid, it is introduced into the cell; its DNA penetrates the genome of the host cell and is replicated. As a result, epithelial cells die, and a significant number of multinucleated cells are formed in the spiny layer of the skin. The development of a local inflammatory process, accompanied by increased vascular permeability, leads to the sweating of serous exudate and the appearance of bubbles on the papillary layer of the dermis against the background of infiltration and edema. Subsequent viremia promotes the penetration of the herpesvirus into the central nervous system, liver, and other organs.

It is believed that one characteristic of this virus is its perineural spreading in the ganglia of the nervous system, where it persists for a long time, periodically activating and again reaching the target tissue along the axons. When HSV is reactivated in the trigeminal or cranial ganglion, the virus spreads along the tympanic string or fibers of the trigeminal nerve; in the first days of relapse, it is detected in the saliva and leads to damage to the facial nerve. With a relapse of herpetic infection, as with the primary infection, the patient is detected for several weeks with immunoglobulin (Ig) M, after which it is replaced by Ig G. The relapse of herpes is promoted by stressful situations, trauma, cooling, neuroendocrine shifts in pregnant women, and acquired immunodeficiency states in oncological, hematological, and infectious diseases during immunosuppressive therapy.

In recent decades, pathological changes in herpetic infection have been intensively studied. At the same time, only necrotic encephalitis caused by herpes simplex virus type 1 is currently sufficiently fully characterized. The incubation of herpetic encephalitis lasts from 2 to 26 days on average. For herpetic encephalitis, the most typical development of necrosis foci is in the parietal-temporal region and the appearance of characteristic intracranial inclusions in nerve cells. It should be noted that the exact mechanisms for necrosis development in this form of encephalitis are not known. But we can assume the significance of both secondary vascular changes and the activation of apoptosis. Obviously, the virus itself is not directly capable of causing necrosis.

Histological and ultrastructural changes in herpetic encephalitis were studied by B. A. Erman et al. in detail [5]. It is shown that the lesions are usually localized in the areas of the brain responsible for olfactory function (temporal and insular cortex, hippocampus, and some other areas of the gray matter of the brain). Acute focal necrotic encephalitis with intracranial inclusions in nerve and glial cells is observed. The inclusions are rounded, eosinophilic, homogeneous, or granular and are more commonly referred to as Cowdry bodies of type A (or 1). For a long time, they were considered the "gold standard" for the diagnosis of herpetic encephalitis in biopsies. Currently, polymerase chain reaction (PCR) is regarded as the most reliable method of clinical diagnosis, which in most cases detects the herpes antigen in the cerebrospinal fluid (CSF). However, in some cases, PCR can give a false-negative result, which is associated with the rapid elimination of the pathogen from the CSF and low viral load. In this regard, in the presence of characteristic clinical manifestations and a negative result of PCR, it is recommended to determine the intrathecal antibodies in the cerebrospinal fluid in comparison with their level in the blood serum.

In recent years, it has been proved that the spectrum of lesions caused by HSV is much wider and includes, along with acute, also subacute and chronic forms of varying severity [3].

Ultrastructural changes caused by HSV in the CNS in patients and in the experiment are characterized by signs of virus reproduction in the nuclei of nerve and glial cells, where virions are arranged in groups. In a small number of cells, the virus is also contained in the cytoplasm. In general, the infectious process is characterized by intensive reduplication and folding of the nuclear membrane due to its hyperplasia, the formation of clumps of nuclear material, as well as the expansion of the tubules and cisterns of the endoplasmic reticulum. In addition, there is a disintegration of the nucleoli and the appearance of network-like worm-like masses in the nuclei. Virions are usually rounded in shape and consist of a centrally located nucleoid with a diameter of 35–40 nm and an outer shell (capsid) with a diameter of 105–130 nm [5].

In an experiment with intraconjunctival and intraperitoneal infection of newborn rabbits, we were able to reproduce a generalized infection with the development of typical lesions in the brain, liver, and spleen [6].

In our large complex experiment [7], 0.1 ml of suspension containing HSV-1 (strain L 2) was administered intraocularly to newborn rabbits. It is believed that when the focus of herpes infection is primarily localized in the structures of the eyeball, the spread of the herpesvirus is mainly along the visual or oculomotor nerves, with damage to the frontal or occipital lobes of the brain. In clinical conditions, with the generalization of infection, such brain lesions can lead to herpetic conjunctivitis, chorioretinitis, and keratitis. Two series of experiments were conducted. In series 1, the animals were infected with a dose of 5 LD50. Of the ten infected animals, six died: one on day 1, three on day 4, and two on day 5; four animals were decapitated on day 2 after infection. In the second series of experiments, a dose of 2 LD50 was used to infect 12 animals. The animals were decapitated on days 3, 4, and 5 after infection. Nine animals from the same litters served as control. Virological, histological, immunohistochemical, electron microscopic, biochemical, and neurochemical studies were conducted. The virological study proved the replication of HSV in the brain tissue, in which the virus titers (in the reverse log) were 1.66 on day 2, 4 on day 3, 5.2 on day 4, and 4.37 on day 5. In histological and immunohistochemical studies, a generalized herpetic infection with damage to the brain, liver, spleen, and kidneys was documented in the first series of experiments. The changes in the brain were very significant. In the experiment, starting from day 2, small basophilic and oxyphilic inclusions were detected inside the nuclei of dystrophically altered and partially dying nerves and glial cells, mainly in the deep parts of the large hemispheres. Along with this, fullness and lymph histiocytic infiltration of the soft meninges were noted. On day 5, the described changes were more pronounced, and moderate focal glial proliferation was also detected near the affected nerve cells and subependimar glial cells (Fig. 5.1). In the soft meninges, pronounced hyperchromatosis and rexis of the cells, lymphohistiocytic infiltration with an admixture of pseudoeosinophilic leukocytes, and sometimes large foci of necrosis were detected. In the second series of experiments, the changes in the brain and internal organs were similar but less pronounced and almost disappeared by the fifth day after infection. The neurochemical study of the content of gangliosides in the brain already on day 2 showed a decrease in the content of glycosphingolipids, which amounted to 50% of the level of these lipids in the controls by day 5. When studying the composition of gangliosides, an almost twofold increase in the GD1b fraction was found on day 5. The remaining fractions of gangliosides were within the limits of the corresponding controls. In the second series of experiments, the content of lipid peroxidation products (TBK-active products and diene conjugates) in the red blood cells and blood plasma of newborn rabbits was determined during biochemical studies. On the third day of infection with the herpesvirus, the content of TBK-active products in the membranes of red blood cells significantly increased, and in the blood plasma, it did not change as compared to the control

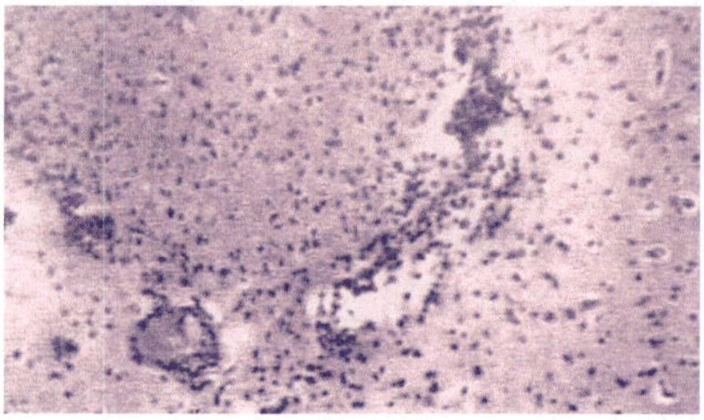

Fig. 5.1 Experimental encephalitis in newborn rabbits in the first series. H-E ×200

(respectively, 18.4 ± 0.6 vs. 15.7 ± 0.5 nmol/ml of red blood cells, $p < 0.001$; 1.40 ± 0.13 vs 1.10 ± 0.20 nmol/ml of plasma), which does not give grounds to associate the intensification of lipid peroxidation (LPO) processes in cell membranes with the possibility of oxidation of plasma lipoproteins, as shown in the case of HSV. The content of diene conjugates in the red blood cells of the infected rabbits was higher than in the control animals (19.8 ± 1.2 vs. 18.3 ± 0.3 nmol/ml of red blood cells, respectively), but the difference was not statistically significant ($p > 0.05$). With the development of herpetic infection in newborn rabbits, there was a further intensification of the processes of LPO. It should be noted that the significant pathological changes of biochemical parameters in the blood of newborn rabbits with experimental herpetic infection developed parallel with rapid hematogenous dissemination and reproduction of the virus in various internal organs. The most pronounced changes were observed in the brain, where, along with intracranial dystrophic changes, both basophilic and oxyphilic, mainly small inclusions were detected, the connection of which with the herpesvirus was confirmed by immunohistochemistry (IHC). In this regard, the activation of LPO processes and the change in the permeability of erythrocyte membranes, which we found, are apparently due to changes in the functional properties of the lipid bilayer during the interaction of viruses with target cells. The ability of the herpesvirus to change the phospholipid and glycolipid metabolism of membranes is known, which leads to the adsorption of more viral particles on the receptors and facilitates the penetration of the virus into the cell. Both histological study and in situ hybridization proved direct lesions of the bone marrow and spleen (Fig. 5.2a, b, c). The immunosuppressive activity of the virus was also shown in parallel immunological studies, primarily against T lymphocytes and neutrophil granulocytes. Against the background of a clearly expressed morphological, virological, and immunological generalized herpetic infection on days 3–15 from the moment of infection of the animals, it was possible to identify a number of changes in the brain, consisting primarily in a significant swelling of the endothelium of blood vessels, sometimes accompanied by inflammatory infiltration. In the subependimar space, there was a slight increase in the number of poorly differentiated cells, some of the nuclei of which were hyperchromic. In the cortex of the large hemispheres, there was also some violation of stratification and ischemic and dystrophic changes in nerve cells. Using the in situ hybridization method, the maximum amount of virus nucleic acid was determined in endothelial and perivascular glial cells. In the form of small islands and stripes, were also found in the neurons of the cortex of the large hemispheres, which allowed us to submit that they were related to the neuronal transport of the nucleic acid of the virus (Fig. 5.3). In some cases, both perivascular and more extended hemorrhages were observed. It should be noted the high frequency of coincidence of the results of histological and molecular biological diagnostics.

Comparative studies were conducted on adult rabbits with generalized herpetic infection. To simulate herpetic infection, animals were intraocularly injected with herpes simplex virus (HSV-1, strain L 2 at a dose of 10TCD50). It should be emphasized that generalized herpetic infection in adult and newborn rabbits was clinically different. So if newborn rabbits, as a result of infection with HSV-1, changed behavior (there was lethargy, restriction of the volume of movement in the limbs; of the ten infected animals, seven fell during the first 5 days, and the rest before the ninth day of infection), then the condition of adult infected rabbits did not significantly change in comparison with the control ones. In microscopic studies of the brain and internal organs of adult rabbits, the degree of severity of changes characteristic of generalized herpes, in contrast to newborn rabbits, was moderate. In adult animals, only a few endothelial cells of the brain, liver, kidneys, and lungs were found to contain small intracellular inclusions, the cellular response to which was minimal or absent. In these experimental animals, the pattern of generalized herpetic infection developed later than in newborn rabbits, by the eighth day of infection; by the 14th day of infection, the histological changes were essentially the same, but

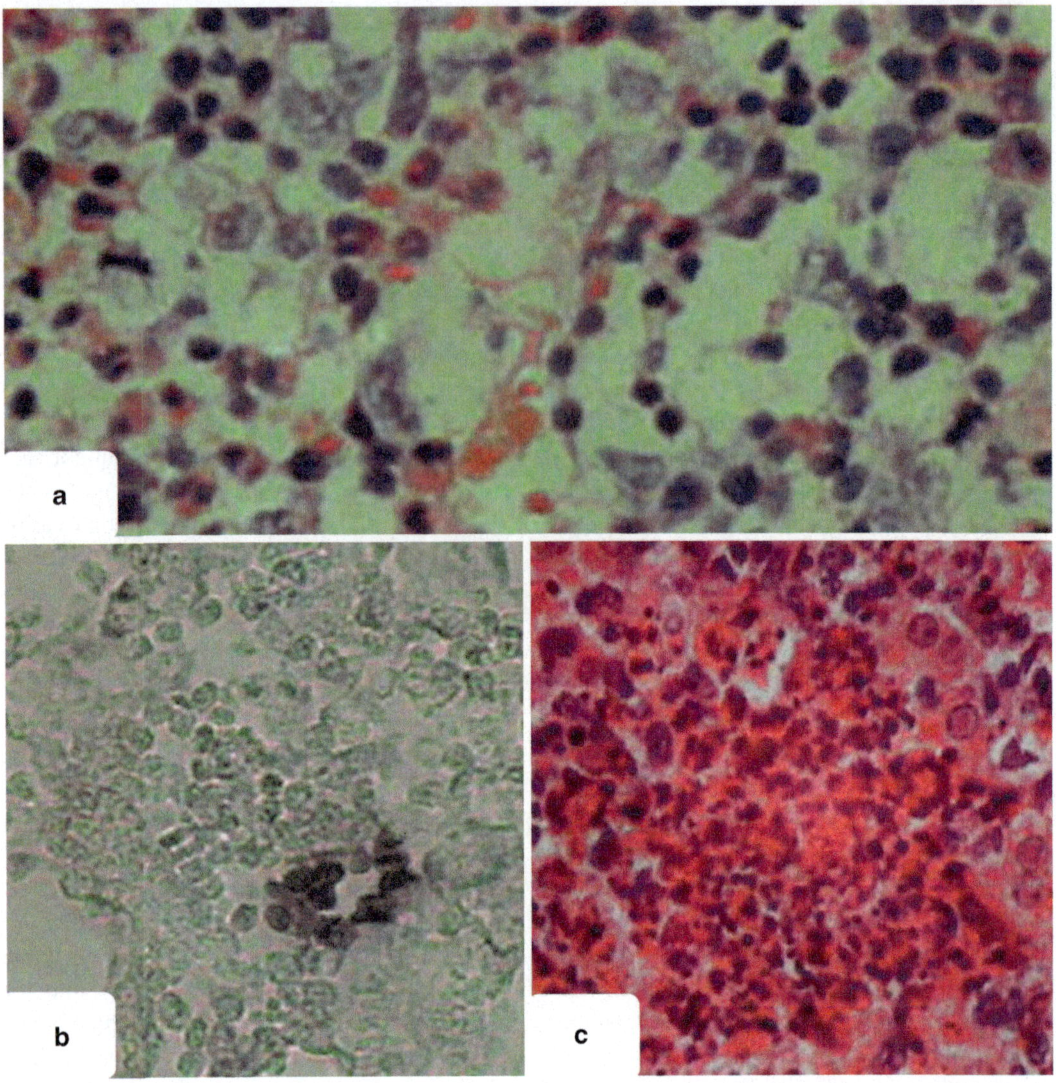

Fig. 5.2 Bone marrow and spleen lesions in the generalized experimental herpes infection in newborn rabbits. (**a**) General view of bone marrow. H-E ×600. (**b**) Expression of HSV-1 DNA in bone marrow. Hybridization in situ. ×600 (**c**) Spleen lesion. Note intranuclear oxyphilic inclusions. H-E ×600

the degree of their severity significantly decreased.

The dynamics of biochemical parameters in adult rabbits with generalized herpetic infection were associated with the data of morphological studies. On the eighth day after infection in adult rabbits with generalized herpetic infection, an increase in the content of TBK-active products in red blood cells was detected; on the 14th day, there was a decrease in these indicators, but the latter exceeded the control values (20.1 ± 0.7, 17.7 ± 0.5, and 16.0 ± 0.5, respectively; $p < 0.05$). There were no significant changes in the content of TBK-active products in plasma and diene conjugates in red blood cells in adult rabbits on the eighth and 14th days of infection with the herpesvirus compared to the control group. The activation of LPO on day 8 of infection was accompanied by a change in the permeability of red blood cell membranes: in the second fraction, the percentage of destroyed red blood cells was significantly reduced compared to that in control

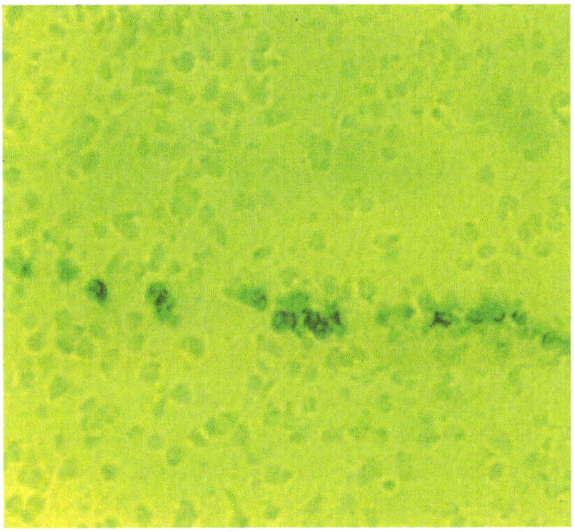

Fig. 5.3 HSV-1 DNA in rabbit brain cortex. Hybridization in situ. ×300

rabbits; on day 14, the TEM indicators in animals with generalized herpetic infection did not significantly differ from the control values. At the same time, the most pronounced pathological changes in adult rabbits with generalized herpetic infection were expressed in the liver.

Consequently, infection with the herpesvirus causes a whole complex of different structural and biochemical changes in the tissues of experimental animals, depending on their age. For a more comprehensive study of the pathogenesis of herpetic encephalitis, we also used the classical "mouse model." To reproduce herpetic encephalitis, CBA mice weighing 10–12 g were administered intracerebral HSV-1, strain L 2, at a dose of 2LD50/0.02. The histological examination of all experimental animals revealed a pattern of focal encephalitis. In the internal organs, against the background of vasculitis, mainly small basophilic inclusions were detected in the nuclei of various cells, including in the spleen and thymus, indicating moderate generalization. Along with the violation of the process of phagocytosis in animals with herpetic encephalitis, a decrease in the spontaneous migration of peripheral blood leukocytes was revealed. At the same time, pronounced metabolic changes occurred in the tissues of the experimental animals. The results obtained in experimental studies indicate that herpetic infection has a multifactorial effect on all body systems, which should be taken into account when managing patients with this pathology.

5.4 Clinical Manifestations of Herpetic Lesions of the Nervous System

Clinical and experimental studies indicate a wide range of lesions of the nervous system in herpes, depending on the type of pathogen, the age of the infected, and their premorbid background.

Currently, it is common to distinguish between congenital (see Chap. 16) and acquired herpetic infection, each of which can be manifest and asymptomatic.

The nature of the spread of herpes infection can be localized, widespread, and generalized. Although neurologists are most often faced with herpetic lesions of the nervous system, the other possible foci of this infection should, however, be remembered. It is necessary to take into account the possibility of simultaneous involvement of various body systems in the pathological process. With regard to localization, herpetic lesions in the skin, mucous membranes, eyes, genitals, and other internal organs are also distinguished. In particular, HSV is the leading cause of keratitis and vision loss caused by an infectious disease. Despite the fact that specialists in infectious diseases distinguish typical and atypical forms of herpetic infection with the development of foci in the central nervous system, it is difficult to separate them due to the polymorphism of both clinical and pathological manifestations. It should also be noted the relativity of the allocation of mild, moderate, and severe forms of damage to the nervous system caused by herpes, due to the frequent rapid generalization and aggravation of the pathological process. The division of neurological diseases of herpetic etiology according to the duration of infection is quite conditional—acute (primary) and chronic (secondary)—since a long-term asymptomatic course is possible. Taking into account the peculiarities of the lesion of the nervous system in children and adults, we will consider the clinical manifestations of herpetic infection, depending on the age of infection.

Long-term monitoring of the structure of death courses in children in Leningrad/St. Petersburg indicates some fluctuations in the frequency of herpes encephalitis. According to modern concepts, the portion of herpetic encephalitis accounts for up to 20% of all cases of viral encephalitis. It seems that with the improvement of the diagnosis of herpes, this indicator can be much higher.

Our studies show that herpetic lesions of the nervous system begin to acquire a defined clinical picture, usually in older children. A detailed study of the clinical and morphological manifestations of herpetic lesions of the nervous system in children was carried out by us together with M. A. Dadiomova et al in the Research Institute of Children's Infections [8]. For 2 years, 125 children with neuroinfections were examined: 56 with serous meningitis, 28 with encephalitis, and 41 with purulent meningitis and meningoencephalitis. Clinical and laboratory analysis made it possible to distinguish three groups of patients with positive results of virological testing for herpesviruses: (1) 17 patients with acute neuroinfections (15 with herpetic encephalitis, one with serous meningitis, and one with myelopolyradiculoneuropathy), (2) one group with central nervous system HSV damage due to the exacerbation of herpetic infection with purulent meningitis, and (3) two children with persistent HSV in the central nervous system with different other neuroinfections.

In group 1, herpetic encephalitis was observed in 11 children under 4 years of age and in four children over 7 years of age. Only three of them had herpetic rashes on the skin or mucous membranes, and five of them had catarrhal changes in the nasopharynx. The disease began acutely—repeated vomiting, high fever, and severe headache appearing—and 2/3 of the patients had a pronounced meningeal syndrome. Leading in the clinical picture were hyperthermia (up to 40–41.5 °C), disorders of consciousness (from somnolence and confusion to stupor and coma), and convulsive syndrome. Convulsions in seven patients were partial; in eight, it was generalized, and they did not respond well to antiepileptic therapy; and in half of the patients, convulsions did not stop for 1–4 weeks. From the very first days of the disease, hemi- and tetraparesis, oculomotor, bulbar, vestibular disorders, and disorders of the respiratory and vasomotor centers were detected. This indicated the involvement in the process not only of the parietal-temporal brain, which is considered the most typical in herpetic encephalitis, but also of the midbrain, upper trunk, and reticular formation.

The pressure of the cerebrospinal fluid in all cases increased to 200–400 mm. Changes in the cerebrospinal fluid were not of the same type: in three cases, it was not changed; in four patients, there was high neutrophil pleiocytosis, in connection with which purulent meningoencephalitis was suspected at the beginning; and in the rest, there was mixed pleiocytosis ($0.3–0.4 \times 10^9$/l) with a predominance of neutrophils or lymphocytes, and in the course of the disease, the cell composition changed. In 1/3 of the children, an admixture of fresh red blood cells was detected. Rehabilitation of the cerebrospinal fluid occurred after 3–5 weeks. Moderate leukocytosis, a slight increase in erythrocyte sedimentation rate (ESR), and a significant rod-shaped shift (up to 30–40%) were detected in the blood. On the fundus of two patients, stagnant nipples of the optic nerves were found. The craniograms of all patients showed clear signs of intracranial hypertension. On the EchoEG, an expansion of the ventricular system was recorded, sometimes a shift of the M-echo by 5–6 mm.

The course of herpetic encephalitis in all cases was severe and extremely severe, requiring a long stay of most patients in the intensive care unit. In seven children, hypertension-hydrocephalus syndrome and gross focal symptoms steadily increased, which significantly complicated the differential diagnosis with the volumetric process; this was not contradicted by the data of additional studies. On the electroencephalogram (EEG) in the early stages of herpetic encephalitis, all patients showed gross diffuse changes, with more than half showing paroxysmal activity and 2/3 showing interhemispheric asymmetry with a predominance of δ-waves. In fatal cases, the severity of slow complexes increased, and then there was a flattening of the EEG in all leads. According to the correlation analysis of EEG, there was a significant decrease in these patients compared to healthy children in the intercentral relationships with an increase of 2.5 times ($p < 0.05$) in the number of negative correlations and 3 times ($p < 0.05$) in the interhemispheric connections, especially in the symmetrical centers of the frontal, inferior parietal and temporal zones. Normalization of the EEG occurred very slowly; single and bilateral bursts of high-amplitude δ-waves, as well as dysrhythmia of oscillations, were recorded for a long time; interhemispheric asymmetry was also preserved. Changes in the interhemispheric organization of potentials depended on the severity and outcome of the disease, but the general pattern was an increase in interhemispheric correlations of the inferior parietal and frontal associative zones in comparison with other centers.

Five children recovered; they had multiple neurological microsymptomatics. Fourteen children died on the 8th–28th day from the onset of the disease. Two patients developed decerebration and decortication, three patients had severe consequences in the form of developmental delay, personality changes, symptomatic epilepsy, and hemiparesis. In one child of 6 years old, herpetic infection occurred as serous meningitis with a favorable outcome, and in one more, as severe meningomyelopolyradiculoneuropathy with residual phenomena.

With computed tomography (CT), the foci are visualized from 2 to 3 days of the disease. After intravenous contrast, the nodal accumulation of the contrast agent is determined. Encephalomalacia with the formation of necrosis foci can be registered from 6 to 9 days.

With magnetic resonance imaging (MRI), the foci are visualized 1–2 days from the onset of the disease; they have an irregular shape, fuzzy borders, a pronounced mass effect, and the accumulation of a contrast agent. Areas of destruction are visible on days 5–6. In the end, after 2–3 months, a rough cystic transformation is formed.

V.A. Zinserling [6] studied in detail 21 autopsy observations. In ten of them, herpetic meningoencephalitis was diagnosed. In these observations, not only were detected morphological signs of infection caused by the DNA virus, but there was also laboratory confirmation of the etiology of the process using at least one additional method (serological, virological, and enzyme immunoassay).

Among the deceased children, there were five boys and five girls aged from 4 to 11 months; the exception was a girl of 12 years. In six out of ten of these observations, there were distinct manifestations of generalized herpetic infection with the development of changes not only in the brain but also in the liver, lungs, and some other organs. In four cases, changes in the internal organs associated with herpes were minimal or practically absent.

The immediate cause of death according to clinical and morphological data in all children was herpetic meningoencephalitis, although bacterial complications, primarily pneumonia, had a certain significance in the thanatogenesis of all the deceased; however, manifestations of microbial lesions in the brain were detected only in one child.

When opening the brain, moderate thickening and sharp fullness of the soft meninges attracted attention, and petechial hemorrhages were also detected in one observation. The brain, in most cases, was very flabby in consistency, and when extracted, it lost its shape. Six children had foci of softening in the frontotemporal or frontotemporal areas, without distinct borders, measuring up to 2 cm in diameter. In one child, it was possible to identify necrotic foci with distinct borders in the absence of significant changes from other parts of the brain. In one child with the maximum duration of the disease, significant cavities with necrotic walls in the parietal-temporal regions were determined, not connected with cerebral ventricles, containing about 200 ml of cloudy whitish-pink fluid. In one child, necrosis was not found macroscopically.

A microscopic examination revealed more or less widespread fields of nerve cell lysis in all the observations, the boundaries of which significantly exceeded the softening foci diagnosed by macroscopic examination. In these fields, however, the vessels in which the hypertrophy of endothelial cells was determined were preserved. Perivascular mononuclear infiltration was also detected. However, in most cases, it was expressed minimally. Only in one child was it intense. The vast majority of the preserved nerve and glial cells underwent pronounced alterative changes; their nuclei were light and swollen, with a marginal chromatin arrangement. In many of them, there were distinct basophilic inclusions, separated by a zone of illumination from the preserved nuclear matter. The nuclei of some of the cells were hyperchromic or had a matte appearance. In two observations, basophilic inclusions were detected in a fairly significant amount in the cytoplasm of nerve cells. Changes similar to those described above were found in the endothelial cells of the soft meninges and the choroidal plexus epithelium. Only two children had distinct glial proliferation. In some cases, the ependymal lining of the cerebral ventricles was exfoliated for a long time and subjected to fine-grained disintegration (Fig. 5.4). The soft meninges of all the deceased were moderately infiltrated by lymphocytes with a slight admixture of neutrophilic leukocytes, and small hemorrhages were regularly detected perivascularly. Similar changes were found in eight more children. However, they were not fully examined by virological methods, and therefore the diagnosis of herpetic encephalitis remained presumptive.

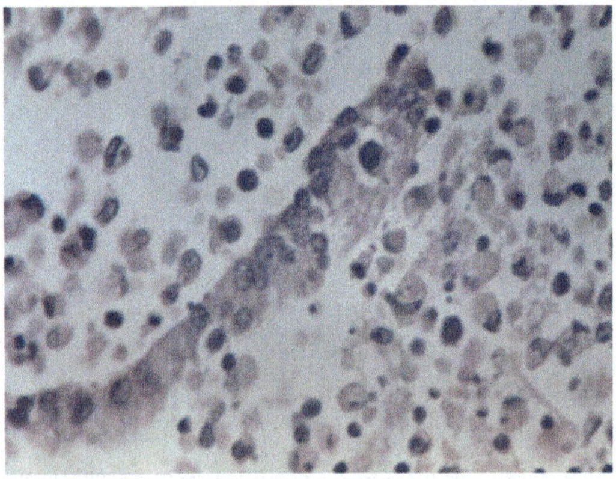

Fig. 5.4 Focal necrotic herpes ventriculitis in 10-month-old girl. Note numerous hyperchromic cell nuclei. H-E ×600

Necrotic changes in one child were subtotal; in four, widespread focal; in one, clearly delineated focal; and in two were detected only microscopically. In addition to acute meningoencephalitis, it was possible to assume the herpetic nature of some changes in the brain in a number of other diseases. Thus, in two cases, a mixed herpetic-meningococcal infection was detected. In addition, our material confirmed the possibility of asymptomatic carriage of the herpesvirus. In one case, a 3-year-old child with repeated intravital and postmortem isolation of the herpesvirus in the absence of antibodies to it was posthumously diagnosed with a hereditary Wilson-Konovalov disease. There were no morphological signs of meningoencephalitis or other manifestations of infection caused by the DNA virus. As an example of a generalized herpetic infection with necrotic meningoencephalitis, one of the observations can be presented.

Ekaterina E., 10 month of age, was born from 3 pregnancy, during which the mother suffered acute viral respiratory infection with otitis media, 2 birth, was born with an umbilical cord entanglement, full-term with normal height and weight indicators. Later, she developed normally and was sane. In mid-February, she had a home contact with a patient with a respiratory infection. She fell ill on the 17th with a rise in temperature to 39 °C, convulsions, and pronounced catarrhal inflammation, in connection with which she was hospitalized and, until the 25th, was treated with a diagnosis of acute respiratory viral infections (ARVI) with febrile convulsions. Until March 1, the girl's condition was compensated, but on this day, the temperature again rose to 39 °C; there was a cough and runny nose. On the night of March 7, repeated clonic-tonic seizures were noted. On the eighth, the girl, with a diagnosis of ARVI (nasopharyngitis) and meningoencephalitis, was transferred to the Research Institute of Children's Infections. Upon admission, her condition in the intensive care unit was regarded as extremely serious, the girl was unconscious, and there were pronounced clonic-tonic convulsions on the left side, floating eyeballs, pronounced meningeal symptoms, hyperthermia, and catarrhal phenomena from the upper respiratory tract. Against the background of active antibacterial, dehydration, and anticonvulsant therapy, the child's condition stabilized during the day, and she began to open her eyes and regain consciousness. However, from the 18th hour on March 9, the girl's condition again deteriorated sharply, she lost consciousness, and she began to have partial seizures in her right limbs, which were refractory to therapy, and this lasted until March 16, when the manifestations of coma began to come to the fore. Since the ninth, she has been constantly on a ventilator. By the 12th, there was a picture of purulent endobronchitis, and from March 14, she had right-sided pneumonia. From the 12th, symptoms of disseminated intravascular coagulation (DIC) syndrome developed; from the same time, pronounced hypothermia was noted. From the 15th, the phenomena of bradiarrhythmia appeared. In the cerebrospinal fluid, cytosis remained about 380/3 throughout the disease with a predominance of neutrophils and protein (0.396 g/l), and all its sowing were negative. In blood tests, in parallel with the development of pneumonia, there was an increase in leukocytosis to 14.4 × 109/l, with a sharp shift to the left of up to 28 rods, and single myelocytes. Subsequently, against the background of active antibacterial therapy, there was a decrease in leukocytosis to 8. 9 × 10^9/l. The blood culture was negative. On the X-ray of the skull, there was a divergence of sutures and finger depressions. On the EchoEG, there were clear signs of intraventricular hypertension without M-echo displacement. On March 18, the child died. The clinical diagnosis was acute viral meningoencephalitis. The following were the complications: edema swelling of the brain, pulmonary edema, DIC syndrome, and myocardiodystrophy. Concomitant diseases found were ARVI; perinatal encephalopathy; bilateral bronchopneumonia, right upper lobe; and DN III. A clinical autopsy (performed by V.A. Zinserling) revealed purulent-necrotic tracheobronchitis and a dark-red-cherry-colored dense focus in the upper lobe of the right lung. The brain has a very flabby consistency, weighing 885 g (with an age norm of 726), and the furrows and convolutions are almost completely smoothed out. In the area of the hippocampal gyrus were noted bilateral spot hemorrhages. On the section, the border between gray and white matter is indistinct; in the area of the left frontal lobe, it is indistinguishable. In all parts of the white matter, sharply dilated vessels and an uneven wet and dull incision surface are detected. On the right, in the parietal lobe, at the border with the temporal and occipital lobes, there is a focus of tissue disorganization of up to 4.0 cm in diameter without clear borders. The cerebral ventricles are moderately dilated, the ependyma lining them is edematous, and the subependymal vessels are dilated. In the kidneys, liver, and heart, there are distinct phenomena of parenchymal degeneration. The thymus is weighing 2.5 g, of very flabby consistency, and hardly distinguishable from the surrounding tissues. Histobacterioscopic and cytological examination revealed a significant number of neutrophilic leukocytes and rods in the tracheal smear. In the lung smears were found mainly altered cells of the alveolar and ciliated epithelium, partially containing fuchsinophilic inclusions, a moderate number of neutrophilic leukocytes and rods. An immunofluorescent (IF) examination revealed moderate positive lighting in lung smears with sera for influenza A3 and parainfluenza. During the serological examination, antibodies to HSV-1 were found in the postmortem blood at a titer of 1:20 and in the CSF1:40; in addition, antibodies to the respiratory syncytial (RS) virus were determined at a titer of 1:80. Antibodies to influenza A3 in the titer were determined in the intravital and postmortem blood samples 1:40/1:40–1:80/1:40. During the virological examination, HSV-1 was isolated from the brain tissue in cell culture. The postmortem determination of interferon content in tissues revealed that it was absent in the lungs; in the blood, it was contained in low titers (0.8); and in the brain, it was contained in quite significant titers (2.1), and by its properties, it could be attributed to viral interferon-α. Bacteriological examination revealed a picture of purulent tracheitis caused by rods. Mononuclears with enlarged hyperchromic nuclei were also detected in the tracheal mucosa. In the lungs, there were massive pillow-like growths of the bronchial epithelium. In the lumen of the alveoli, especially in the area of compaction, were seen red blood cells and protein-rich fluid, "influenza" cells. Many cells in both the alveolar wall and the alveolar lumen have enlarged hyperchromic nuclei. Similar changes were also detected in lymphocytes in various groups of lymph nodes, the spleen, the adrenal glands, epithelial cells and interstitial cells in the kidneys, hepatocytes and Kupffer cells in the liver, and enterocytes. In addition, expressed alternative and sometimes necrobiotic changes were found in all these organs. There was a suppression of the central and peripheral immune organs. The soft meninges are significantly thickened due to lymph-mononuclear infiltration, many cells in which have enlarged hyperchromic nuclei. In the wall and around individual vessels, mainly lymphocytic infiltration is detected, including cells with enlarged hyperchromic nuclei. Perivascular hemorrhages in the hippocampus region are surrounded by a significant number of cells typical of herpes. Here, as well as in other departments, there are clusters of cells of the macrophage lineage, as well as poorly differentiated glia, usually with enlarged nuclei containing hyperchromic inclusions. Were noted as well common alterative changes in nerve cells, many of which had a typical appearance for herpes, lysis of many neurons with the appearance of extensive fields of prolapse. The ependyma is sloughed for a considerable length, and in its place are rather massive mononuclear infiltrates with hyperchromic cells, often subjected to fine-grained decay (see Fig. 5.4). In the choroidal plexuses, there are distinct growths of the epithelial cells of their lining. The final pathological diagnosis is necrotic herpetic meningoencephalitis on the background of generalized herpes with damage to the respiratory system, kidneys, liver, intestines, spleen, lymph nodes, and heart. Complications of the main disease are cerebral edema, bilateral hemorrhages in the hippocampal gyrus area, accidental involution of the thymus gland IV with pronounced suppression of peripheral immune organs, tracheal intubation, purulent tracheobronchitis caused by *Klebsiella,* and hemorrhages in the upper lobe of the right lung. The following are the concomitant diseases: mixed viral respiratory infection (influenza A3 + parainfluenza), respiratory syncytial infection with predominant brain damage, and pathological epicrisis. Ekaterina E., 10 months old, died from a generalized herpetic infection and was diagnosed on the basis of the clinical picture, characteristic structural changes in a number of internal organs, the results of the serological examination of the blood and cerebrospinal fluid, and the isolation of the HSV-1 virus from the brain. The most important manifestation of this infection was necrotic meningoencephalitis with severe changes characteristic of this infection in the meninges, brain matter, and ependyma, which served as the direct cause of the child's death. Herpesvirus lesions of other organs, primarily the lungs, spleen, and kidneys, also had a certain significance in thanatogenesis. The severe course of the main disease, as well as the direct impact of the herpesvirus, led to a pronounced secondary immunodeficiency condition in the child.

Significant difficulties were also presented by the clinical diagnosis of the fatal follow-up of child X, 9 years old, who was clinically suspected of having a brain tumor (Figs. 5.5, 5.6, 5.7, 5.8).

Among the causes of mortality in nonepidemic encephalitis and herpetic encephalitis in adults is the main one. The mortality rate in herpetic encephalitis is 70–90% in cases of late diagnosis. In adults, as well as in children, the onset of herpetic encephalitis is in most cases acute

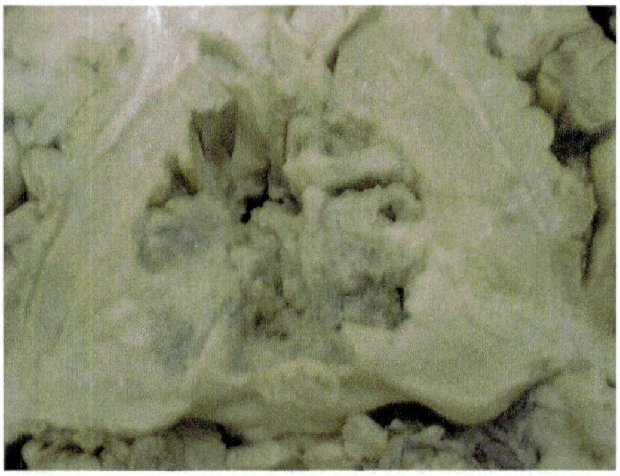

Fig. 5.5 Macroscopic changes in tumor-like course of herpetic encephalitis in a boy 9 years old

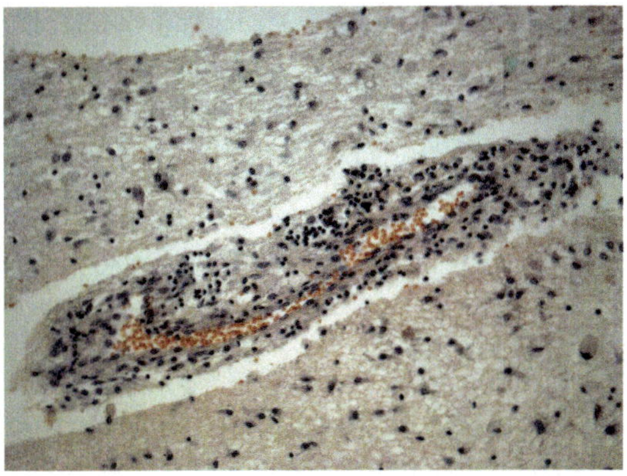

Fig. 5.6 Expressed vasculitis and perivasculitis with mononuclear cuffing in the same case. H-E ×200

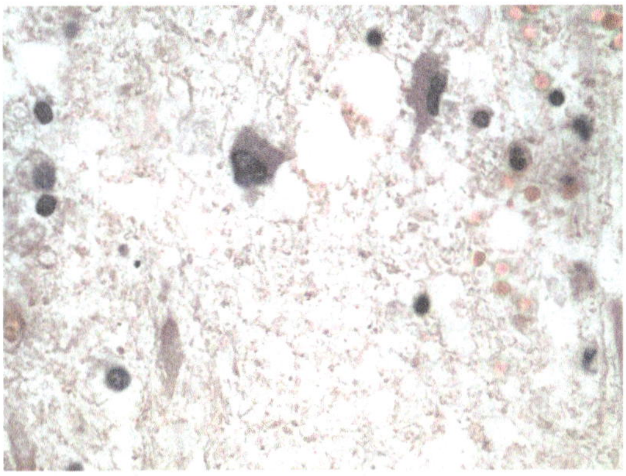

Fig. 5.7 Focal necrosis and intranuclear basophilic inclusion in neuron in the same case. HE ×600

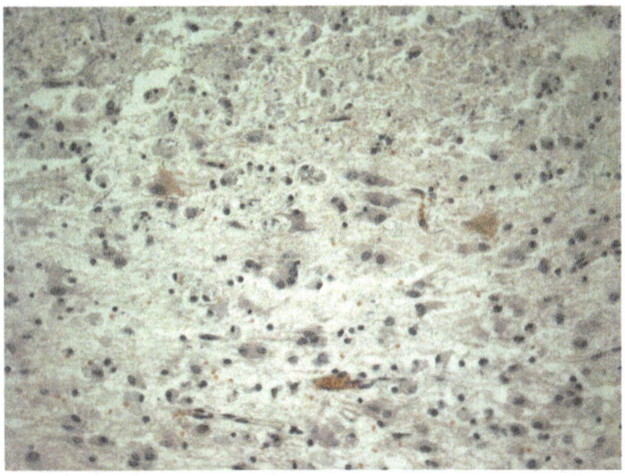

Fig. 5.8 Focal necrosis and moderate glial proliferation in the same case. H-E X300

with a rapid rise in temperature. There are early disorders of consciousness in the form of sopor, coma, characterized by focal and generalized convulsive seizures. Hemiparesis and speech disorders of the type of aphasia are detected, and meningeal symptoms can be determined. Due to the fact that herpetic rashes on the skin in such patients are rare, carrying out a differential diagnosis causes significant difficulties. Quite often, these patients with directional diagnoses (acute cerebrovascular disturbance, subarachnoid hemorrhage) are hospitalized in neurological departments instead of infectious hospitals. As a result, modern laboratory diagnostics of herpes are not carried out at an early stage, which does not allow the timely prescription of antiviral drugs.

We conducted a comprehensive clinical, laboratory, and morphological analysis of 14 cases of patients who died at the S.P. Botkin Infectious Diseases Hospital, No. 30, in St. Petersburg [6]. The diagnosis was made on the basis of clinical and laboratory data and the results of postmortem histological and immunohistochemical studies. Among the deceased were seven men (aged 40 to 93 years) and seven women (aged 19–86 years).

In the literature, the most complete information is about the structural changes in the adult brain with necrotic encephalitis [1, 2]; in other numerous variants of herpetic lesions, it is rare. It is possible to distinguish between acute and chronic meningoencephalitis and herpetic encephalopathy. Acute herpetic encephalitis was clinically characterized by fever, headache, small CSF cytosis, and increased ESR. In the terminal period, there were symptoms of deafness, coma, sopor, generalized convulsions, and acute multiple organ failure. A morphological examination revealed extensive foci of cortical necrosis, hemorrhages, and pronounced perivascular mononuclear infiltrates. In the preserved neurons, glia, and endothelium, inclusions of Cowdry types 1 and 2, the "mulberry" phenomenon, were determined. In chronic herpes meningoencephalitis (HME), a recurrent course with a tendency for progression was noted in the clinic. The morphological examination revealed perivascular mononuclear infiltrates in the cortex and white matter of the brain; sclerosis of the soft meninges with lymph-histiocyte-plasma cell infiltration, occasionally with an admixture of segmental neutrophil granulocytes; deposition of calcium salts in the walls of blood vessels; sclerosis of perivascular spaces; and single hemosiderophages in the membranes and the substance of the brain. In the cortex, there was shrinking and hyperchromia of neurons and their focal loss mainly along the third layer, satellitosis, neuronophagy, foci of gliofibrosis and microglial nodules, and proliferation of capillary endothelium. With exacerbation, necrosis of various sizes also occurred. In 90% of cases, there was a correspondence between the clinical picture and morphological data. Herpetic infections were characterized by a combination of neurological and somatic symptoms. In the morphological examination, foci of necrosis, hemorrhages, and "signs of inflammation" were not found. Mainly, severe dystrophic (swelling of the cell body, uneven chromatolysis, melting of the cytoplasm, hyperchromatosis of the nucleus and its shrinking) and hypoxic changes in the nerve cells; satellitosis and neuronophagy; as well as the presence of intracranial inclusions, mainly type 1, were determined. It should be noted that this diagnosis in the world of pathological practice is extremely rare, mainly in single centers. These circumstances certainly open up prospects for further research. Based on our material, the analysis of variants of changes caused by herpes simplex virus type 1 showed that it can be associated with various necrotic foci, surrounded by a moderate number of cells with hyperchromic nuclei, some of which are usually contoured with basophilic inclusions. The degree of severity of the predominantly astroglial cell reaction varies sharply in individual observations. The involvement of blood vessels with the development of vasculitis was also very characteristic.

A consultative observation from a large multispecialty hospital was of considerable interest. A middle-aged patient was examined for a long time in connection with a brain lesion of unknown origin, and an atypical course of stroke was not excluded. A histological examination revealed focal necrotic encephalitis (with distinct intracranial basophilic and oxyphilic inclusions). An IHC study demonstrated HSV antigen (Fig. 5.9).

When studying individual advisory observations of biopsy material, it is occasionally possible to establish the herpetic etiology of focal encephalitis. In these cases, patients were operated on due to an erroneous diagnosis of a brain tumor. The latter is due to the fact that herpetic necrotic encephalitis can occur under the guise of glial brain tumors (see Chap. 19).

There are generalized and local forms of necrotic encephalitis. The local form is usually associated with a lesion of the temporal lobes. The development of sensory aphasia is characterized by focal necrotic encephalitis with distinct intracranial involvement of the left temporal lobe; auditory, olfactory, and taste hallucinations; and focal convulsive seizures. The manifestation of the generalized form includes the addition of general cerebral symptoms.

Pathological diagnosis is based upon an evaluation of necrotic foci at autopsy (Fig. 5.10) and typical histological changes, including intranuclear basophilic inclusions (Fig. 5.11) and widespread inflammatory changes (Fig. 5.12). Confirmation by IHC is necessary (Fig. 5.13).

We can present the following example. Man A, 39 years old, died on the 11th day of his stay in the hospital, in the third week of the disease. From the anamnesis, it is known that he suffered from vasomotor rhinitis and infrequent acute respiratory infections and smoked. He fell ill on December 30, acutely with a temperature of 39 °C. The next day at work, he had a convulsive seizure and was hospitalized in a somatic hospital, from where he was discharged home. Since 3/01, a series of convulsive seizures occurred, he was taken to the neurological department of another somatic hospital in a serious condition, with a temperature of 39 °C, tachycardia with pulse up to 150 in min, in the cerebrospinal fluid, lymphocytic cytosis 114/3. With a diagnosis of viral meningitis and probable myocarditis 4/I in an extremely serious condition, unconscious, with positive meningeal symptoms, he was transferred to the intensive care unit of the S. P.

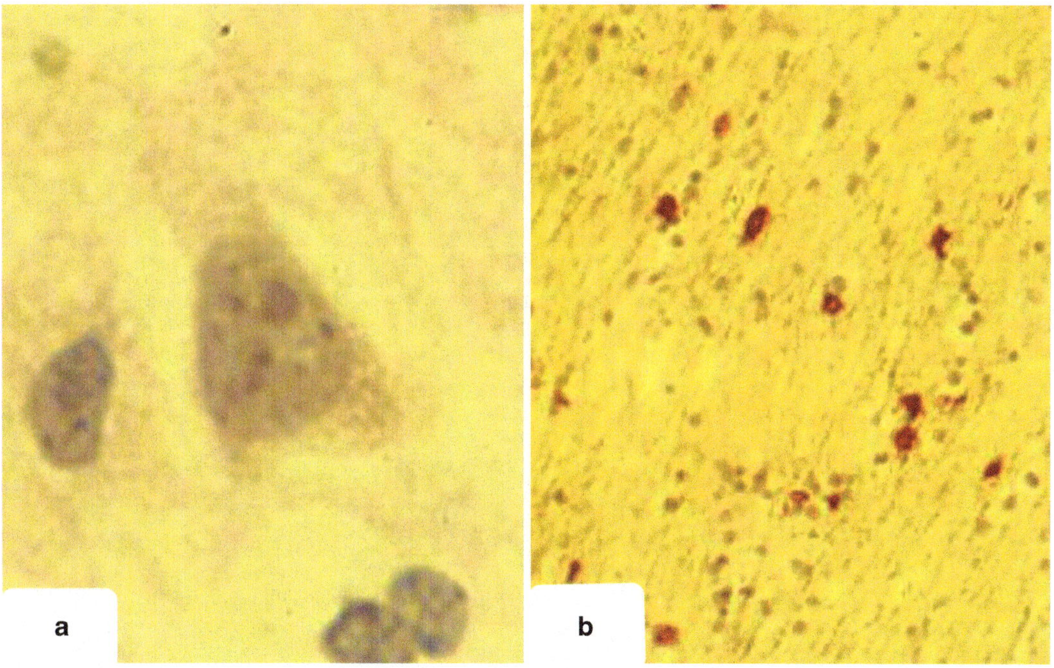

Fig. 5.9 Focal herpes encephalitis with atypical clinical course in adult patient. (**a**) Typical intranuclear inclusion. H-E X 600. (**b**) Antigen of HSV in numerous nervous cells. IHC X 200

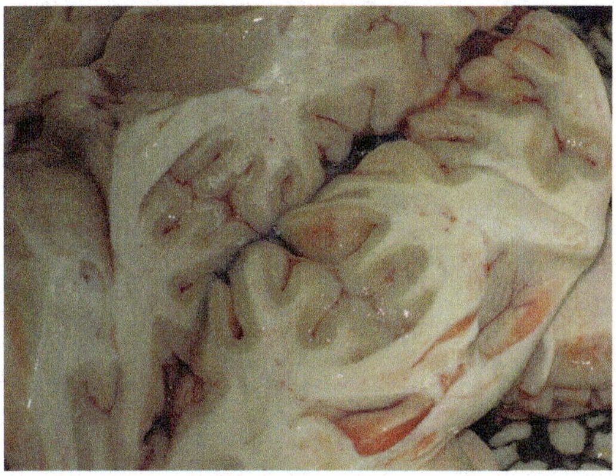

Fig. 5.10 Focal necrotic encephalitis in adult. Courtesy of A.N. Isakov

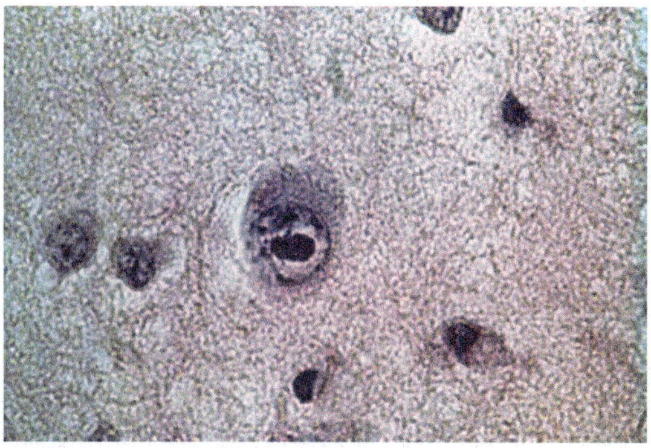

Fig. 5.11 Typical for herpes encephalitis intranuclear inclusion in adult. H-E X600

Botkin infectious hospital. During the entire time of unconsciousness, he had left eye paresis, horizontal nystagmus, and subfebrile fever. Eventually, the development of dislocation syndrome, secondary pneumonia, and death was noted. In the CSF, the fluctuations are mainly lymphocytic in the range of 252–992/3 cytosis. In the blood test, there was moderate leukocytosis with a shift to the left. A herpes simplex virus antigen was detected in the blood.

The macroscopic examination of the brain revealed small-focal hemorrhages in dull soft meninges. The brain is large and flabby with a smoothed surface. The left hemisphere spreads out more than the right. The tissue on the incision is bulging with many reddish-greenish foci of different sizes from petechial to 1.0 cm

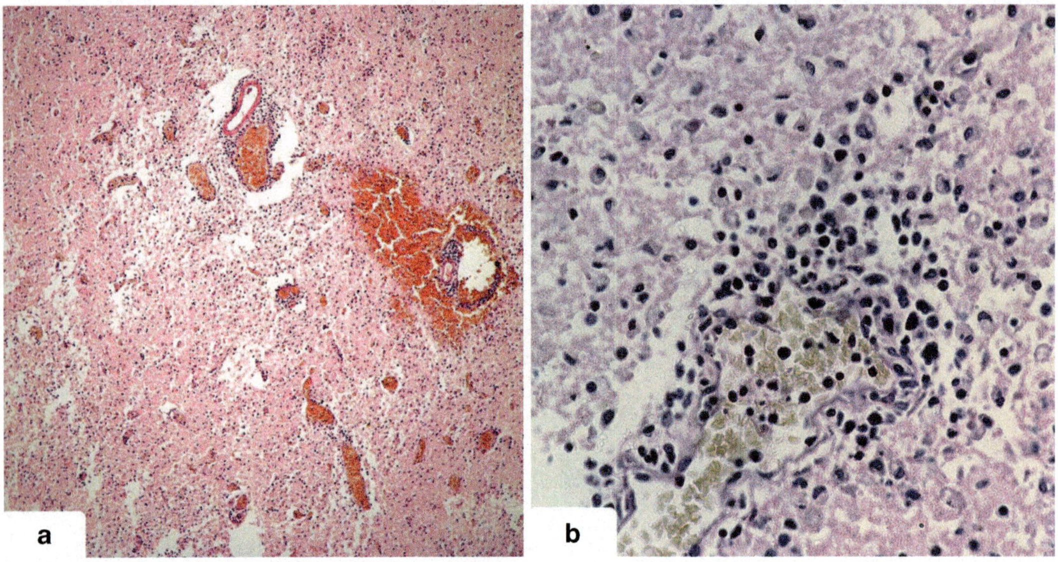

Fig. 5.12 Different types of inflammatory reactions in herpes encephalitis in adult. H-E. (**a**) Acute necrosis, hemorrhage, loose mononuclear cell infiltration. X 100. (**b**) Dense perivascular infiltration, including hyperchromic cells. X 200

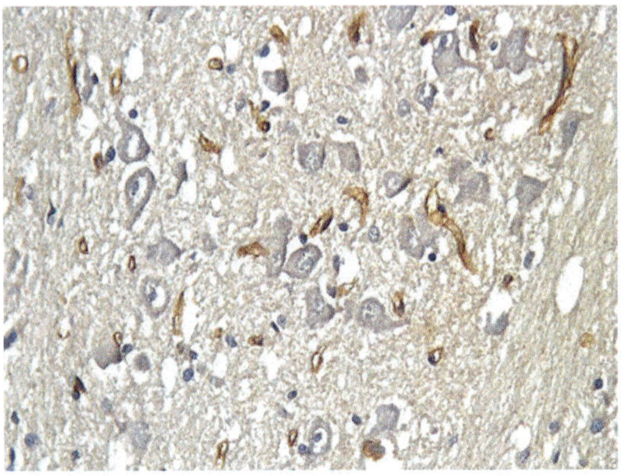

Fig. 5.13 HSV antigen in different parts of neurons with moderate inflammatory reaction. IHC X200

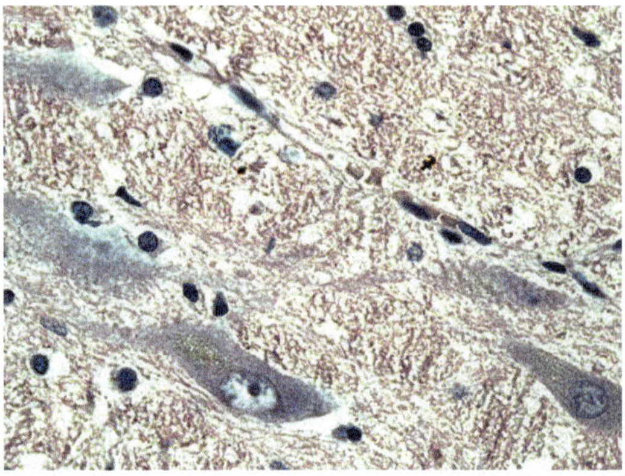

Fig. 5.14 Severe degenerative changes in neurons of brain stem in necrotic encephalitis in 39-year-old man. H-E X600

in diameter. In the temporal-parietal region of the left hemisphere was found large foci of mush-like grayish-reddish-cyanotic spreading tissue up to 8.0–9.0 cm in diameter. The microscopic examination shows a picture of necrotic encephalitis (Fig. 5.14), serous-hemorrhagic leptomeningitis, and ventriculitis. On the part of the internal organs, purulent-necrotic tracheitis (on the background of mechanical ventilation) and focal abscessing pneumonia had some significance to the unfavorable outcome of the disease.

The complexity of the clinical-computer-tomographic differential diagnosis of acute necrotic encephalitis and glial brain tumor is known. It should be emphasized that in the early stages of the development of herpetic encephalitis, CT and MRI manifestations correspond to brain edema, a hyperintensive signal on T2-VI is

Table 5.2 Distribution of children by age and study group

Age	Group I	Group II	Group III	Group IV	Total
2–5 months	1	7	2	2	12
6–11 months	1	0	1	1	3
1 year	0	0	2	1	3
2–3 years	1	1	1	1	4
Total	3	8	6	5	22

typical, and foci of hemorrhage are possible; when contrast is introduced, a gyral or parenchymal type of change in signal intensity is observed [8]. Only later on were there foci of necrosis, typical for herpetic infection, in the projection of the medial parts of the temporal lobes and the lower frontal gyri. Herpetic infection often causes not only CNS lesions but also diseases of the peripheral nervous system. In recent years, a connection with herpesviruses of facial nerve lesions has been established. The etiological heterogeneity of this pathology is known. The spectrum of nervous system lesions caused by herpesviruses is quite wide; they differ in the polymorphism of clinical manifestations and in the outcomes, depending on the nature of the pathogen, the age of the patients, and their premorbid background. Herpes is diverse and insidious, often persisting in the body for decades, and it is activated, causing severe damage to the nervous system. It is proved that a good therapeutic effect in herpetic encephalitis is possible only with early diagnosis and the timely appointment for etiotropic and pathogenetic therapy.

5.5 Chronic Course of Herpetic Brain Lesions in Children

The literature has repeatedly described and analyzed how the relationship between intrauterine infections and such diseases of the nervous system as perinatal brain damage and encephalopathy (PEP), cerebral palsy (cerebral palsy), and others demonstrated a significant role of inflammatory reactions within the central nervous system in fetuses and newborns (for example, by the activity of certain cytokines in the CSF in the occurrence of neurological pathology. The pathology of intrauterine herpes has been described in sufficient detail to date (see Chap. 16), but the features of the morphological manifestations of chronically current herpetic intrauterine infection in the central nervous system in the postnatal period and its relationship with neurological pathology in children of different ages have been studied to a much lesser extent.

We (P.V. Antonov, V.A. Zinserling, S.P. Vydumkina) conducted special studies in this direction [9]. The subjects of the study were CNS tissues (brain matter, soft meninges, choroidal plexuses), CSF, and blood serum of 22 deceased children aged 1 month to 3 years with clinically unrecognized herpetic infection (Table 5.2). All major parts of the brain were examined: the cortex and the periventricular parts of the major hemispheres in various lobes, the basal ganglia, the hippocampus, the thalamus, the brainstem (medulla oblongata and midbrain), and the cerebellum (cortex and dentate nucleus). In 17 cases, the afterbirth of deceased children was examined.

Most of the children from the neonatal period suffered from persistent neurological pathology of varying severity. According to the severity of the neurological symptoms diagnosed during life, all children can be divided into the following groups:

- Group I (three children): no manifest clinical manifestations of nervous system damage.
- Group II (eight children): mild and moderate manifestations of perinatal encephalopathy (PEP)—disorders of muscle tone, moderate hypertension-hydrocephalus syndrome were registered.
- Group III (six children): diagnoses of severe PEP, organic brain damage, hydrocephalus, delay in psychomotor development, convulsive seizures, and pyramidal or extrapyramidal insufficiency.

Table 5.3 The number of children with unfavorable factors of anamnesis

Factors	Group I	Group II	Group III	Group IV	Total
Gestosis	1 (33)[a]	2 (25)	1 (17)	No information	4 (18)
Infections of genitourinary system in mothers	1 (33)	2 (25)	2 (33)	3 (60)	8 (36)
Prematurity	2 (66)	3 (38)	3 (50)	3 (60)	11 (50)
Prenatal hypotrophy	0 (0)	3 (38)	2 (35)	4 (80)	9 (41)
Asphyxia	1 (33)	4 (50)	1 (17)	3 (60)	9 (41)
Retardation in psychomotor development	1 (33)	4 (50)	6 (100)	5 (100)	16 (73)

[a]In brackets is presented percentage of children in the group, in the graph «Total» percentage to the general number of children

- Group IV (five children): severe organic brain damage and cerebral palsy—spastic paralysis, pseudobulbar syndromes, epileptic seizures.

Many children had an unfavorable medical history, including the obstetric and gynecological history of their mothers (Table 5.3).

In all the observations, an IF study of smears from the soft meninges of the cerebral hemispheres and vascular plexuses, a serological examination of blood serum and cerebrospinal fluid (complement binding reaction), as well as a macroscopic and microscopic (cytological and histological) examination of CNS tissues were performed. In 20 cases, an IHC study was conducted with the detection of HSV 1/2 antigen. The specimen were fixed in a 10% solution of neutral formalin, wired according to the standard scheme, embedded in paraffin, stained with hematoxylin and eosin, according van Gieson, methylene blue - basic fuchsin according to Seller.

The results of the virological examination according to at least one method were positive in all cases (Table 5.4). As can be seen from Table 5.4, HSV antigens were most often detected in children of groups 3 and 4. In children of groups 1 and 2, they were detected, as a rule, in the vascular plexuses.

Macroscopically, the brain mass in the children of group I corresponded to the age norm, the convolutions of the large hemispheres were convex, the furrows were deep enough, the ventricles had a slit-like shape, the differentiation into white and gray matter was clear, and no focal changes were detected. In group II, three children had reduced brain mass, two had disturbed differentiation of brain tissue, and two had a relative expansion of the lateral ventricles. Of the children of group III, three had a reduced brain mass, five were diagnosed with the initial stages of internal hydrocephalus, and occasionally indistinct differentiation of the brain substance was detected. In all cases in group IV, there were pronounced macroscopic changes, consisting of internal hydrocephalus of varying severity, focal microgyria, false porencephaly, and weak differentiation of the cerebral cortex.

A microscopic examination revealed a number of changes that were considered specific for the HSV lesion. First of all, these were oxyphilic and basophilic intracranial inclusions (Fig. 5.15), of which the latter were often surrounded by a rim of enlightenment. The size of the inclusions ranged from 2 to 7 microns; sometimes, several inclusions were observed in one core. Along with having a rounded shape, there were inclusions with an uneven border, oval, or irregular star shape. In many cells, hyperchromatosis and enlargement of the nuclei were noted, they were of uneven color, had matte appearance, chromatin was often located in large clumps, frequently on the periphery of the nuclei. The described inclusions were detected in different cells of the central nervous system (located by decreasing the frequency of occurrence): neurons, astrocytes, oligodendrogliocytes, and meningocytes; in the epithelium of the vascular plexus, ependymocytes and endotheliocytes were detected. Often, the inclusions were localized in the cerebral cortex, less often but also quite regularly in the basal ganglia and thalamus, and even less often in the brain stem and cerebellum.

From nonspecific changes, inflammatory infiltrates were identified, consisting mainly of

Table 5.4 Results of virological and IHC research (In each group, observations are arranged from top to bottom according to the increase in the age of the children)

	IF meninges		IF plexus chorioideus		IHC		Blood serology		Liquor serology	
Group	HS1	HS2	HS1	HS2	Cortex	Basal ganglia	HS1	HS2	HS1	HS2
I (without manifest clinical manifestations)	–	–	+	–	+	–	20	0	0	0
	–	–	+	–	No inf.	+ –	0	0	20	40
	+	+	–	–	+	–	0	0	0	0
II (mild-degree PE)	–	–	–	+	–	–	0	0	0	40
	–	–	+	–	No inf.	No inf.	0	0	0	0
	–	–	+++	–	–	+ –	40	20	0	0
	–	–	–	–	+ –	+	10	0	10	0
	–	–	–	–	+ –	+ –	20	40	0	20
	–	–	+	–	+ –	+ –	0	0	20	20
	–	–	+	–	–	+ –	10	0	0	0
	–	–	–	–	+ –	–	0	10	0	0
III (moderate PE)	+	–	++	–	+	+	0	0	40	40
	–	–	–	–	–	–	20	20	0	0
	+	–	+	–	+ –	–	40	10	10	0
	+	–	+++	–	+	–	20	40	0	20
	–	+	–	+	+ –	+	80	40	0	0
	+	–	+	–	+ –	+ –	0	0	0	0
IV (severe PE)	++	+	++	+	–	–	0	0	0	0
	+	–	+++	–	+	–	20	0	0	0
	++	–	++	–	–	–	0	0	0	0
	–	–	+++	–	No inf.	No inf.	0	0	0	0
	+	–	+	–	+ –	–	0	40	0	20

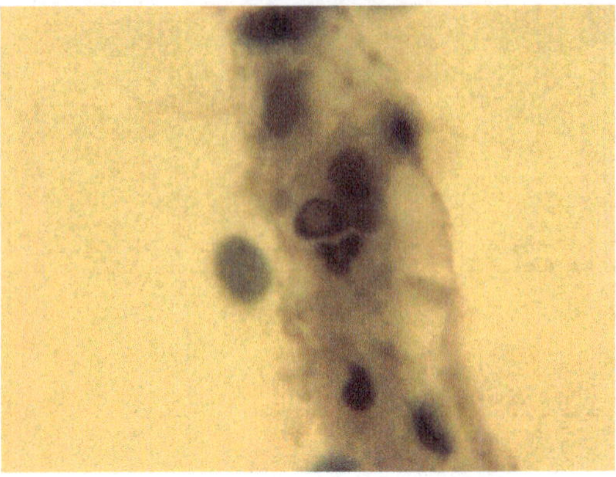

Fig. 5.15 Oxyphilic intranuclear inclusion in brain meninges in a child with chronic course of herpes encephalitis. H-E X 1000

lymphocytes, occasionally with an admixture of histiocytes. In the meninges, they were, as a rule, focal or small focal in nature; in some cases, they were located over a fairly large length, while sometimes there were areas of fibroblastic changes. The cell concentration was low. Also, weakly or moderately pronounced infiltration was detected in the vessel walls and perivascularly; sometimes, it was accompanied by vascular fibrosis, swelling and proliferation of endothelial cells, and loss of their connection with the vessel wall. Most often, such changes occurred in vessels of medium and small calibers, usually arteries and arterioles, and less often in veins. Their localization was diverse (including the brainstem and cerebellum) but still somewhat more common in the cerebral cortex. Separate infiltrates and focal fibrosis were also observed in the vascular plexus tissue.

In most cases, gliosis of brain tissue was detected. Often, it was located in subperpendicular sections, representing a narrow or wider band. Sometimes, focal and diffuse-focal gliosis was detected in the deep layers of the large hemispheres; the size of the foci ranged from 50 to 100 microns. Often, the glial elements were located near or close to the blood vessels. In some cases, gliosis was mainly found in the basal ganglia, thalamus, and hippocampus and in others, in the cortical and subcortical parts of the brain.

In many observations, changes in the ependyma were found in the form of its folding, often quite deep, and on some sections having the appearance of small cysts lined with ependymocytes. The study of serial sections convincingly showed that these are ependymal folds. In addition, small calcifications; increased satellite formation, often with separate neuronophagic nodules; and a violation of the cytoarchitectonics of the cerebral cortex were also detected. The described changes occurred in all cases, but their frequency and severity tended to be directly related to the severity of the clinical picture. There was no convincing correlation with the age of children; in different age groups, there was either an active process (intracranial inclusions, vasculitis) or a torpid current (gliosis). This circumstance may indicate that the persistence of viruses proceeds in waves. Changes characteristic of herpetic infection were found in all the studied aftereffects in varying degrees of severity [10], namely, giant cell metamorphosis with enlargement and hyperchromatosis of the nuclei, basophilic intracranial inclusions with a rim of enlightenment, and foci of fine-grained cell decay. Such changes were detected in the basal lamina, syncytiotrophoblast of the villous chorion, amniocytes, as well as extraplacental membranes. The presence of such changes in the afterbirth confirms the fact of intrauterine infection of the studied children. The presence of antibodies not only in the blood serum but also in the cerebrospinal fluid strongly indicates both the duration of the infectious process and the localization of the antigens of these viruses within the central nervous system. In the IHC study, which detected replicating viruses, HSV antigens were detected mainly during active infection or its activation in the walls of blood vessels, on the surface of blood cells, in soft meninges, and in single nerve and glial cells. In the area of glial nodules, the virus antigen was not detected in any observation. Taken together, the described changes can be considered manifestations of a weakly (rarely moderately) pronounced inflammatory reaction caused by HSV. There were no fundamental differences in the morphological picture in HSV types 1 and 2. Thus, it can be assumed that herpes simplex viruses types 1 and 2, which infected the fetal central nervous system in utero (often hematogenically), can persist for a long time, causing characteristic morphological changes; the course of such an infectious process is undulating. The persistence of HSV in the central nervous system is often accompanied by clinical manifestations similar to those described in encephalopathy and cerebral palsy in children, since most of the detected morphological changes indicate a viral lesion of the central nervous system and correlate with the severity of the clinical picture; changes associated with other etiological factors of neurological pathology were significantly less pronounced. However, the patterns of pathogenesis of such lesions require further study. Comparisons between the results obtained using different methods prove that in many cases, signs of chronic (latent) infection can only be detected with a very thorough and comprehensive study.

References

1. Kradin RL, editor. Diagnostic pathology of infectious diseases. Elsevier; 2018. p. 698.
2. Hofman P, editor. Infectious disease and parasites. Springer Reference; 2016. p. 343.
3. Herpes Simplex Virus/R. Diefenbach, C. Fraefel/ Springer, p. 457, 2020.
4. Agut H, Bonnafous P, Gautheret-Dejean A. Laboratory and clinical aspects of human herpes virus 6 infection. Clin Microbiol Rev. 2015;28(2):313–35.
5. Frye TD, Chiou HC, Hull BE, Bigley NJ. The efficacy of DNA vaccine encoding herpes simplex virus type1 (HSV-1) glycoprotein D in decreasing ocular disease severity following corneal HSV-1 challenge. Arch Virol. 2002;147(9):1747–59. https://doi.org/10.1007/s00705-002-0830-6.
6. Zinserling VA, Chukhlovina ML. Infectious lesions of nervous system. Issues of etiology, pathogenesis and diagnostics. Saint-Petersburg: ElbiSPb; 2011. p. 583. (In Russian)
7. Tsinzerling VA, Popova ED, Baikov VV, et al. Experimental model of generalized herpetic infection in newborns. Arkh Patol. 1993;55(5):28–32.
8. Dadiomova MA, Sorokina MN, Tsinzerling VA, Zinchenko AP, Kogan IL. Herpetic lesions of the nervous system in children. Zh Nevropatol Psikhiatr im SS Korsakova. 1987;87(10):1473–9. (in Russian)
9. Antonov PV, Vydumkina SP, Tsinzerling VA. The role of intrauterine infection of the central nervous system with herpes simplex viruses in development of encephalopathies in infants. Arkh Patol. 2003;65(4):43–6. (in Russian)
10. Zinserling VA, Melnikova VF. Perinatal infections: issues of pathogenesis, morphological diagnostics and clinico-pathological correlations. SPb, Elbi SPB 2002, (in Russian).

6 Acute Viral Encephalitis of Other Etiology

6.1 Enterovirus Infections

Enteroviruses are widespread pathogens with antigenic polymorphism, polytropism, and the ability to cause various degrees of disease severity.

The genus of enteroviruses of the picornavirus family includes primarily polioviruses, Coxsackie viruses (A and B), enteric cytopathic human orphan (ECHO) group viruses, and hepatitis A. All of these pathogens (except for the hepatitis A virus, for which this issue is insufficiently studied) have a tropism to the nervous tissue and are able to cause a wide range of neuroinfections at different ages. They play the greatest role during childhood.

6.1.1 Polio

Polio has been known to exist on Earth for thousands of years [1]. An image of a man with a paralyzed leg with pronounced atrophy has been found on an ancient Egyptian tombstone. The description of the outbreak of the disease with paralysis and atrophic changes on the Greek island of Phasos is found in the works of Hippocrates. In the 1840s, the German orthopedist J. Heine described a disease with an acute febrile onset, affecting the spinal cord, leading to the development of paralysis, atrophy, and deformities of the limbs in children. At the end of the nineteenth century, the first polio epidemics were recorded in Northern Europe. A description of the epidemic of this disease in Stockholm in 1887 by K. Medin was the most complete; the disease was called epidemic childhood polio.

In 1908, K. Landsteiner and E. Popper created an experimental model of polio by injecting monkeys with an extract of the spinal cord of a patient who died from polio. At a meeting of the Royal and Imperial Medical Association in Vienna on December 18, 1908, K. Landsteiner said that the pathogen of polio belongs to the group of filtered microorganisms; four years later, he wrote about the possibility of creating a vaccine against this serious disease. Indeed, in 1955, Salk first prepared a formalin-inactivated polio vaccine. In 1960, Sabin created a live vaccine.

6.1.2 Etiology and Epidemiology

Numerous studies have established that polio (Heine-Medina disease) is an acute infectious disease caused by the poliovirus. Three serotypes of the virus were identified: I—Brunhilda, II—Lansing, III—Leon, which differ in antigenic properties. It is believed that the Brunhilda virus more often causes epidemic outbreaks of paralytic forms of the disease, the Lansing virus sporadic cases, and the Leon virus-vaccine-associated polio. The poliovirus belongs to the picornavirus family, a genus of enteroviruses, and contains

V. Zinserling, *Infectious Lesions of the Central Nervous System*,
https://doi.org/10.1007/978-3-030-96260-9_6

ribonucleic acid (RNA). It is destroyed when heated to 56 °C after 30 min, under the action of chloramine, hydrogen peroxide in normal concentrations, and ultraviolet irradiation. The virus is resistant to environmental factors. When frozen, the activity of the poliovirus persists for many years; at room temperature, it lasts for several days, tolerates drying well, and is not destroyed by digestive enzymes.

The source of the spread of infection is sick and healthy virus carriers that secrete the virus to nasopharyngeal and intestinal contents, allowing alimentary and airborne pathways of infection. In the first 7–10 days of the disease, the virus can be isolated from pharyngeal flushes. For a longer period (6 weeks, sometimes several months), the virus is released in the fecal masses. The disease can be transmitted through dirty hands, food, or toys. There is evidence of a wide spread of enteroviruses, including polio, in the external environment and in food.

Polio is classified as a seasonal infection with a pronounced increase in incidence in the summer-autumn period (July–September). Acute polio is highly contagious; people of any age are affected but most often children under 7 years of age (70–90%).

Acute polio has been registered in all countries of the world. The use of polio vaccines has dramatically reduced the incidence. Currently, sporadic cases and epidemic outbreaks continue to be reported in some countries.

Currently, the World Health Organization (WHO), developing the concept of polio eradication, has paid special attention to the epidemiological surveillance of cases of acute flaccid paralysis, among which patients with polio may be hiding.

6.1.3 Pathogenesis and Pathology

Infection with polio occurs by fecal oral and airborne droplets: by eating contaminated food or by contact with a patient. Most often, the disease occurs in the summer-autumn period. The entrance gates of the virus are the upper respiratory and gastrointestinal tracts. The virus multiplies in the lymphatic structures of the posterior wall of the pharynx and intestine, then viremia occurs; during this period, the virus can be isolated from the patient's blood. During the circulation of the virus in the blood, intoxication develops, and the body temperature rises. The poliovirus has a high rate of replication; its reproduction is detected in the lymph nodes, spleen, liver, and lungs.

In most infected people, as a result of the activation of the immune system, the virus is released from the body, and the disease ends with recovery. Nonparalytic forms account for up to 99% of all cases of polio; in 1% of infected patients, the virus penetrates the blood-brain barrier from the blood.

The penetration of the poliomyelitis virus into the nervous system can occur through the endothelium of small vessels, choroidal plexuses, and ventricular ependyma; virion transmission through intercellular spaces and the axoplasm is possible; virus replication in lemmocytes and fibroblasts of the endothelial and perineural membranes is not excluded.

When the virus interacts with the cells of the nervous system, the motor neurons undergo the most intense changes, in which tigrolysis occurs; the process of neuronophagy is expressed significantly already in the early stages of the disease. Experimental studies show that the severity of structural changes in polio also depends on the way in which the virus enters the body. It is believed that the introduction of drugs or vaccines in the incubation period of polio can serve as a provoking factor for the development of paralytic forms of polio.

The virus multiplies in the central nervous system (CNS), mainly in nerve cells. It should be noted that the virus is very similar in structure to the information RNA of the cell. The initial phase of infection is the binding of the virus to a specific cellular receptor, a transmembrane protein of the immunoglobulin superfamily. In addition, the CD44 antigen is also associated with the sensitivity of human cells to the poliovirus, although the poliovirus does not bind directly to it. It is also shown that on the part of the virus, tropism to nerve cells is associated with a section of the

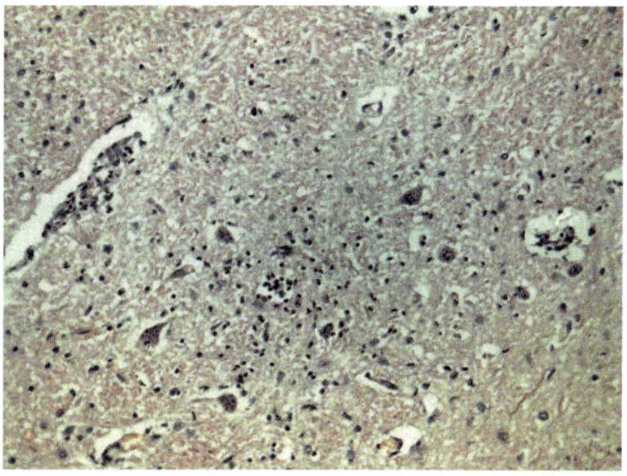

Fig. 6.1 Changes in the spinal cord in polio. Vasculitis, focal loss of nervous cells and neuronophagy. H-E, ×300

genome 5'NTR (nontranslated region). The affected cells swell, and there is a dissolution of tigroid substance and pyknosis of the nucleus. After the death of such cells, neuronophagic nodules are formed, passing through a number of stages in their development. In the first 2 days, clusters of neutrophilic leukocytes appear around the affected cells. Then there is a focal and then a more diffuse reaction of micro-, oligo-, and astrocytic glia (Fig. 6.1). Phagocytosis of the decay products occurs. Cells with a sharply enlarged foamy cytoplasm are called grainy balls. In the acute phase of the disease, in addition, there is a violation of the permeability of the walls of blood vessels, plasmorrhagia, and diapedesis hemorrhage. In parallel with the development of lesions of the spinal cord and brain, changes occur quite naturally in their membranes, where acute inflammation develops with edema and plethora. There is also short-term moderate infiltration by neutrophilic leukocytes and later is more pronounced by lymphoid cells. The amount of protein in the cerebrospinal fluid (CSF) increases. The described changes gradually progress, reaching their maximum by the fourth day of the disease. In the event that 1/3 or more nerve cells are damaged, paralysis of those muscles that are innervated by the affected area of the nervous system develops. Later on, there is gradual resorption of necrotic areas of nervous tissue with the formation of glial scars. Macroscopic changes in the nervous system are insignificant. In the first days of the disease, they consist of moderate hyperemia of the meninges, as well as of the spinal cord and brain. Later, small hemorrhages and areas of yellowish necrosis are sometimes visible. After a few weeks, the borders of the anterior horns begin to change. They become indistinct and sink in on the cut. Later on, small cysts appear at the site of necrosis. Ultrastructural studies of experimental materials have shown that the pathological process of nerve cells in poliomyelitis can be divided into three stages [2]. Stage 1 corresponds to the eclipse phase of infection and is associated with the suppression of the virus synthesis of the cell's own proteins. It is characterized by dystrophic changes on the part of the granular endoplasmic network and vacuolization of the cytoplasm. Stage II corresponds to the period of intracellular reproduction of the virus and the composition of viral particles and is characterized by an increase in the processes of dystrophy and necrobiosis of ultrastructures with the simultaneous appearance of various viral inclusions and an increase in RNA-containing granules in mitochondria that are atypical for nerve cells. The viral matrix and clusters of mature virions with a crystal-like character of virion stacking are localized in the cytoplasm of cells. Mature virions have the form of electron-dense rounded formations with dimensions of 24–27 nm. The distances between the centers of adjacent virions in crystal-like clusters are between 27 and 30 mm. At the third stage of the pathological process (after the release of the virus), severe necrotic changes occur in the cell with the complete disintegration of all its ultrastructures, including the nuclear matrix. In some cells, a large accumulation of lysosomes and lipids was observed before death, which was apparently associated with pathological regenerative processes in the dying cells. Viral inclusions in the lesions were also found in astrocytes, oligodendrocytes, endothelial, and mononuclear cells of inflammatory infiltrates. With polio, other manifestations of the generalization of the infection can also be noted, in particular, lesions of the spleen and lymph nodes, as well as interstitial myocarditis. Among secondary changes, the most frequently are described lesions of the motor and sensory nerves with the collapse of the axial cylinders and the subsequent proliferation of lemmocytes, leading to a sharp atrophy of the corresponding muscle groups, impaired joint function. As a result of violations of the nervous regulation of the respiratory system, lung atelectasis and aspiration pneumonia were often observed. Currently, polio diseases in St. Petersburg have not been registered for a long time, and documented deaths have not been observed since 1958.

6.1.4 Clinical Forms of Polio

The classification of polio is based on pathomorphological data, pathogenetic mechanisms, and clinical manifestations. There are paralytic and nonparalytic forms of polio. The ratio of the first and second epidemic areas corresponds to 1:100. Among the nonparalytic forms of polio, inapparent, abortive, and meningeal are distinguished. Inapparent, or asymptomatic, form of polio is characterized by a brief mild malaise and lethargy. The temperature usually remains normal, and after 2–3 days, the child feels healthy. In some cases, dyspeptic or catarrhal phenomena are noted. The pathogen of poliomyelitis in this case penetrates only into the epithelial cells of the pharynx and intestines, without going beyond these organs. Children with an inapparent form are a source of infection for others as they secrete the poliovirus into fecal masses, and they have a high level of specific antibodies in their blood.

The abortive form of polio is characterized by an acute onset with fever, catarrhal phenomena, and moderate headache; often, especially in young children, gastrointestinal disorders (abdominal pain, nausea, frequent loose stools) are observed. There is pallor, adynamia, and hyperhidrosis. This form proceeds favorably; within a week, recovery usually occurs.

It should be noted that the diagnosis of unapparent and abortive forms of polio is quite difficult, and it is carried out only on the basis of epidemiological and laboratory data.

The meningeal form of poliomyelitis is a type of serous meningitis with an acute onset, high fever, severe headache, and repeated vomiting. The two-wave nature of the temperature curve is often noted.

Among the paralytic forms of polio, there are spinal, bulbar, bulbospinal, pontine, and pontospinal forms. During the spinal form of poliomyelitis, there are four periods: preparalytic, paralytic, restorative, and residual. The clinical picture of the disease develops after an incubation period of 10 days on average (fluctuations from 5 to 40 days are described). During this period, the poliovirus is present in the body; it can be detected in the fecal masses 10–12 days before the first symptoms of the disease. The onset of the disease is acute, the temperature rises to 38–40°C, often with a double rise for 5–7 days. Patients are concerned about headaches, frequent vomiting, and pain in the limbs and back. Neurological symptoms often appear on the second rise in temperature; there is rigidity of the occipital muscles and positive symptoms of Brudzinski and Kernig. The duration of the preparalytic period is 1–6 days, but in some patients, paralysis develops without a clear preparalytic period. Paralysis usually occurs at the end of a feverish period or in the first hours after a temperature decrease.

The spinal form, according to the initial localization, can be cervical, thoracic, or lumbar, depending on which part of the spinal cord the motor cells of the anterior horns are affected. The most severe are the spinal forms with damage to the diaphragm and respiratory muscles of the chest. The recovery period usually lasts 1–3 years, especially active in the first months of the disease, then comes the period of the residual phenomenon.

The bulbar form of poliomyelitis occurs with the defeat of the IX, X, and XII pairs of cranial nerves. If the fatal outcome does not occur, the process is stabilized. In such cases, the recovery period begins at the third week of the disease.

In the bulbospinal form of polio, in the clinical picture, along with bulbar symptoms, peripheral paresis and paralysis of the muscles of the trunk and limbs are detected. In this regard, there is a need for a differential diagnosis between the bulbospinal form of polio and Guillain-Barre syndrome.

According to the International Classification of Diseases (ICD) tenth revision, the diagnosis of acute paralytic poliomyelitis is made in the presence of a characteristic clinical picture and the release of poliovirus from fecal masses with the specification of the virus (vaccine-associated, wild imported, or wild indigenous respectively codes A. 80. 0; A. 80. 1; and A. 80. 2).

The laboratory diagnostics of poliomyelitis include virological and serological methods.

6.1.5 Other Enterovirus Infections

The clinical picture and morphological changes caused by all pathogens are similar, which allows us to consider these two infections in total [1]. In addition, in both clinical and morphological practice, accurate virological identification is usually not provided.

6.1.6 Etiology and Epidemiology

Coxsackie A (23 serotypes), Coxsackie B (six serotypes), and ECHO (33 serotypes) viruses, together with the poliovirus, belong to the enterovirus group since they can often be isolated from the intestine. The Coxsackie and ECHO viruses differ in their small size (diameter from 18 to 30 nm), contain RNA, and are stable in the environment: they persist in fecal mass at room temperature for 2–3 weeks and do not die during freezing for several years. However, these viruses are easily destroyed by boiling under the influence of ultraviolet rays.

The infection is transmitted by droplets and fecal-oral route from a patient or a virus carrier and has a peak incidence in summer and autumn. Children get sick more often from 3 to 10 years, and adults at any age. It is believed that enterovirus infection manifests itself differently depending on the age of the patient. Newborns rarely get sick and develop a picture of encephalomyocarditis, children of the first months of life often have enterovirus diarrhea, and at the age of 1–3 years, there are paralytic forms, the so-called polio-like diseases.

6.1.7 Pathogenesis and Pathology

After the virus passes through the mucous membranes of the nasopharynx and small intestine, it multiplies in the lymphoid cells of the lymph nodes and in the epithelium and penetrates into the blood, with the current of which it spreads throughout the body, showing neurotropy and myotropy. Pathologically, edema and infiltrative changes in the pia mater of the brain are detected; in the cortex, trunk, and cerebellum, diapedesis hemorrhage, glial proliferation, and dystrophic changes in the nerve cells are observed. In the striated muscles, the transverse striation disappears, and individual muscle fibers swell and necrotize.

Morphologically, edema, hyperemia, and mainly lymphocytic monocytic infiltration are detected in the soft meninges of the brain and spinal cord. A similar infiltration can be detected in the choroidal plexus. In cases of meningoencephalitis in the brain substance, in addition, diapedetic hemorrhage, mild lymphomacrophagal infiltration, and focal glial proliferation are detected. It is also possible, in particular with Coxsackie B5 infection, the development multiple foci of colliquative necrosis not associated with cellular infiltrates nor lying near vessels.

In our material, the combination of various CNS lesions with at least minimally pronounced lesions of the myocardium, skeletal muscles, intestinal mucosa, as well as other organs with similar morphological changes was also very characteristic.

In the experimental studies previously conducted at our department (N.I. Andrushchenko Yu. V. Matveev), the most severe changes were found in the cerebral cortex. During the first day after the infection of pregnant mice, against the background of increasing circulatory disorders, dystrophic and necrobiotic changes in nerve cells and a weak glial reaction were quite commonly detected for 4–6 s. After infection, pronounced perivascular and pericellular edema, dystrophic changes in nerve cells with lysis of some of them, and a pronounced glial reaction with the formation of small nodules were observed. There were small lymphohistiocytic infiltrates around individual vessels. By the end of 2 weeks, these changes decreased and disappeared by 30 days.

6.1.8 Clinical Manifestations

Lesions of the nervous system most often occur in the form of serous meningitis with a sudden onset, a rise in temperature to 39°C, with intense headache, accompanied by nausea, vomiting, development of a convulsive syndrome, or a sopor or comatose state. During a neurological examination, meningeal symptoms are usually expressed, CSF flows out under high pressure, pleocytosis is determined to be 200–500 cells in 1 μl; at first, it can be neutrophilic, and then lymphocytes predominate.

Encephalitic (stem, cerebellar, hemispheric) or meningoencephalitic forms can develop. The most severe is the stem form with bulbar syndrome and respiratory and cardiac disorders. In the cerebellar form are detected coordination disorders; the severity of the condition does not correspond to the severity of motor disorders and changed speech. Hemispheric forms are characterized by psychotic manifestations, accompanied by epileptic seizures, and the development of central paralysis. The severe course has a paralytic spinal form similar to that of polio. Previously, it was believed that Coxsackie viruses are not characterized by paralytic spinal forms, but the outbreak of this infection in 1975 in Bulgaria was accompanied by the development of such forms.

Based on the material of the pathology department of the S.P. Botkin Clinical Infectious Hospital, we analyzed a number of observations in which, on the basis of clinical and morphological and, in some cases, virological data, a generalized enterovirus infection with severe brain lesions was diagnosed. In isolated cases, brain lesions were isolated.

Clinically, the disease was usually not recognized.

As an example, we present one of our observations.

Vladimir O, 38 years old, is homeless, eats from garbage dumps, and abuses alcohol substitutes. He was ill for 3 weeks: loose stools, lower abdominal pain, tenesmus, and fever. He was hospitalized by ambulance transport to the S.P. Botkin Hospital from the street with a diagnosis of acute gastroenterocolitis on December 7. On admission, the condition is of moderate severity, disoriented, and abdominal pain on palpation on the glove during a rectal examination of feces with mucus. His stool was liquid with mucus on admission, and in the following days, there was no stool. All days of delirium sedation was without effect. On December 13, he was transferred to the intensive care unit with a diagnosis of dysentery, complicated by cerebral edema. The neurologist recorded a toxic (metabolic) coma. The temperature in the first days is subfebrile and later normal. In the blood at the admission - Hb-116 g / l (on 16/12–140), leukocytosis 18.7 (on 16/12–7.5), including rods –21 (32), lymphocytes 12 (28), ESR-53 mm / h. Amylase 44–105. 6, creatinine 0.094, urea 13.37, protein-76.1. ALT-13, AST-46. Serological test with intestinal pathogens is negative. Fecal cultures are negative. On December 16, death occurred.

Clinically, the disease was regarded as a severe form of acute dysentery, complicated by multiple organ failure and cerebral edema. As a concomitant pathology, chronic alcoholism, chronic adrenal insufficiency, myocardiodystrophy, bilateral pneumonia, and hypertension 2 in combination with general atherosclerosis were considered.

At the clinical autopsy, there is the corpse of a middle-aged man of reduced nutrition.

The soft medulla is full blooded, dull with a few small hemorrhages up to 0.2 cm in diameter. There is a convolution of the brain with slight smoothness. On the incision, the brain tissue is wet. The white substance is slightly sunken throughout, and the gray substance is bulging; the border between them is clear. The brain tissue is unevenly full blooded. In the central part of the medulla oblongata was noted a slightly sinking subependimal focus 0.8 cm in diameter, with the ependyma of the 4th ventricle slightly sinking above it. The ventricles of the brain are not dilated; they contain clear cerebrospinal fluid, and their ependyma is full blooded, smooth, and shiny. Vascular plexuses are of large size and gray-pink in color.

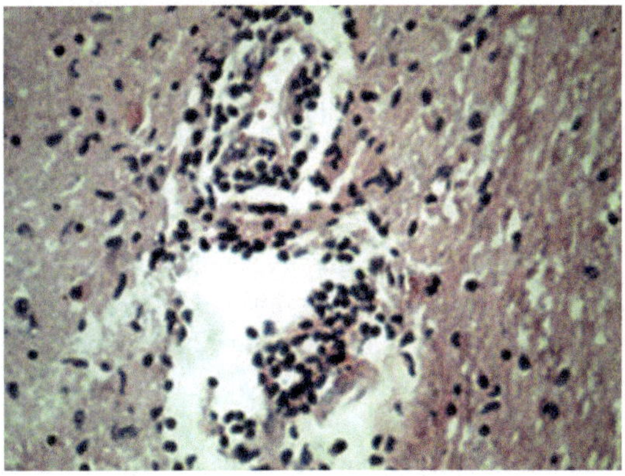

Fig. 6.2 Brain changes in ECHO encephalitis in a patient, V.O., 36 years. Vasculitis, perivascular edema, and prominent lymphocytic infiltration. H-E, ×500

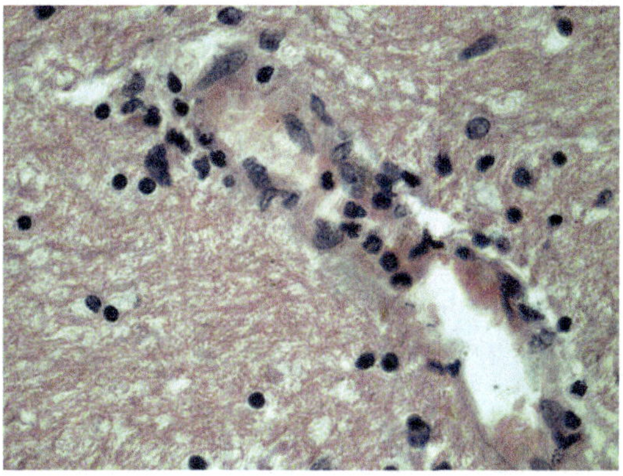

Fig. 6.3 Brain lesions in the same patient. Moderate perivascular infiltration. H-E, ×500

The macroscopic examination of the internal organs revealed widespread catarrhal enterocolitis; hyperplasia of the mesentery lymph nodes; acute spleen hyperplasia; parenchymal dystrophy of the kidneys, liver, and myocardium; focal hemorrhages in the skin, lung tissue, gastric mucosa, bladder, and renal pelvis; mild pulmonary edema; and uneven fullness of the internal organs.

The microscopic examination of the soft meninges revealed edema, fullness, moderate uneven lymph-leukocyte infiltration, and proliferation of arachnoendothelial cells. In the substance of the brain, there is uneven perivascular and pericellular edema. The cells of the endothelium of blood vessels have large light swollen nuclei, sometimes leading to a narrowing of their lumen. There is moderate perivascular lymphohistiocytic infiltration, small focal perivascular hemorrhages, and severe dystrophic and necrobiotic changes in the nerve cells (Figs. 6.2, 6.3, 6.4) with pronounced phenomena of satellite disease. In one of the fields of view, there is a focus of gray softening of the brain tissue.

The internal organs showed signs of moderate viral lesions of the stomach, small and large intestines, liver, kidneys, and myocardium (Fig. 6.5) and bilateral small focal bacterial pneumonia.

These materials allowed us to conclude that this patient was suffering from severe viral encephalitis with secondary circulatory disorders

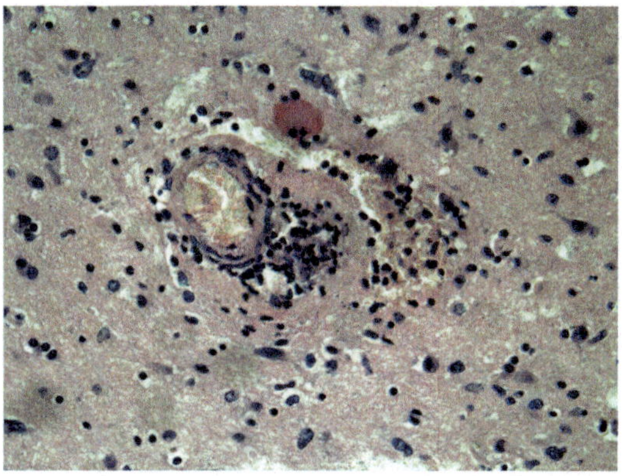

Fig. 6.4 Brain lesions in the same patient. Focal perivascular infiltration and hemorrhage, degeneration of the nervous cell. H-E, ×600

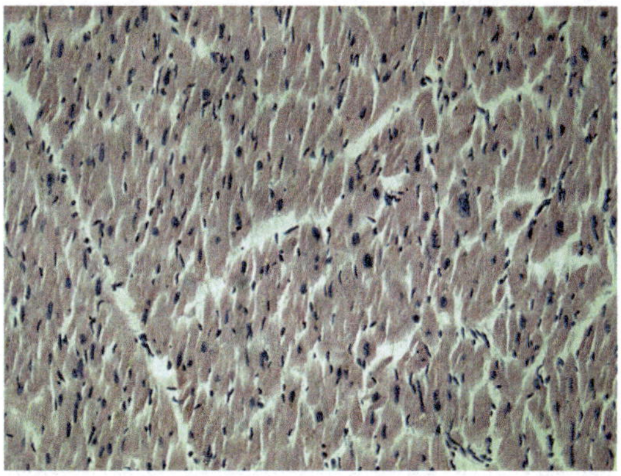

Fig. 6.5 Moderate myocarditis in the same patient. H-E, ×100

in the brain stem, which became the leading manifestation of generalized enterovirus infection (ECHO 30), the entrance gate for which was the gastrointestinal tract. This observation is regarded as a discrepancy between the clinical and pathological diagnoses.

In another example, it was extremely difficult to diagnose the observation of clinically isolated meningoencephalitis of enterovirus etiology. Patient E. Sh., 39 years old, did not work. From the anamnesis, at the age of 11, she had brain injury; otitis media at the age of 16; and in childhood, sinusitis, repeated acute respiratory infections, and angina. Her husband had tuberculosis. This disease started on January 3, with headache and subfebrile fever. The next day, the temperature rose to 39 °C, with chills, body aches, and nausea. She was hospitalized on January 6 with a diagnosis of acute meningitis(?) and acute respiratory viral infection (ARVI). On admission, the condition was moderate, her temperature was 38.9 °C, and she appeared flaccid, pale, and without rash. The heart tones were clear, the breathing in the lungs was hard, she had pharyngeal hyperemia, and the liver and spleen were not palpated. Focal and meningeal signs were not detected. On the morning of January 8, the appearance of meningeal symptoms was noted, in connection with which the CSF was punctured and transparent. She was transferred to the neuroinfection department. The condition was regarded as "closer to bad," contact, adequate, and oriented, and she was answering questions correctly. There was rigidity of the occipital muscles++, Kernig's symptoms+, with no gross focal symptoms. The patient worried about a severe headache. After five days of hospitalization, the febrile fever stopped, the temperature became subfebrile, and then it became normal. On January 11, a deterioration of the condition was noted: the patient became poorly oriented, and there were repeated vomiting and involuntary twitching of the limbs. In a serious condition, she was transferred to the intensive care unit. On the 18th, hypoventilation phenomena were noted. Death occurred on January 19 at 22 hours. During her stay, lumbar puncture was repeatedly done. Cytosis was in the range of 230–470/3 with a predominance of lymphocytes (67–97%), sugar 1.6, protein 0.99. In blood tests, leukocytosis is 7–16 × 109/L with a shift to the left. Blood and CSF cultures were negative. Tests for tick-borne encephalitis, borreliosis, and leptospirosis were negative. The final clinical diagnosis was formulated as serous (tuberculosis?) meningoencephalitis, complicated by edema, swelling and dislocation of the brain, and acute cardiovascular and respiratory failure. At the clinical autopsy of the corpse of a middle-aged woman of medium height, asthenic constitution was examined. The soft medulla is full blooded, swollen, dull, with uneven redness. At the base of the brain at the intersection of the optic nerves, slight thickening and whitishness were noted. The convolutions of the major hemispheres are flattened, the furrows are narrow, and the brain tissue in all parts is slightly flabby. On the incision, the gray matter is unevenly full-blooded, gray-bluish, focally its border with white matter is smeared with several petechial hemorrhages. White substance fading with a dull, unevenly expressed fullness of vessels. In the right hemisphere of the cerebellum above the fourth ventricle, a clearly defined focus of hemorrhage is dark red, up to 0.8 cm in diameter. There were indistinct hemorrhages in the wall of the fourth ventricle. Cerebral ventricles were of the usual lumen, but their ependyma was unevenly reddish, dull. Vascular plexuses are sharply full blooded, reddish, and shiny. On the part of the internal organs, only subpleural atelectasis of the lower lobe of the right lung, post-traumatic (after artificial ventilation) laryngotracheobronchitis, right-sided lower lobe small focal pneumonia, parietal thrombophlebitis of the superior vena cava during cava catheterization, and parenchymal dystrophy of the liver, kidneys, and myocardium were noted. The microscopic examination of the brain revealed serous meningitis with perivascular lymphocytic coupling. In the substance of the brain, there are distinct lymphocytic perivascular couplings. There is moderate hypertrophy of glial cells, sometimes forming glial nodules; necrobiotic changes in the nerve cells with distinct phenomena of satellite disease (Fig. 6.6); foci of fresh hemorrhage; severe viral ventriculitis with a focal

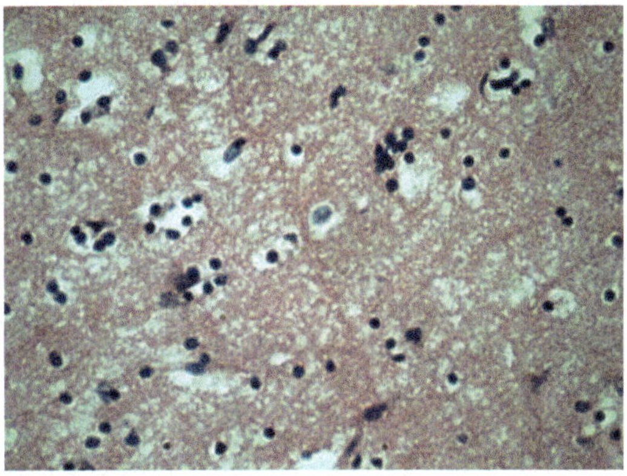

Fig. 6.6 Brain lesions in ECHO encephalitis in a patient, E. Sh., 39 years. Necrobiotic changes of nervous cells and satellitosis. H-E, ×300

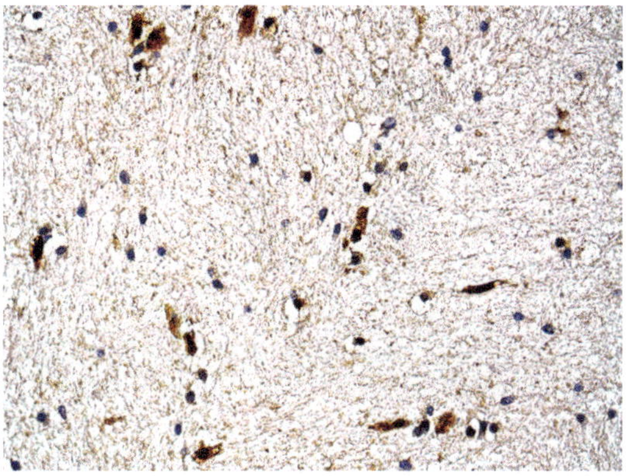

Fig. 6.7 Enterovirus common antigen in nervous cells. IHC, ×100

proliferation of ependymal cells; in the choroid plexus, focal lymphocytic infiltration with the proliferation of ependymocytes; viral neuritis of the cerebrospinal nerves with partial demyelination; pronounced viral ganglionitis of the semilunar ganglia; and distinct productive neuritis. The microscopic examination of the internal organs confirmed the presence of secondary respiratory lesions detected during macroscopic examination and revealed nonspecific circulatory and dystrophic changes. No data were obtained for the presence of a generalized viral infection. A comprehensive virological study revealed enterovirus ECHO 30. No diagnostically significant microflora was isolated in bacteriological cultures. The given data allowed to state in the final pathological diagnosis in the patient the presence of enterovirus meningoencephalitis, complicated by a cerebral coma. The disease was also accompanied by iatrogenic episodes.

There are cases of Guillain-Barre syndrome of enterovirus etiology with an acute onset, the development of peripheral tetraparesis, of the ascending Landry type, with sensitive disorders in the distal extremities, symptoms of tension of nerve trunks, and protein cell dissociation in the cerebrospinal fluid. Laboratory diagnostics of enterovirus infection include the isolation of viruses from the nasopharyngeal mucus, fecal masses, serological methods – an increase in the titer of specific antibodies by more than 4 times in the reactions of neutralization and binding of complement), enzyme immunoassay, determination of viral antigen by PCR, taking into account that healthy individuals may carry enteroviruses. During neuropathological studies, the detection of virus antigen by IHC is helpful (Fig. 6.7).

6.2 Tick-Borne Encephalitis

6.2.1 Etiology and Epidemiology

The history of the study of tick-borne encephalitis is interesting and instructive [1]. In recent years, the urgency of the problem of improving the diagnosis and treatment of tick-borne encephalitis is due to the sharp rise in its incidence on the Eurasian continent in the 1990s of the twentieth century. This is associated with the development of new land in the area of this infection, the influx of nonimmune populations, and the reduction of acaricide measures. The incidence of tick-borne encephalitis corresponds to the distribution zones of the main vectors of the disease, Ixodes ticks in the taiga zone of Asia and Europe, in the forests, shrubs and meadow pastures it depends on the number of ticks and their virus load. The increase in the frequency of tick-borne encephalitis in Russia continues: in the classical works of A.G. Panov and A.N. Shapoval [3], it is shown that the clinical manifestations of tick-borne encephalitis differ in different regions. In the ICD tenth revision, in the section "Viral infections of the Central nervous system," Far Eastern tick-borne encephalitis and Central European tick-borne encephalitis are separately distinguished.

Tick-borne encephalitis is also called spring-summer endemic encephalitis. The main carriers of the pathogen in nature are *Ixodes* mites (*Ixodes ricinus*, *Ixodes persulcatus*). Their biology determines the seasonality of the disease. At this time of the year, they appear in large numbers. In ticks, there is transovarial transmission of the virus. It was found that the reservoirs of the tick-borne encephalitis virus, in addition to ticks, are the host animals of ticks: voles, hamsters, hedgehogs, chipmunks, hares, squirrels, badgers, foxes, house mice, goats, and sheep.

Tick-borne encephalitis virus—a small, enveloped RNA-containing *Flavivirus*—has the ability to cause acute, latent, and persistent forms of tick-borne encephalitis. There are a large number of strains of the tick-borne encephalitis virus. As A.N. Shapoval [3] emphasizes, they differ significantly from each other in many indicators, including the degree of pathogenicity for humans. Currently, the strains of the tick-borne encephalitis virus are divided into four genetic types: Far Eastern, Western, East Siberian, and Ural-Siberian. When studying the genomes of 46 West Siberian strains of the tick-borne encephalitis virus, the stability of genomic RNAs was shown, which, apparently, is provided by natural selection through the elimination of defective virions.

The tick-borne encephalitis virus enters the human body through a tick bite or alimentary route when eating raw milk from infected goats, sometimes cows, or dairy products made from it. Isolated cases of contact or airborne infection have been described when the tick was crushed by fingers and the pathogen got on the skin and mucous membranes. When working with cultures of the pathogen in laboratories, cases of tick-borne encephalitis have also been noted.

6.2.2 Pathogenesis and Pathology

A histological examination of the brain of people and experimental animals reveals diffuse, widespread meningoencephalitis. Mainly gray and, to a lesser extent, white matter is affected. The process is characterized by an inflammatory reaction of the exudative-proliferative type and dystrophic-necrotic changes in neurons. Edema of the brain tissue is pronounced, and the number of oligodendrocytes is increased. In addition to full blood, severe vascular changes are detected with stasis, thrombosis, homogenization, and even necrosis of the walls. Perivascular infiltrates consisting of lymphocytes, monocytes, histiocytes, and plasmocytes as well as diapedesis hemorrhage are naturally detected. There is a diffuse and focal proliferation of microglia and astrocytes, partially undergoing destructive changes. On the part of neurons, acute swelling, chromatolysis, cytoplasmic vacuolization, karyocytolysis, and pycnomorphic changes are usually observed, sometimes accompanied by neuronophagy. In the outcome of the described lesions, small foci of necrosis may develop. With a progredient course in the CNS of the deceased, necrotic changes in the nerve cells, perivascular lymphoplasmocytic infiltration, and significant proliferation of microglia are noted. A sign of progression is the appearance of fresh foci and the spread of changes to previously unaffected areas. With a prolonged course of infection in the central nervous system, there is fibrosis of the meninges, dystrophic changes in the nerve cells, spongious degeneration, and circulatory changes, in the absence of inflammation. In recent studies, B.A. Erman et al. [2] proposed to distinguish three types of pathological changes: alterative productive inflammation, alterative exudative inflammation, and alterative inflammation in patients with immunodeficiency. The authors note that along with the typical forms, numerous intermediate variants are also noted. In the alternative-productive variant of inflammation, the process is diffuse and is observed throughout the brain and spinal cord and consists of vasculitis, focal proliferation of glia, and areas of alteration of nerve cells, most pronounced in the motor nuclei of the spinal cord and brain. According to B.A. Erman et al. [2], the alternative-exudative variant of CNS lesions is characterized by mass loss of nerve cells throughout the spinal cord; dystrophic and necrobiotic changes in the nerve cells of the brain stem and cerebellum, as well as other parts of the brain; necrobiotic and necrotic changes in the walls of the blood vessels of both white and gray matter with a weak glial reaction; and the absence of perivascular cellular inflammatory infiltration. In some cases, there is a pronounced destruction of the tissue. The authors associate the development of this form with the virulence of the pathogen. In the deceased with a predominantly alterative variant of inflammation against the background of congenital or acquired immunodeficiency, widespread degenerative-necrobiotic changes in nerve cells with their mass loss are described, against the background of moderate dyscirculatory changes and a weak diffuse glial reaction, are noted small cell proliferations of adventitial cells around the vessels. Macroscopically, the brain and its membranes in tick-borne encephalitis are sharply hyperemic and edematous, and the substance of the organ is moderately flabby. With the incision in the brain tissues, multiple point hemorrhages are found, especially in the area of the basal ganglia and the gray matter of the brain stem.

According to B.A. Erman et al. [2], who conducted experimental studies on mongrel white mice and Macaca rhesus monkeys, virus particles are localized mainly in nerve cells, especially on the membranes of the endoplasmic reticulum. In addition, the decay and reduction of cell organelles with pronounced hyperplasia of smooth membranes and moderate vacuolization of the cytoplasm are detected. At a later stage of the disease, severe destructive changes occur in nerve cells with the disintegration of the nuclear and plasma membranes and the release of organelles and virus residues into the intercellular space. Around the decaying nerve cells, the destruction of the processes of glial cells, blood vessels, and inflammatory infiltrate cells is observed. Interesting data were obtained in the study of cerebrospinal markers of glial and neuronal destruction in patients with tick-borne encephalitis. The tick-borne encephalitis virus can cause neuronal degeneration and a pronounced inflammatory response. Commenting on the presented data, it can be noted that the materials presented by the authors, including experimental material, on the influence of the virulence of the pathogen on the nature of the clinical and morphological manifestations of the disease are most interesting and absolutely convincing. In patients with paralytic forms of tick-borne encephalitis, a significant increase in the level of neuron-specific enolase, a marker of neuronal damage, and neurofilament protein, the main structural component of axons, was found in the cerebrospinal fluid, which indicates the cytolysis of neurons. In these patients, the content of S-100 protein, a marker of astroglial cells, was also significantly increased in the cerebrospinal fluid, while in the remaining patients with tick-borne encephalitis, only small changes in this indicator were noted. For the development of tick-borne encephalitis, the bite of a tick containing a pathogenic strain of the causative agent of the disease is insufficient; it is necessary that the human body has a susceptibility to this disease. It turned out that only 2% of people who were bitten by mites acquired a disease [3]. In the acute period of tick-borne encephalitis, T lymphocyte deficiency is expressed, the content of B lymphocytes is increased, and the level of immunoglobulins (Ig) A, G, and M is increased. People with a genetically determined early production of IgG antibodies with a high affinity for the tick-borne encephalitis antigen have a favorable outcome of the disease.

After the bite of a tick carrier virus, the virus located in its salivary glands immediately enters the blood, then into the central nervous system, where it penetrates as a result of hematogenic dissemination, a violation of the permeability of the blood-brain barrier. There are also possible lymphogenic and perineural ways of spreading the virus, which can be detected in the brain tissue within a few days after the bite. In the alimentary pathway of infection (drinking raw goat's milk), the tick-borne encephalitis virus passes through the barriers of the gastrointestinal tract and spreads through the lymphatic system. It is proved that the reproduction of the tick-borne encephalitis virus on the first day of infection occurs in immunocompetent peripheral blood cells. It is believed that the virus first multiplies in the lymphoid organs and then in the nervous tissue. To date, no laboratory indicators have been developed that allow us to predict the course of tick-borne encephalitis.

Experimental studies indicate that the clinical manifestations of tick-borne encephalitis depend on the way of challenge. It was found that the introduction of the virus into the brain of monkeys leads to the development of CNS lesions with a fatal outcome; oral, subcutaneous, intramuscular infection is accompanied by the occurrence of a benign acute or asymptomatic infection.

We analyzed 13 observations of deceased persons in S.P. Botkin Infectious Hospital. Among them, there were seven men aged 49 to 75 years and six women aged 39–75 years. The duration of hospitalization ranged from 2 to 77 days. All these observations fundamentally correspond to the descriptions available in the literature. It should only be noted that not all medical records had information about tick bites. The diagnosis was confirmed by the results of lifetime and/or postmortem serological studies.

As an example, we give a few of our observations. Valery P., 33 years old, fell ill on May 30, with a rise in temperature to 39 °C, repeated vomiting, and dizziness. There was no information about a tick bite. On May 31, there was a frenzy of the tongue, the eyelids did not rise, and the lower lip was numb. He was admitted to a multidisciplinary hospital in a serious condition, with continued vomiting and dizziness. Temperature was 40 °C; she had slurred speech and was delirious at night. After an examination by a neurologist on June 1, a lumbar puncture was performed, in which the cytosis was 165/3, including 165 neutrophils. On June 3, he was transferred to a station of artificial ventilation. With a diagnosis of meningoencephalitis on June 4 in an extremely serious condition, in a coma, he was transferred to the S.P. Botkin Hospital. A differential diagnosis was made between tick-borne encephalitis and local epiduritis. Antitick gammaglobulin, antibiotic, and hormone therapy were introduced. After a short-term improvement in the condition, the patient again fell into a cerebral coma, and with an increase in the phenomena of cardiovascular and respiratory failure, the patient died on the night of June 9. The clinical diagnosis was formulated as purulent meningoencephalitis of unclear etiology, complicated by ventriculitis and edema swelling of the brain. The final pathological conclusion was as follows. Patient Y, 33 years old, with a severe course of tick-borne meningoencephalitis (IgM to the tick-borne encephalitis virus was detected in the cerebrospinal fluid), histologically corresponds to an acute form with widespread neuron lesions and proliferation of glia, including rod-shaped microglia, pronounced serous meningitis, epiduritis, and ependymatitis (Figs. 6.6, 6.8, and 6.9), dies in the phenomena of brain coma associated

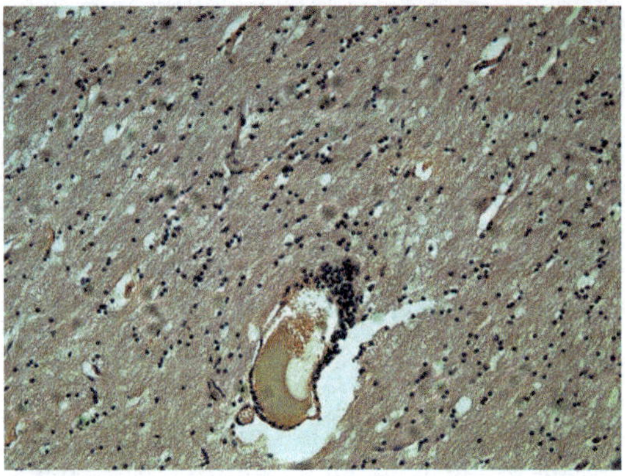

Fig. 6.8 Brain lesions in acute tick-borne encephalitis. Focal perivascular infiltration. H-E, 200

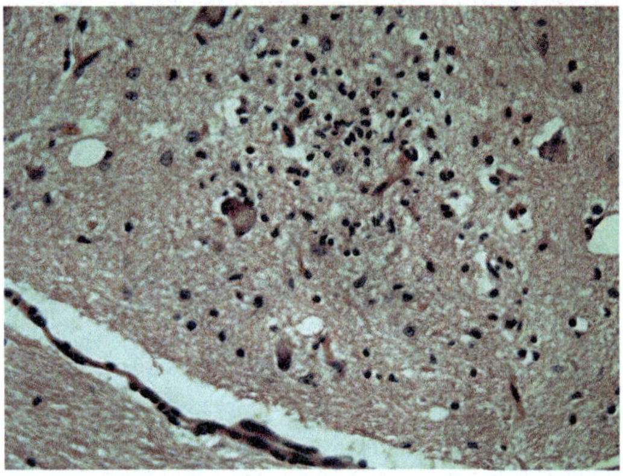

Fig. 6.9 Brain lesions in acute tick-borne encephalitis in a patient, V.P., 33 years. Degeneration of nervous cells, glia proliferation. H-E, ×300

with the progression of meningoencephalitis with the development of edema swelling of the brain and the addition of pulmonary insufficiency due to right-sided large- and small-focal purulent bronchopneumonia caused by rod microflora (*Citrobacter*, according to a bacteriological study), which developed a few days before death. In addition, preexisting changes in the lung tissue were also identified, probably associated with a chronic deoxyribonucleic acid (DNA) viral lesion. In addition, a histological examination revealed purulent sphenoiditis, no more than a few days old, with the seeding of *Salmonella* group D enteritidis in the contents of the pterygoid sinus.

As the example can serve observation of A. S., 30 years old, who died on the 6th day of his illness and the third day of his stay in the Botkin hospital. Diagnosis of the direction was: acute meningitis? The final clinical diagnosis: serous meningoencephalitis of unclear etiology. Preliminary (after autopsy) pathological diagnosis: left-sided lower lobe large focal pneumonia, complicated by purulent leptomeningitis. The final pathological diagnosis is acute tick-borne meningoencephalitis (tick-borne encephalitis virus was detected in the blood; IgM-a was detected in the blood and CSF), complicated by unrecognized large-focal pneumonia during life, which contributed to the onset of death.

R.P., 69 years old, a pensioner, was bitten by a tick on July 7 in the Leningrad region. 8/07 himself removed the tick, which was taken to the virology center, where it was detected by the antigen of the tick-borne encephalitis virus. Prevention was carried out in the polyclinic of the S.P. Botkin Hospital. On July 22, there was a rise in temperature to 37.2 °C, headache, and vomiting. On July 23, in a serious condition with a diagnosis of tick-borne encephalitis, he was hospitalized in Botkin Hospital. On July 25, due to the development of stem symptoms, she was transferred to the intensive care unit, where a tracheostomy was performed, and he was on a ventilator. He received antitick gammaglobulin and had a constant fever. In the cerebrospinal fluid at the admission cytosis, 148/3, 86% lymphocytes. IgM antibodies are detected in the blood and cerebrospinal fluid. The test for tick-borne borreliosis was negative. Death occurred on the 20th day of hospitalization on August 12. In the clinical diagnosis, brain edema, bilateral bronchopneumonia, bilateral bronchopneumonia, hemorrhagic cystitis on bedsore of the bladder, and thrombophlebitis of the superior vena cava were considered as complications of meningomyelopolyomyelitis form of tick-born encephalitis.

At the clinical autopsy is the corpse of an elderly woman with high nutrition. The soft meninges are full blooded, sharply edematous, and transparent, with uneven, sometimes barely noticeable dullness. On the cut, the fabric is unevenly full blooded, with areas of bluish color and sinking; the pattern is preserved. The ventricles of the brain of the usual form are not expanded; they contain a clear cerebrospinal fluid. Their ependyma is smooth and shiny throughout. Vascular plexuses are red-bluish in color. On the part of the internal organs, the most significant changes were thromboembolism of the large and small branches of the pulmonary artery, focal hemorrhages in the lung tissue, gastric mucosa, and duodenum. On the background of tracheostomy, purulent tracheobronchitis was detected (during bacteriological examination of proteus seeding), after catheterization of the superior vena cava - its thrombophlebitis, after catheterization of the bladder hemorrhagic cystitis. In addition, there was a pronounced atherosclerosis of the aorta and coronary arteries and moderate of the arteries of the base of the brain, hypertrophy of the left ventricular wall, arteriolosclerotic nephrosclerosis, atherosclerotic cardiosclerosis. A microscopic examination of the brain reveals widespread dystrophic and necrobiotic changes in the nerve cells and proliferation of the endothelium of small blood vessels and ependyma. In some places was noted productive vasculitis with significantly pronounced perivascular infiltration (Fig. 6.10). Thus, this case demonstrates the possibility of a fatal outcome from acute tick-borne encephalitis in the late stages of the disease against the background of regression of clinical symptoms. The immediate cause of death of the patient was a massive pulmonary embolism.

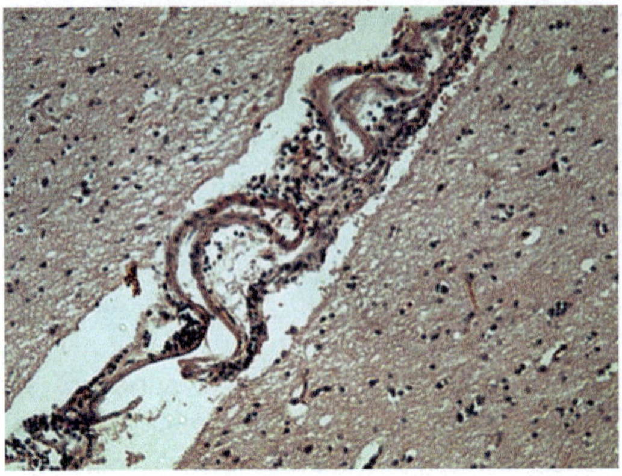

Fig. 6.10 Brain lesions in the prolonged course of acute tick-borne encephalitis in patient, R.P., 69 years. Productive vasculitis. H-E, ×300

6.2.3 Clinical Manifestations

It should be emphasized that, often, patients with tick-borne encephalitis deny the fact of tick suction since, for many, it goes unnoticed. The duration of the incubation period after a human tick bite is from 3 to 30 days, more often about 2 weeks; with alimentary infections, it is shorter—up to 4–6 days. However, cases have been described where the incubation period was measured for several hours or, conversely, exceeded 40 days. It is believed that the duration of the time interval between infection by the tick-borne encephalitis virus and the onset of the disease is determined by the virus load in the tick and the state of the human body, primarily its immune status. In addition, the place of suction of the tick is important. It is established that the favorite place of fixation of the tick is the area of the neck, head, arms, and shoulder girdle. With this localization of tick suction, the incubation period is often short (1–10 days); in the case of a bite in the trunk and lower extremities, it is extended by two times. In the prodromal period, which occurs infrequently, patients complain of malaise, general weakness, pain in the muscles of the back and limbs, and moderate headache. In most cases, the onset is acute: severe headache, vomiting, and chills with an increase in temperature to 39–40 °C and sometimes higher. This temperature can last from 4 to 10 days and then lytically decreases; subfebrility is maintained for a long time. On the background of fever, in addition to pronounced general cerebral symptoms, meningeal phenomena occur. In some cases, there are pronounced mental disorders (visual and auditory hallucinations, delirium, or depression). There are nonfocal and focal forms of the disease. The first includes feverish, erased, and meningeal. The second, depending on the predominance of certain symptoms and the predominant damage to certain nervous structures, includes poliomyelitic, meningoencephalitic, polioencephalomyelitic, and polioencephalitic forms. In the poliomyelitic form, there is a predominant lesion of the cells of the anterior horns of the cervical spinal cord, sometimes also of the thoracic. This form of lesion is the most typical in the clinical picture. After 3–4 days from the onset of the disease, flaccid paresis or paralysis appears in the muscles of the neck, shoulder girdle, and proximal parts of the upper extremities; a typical picture develops: "hanging head." The polioencephalitic form is characterized by a rapidly developing comatose state, bulbar paralysis, increased respiratory disorders, cardiac disorders, and mortality reaching 60–65%. The polioencephalomyelitic form is also severe. In addition to damage to the cells of the anterior horns of the spinal cord, the nuclei of the medulla oblongata suffer from the development of bulbar syndrome; there are violations of respiratory and cardiac activity. The acute period lasts for 4–6 weeks, high temperature lasts 7–8 days, there are violations of consciousness, and manifestations of bulbar paralysis are combined with the paralysis of the muscles of the neck, diaphragm, and upper extremities. Mortality rate reaches 20–30%.

The meningoencephalitic form is characterized by general cerebral symptoms, meningeal symptoms, and predominant brain damage, which leads to impaired consciousness and, in some cases, causes epileptic seizures, pseudobulbar syndrome, and central hemiparesis; also, cerebellar syndromes can develop. Among the nonfocal forms of tick-borne encephalitis, one of the most frequent is feverish. Diagnosis is based on epidemiological data, general infectious manifestations, and the results of serological studies.

With the erased form, anisoreflexia, central paresis of the facial muscles, tongue, slightly pronounced, nystagmus, meningism can be detected. The meningeal form is characterized by a symptom complex of acute serous meningitis with pronounced general cerebral and meningeal symptoms. Along with the erased form, there are also forms of tick-borne encephalitis with a pronounced clinical picture. There is a comatose form of tick-borne encephalitis with an extremely violent onset: a sharp increase in temperature to 41 °C with a deep violation of consciousness. A polyradiculoneuritic form of tick-borne encephalitis is described separately. In this form, the leading complaints are pain along the nerve trunks, which is dull or burning, and a feeling of numbness, tingling, and "crawling goosebumps." Various sensitivity disorders are described: at the same time, there may be expressed decrease in pain, temperature, tactile, deep sensitivity, and symptoms of tension of the nerve trunks. The development of acute polyradiculopathy with an ascending type of Landry's palsy is possible; when motor disorders begin with the lower extremities, then the upper extremities and the medulla oblongata are involved in the pathological process. As a result, flaccid tetraparesis develops with radicular symptoms, sometimes with a peripheral type of sensory disorders, bulbar syndrome, and protein cell dissociation in the cerebrospinal fluid. It should be noted that since the first descriptions of tick-borne encephalitis, the frequency of its various forms has changed.

Radiation semiotics of disseminated encephalitis caused by tick-borne encephalitis virus in the acute phase of the process in most cases inludes a multifocal lesion of brain structures (66.7%), but the presence of a single focus is not a rarity (25% of cases). In 8.3% of cases, there are no structural changes in the acute phase of the process. The foci are characterized by a hyperintensive signal on T2 VI and FLAIR IP. Only single changes in the form of sections of the hypointensive MR signal are visualized on the T1 VI. The size of the foci varies from a few millimeters to 2 centimeters. The structure of the foci is uniform, and the contours are clear. The presence of perifocal edema is not characteristic. Signs of volumetric impact are not expressed. The characteristic localization of foci is the basal ganglia (66.7%). In addition, the pathological process often involves the white matter of the hemispheres of the brain (41.7%); much less often, changes affect the gray matter of the cortex (16.7%). The presence of focal changes in the corpus callosum, stem structures, and structure of the posterior cranial fossa is relatively rare (8.3%). Course of encephalitis caused by the tick-borne encephalitis virus is monophasic and a has tendency to rapid (1 month – 10 months), total (71.4%) regression of focal changes. In a small percentage of observations, residual changes in the form of gliosis zones are determined (28.6%). As the disease develops against the background of a gradual decrease in focal changes, atrophy occurs and progresses in the brain substance, which is extremely characteristic of the pathological process of this etiology. Residual changes after tick-borne encephalitis are usually represented by diffuse atrophy in the brain substance (63.63%); in 18% of cases, there is the formation of hemiatrophy. With the same frequency, on the background of unchanged matter of the supratentorial parts of the brain, isolated atrophy of the structures of the posterior cranial fossa is determined.

6.2.4 Chronic Forms

Among the chronic forms of tick-borne encephalitis, there are recurrent and continuously progressive ones. The main clinical manifestation of recurrent forms is the symptoms of an increasing focal lesion of the nervous system. In most patients, the progredient course is accompanied by an increase in previously occurring paresis of the muscles of the shoulder girdle, as well as the neck. Chronic forms of tick-borne encephalitis in the vast majority of cases are not accompanied by changes in the cerebrospinal fluid. When chronic forms of tick-borne encephalitis occur without a previous acute period, diagnostic difficulties are often noted. The difficulty also lies in the fact that serological reactions in the progredient course of tick-borne encephalitis often become negative.

At the same time, overestimation of the results of paraclinical methods with shortcomings in collecting anamnesis and in analyzing the features of the clinical picture of the disease also leads to diagnostic errors.

The problem of the chronic forms of tick-borne encephalitis has been repeatedly highlighted in the fundamental works of Professor A.N. Shapoval [3], in which a large number of clinical and pathological comparisons are given. According to A.N. Shapoval, chronic infections can be divided into the following groups:

- Diseases that were preceded by an acute period of the disease, regardless of its duration.
- Diseases in which the acute period is not established: they are classified as primary progredient forms of tick-borne encephalitis. The vast majority of patients in this group had a latent infection that could last for many years, so such patients are referred to as primary progredient forms only conditionally.
- A combination of chronic forms of tick-borne encephalitis with other organic diseases of the nervous system.

Within each group (or form), the following clinical syndromes may occur: asthenia, cortical syndrome (spastic hemiparesis, speech disorders, etc.), subcortical syndrome (parkinsonian, hyperkinetic), Kozhevnikov epilepsy, Jackson's epilepsy, polioencephalitic syndrome with a predominant lesion of stem structures (mesencephalic, bulbar), polioencephalomyelitis (bulbo-spinal), polio (upper and lower spinal), poliomyeloradiculoneuritic, amyotrophic lateral sclerosis syndrome, and psychosis.

In the second group of diseases, there may also be recurrent and continuously progressive forms with the same clinical syndromes.

The third group of diseases, both then and in recent years, has not yet been sufficiently studied. There is a combination of chronic forms of tick-borne encephalitis with other organic diseases: syringomyelia and amyotrophic lateral sclerosis.

According to A.N. Shapoval, the transition of the acute stage of tick-borne encephalitis to subchronic (subacute) is a frequent phenomenon (the researcher observed it in 14% of patients), then the progredient course is relatively rare (in 1–3% of patients). Thus, in the long-term observations of A.N. Shapoval, only 87 patients with a progredient course were identified.

It has been established that the chronic forms of tick-borne encephalitis are heterogeneous in their clinical manifestations, course, and outcomes and can be conditionally divided into recurrent and continuously progressive forms of the disease.

Recurrent chronic forms of tick-borne encephalitis were described by many authors in the 1950s and 1960s. According to A.N. Shapoval, a relapsing course was established in 41 patients who had a previous acute period of the disease. In the vast majority of them, the infection occurred in a vector-borne way. Only in three patients was the disease associated with the consumption of raw goat's milk. Chronic forms were usually found in rural residents in natural foci, while in urban residents, they were observed in isolated cases.

In the literature, there are many reports of the development of chronic forms a number of years after the acute period. The main clinical manifestation of the recurrent forms is the symptom of an increasing focal lesion of the nervous system, which can develop over several weeks, months, and often up to 20 years or more. The clinical picture of the disease largely depends on the localization of the lesion in the nervous system.

Of the cranial nerves, disorders of the function of the facial, sublingual motor portion of the lingopharyngeal and vagus nerves were most often noted, and there are cases of a decrease and perversion of the sense of smell, with stagnant nipples of the optic nerves and paresis of upward gaze.

In most patients, the progredient course is accompanied by an increase in previously occurring paresis of the muscles of the shoulder girdle, as well as the neck. In some cases, this happens even in the absence of these symptoms in the acute period of the disease. This paresis with amyotrophy has the features of a peripheral lesion but can sometimes be spastic. Cases of flaccid lower paraparesis are also described.

Often there are also sensitive disorders, such as flaccid paresis. In these cases, pain hypesthesia is found according to the segmental type. In some cases, there is a decrease in deep sensitivity in the hands, as well as a disorder of two-dimensional and discriminatory feelings.

Disorders of the autonomic functions of the nervous system, expressed through the lability of the cardiovascular system, fluctuations in blood pressure in general, or regional hyperhidrosis, were very characteristic. Some patients complained of urinary incontinence and nocturnal enuresis.

Among the chronic forms of tick-borne encephalitis, Kozhevnikov epilepsy occupies a special place. To recall, this syndrome was identified by A. Ya. Kozhevnikov in 1894, and he called it "Epilepsia partialis continua." It was characterized by constant or repeated myoclonia at short intervals, which sometimes intensified and ended in a generalized convulsive seizure. A. Ya. Kozhevnikov suggested that the main cause of this syndrome is encephalitis.

Currently, the criteria for the diagnosis of Kozhevnikov epilepsy have been developed: the presence of simple partial motor paroxysms, focal myoclonia, focal neurological disorders (hemiparesis), and a nonprogressive course. Electroencephalographic studies have shown that in the interattack period, patients with Kozhevnikov epilepsy show normal basic activity and the presence of spikes or "spike-wave" complexes with clear localization in the central areas, which are detected at the time of the attack. It should be noted that in recent years, within the framework of epilepsia partialis continua, two syndromes have been distinguished: (1) Kozhevnikov syndrome, which has been known since 1894 and covers most of the cases, and (2) Rasmussen's syndrome, which was isolated in 1958, and 51 cases of the disease were described over 35 years. It is believed that Rasmussen's syndrome is characterized by the onset of the disease mainly in 2–10 years, manifested by treatment-resistant partial seizures, combined with focal neurological symptoms (hemiparesis, hemianopsia, speech disorders), and a decrease in intelligence. Computed tomography (CT) and magnetic resonance imaging (MRI) scans of the brain reveal focal cortical atrophy. Histological studies of brain tissue reveal perivascular infiltrates and glial proliferation, which is similar to the picture of encephalitis, although the virus is not detected. The criteria for the diagnosis of Rasmussen syndrome are the following cardinal signs: debut before the age of 10, simple partial motor and somatosensory seizures, diffuse myoclonia, progressive focal neurological disorder (hemiparesis), progressive course, and resistance to anticonvulsant therapy. The detection of Rasmussen's syndrome changes the treatment tactics since this disease shows the effectiveness of neurosurgical interventions like subtotal functional hemispherectomy.

In conclusion, it should be emphasized that chronic forms of tick-borne encephalitis without a previous acute period of the disease, according to various authors, account for 4–20% of the number of identified progredient forms. In other words, they occur tens and hundreds of times less often than in cases of tick-borne encephalitis with pronounced clinical symptoms. The latter suggests that improving the early diagnosis of acute forms of tick-borne encephalitis will help reduce the frequency of chronic forms characterized by a severe progredient course. Since the formation of Kozhevnikov epilepsy can occur at different terms after an acute form of tick-borne encephalitis, patients who have suffered this infection should be under the supervision of a neurologist. Chronic forms of tick-borne encephalitis also include amyotrophic lateral sclerosis (ALS) and amyostatic syndrome. The ALS syndrome associated with tick-borne encephalitis is characterized mainly by the same clinical manifestations as in cases of its different genesis. Patients gradually develop mixed paresis of the hands (increased deep reflexes, pathological hand signs combined with muscle hypotrophy and fasciculations) and central paresis of the legs with increasing bulbar disorders. Later on, respiratory disorders are added, and after a few years, a fatal outcome occurs. Amyostatic syndrome is characterized by amymia, hypokinesia, oligokinesia, bradykinesia, rest tremor, increased muscle tone in the case of the extrapyramidal type, unsteadiness, uncertainty when walking, mental features in the form of slow thinking, and cognitive disorders. Clinical observations indicate that the diagnosis of tick-borne encephalitis at the onset of the disease is quite difficult, especially in cases of erased meningeal forms. In this regard, the diagnosis of tick-borne encephalitis should be carried out on the basis of epidemiological data, the clinical manifestations of the disease, and the results of virological and serological examinations. In the acute period of tick-borne encephalitis, it is possible to isolate the virus from the patient and detect its antigen or the specific antibodies in the blood. Among the serological methods, serological tests are used, which are carried out in paired sera in the first days of the disease and after 2 weeks. The most accurate confirmation of the diagnosis of tick-borne encephalitis is the detection of specific IgMs in the blood and/or cerebrospinal fluid. It is shown that enzyme-linked immunosorbent assay (ELISA) is more sensitive at detecting the tick-borne encephalitis virus antigen in the early stages of the disease, and serology is more sensitive in the late stages of the disease. Special attention should be paid to the differential diagnosis of tick-borne encephalitis. Diagnostic faults can be divided into three groups. The first group of misdiagnosis: tick-borne encephalitis was mistaken for other diseases – influenza, tonsillitis, acute pneumonia, bronchitis, typhoid fever, acute respiratory infections, acute polyarthritis, acute colitis, acute poisoning, "fever", tuberculosis meningitis, cerebrospinal meningitis, brain abscess, ischemic stroke, subarachnoid hemorrhage. Sometimes patients were sent for examination with infections of an unknown nature.

6.2.5 Features in Children

Both adults and children suffer from tick-borne encephalitis. Meanwhile, there is an increase in the number of cases of tick-borne encephalitis in children in older age groups: from 1 to 3 years, 2–5% of cases occur; from 4 to 7 years, up to 25%; and from 8 to 15 years, up to 70% [4]. It is emphasized that the most common is meningeal form with pronounced general infectious, general cerebral, meningeal symptoms, and meningoencephalitic form; very rarely there is a polio form. There is a characteristic manifestation of tick-borne encephalitis in children – a violation of consciousness up to coma, a high frequency of convulsive seizures, generalized and partial, (especially in preschool age), the severity of autonomic disorders. With the progression of the pathological process, children develop various hyperkineses (myoclonia, choreoathetosis, torsion, dystonia, and tremor); Kozhevnikov epilepsy is formed, and deep disability occurs.

It should be noted that there have been no deaths from tick-borne encephalitis in children over the past few years in St. Petersburg. Due to the high incidence and severity of clinical manifestations and the outcomes of tick-borne encephalitis, the development of new methods for the early diagnosis of its acute forms using modern serological and molecular genetic methods continues, which will contribute to timely rational therapy, reduced mortality, the frequency of development of chronic forms with a progressive course, and reduced degree of disability. Currently, special attention is paid to the prevention of tick-borne encephalitis, which goes in two directions: improving the health of endemic territories (destruction of vector ticks, strengthening individual protection against tick attacks) and creating or increasing immunity to this disease.

6.3 West Nile Fever

The most important manifestation of this disease is encephalitis. West Nile viral encephalitis belongs to the group of arbovirus encephalitis, the virus that causes it is transmitted by arthropods, belongs to the group of flaviviruses, which also includes Japanese encephalitis, tick-borne encephalitis, yellow fever. Wild birds are the natural hosts for the West Nile fever (WNF) virus and spread it during migration. A person is infected with WNF through the bites of culicine mosquitoes. Not only people and birds but also horses suffer from WNF [5]. The WNF virus's envelope protein induces immunological responses in infected hosts and causes the formation of virus-neutralizing antibodies. E protein domain III (DIII) contains a panel of epitopes that are recognized by virus-neutralizing monoclonal antibodies. In the pathogenesis of the disease, a certain role is assigned to toll-like receptors (TLRs). Thus, TLR3, according to some authors, mediates WNV's entry into the brain, causing lethal encephalitis, but due to other data, it plays a protective role. MyD88 and the selective androgen receptor modulator (SARM) both seem to restrict viral replication.

In 93% of patients, the debut of WNVE occurs in June–September. In recent years, outbreaks of WNVE have been reported in Austria, Hungary, and Italy [6]. In 1999, an outbreak of West Nile viral encephalitis was reported in New York in the United States. From 1999 to 2008, there were 28,961 cases of WNF in 47 US states, including 11,822 (41%) cases involving the nervous system (Lindsey NP et al., 2010). In the United States, WNVE is the most common of arbovirus encephalitis, with 720 cases reported in 38 states in 2009, with the most common cases occurring in Mississippi and South Dakota. In 80% of people, the disease can be asymptomatic; in the rest, fever, headache, myalgia, arthralgia, rash, and gastrointestinal disorders are detected. Approximately 1% of patients develop lesions of the nervous system: encephalitis, meningitis, and acute flaccid paralysis. The degree of severity of lesions of the nervous system in this disease depends on the age of the patients: the most significant injuries occur in persons older than 70 years, and fatal outcomes are described. Severe forms of the disease develop in patients who have undergone internal organ transplantation operations with chronic immunosuppression. The recovery period is usually long, with the patient often developing depressive states and increased fatigue. The diagnosis of WNVE includes anamnesis data, complaints, results of clinical examination, neuroimaging, serological methods for the determination of specific IgM and IgG, and polymerase chain reaction for the detection of WNV virus antigens. Currently, vaccines against WNF are under development. It is recommended to monitor mosquitoes and wild birds, destroy infected individuals, and use personal protective equipment against mosquito bites. In Russia, an outbreak of WNF was registered in 1999–2001, with the maximum number of cases in the Volgograd region, with a mortality rate of 10–12%.

A number of studies previously carried out by V.B. Pisarev et al. [7] are devoted to the pathological anatomy of West Nile encephalitis. No noticeable changes were observed during the macroscopic examination. The microscopic examination of the soft meninges revealed edema, fullness of blood, stasis in small vessels, and lymphoplasmacytic infiltration with an admixture of eosinophils and neutrophils. In the middle and medulla oblongata, the phenomena of exudative vasculitis are noted. In the nerve cells, the phenomena of swelling, tigrolysis, chromatolysis, vacuolization, and neuronophagy were noted in various parts of the brain. The formation of lymph-glial infiltrates was noted in the medulla oblongata (Fig. 6.11). During immunohistochemistry (IHC), the greatest expression of virus antigens was observed in the vascular endothelium, and they were insignificant in the neurons of the medulla oblongata.

From the side of other organs, the phenomena of serous pneumonia and focal myocarditis were noted. In the kidneys, fibrinoid necrosis in the

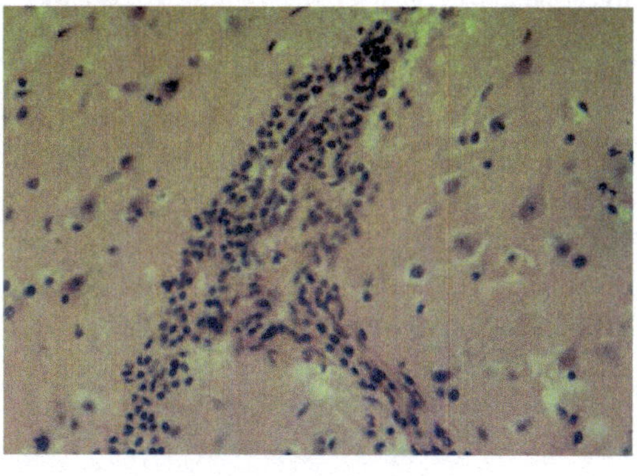

Fig. 6.11 Brain lesion in West-Nile encephalitis. Expressed perivascular infiltration. H-E, ×600

glomeruli and tubule karyolysis were observed. The virus antigen was detected in the endothelium of the renal capillaries and the area of the basal membrane of the tubules. In the liver, there is diffuse mononuclear infiltration of the perisinusoidal and periportal spaces; the antigen was expressed in both hepatocytes and endothelial cells.

In our material, there were no clinical or pathological observations of this disease.

6.4 Rabies

Rabies is an acute infection, the most characteristic signs of which are severe neuropsychiatric disorders, convulsions, spasms of the pharynx when swallowing, and attacks of hydrophobia.

The rabies virus belongs to the family *Rhabdoviridae* and is an RNA-containing virus with characteristic bullet-shaped particles 170–180 nm long and 75–80 nm in diameter. Inside the cylinder, a nucleocapsid helix is enclosed, which is revealed in the form of a striated structure during Electron microscopy (EM). On the outside, the particles are covered with capsomers about 10 nm long, resembling clubs.

The reservoir of the virus in nature is various animals: wolves, jackals, foxes, bats, squirrels, dogs, and large and small cattle, which, along with an acute infection, can also have asymptomatic forms of the disease. The virus spreads to the saliva from the bites of sick animals.

In Russia, there are natural foci of wild animals everywhere. It is shown that foxes, dogs, ferrets, and hedgehogs are the source of rabies in 58.9% of cases while domestic animals (dogs, large and small cattle) in 41.1%. It was found that the number of persons affected by bites from rabies-infected animals increased from 1994 (0.02%) to 1998 (0.29%). In the UK, rabies was eliminated in the 1920s. However, in 2002, in Dandin has been reported the first death from rabies since 1902 in a man who sold bats [8]. The authors emphasize the need for vaccination against rabies in persons whose profession involves contact with animals, which are the source of this infection.

6.4.1 Pathogenesis and Pathology

In the area of the entrance gate, the virus contacts the endings of the peripheral nerves and begins to move in a centripetal direction. In the central nervous system, the virus penetrates through the perineural spaces, which do not exclude the hematogenic and lymphogenic pathways of distribution. The virus reproduces mainly in the brain and spinal cord. In experiments on mice, rats, and hamsters, it was shown that the passage of the virus from the lumbar spinal cord to the brain stem takes only a few hours, which is accompanied by a pronounced expression of the virus antigen. Axoplasma is the main route of viral genome transport. With centripetal spread, the virus additionally multiplies on the axon membranes, as well as in the nerve cells of the spinal ganglia. From the central nervous system, the virus moves in a centrifugal direction to the peripheral organs and tissues, primarily the salivary glands and oral and nasal cavities, where it continues to accumulate, creating prerequisites for the infection of other hosts. The intracellular virus has little access to immunocompetent cells. It is only immediately before the death of sick animals that antibodies appear in the blood in high titers.

Histological examination usually reveals a picture of diffuse encephalitis, characterized by a perivascular inflammatory reaction, neuronophagy, and various alternative changes in the nerve cells (Fig. 6.12). In addition, degenerative inflammatory changes in the spinal ganglia, as well as cranial nerve ganglia, are evident. Many authors note a discrepancy between the clinical picture of severe rabic encephalitis and relatively weak histological changes.

For many decades, the Babesh-Negri calf has been considered the most important diagnostic sign of rabies infection. On a histological examination, they look rather like large formations with a diameter of 0.5–10 microns and consist of a homogeneous basic substance containing a certain number of basophilic grains. Homogeneous eosinophilic inclusions are also described.

In EMR, viral particles are usually detected in the nerve cells or their appendages. Some authors

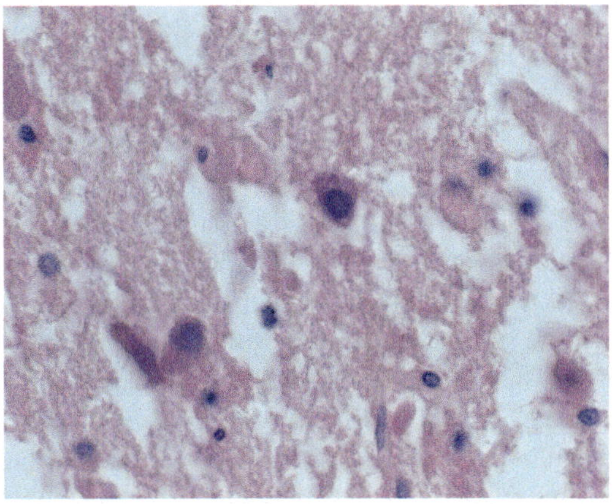

Fig. 6.12 Brain lesions in rabies. Degenerative changes of nervous cells, unclear intranuclear inclusion. H-E, ×600

also point to the possibility of reproduction of the rabies virus also in astrocytes. The accumulation of the virus occurs primarily in the neurons of the Ammonian horn and the cells of the cerebellum. In some cases, almost all neurons in most parts of the central nervous system can be infected. The virus titer can reach 106 infectious units per gram of the brain. The most characteristic ultrastructural sign of rabies is the appearance in the cytoplasm of polymorphic homogeneous inclusion matrices consisting of clusters of fibrous materials of moderate electron-optical density, which are clusters of viral nucleocapsids. Such matrices are freely located in the cytoplasm of infected cells. As the process progresses, there is an increase in the number and size of the matrices, as well as an increase in the condensation of their constituent filaments. These structures look like the eosinophilic substance of Babesh-Negri bodies under light microscopy. The formed rabies virus virions are detected only in the cytoplasm, either in association with the matrix substance or on the cell membranes, mainly of the granular endoplasmic reticulum. They look like basophilic particles under light microscopy. The maturation of virions occurs by budding into the lumen of the reticulum or on the cell membrane. Numerous EMRs of experimental rabies have described several types of virus-like particles that differ slightly when animals are infected with "wild" or "fixed" virus strains and in the time elapsed after their isolation [9]. The significance of the different types of inclusions in rabies is not clear enough. After the bite of an animal with rabies, an incubation period (20–180 days) usually occurs, which is followed by a prodromal period (2–10 days). At this time, there are burning sensations, pain at the bite site, an increase in body temperature (37.3–37.50 °C), headache, nausea, vomiting, a feeling of fear, irritability, sometimes apathy, and insomnia. Then the patient gradually develops a period of excitement, which lasts 2–5 days, and develops hydrophobia, which is pathognomonic for rabies; even at the sight of water, there are spasms of the muscles of the pharynx; the patient rushes to bed and bites; and there may be violations of breathing and heart activity, which often lead to death. During the next period of paralysis, the manifestations of hydrophobia disappear; however, after the temperature rises to high numbers, pelvic motor disorders develop. Soon there is a fatal outcome in the phenomena of respiratory and heart failure circulatory disorders. Clinical manifestations of neurological disorders in rabies are usually characterized by a picture of fatal encephalomyelitis. The differential diagnosis is carried out with another serious disease—tetanus, in which there are convulsive seizures like tetany, and with a "sardonic smile," there is no hydrophobia. Epidemiological history, absence of pain, and hydrophobia allow us to distinguish the neurological manifestations of rabies from encephalomyelitis of a different etiology. In some cases, it is necessary to make a differential diagnosis with hysteria, taking into account the features of the epidemiological history, characteristic personality traits, and the absence of symptoms typical of rabies. In our material, rabies was observed extremely rarely. We present an observation of previous years based on the materials of the pathology department of S.P. Botkin Hospital. A 64-year-old woman was bitten by a cat in late August. A week before the onset of the disease, she noted malaise. On October 19, there was a severe headache and fever. In the morning of October 21, she started experiencing difficulty in breathing, aerophobia, difficulty in swallowing, and fear of water. She was admitted to the infectious diseases hospital on October 21 at 19:30 and died on the 23rd at 2:00. At the clinical autopsy, the macroscopic changes turned out to be of little character. The microscopic examination of the brain revealed fullness, perivascular edema, and dystrophic changes in the nerve cells with tigrolysis. There is pronounced perivascular lymphoid infiltration in the medulla oblongata. In the spinal cord, lymphoid infiltration is most pronounced in the area of cervical thickening. Negri bodies and other inclusions were not detected. In the antirabies department of Pasteur Institute (Leningrad). In the antirabies department of the Institute Pasteur (Leningrad) was isolated street rabies virus; focal bronchopneumonia with purulent exudate also played a role in the genesis of death.

6.5 Other Encephalitis Due to Neurotropic Viruses

In the case of ***mosquito (Japanese) encephalitis***, perivascular lymphoid infiltrates are observed in the white and gray matter of the brain. There is evidence that, unlike tick-borne encephalitis, there are no neutrophilic leukocytes in the infiltrates. It is characterized by foci of destruction with neuronophagy and diapedetic hemorrhage. The greatest changes are observed in the basal ganglia, the Varolian bridge, and the medulla oblongata, where granulomas can form around small vessels and dying nerve cells. The cortex of the large hemisphere and the vegetative centers are also affected.

The small number of observations of ***Powassan encephalitis*** with a fatal outcome does not allow us to analyze in detail the pathomorphology of this disease in humans. In an experiment on hamsters, an intense inflammatory process develops in the vascular plexuses and membranes of the cerebral hemispheres of the brain and cerebellum; signs of destructive meningoencephalitis were determined [10].

Dengue virus infection of the nervous system is caused by *Flavivirus*, transmitted by mosquitos *Aedes* spp. Through the bite of an infected insect, the virus enters the bloodstream and invades the macrophages, which transport it via the lymph channels to the lymph nodes, the site of their replication. The viremia lasts 4–5 days on average. Endothelial and possibly also bone marrow cells are susceptible to infection. The incubation time ranges from 3 to 14 days. Dengue infections are usually clinically mild or even often asymptomatic. Patients initially present with fever, headache, muscle and joint pain, and rash. Usually, there is a sudden increase in fever. It may come to a second fever peak with body exanthema as well as petechiae. In general, the course of the disease is short and favorable, but in about 10%, there is the involvement of the nervous system. The most common presentations are encephalitis, meningitis, strokes, cerebellar hemorrhage, and Guillain-Barré syndrome [11]. Detailed descriptions of neuropathology are absent in the literature; we do not have our own experience either.

Nipah virus is an emerging bat-borne virus and belongs to the paramyxoviruses. In Southeast Asia, fruit bats (*Pteropus* species) transmit the virus, but human-to human transmission is also possible. The incubation period ranges from 3 to 31 days. Most patients present with acute encephalitis, fever, headaches, and alteration of consciousness. The mortality rate for the last outbreak in Kerala, India, was 86%. Data on pathological changes are very scarce. Blood vessels are affected in the brain, lungs, heart, and kidneys with the development of secondary changes till fibrinoid necrosis. As indicated by IHC, neurons are also clearly infected [12]. There are several animal models of the infection on Syrian hamsters, ferrets, African green monkeys, cats, and mice [13]. The most common described changes in the brain are vasculitis with perivascular cuffing and meningeal inflammation. We have not seen appropriate cases.

Zika virus belongs to the flaviviruses, entering host cells through endocytosis initiated upon the interaction of the virus envelope glycoprotein with cell surface receptors. The virus can be transmitted by *Aedes* mosquitoes (mainly *A. aegypti*), vertically from mother to the child, and through sexual contact, blood transfusion, or organ transplantation. Its estimated incubation time is

3–14 days. Generally, the symptoms are mild (or even absent): fever, rash, conjunctivitis, muscle and joint pain, malaise, or headache. Neurological complications include Guillain-Barré syndrome; neuropathy and myelitis can occur in adults as well as in children and infants. Histopathology was descibed in human and animal embryo and fetus (see Chap. 16).

Borna disease virus is a member of the family *Bornaviridae* with a negative single-stranded nonsegmented RNA. The most likely natural route of entry is nerve endings in the nasal and pharyngeal mucosa. Borna disease has been first described in European veterinary textbooks in the eighteenth and nineteenth centuries as a disease with high lethality in horses. The virus can cause CNS disease in a broad range of vertebrate animal species, which is manifested by behavioral abnormalities and diverse pathology. Within the CNS, the virus exhibits preferential tropism for the limbic system, including the hippocampus, but also it can be detected in the hypothalamus, thalamus, and cerebral cortex. Viral antigen accumulates in the nucleus, the perikaryon, and the processes of infected neurons. Virus-specific materials form intranuclear Joest-Degen inclusion bodies. It is supposed that the virus can interfere in the metabolism of glutamate and neurotransmitters. Virus antigen and RNA appear rather early in astrocytes, followed by oligodendrocytes, Purkinje cells of the cerebellum, and Schwann's cells at the periphery.

In humans, clinical, epidemiological, and virological data indicate that the virus can persist in the CNS and induce progressive neurological disorders, which are associated with diverse pathological manifestations, including alteration in behavior and cognition (see also Chap. 20). The virus has been detected also in clinical samples of brain tumors. Possible relationship of immunosuppression and level of virus expression has been postulated [14]. The histopathology of Borna disease in men remains undescribed and we have no own experience as well.

Chikungunya virus also belongs to arthropod-borne viruses (family *Togaviridae*, genus *Alphavirus*) and causes endemic infections in Africa, Asia, and South America. It is transmitted by mosquitoes *Aedes aegypti* and *A. albopictus* and also from the viremic mother to the infant. Several outbreaks have been reported also in Europe. The disease manifests with high fever, headache, maculopapular rash, and painful arthralgia, with a typical incubation time of 3–7 days. In several outbreaks, in 12% of patients, there were neurological signs, including quantitative and qualitative alteration of consciousness, and focal neurological signs, such as cranial nerve deficits, seizures, hemi-/paraparesis, and involuntary movements [15].

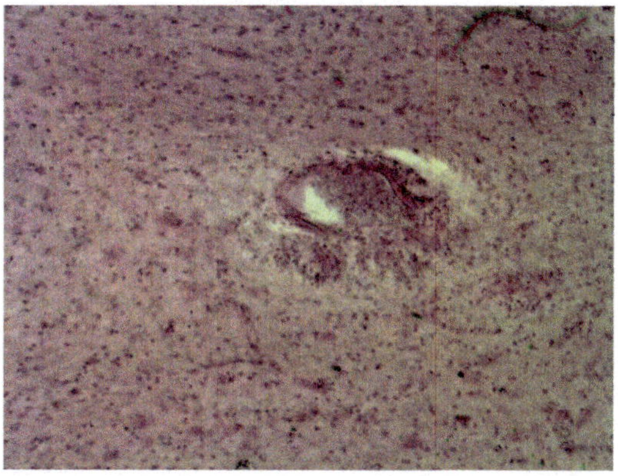

Fig. 6.13 Brain lesion in lethargic encephalitis. Preparation from collection of L.V. Blumenau. Courtesy of S.V. Lobzin. Embedding in celloidine. ×100

In the classical neurological and neuropathological literature lethargic (Economo) encephalitis was described, nowadays not diagnosed any more for many decades. Thus, it is impossible to give its characteristics based upon modern data, nevertheless we present the image from original slide from the 30th of XX century with diagnosis of lethargic encephalitis (Fig. 6.13).

References

1. Zinserling VA, Chukhlovina ML. Infectious lesions of nervous system. Issues of etiology, pathogenesis and diagnostics. Saint-Petersburg: ElbiSPb; 2011. p. 583. (In Russian)
2. Erman BA, Shestopalova NM, Bocharov AF. Ultrastructural pathology of neuroviral infections. Novosibirsk: Nauka; 1984. p. 92. (in Russian)
3. Shapoval AN. Tick-borne encephalomyelitis. Leningrad: Meditsina (In Russian); 1980.

4. Sorokina MN. Tick-borne encephalitis. In: Zinchenko AP, editor. Acute neuroinfections in children. Leningrad Meditsina; 1986. p. 126–37. (in Russian).
5. Rossi SL, Ross TM, Evans JD. West Nile virus. Clin Lab Med. 2010;30(1):47–65. https://doi.org/10.1016/j.cll.2009.10.006.
6. Ziegler U, Seidowski D, Globig A, et al. Sentinel birds in wid-bird resting sites as potential indicators for West Nile virus infections in Germany. Arch Virol. 2010;155(6):965–9. https://doi.org/10.1007/s00705-010-0.
7. Pisarev VB, Grigor'eva NV, Petrov VA, Butenko AM. Pathomorphology of West Nile fever. Arkh Patol. 2004;66(5):15–7. (in Russian)
8. Pounder D. Bat rabies. BMJ. 2003;326(7392):726. https://doi.org/10.1136/bmj.326.7392.726.
9. Selimov MA, Korolev MB, Tatarov AG. Morphology of the Arctic rabies virus. Vopr Virusol. 1984;29(2):253–6. (in Russian)
10. Isachkova LM, Shestopalova NM, Frolova MP, Reingold VN. Light and electron microscope study of the neurotropism of Povassan virus strain. Acta Virol. 1979;23(1):40–4.
11. Meyding-Lamadé U, Craemer E, Schnizler P. Emerging and re-emerging viruses affecting the nervous system. Neurol Res Pract. 2019;1:20. https://doi.org/10.1186/s42466-019-0020-6.
12. Wong KT, Shieh WJ, Kumar AS, et al. Nipah virus infection: pathology and pathogenesis of an emerging paramyxovirus zoonosis. Am J Pathol. 2002;161:2153–67.
13. de Wit E, Munster VJ. Animal models of disease shed light on Nipah virus pathogenesis and transmission. J Pathol. 2015;235(2):196–205.
14. Gonzalez-Dunia D, Sauder C, de la Torre JC. Borna disease virus and the Brain. Brain Res Bull. 1997;44(6):647–64.
15. Waggoner JJ, Gresh L, Vargas MJ, et al. Viremia and clinical presentation in Nicaraguan patients infected with Zika virus, Chikungua virus, and Denge virus. Clin Infect Dis. 2016;63:1584–90. https://doi.org/10.1093/cid/ciw589.

Lesions of the Nervous System in Generalized Viral and Related Infections

7

Lesions of the nervous system can occur in many viral and close to them mycoplasma infections and are caused by both direct injury associated with the location of pathogens, and be associated with a number of secondary mechanisms (autoimmune and others). Among the large number of diseases, we consider only those in respect of which we have sufficient experience of our own. Taking into account the fact that the last decade's pathological issues have not been popular in the literature, we preferably cite our older publications, where they were analyzed in detail. Our research in children has been provided several decades when the lethality in respiratory infections was rather high.

7.1 Influenza

Brain damage in influenza in the sense that it has been understood in various years, is constantly described by hundreds of authors for several centuries, starting with the epidemics of the XVI century. The first most detailed generalized study on this topic was made in 1904 in the doctoral dissertation of N.P. Postovsky, who considered it necessary to isolate the nervous form of influenza, which, according to his data, proceeded in the form of pseudomeningitis, true meningitis, or hemorrhagic encephalitis. Subsequently, a number of monographs were devoted to this issue, which covered the clinical aspects of the problem in more detail. According to various authors, in influenza, the frequency of damage to the nervous system varies widely (from 0.3% to 32%) [1].

Neurological complications were described both in influenza A of various serotypes and in influenza B. The literary data were recently updated [2, 3]. Clinically, there are meningeal and meningoencephalitic syndromes, serous meningitis and meningoencephalitis, hemorrhagic syndrome, meningitis and meningoencephalitis, diencephalitis, encephalomyelitis and encephalomyelopolyradiculoneuritis, and mono- and polyneuritis. Significantly less frequently described are ischemic syndrome; Guillain-Barre syndrome; psychotic disorders in the acute period of the disease and, soon after its end, hypomanic, hallucinatory-paranoid, delirious syndromes; Parkinson's syndrome; cerebral arachnoiditis; optochiasmal arachnoiditis; and angiitis of the cerebral vessels.

Neurotoxic syndrome in influenza is manifested by headache, pain when moving the eyeballs, intestinal and joint pain, general weakness, lethargy, adynamia, sleep disorders, low mood, apathy, dizziness, nausea, vomiting, changes in pulse rate and blood pressure, and other autonomic disorders. Sometimes the manifestations of neurotoxic syndrome also include convulsions and changes in consciousness, although other authors consider these symptoms as manifestations of encephalitic syndrome.

V. Zinserling, *Infectious Lesions of the Central Nervous System*,
https://doi.org/10.1007/978-3-030-96260-9_7

Meningeal syndrome often develops at the height of intoxication against the background of general brain disorders and is characterized by moderately pronounced meningeal symptoms in combination with signs of increased intracranial pressure. During lumbar puncture, the pressure of the cerebrospinal fluid is increased to 300 mm water column. With unchanged cell number in CSF or pleiocytosis with dozens of cells in mm^3 of a predominantly mononuclear nature with a moderate increase in protein. Based on the results of the CSF study, a differentiation is made between meningism and serous meningitis.

Encephalitic syndrome develops most often at the height of intoxication, but sometimes in later stages, usually in combination with meningeal syndrome. It is characterized by the predominance of general brain disorders in the form of varying degrees of changes in consciousness and psychotic disorders over focal symptoms. Some authors identify stem, vestibular, diencephalic, and other forms of these conditions.

Hemorrhagic encephalitis is most often diagnosed in the acute period of the flu or with a repeated rise in temperature. Hemorrhagic encephalitis is characterized by pronounced general cerebral syndromes in the form of convulsive seizures and comatose state, paresis, paralysis, stem symptoms, and meningeal syndrome. In the CSF, this disease is characterized by an admixture of significant amounts of blood pleiocytosis and an increased protein content. The mortality rate in this form reaches 30%.

The neurological complications of influenza in the vast majority of studies are diagnosed on the basis of the above-described clinical symptoms detected in patients on the background of respiratory infection occurring based on the type of influenza, which are confirmed most often by a serological examination of paired sera. In some studies, to prove the direct connection of the above-described symptoms with influenza viruses, serological studies of CSF are also carried out [1].

Most pathologists of previous years describe diffuse circulatory changes in various parts of the brain in the form of a sharp fullness of the soft meninges and white matter of the brain, stasis, and different sizes of hemorrhages, from petechial to very massive. They also observed swelling and alternative changes in nerve cells in the form of diffuse tigrolysis of the Nissl substance, hyperchromatosis of the nuclei, and demyelination of nerve fibers. Part of the work describes, in addition, lymphocytic and plasmocytic perivascular infiltrates in the form of "couplings" and "rings," proliferation and swelling of the endothelium of small vessels of the soft meninges and mainly white matter of various parts of the brain and spinal cord, and proliferation of astrocytes, oligodendroglia, and microglia. The majority of morphological works devoted to brain changes in neurological complications of influenza do not describe the state of the ependymocytes of the choroidal plexus and cerebral ventricles.

In the scientific literature in 2009–2016, much attention was paid to the pandemic of the A (H1N1) virus. It is emphasized that cases of suspected H1N1 influenza virus disease are characterized by the following signs: fever rise to 38 °C or above, with cough or inflammatory changes in the throat, headache, vomiting, and myalgia with the onset of symptoms within 7 days after a trip to the affected regions and close contact with persons infected with influenza [2–4]. The age of patients with H1N1 flu ranged from 3 months to 81 years; about 40% of patients were aged 10–18 years, and only 5% of the examined were older than 51 years. The role of the immunodeficiency state in the occurrence of central nervous system (CNS) lesions in such patients has been established.

The examined patients often had epileptic seizures, encephalopathy, and epileptic status; after discharge from the hospital, focal neurological symptoms persisted in 22% of children. It was found that patients with A/H1N1 influenza were more likely to develop encephalopathy, focal neurological symptoms, aphasia, and changes in electroencephalogram (EEG).

7.1.1 Brain Lesion in Children

We [1] conducted a comprehensive clinical, viral, and morphological analysis of 78 sectional observations of children who died from acute respiratory infection (ARI) with varying degrees of neurological symptoms. The existence of several pathogenetic forms of CNS damage was shown: (1) hemo- and cerebrospinal fluid disorders without signs of direct viral damage, (2) brain damage on the background of generalized viral infection, and (3) isolated brain damage by respiratory viruses. It should be noted that although the causative agents of these forms can be various viruses of the respiratory group, often in combination, it is necessary to emphasize the special role of influenza viruses of various types. The etiological diagnosis in all observations was based on the results of the study of smears from the lungs and soft meninges, a serological examination of the blood and CSF, and, in some cases, the isolation of the virus.

The first group included 15 children who died from ARI with neurological symptoms. Neurotoxicosis was diagnosed clinically in eight cases, encephalitis or encephalitic reaction in four cases, meningoencephalitis in two cases, and epileptic status in one case. The duration of the disease in all cases did not exceed 3 days. The average age of children in this group was 13.5 ± 3.6 months. Respiratory infection in 85% of cases was mixed; influenza (more often A1 and A2) was diagnosed in all cases. Macroscopic changes were mainly reduced to edema—the mass of the brain increased by an average of 15–20%. A histological examination revealed edema and fullness of the soft meninges (Fig. 7.1) and the substance of the brain. Nerve cells of various parts of the brain and spinal cord were subjected to "severe" and "ischemic" changes (Fig. 7.2); occasionally there were small areas of neuron's loss. Parts of the ependymal cells of the lateral ventricles and vascular plexuses were exfoliated; the remaining ones were subjected to dystrophic changes. On various types of glia, mainly moderate swelling was noted, and its proliferation could not be detected in any of the observations. In all cases, changes were detected on the part of small blood vessels, consisting of thickening and disorganization of their walls (Fig. 7.3), swelling of the endothelium, and violation of the integrity of elastic membranes.

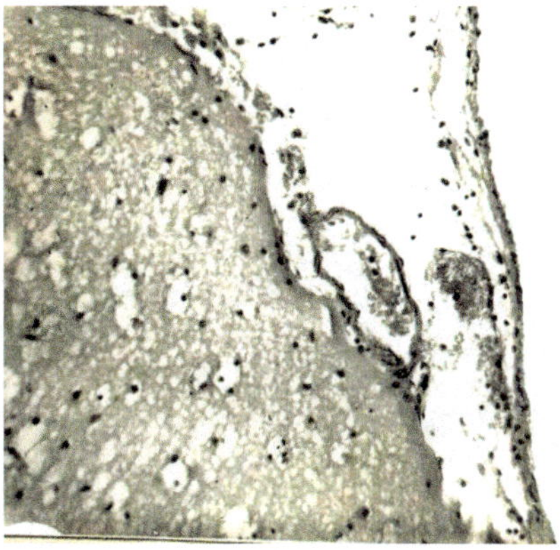

Fig. 7.1 Edema and full blood vessels in meninges of a child who died from influenza with clinical picture of neurotoxicosis. H-E ×250

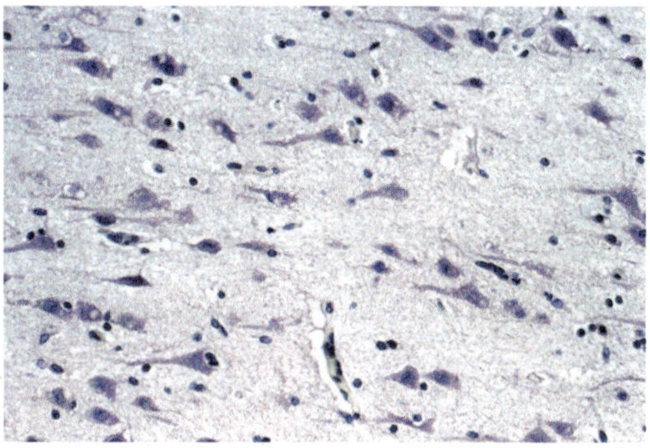

Fig. 7.2 "Severe" and ischemic changes of nervous cells in child with mixed respiratory infection with clinical picture of neurotoxicosis. Stained by thionin according to Nissl ×600

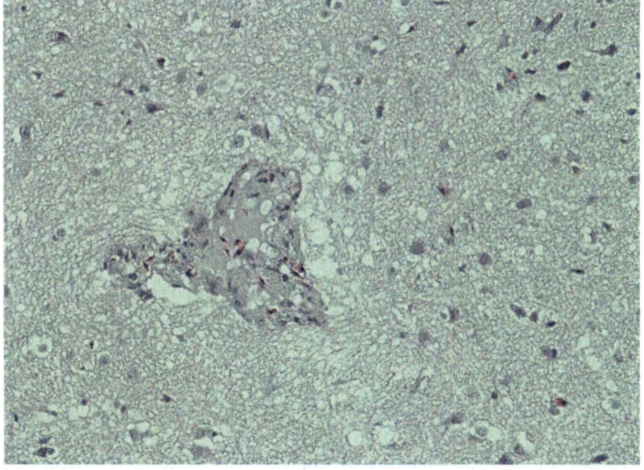

Fig. 7.3 Swelling of endothelial cells in child with mixed respiratory infection with clinical picture of neurotoxicosis. H-E ×200

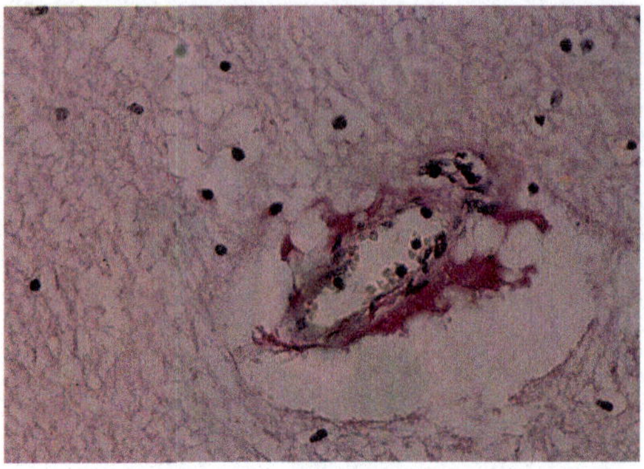

Fig. 7.4 Increased permeability of small vessel in brain matter with mixed respiratory infection with clinical picture of neurotoxicosis. PAS, ×350

These changes led to the increased permeability of blood vessels in the form of a release of fluid rich in proteins (Fig. 7.4) or focal hemorrhage. It should be noted that similar changes were detected in these children and in the vessels of the microcirculatory circle of other organs, although they were significantly smaller.

We [1] also studied 17 observations of generalized influenza with brain damage. The diagnosis of influenza in all cases was made on the basis of immunofluorescent and histological studies; in five cases, it was confirmed by the isolation of the virus (including twice from the brain) and in 12 cases by the results of serological studies (including in four, CSF). Influenza A1 was diagnosed in eight cases, influenza A2 in eight cases, and influenza B in one case. Due to the lack of significant differences in the clinical and morphological manifestations of the disease, depending on the serotype of the virus, all observations were considered by us in total. The deceased children (ten boys and seven girls) were aged 15 days to 2.5 years, and only one child died at the age of 8 years.

In a significant part of the cases, the disease developed on an unfavorable background in the form of encephalopathy (in six children), congenital heart disease, brain disease, spasmophilia, and congenital lipid metabolism disorders (one child). Generalized intrauterine infections (mycoplasmosis and cytomegaly) were detected in three children during a pathological examination. One child developed influenza on the background of residual changes after purulent meningoencephalitis, and one was convalescent of acute viral hepatitis. Only in four children was a significant background pathology not found during the pathological examination, although the parents of one of them were chronic alcoholics, and the mother of the other suffered from a mental illness.

In eight children, the flu was complicated by focal bacterial pneumonia caused by various pathogens. In the majority of cases, influenza was a monoinfection; only in five cases were moderate manifestations of parainfluenza and adenovirus (Ad) infection observed in the respiratory organs without clear signs of generalization. Changes characteristic of influenza [4] were detected in the lungs and brain and sometimes in other internal organs (liver—three times, kidneys and intestines—two times). In the morphological study of the brain, main attention was paid to clear signs of direct brain damage by influenza viruses. The analysis showed that the macroscopic changes in the brain were not fundamentally different from those observed in children who died from neurotoxicosis.

The changes considered as characteristic of influenza were of the greatest interest during microscopic examination. Most naturally (in all observations), they were detected in the soft meninges and consisted of an increase in size (from very moderate to several times) and pronounced basophilia of the cytoplasm of meningocytes and the appearance of cells that could be regarded as macrophages (Fig. 7.5). In some observations, such cells were clearly grouped around vessels with damaged walls. In three observations, meningocytes with enlarged light nuclei were detected in the soft meninges in the presence of influenza virus antibodies in the cerebrospinal fluid. Ependymocytes of vascular plexus in all observations were dystrophic, altered, and often exfoliated. In six observations, in addition, cells with an enlarged basophilic stained cytoplasm appeared, which were regarded as influenza. Some ependymocytes of the cerebral ventricles also acquired a similar appearance in these observations. Changes in nerve cells,

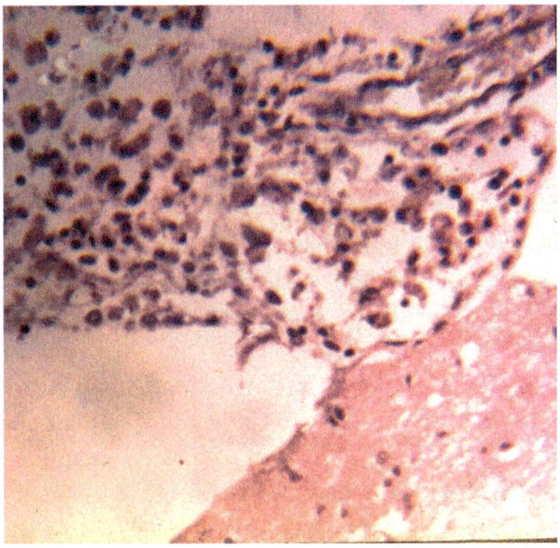

Fig. 7.5 Serous meningitis with numerous macrophages with enlarged intensive stained cytoplasma in a child with influenza. H-E ×600

presumably associated with exposure to the influenza virus, in most cases had the character of a "severe lesion," with or without a moderate glial reaction. However, in several observations with a long course of influenza, documented by clinical, laboratory (repeated serological, immunofluorescent, virological), as well as morphological data, some neurons, especially clearly in the area of the basal nodes, acquired an external pitchfork similar to "influenza cells." Changes on the part of glial cells in most cases were minimal and were reduced to a moderately pronounced swelling. Only in some cases, mostly with long-term clinical manifestations, that moderate hypertrophy of oligodendroglia and astrocytic glia was noted. In the same observations, there was a moderately pronounced demyelination in the white matter of the brain. In addition, hemodynamic changes were observed that were fundamentally similar to those described in the previous group. In all observations, there was a swelling of the endothelial nuclei with a thickening of the walls of blood vessels. Three children also had lymphoid infiltration of their walls. In four observations, mononuclear cells with enlarged intensely stained cytoplasm, most likely perivascular macrophages, were detected around the vessels in the brain substance. Hemorrhages in the soft medulla were determined in two observations: in one diapedesis and in the other extensive. In one case, diapedesis hemorrhages were detected in the area of the brain stem. In four children of this group, the content of interferon in the brain tissue was determined. Its amount ranged from about 1.1–2.7 lg (normally, interferon is not detected in the brain tissue), which, of course, indicates the reaction of the brain to the pathological process. The properties of interferon were studied in two observations. In one deceased child (who developed flu on the background of intrauterine mycoplasmosis), interferon was immune, and in the other viral. The content of interferon in the CSF also fluctuated but at slightly lower amounts (from 0.9 to 2.2 lg). In the lungs of two children, interferon was absent, and in two other children, it was determined in an amount greater than 2 Lg.

The clinical, laboratory, and morphological analysis made it possible to divide the studied observations into three groups. The first group included seven children who died within the first 3 days of the onset of the disease. The clinical picture of their disease was regarded clinically as neurotoxicosis. The second group included five children in whom the presence of distinct neurological symptoms within 5–15 days before death caused these observations to be regarded as acute encephalitis. Group 3 included five children whose generalization of influenza with brain damage occurred shortly before death on the background of severe preexisting pathology and therefore did not give new distinct clinical symptoms. An example of the observations on the first group (rapid development of generalized influenza with a clinical picture of neurotoxicosis) is presented below.

Oleg S, 11 months old, was born prematurely, with a weight of 2900 g and length of 48 cm. The mother has nephropathy during pregnancy. The boy was retarded in development; an unclear subfebrility was noted. He became acutely ill on December 20, with a rise in temperature to 38 °C, a cough, and a runny nose. Despite the symptomatic therapy, the child's condition worsened, and twice there was vomiting. On December 28, he was hospitalized with a diagnosis of "serous meningitis(?)." Upon admission, the condition is preagonal, he does not react to pain stimuli, pupils are wide, $D = S$, there is no reaction to light, and there is general muscle hypotension and a sharp violation of peripheral blood circulation. The pharynx is loosened and hyperemic, moaning breath up to 80 in 1 min, with the participation of auxiliary muscles, auscultative hard breathing, and intermittent wet wheezing. Blood pressure and pulse in the peripheral vessels are not determined. The heart tones are muffled. The abdomen is swollen and soft; the liver protrudes from under the edge of the costal arch by 3.5 cm and the spleen by 1 cm. There are several elements of petechial rash on the skin near the ankle joint. In CSF cytosis was $2{,}3 \times 10^6$/l. Despite the actively initiated treatment measures, the child's condition continued to deteriorate progressively, and in 1 h 15 min. After admission, he died. Clinically, the disease remained unclear. A differential diagnosis was made between acute respiratory viral infection with neurotoxicosis and meningococcal infection with toxic shock.

At the autopsy (V.A. Zinserling), catarrhal laryngotracheobronchitis and focal viral pneumonia were revealed. The brain weighs 850.0 g (with an average age norm of 960.0 g), with a relatively dense consistency. The soft meninges are thickened, mainly due to the transparent fluid located between their leaves. The gray matter has a slightly bluish tinge, and the vessels of the white matter are dilated and gaping. There were no changes in other parts of the brain. During the bacteriological study, the growth of microflora was not obtained. The immunofluorescence (IF) study of smears from the lungs and soft meninges revealed antigens for influenza A1 and *Mycoplasma hominis*. The serological examination of the blood revealed antibodies to influenza A1 in the titer 1:320 and CSF antibodies to influenza A in titer 1:160. The results of the virological examination are negative. Interferon was detected in the CSF in the titer of 1.0 lg, in the brain-2.7 lg, choriodal plexus-0.9 lg, lung –0, and was classified as immune. During cytological examination, lung smears contain numerous large fuchsinophylic inclusions (FI), "influenza" cells, as well as cells with an enlarged foamy cytoplasm (for explanations, see [4]). Smears from the soft meninges contain a large FI in the nuclei and cytoplasm of individual meningocytes. The histological examination of the central nervous system revealed distinct specific and nonspecific changes. The soft meninges are moderately, in some places more significantly, infiltrated by mononuclear cells, among which there are those with enlarged light nuclei, enlarged dark-colored cytoplasm, and enlarged foamy cytoplasm. The endothelium of many small blood vessels in the substance of the brain is swollen; in some places, it proliferates. Around some vessels, mainly medium-sized veins, there is moderate, mainly lymphocytic infiltration. The nerve cells, especially clearly in the caudate nucleus, thalamus, and quadruple underwent changes of "severe" type, lysis, and to a lesser extent "ischemic". The phenomena of satellite formation, some diffuse increase in oligodendroglia cells, some of which have slightly enlarged light nuclei, are clearly expressed. Single nerve cells have an enlarged vacuolated cytoplasm with small periodic acid-Schiff (PAS)-positive and azur-positive inclusions. The ependymocytes of the vascular plexus have predominantly dark, incorrectly oriented pycnotic nuclei. The vascular plexuses are full blooded, and the cells lining them are dystrophic. Some of them have an enlarged vacuolated cytoplasm with small inclusions. Only moderate degenerative changes in large nerve cells were detected in the spinal cord. Serous pneumonia due to influenza and mycoplasma was detected in the lungs. In the liver and kidneys, alterative changes in epithelial cells were detected. In conclusion, the boy died from generalized influenza A1, which occurred with lesions of a number of internal organs, including the brain in the form of serous meningitis, and was accompanied by severe violations of hemo- and cerebrospinal fluid dynamics and brain edema. The unfavorable course of the underlying disease was promoted by mycoplasmosis, which probably occurred in utero, which can be associated with a delay in the development of the child and prolonged subfebrility.

The clinical and morphological manifestations of influenza in six other children of the first group were fundamentally similar to those described above.

As an example of group 2 observations (acute influenza encephalitis), the following can be presented.

Olga S., 2.5 years old, from normal pregnancy and childbirth, in development corresponded to age. She became acutely ill on December 6 with a temperature of 37.3 °C and convulsive twitching of the facial muscles. Later on, the child's condition worsened, her temperature increased, generalized convulsive seizures occurred, and she lost consciousness. On the fourth day of the disease, she was transferred to the clinic with a diagnosis of encephalitic syndrome. Upon admission, there was a lack of consciousness, generalized clonic convulsions, lack of reaction to light, anisocoria, $D > S$, trism, general muscle hypotension, and deep reflex inhibition. At lumbar puncture, cytosis 14.3 × 10^6/l, in the sediment predominace of mononuclears, protein 0.825%. The IF study revealed the antigen of influenza A2 virus. Despite active therapy, the child's condition continued to be severe, tonic seizures were periodically repeated, and the girl was feverish. Due to cardiovascular insufficiency, the child died on December 15 (on the ninth day of the disease). Clinically, the disease was regarded as acute viral encephalitis associated with influenza A2. The autopsy revealed the phenomena of catarrhal laryngotracheobronchitis, focal viral pneumonia, and venous fullness of internal organs. The brain weighs 990.0 g (with an average age norm of 1050 g) and is of flabby consistency. The soft medulla is thin and transparent throughout, and its vessels are sharply full blooded. The border between gray and white substances is blurred. The vessels of the white matter are dilated and full blooded. The cerebral ventricles are narrow and contain a small amount of clear liquor, and the vascular plexuses are full blooded. In the right temporal lobe, the focus of softening is 5 × 5 cm in size. During the bacteriological study, hemolytic streptococcus, *Staphylococcus aureus*, and *Escherichia coli* were isolated from the lung. *E. coli* was isolated also from CSF. The IF examination of tracheal and lung smears revealed influenza A2 antigen. The serological examination of paired blood sera showed a twofold increase in influenza A2 antibodies. During virological research on chicken embryos, the A2 influenza virus (Hong Kong) was isolated from the trachea and brain. The histological examination revealed that soft meninges were thickened due to edema and perivascular mononuclear infiltration among the cells, of which many had enlarged intensely stained cytoplasm. In the cortex of the large hemisphere, there are many dystrophic altered nerve cells, some of which have a dark-colored cytoplasm. The walls of the vessels in the substance of the brain are thickened, and there is a disorganization of their muscle layer and swelling of the nuclei of endotheliocytes. There is a rather distinct, mainly lymphocytic, infiltration of the walls of blood vessels and perivascular spaces and pronounced perivascular and pericellular edema. Ependymocytes, especially clearly in the region of the posterior horns of the cerebral ventricles, are flattened; subependimar, there is a small mainly macrophage infiltration among the cells, of which there are enlarged intensely colored cytoplasm. In the cells of the ammonic horn and the lining of the vascular plexus, there are distinct degenerative changes. Glial cells show signs of moderate hyperplasia and proliferation. The histological examination of the internal organs revealed influenza lesions in the lungs and epithelial cell degeneration in the kidneys, liver, and intestines. In conclusion, the girl died from generalized influenza A2, among the manifestations of which acute encephalitis was the most important.

Similar clinical and morphological manifestations of the disease were observed in three children. In a girl, Irina P., 3 months old with a disease duration of about 1 month, influenza-specific cells were detected in the meninges, as well as in the brain substance, along with microglial nodules in the basal nodes. In the boy Pavel, A., 10 months old with a disease duration of about 15 days, typical flu cells were detected only in the meninges and vascular plexuses. Only nonspecific necrobiotic changes were observed on the part of the nerve cells. The clinical and morphological manifestations of the disease were different from those described in Vera M, 11 months old, in whom the combination of acute encephalitis with toxic hepatitis, lasting for 5 days, allowed clinicians to diagnose Rey's syndrome. A postmortem morphological and laboratory examination revealed generalized influenza A1, including brain lesions. In the brain, along with hemodynamic changes among the cells of mononuclear leukocyte infiltration of the soft meninges, there were typical flu-like changes. A special feature of this observation was pronounced fatty liver dystrophy and a sharply increased content of sphingomyelin in the brain tissue, detected by a special neurochemical study, which was determined in the gray matter in the amount of 186 mcg/g (at a norm of 120 mcg/g). When analyzing this observation, it was decided to consider the disease as a peculiar course of influenza against the background of a congenital disorder of lipid metabolism (neurochemically, according to the type of Niemann-Pick syndrome).

In the third group of five children, the generalization of influenza with brain damage occurred shortly before death on the background of severe preexisting pathology, and therefore new clinic manifestations were not recorded by the attending physicians. In three children (Dmitry F., 1 year 7 months; Sergey M., 6 months; Vyacheslav M., 10.5 months), this was a pronounced perinatal brain lesion to varying degrees; in the boy F., the latter was combined with congenital endocrinopathy. Vladimir D, 6 months old, was in the clinic for the consequences of birth trauma, and Vladimir R, 8 years old, had residual changes after purulent meningoencephalitis. A histological examination of the brain in all these children, along with changes typical of their background sufferings, revealed, mainly in the soft meninges, cells typical of influenza with an enlarged intensely colored cytoplasm or enlarged light nuclei.

These materials indicate the possibility of the development of lesions typical for influenza against the background of circulatory changes. They consist in the appearance in the soft meninges, the vascular plexuses, and, much less often (with a long course of the process), the substance of the brain of cells of different origin with an enlarged, intensely colored cytoplasm or, less often, enlarged light nuclei. Such changes are fundamentally similar to those detected in influenza in the lungs, kidneys, intestines, and other organs [4]. It can be assumed that these changes are directly related to the presence of the virus or its components in the altered cells.

The degree of severity of the hemorrhagic syndrome was small; we did not observe any hemorrhagic encephalitis described in the literature. Perivascular infiltration and glial reaction were weakly expressed. Confirmation of the presence of an inflammatory process in the central nervous system was the detection of anti-influenza antibodies in the CSF and interferon in the brain tissue.

Many of the propositions we put forward were confirmed in subsequent studies. Thus, a team of Japanese authors [5] conducted a comprehensive clinical, virological, molecular biological, and immunohistochemical (but not histological!) examination of the internal organs and brain of a 2.5-month-old girl who died from influenza A (H3N2) with a picture of acute viral encephalitis. Death followed after 6 days of being on a ventilator. Polymerase chain reaction (PCR) detected the hemagglutinin gene of the virus, which was found in the CSF, frontal lobe, hippocampus, cerebellum, lung, kidney, and liver. In a similar study of peripheral blood mononuclear cells taken at admission, the virus was not detected. In immunohistochemistry (IHC), viral hemagglutinin was detected in the lung, lining the alveoli (according to the authors, the lesion of alveolocytes) and $CD3^{+}T$ lymphocytes. The same antigen was detected in the beta cells of the pancreas and $CD\text{-}8^{+}$ lymphocytes of the spleen. In the brain, the viral antigen was detected in the Purkinje cells of the cerebellum and the bridge neurons. It was not detected in the hippocampus, midbrain, and cortex. The soft meninges and choroidal plexuses were not examined. To study the pathogenesis of this observation, an intracerebral infection of cynomolgus monkeys with a strain isolated from the girl was performed. During the study, the virus remained only in the injection area for a week, which allowed the authors to conclude that in the pathogenesis of the neurological symptoms that quickly developed in the girl, in addition to replication and dissemination of viruses, inflammatory cytokines that contributed to the violation of the blood-brain barrier (BBB) should have played a significant role. Unfortunately, the absence of any, primarily histological, data on the changes in the soft meninges and choroidal plexuses does not allow us to express a definite opinion about the pathogenesis of brain damage in this observation. Later on, no publications on the topic were found.

7.1.2 Lesions of the Nervous System in Adults

The clinical characteristics of CNS lesions in influenza in adults are most fully presented by V. A. Isakov et al. [6]. The study analyzed almost 19,000 observations over 20 years. According to its data, hypertoxic forms of influenza are observed on average in 5% of patients, and the mortality rate among hospitalized patients is from 0.6% to 2.5%. The frequency of neurological complications in different years ranged from 0.3% to 30%. During the period of the maximum epidemic rise in the incidence of influenza (1974–1975), the author examined 160 patients in detail. Neurotoxic syndrome was detected in 56 people, meningoencephalitic syndrome in seven, cerebrovascular disorders in four, and polyradiculoneuritis of the Landry type in one. When using biophysical methods based on light scattering, structures of more than 500 nm in diameter were found in the CSF, which were regarded as virus-containing immune complexes. The level of antibrain antibodies detected in the blood correlated with the severity of the disease.

The literature data concerning the pathology of brain lesions in influenza are almost exclusively based on past autopsy observations when there was no possibility of verifying the etiology of the disease. In this regard, quite common ideas about the development of "hemorrhagic meningitis" and "hemorrhagic encephalitis" in influenza cannot be considered convincing today. The polar point of view that the brain is not affected by influenza in adults also remains without any weighty arguments.

Due to the lack of recent literature materials, we present the data related to different influenza outbreaks.

The beginning of 1999 was characterized by a significant increase in the number of cases of viral respiratory infections, primarily influenza.

To assess the severity of the 1999 influenza epidemic in comparison with previous periods, we have analyzed data from the reports of the pathological department of S.P. Botkin Infectious Hospital (representative for the city) since 1965. Depending on the epidemic situation, the number of deaths diagnosed with influenza varied significantly. The highest rates were recorded in 1973 (41 people), 1975 (40 people), 1970 (22 people), 1969 (20 people), and 1984 (15 people). Since 1985, the annual number of deaths has ranged from one to ten.

All 27 cases of fatal outcomes in adults were subjected to special analysis, in which the flu could be diagnosed according to clinical, epidemiological, virological, or morphological data. Virological (blood serology and immunofluorescence smears from the trachea and lungs), bacteriological, and detailed histological studies were performed in almost all cases. Based on the principles of the influenza infection assessment made by A.V. Zinserling [4], all observations were divided into three groups.

The first group included 15 observations, in which there was a clear clinical and morphological picture of active influenza in the respiratory organs, often with signs of generalization of influenza infection, primarily in the soft meninges, with varying degrees of severity of the bacterial process in the lungs. In this group, the patients were aged 17–74 years, and the duration of the disease ranged from 5 to 20 days. During virological examination, the diagnosis of influenza A2 was verified in two cases by immunofluorescence, according to serological data; in three cases, it was possible to talk about influenza A1 + A2, in three cases A2, and in two cases A2 + B and B1–A1 + A2 + B; in five cases, the results of laboratory tests gave an uncertain result. Of crucial importance is the fact that in almost all observations it was possible to detect the presence of mixed respiratory infections:

DNA - virus unspecified infection-2 times, probably enterovirus infection-2 times, parainfluenza and mycoplasmosis according to morphological data (1 time each). One or another degree of bacterial superinfection was determined in all observations: bronchiolitis (two times), small focal pneumonia (two times), large focal pneumonia (six times), confluent (four times), and abscessing (two times). During bacteriological studies, the following pathogens were isolated: in four cases, staphylococci; in three, streptococci; in two, pneumococci; and in eight, various gram-negative rods, including in seven observations in which mixed microflora was isolated from the respiratory system. Hypertension in combination with atherosclerosis, alcoholism (twice), drug addiction, viral hepatitis C, progressive pulmonary tuberculosis, Down's disease, acute sphenoiditis, bronchial asthma, and cholelithiasis (one time) were identified as the most important background and concomitant diseases in 11 cases. When retrospectively assessing the factors that influenced the unfavorable outcome of the disease, late admission, short-term stay, and lack of antiviral therapy were noted. There was no uniformity in the clinical diagnoses of patients in this group, and neurotoxicosis, encephalopathy, and brain coma (twice) were reported as flu complications. In a special study of the brain, nonspecific disorders of hemo -and cerebrospinal fluid dynamics, described in the previous sections, prevailed. Special attention was paid to the condition of the soft meninges, in which moderate mononuclear infiltration was determined, among the cells of which typical influenza was determined according to our ideas.

The second group included eight observations in which, while maintaining moderate or slightly pronounced signs of influenza infection activity, bacterial pneumonia associated with influenza was of the greatest importance for the onset of death. In the brain, there were no lesions characteristic of influenza; only moderately pronounced hemo- and cerebrospinal fluid changes were detected. The age of the deceased ranged from 15 to 86 years, and the duration of the disease ranged from 9 to 21 days. In the virological study, the immunofluorescence study in all observations gave negative results, serologically, and in two cases high titers to A1 + A2, 1, A2 and A2 + B, B, and A1 + A2 + B; in one observation, the laboratory data were uninformative. In the etiology of bacterial pneumonia (large focal or confluent), the role of various cocci and rod pathogens has been shown. In addition, in two cases, it was possible to talk about the addition infection of parainfluenza and in one of respiratory chlamydia. The most important background and concomitant diseases were identified as atherosclerosis in combination with hypertension (six times) and chronic viral hepatitis of unspecified etiology and mental retardation (one time each). One woman, 28 years old, died in the postpartum period (after cesarean section). When retrospectively assessing the factors that influenced the unfavorable outcome of the disease, first of all, late admission and short-term stay were noted.

The third group included 23 observations, in which the role of influenza in the onset of death was not obvious and was documented only by the results of serological and/or histological studies. Changes characteristic of influenza in the deceased in this group were also not determined. The main diseases of the deceased in this group were pneumonia (five times), polysinuitis (four times), hypertension (three times), purulent otitis (two times), chronic viral hepatitis (three times), gastroenterocolitis, diabetes mellitus, stomach cancer, human immunodeficiency virus (HIV) infection, purulent prostatitis, and ovarian cysts. The age of the deceased was from 21 to 76 years. Information about respiratory infection in anamnesis was available in 15 cases, its duration ranged from 5 days to 1 month, and in eight, cases there was no information about it in the medical history. The specific role of influenza viruses (more often A2 according to serological data) is not completely clear. In one case, a 50-year-old man with a 4-day picture of acute respiratory infection and negative results of virological examination revealed a distinct morphological picture of generalized parainfluenza with respiratory and brain damage with the addition of small focal pneumonia of pneumococcal etiology.

The presented data do not exclude the possibility of developing other, more severe brain lesions in adults with influenza caused by strains with more pronounced neurotropic properties. Presumably, this could have occurred in 1918–1920 during the "Spanish" epidemic. Unfortunately, it appeared not possible to decipher the essence of the defeats in those years.

The few deaths from influenza observed in recent years suggest significant differences in the thanatogenesis of individual cases. It can be assumed that the diagnosis of influenza is completely indisputable in observations in which death occurred during the active course of this viral infection. According to our data, one of the most reliable signs of generalization of influenza in adults is the appearance of a characteristic transformation of the cells of the soft meninges. Unfortunately, we have to state that a similar analysis of deaths from influenza is not carried out anywhere in the world.

The 2009–2010 H1N1v influenza A pandemic was characterized by a wide coverage of the population of many countries of the world, a severe clinical course, and high mortality. Lethal outcomes were most often observed, not only in people with concomitant chronic diseases but also in young people without significant previous pathology, including pregnant women. In St. Petersburg, 31 deaths were registered among adults, and it can be assumed that the true number of deaths was higher. There were no deaths among children in St. Petersburg and the Leningrad Region. They were practically absent in other regions of the country. In most publications devoted to the clinical and pathological anatomy of the most severe forms of this disease, the main attention is paid to respiratory diseases, while there are indications of the possibility of developing diseases caused by different strains of the influenza virus and generalized infection. We present the results of our complex analysis [4]. The age of the deceased patients ranged from 15 to 58 years (19 men and 10 women). The influenza A/H1N1v virus was confirmed in 28 cases. In the first case, the flu virus was not detected, but clinical epidemiological and pathologic analysis allowed to diagnose the flu. All patients were hospitalized at different times from the onset of the disease. Prior to hospitalization, 21 patients did not seek medical care, and eight patients were on outpatient treatment. All patients at admission had a pronounced intoxication syndrome: fever (38.7 ± 0.6 °C), weakness, and headache. All patients complained of severe cough, shortness of breath, and runny nose. Some patients had symptoms probably associated with CNS damage. Headache was observed in 15 (51.7%) patients, pain in the eyeballs in 24 (82.8%) patients, vomiting in five (17.2%) patients, and manifestations of meningism in one (3.4%) patient; dizziness was reported in 11 (38%) patients. Their condition was regarded as serious. Twenty patients had two or more concomitant chronic diseases: diseases of the cardiovascular system in four people, chronic kidney failure in six, alcohol disease in four patients, chronic obstructive pulmonary disease in four, obesity in nine patients, and anemia of mixed genesis in five patients; three patients had no comorbidities. In the hospital, all underwent massive antibacterial therapy. Antiviral therapy using the drug "Tamiflu" was received only by five patients (16.6%), who were admitted at a late stage of the disease. All patients were treated in the intensive care unit. Death occurred from the fourth day till the 38th day of the disease. The cause of death in 25 cases (86.2%) was acute respiratory failure, in two cases (6.9%) acute cardiovascular failure, and in one (3.4%) case pulmonary heart failure. A pathological diagnosis of "Viral total hemorrhagic pneumonia" was formulated in 16 patients and "Community-acquired hemorrhagic viral-bacterial pneumonia" in 13 patients. According to PCR diagnostics, H1N1v influenza virus ribonucleic acid (RNA) was identified in 28 autopsy lung samples. In all fatally ended observations, severe lesions are noted mainly in the respiratory parts of the lungs, as well as in the bronchi of different calibers and the trachea, and "flu-like" changes in epithelial cells; alveolar macrophages are observed. The general nature of the morphological changes caused by the current strain of the influenza virus is similar to the descriptions made by A.V. Zinserling and his school [4]. In contrast to the descriptions of previous years, such changes were traced up to the third week from the onset of the disease. At the same time, epithelial, macrophage, and endothelial cells with large light nuclei, which were not previously described in detail, were also noted. Some of these cells had two or more nuclei, and the presence of symplastic structures was noted in the late stages from the onset of the disease. We have conditionally designated such cells as influenza type 2. The ciliated epithelium of the respiratory tract was predominantly preserved. Foci of neutrophilic infiltration, regarded as signs of bacterial superinfection, were observed only in 13 dead patients and had no significant significance in thanatogenesis. The leading role in the formation of acute respiratory failure was respiratory distress syndrome, which manifests itself in a sharp fullness of blood vessels, serous exudates in the lumen of the alveoli, and their uneven airiness. Hyaline membranes and disseminated intravascular coagulation were also detected naturally. In addition, some observations showed a swelling of endothelial cells and moderate perivascular lymphocytic infiltration in the myocardium, brain (Fig. 7.6), liver, and kidneys, similar to those previously described as manifestations of influenza generalization. When analyzing the autopsy material of patients who died from influenza A (H1N1v), hemagglutinin (NA) and nucleoprotein (NP) were detected in the tissues of the lungs, heart, and brain (Fig. 7.7). Viral antigens were found in the lungs, the epithelium of the alveoli and bronchioles, the endothelium of blood vessels of different calibers (capillaries and arterioles), and individual tissue macrophages. In the brain, HA and NP were detected in glial cells, neuronal bodies, and the endothelium of some microvessels. It should be noted that the localization of viral antigens in the epithelium of the alveoli and bronchioles and in the endothelium of blood vessels was noted in all analyzed lung autopsies, while lesions of the heart vessels and brain tissues were recorded only in isolated cases.

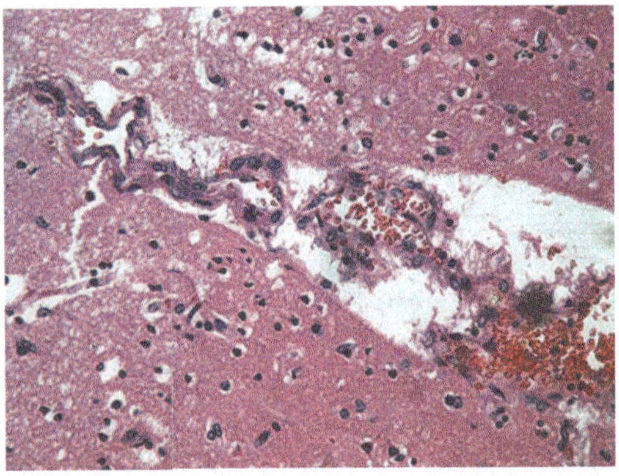

Fig. 7.6 Full blood and swelling of endothelium, perivascular edema in brain matter in an adult who died from influenza H1N1v (swine). H-E, ×320

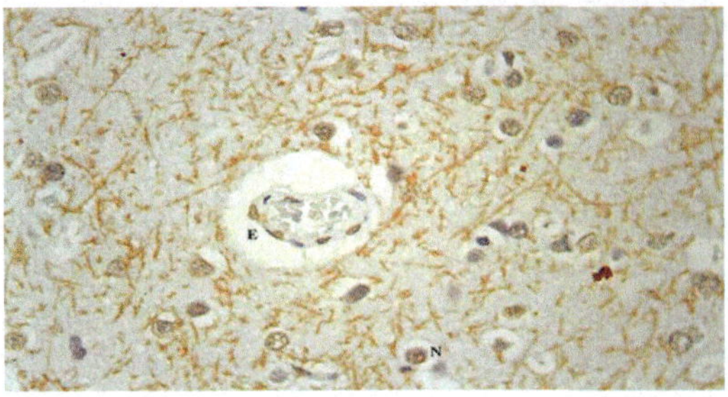

Fig. 7.7 Neuroaminidase of influenza virus A(H1N1) in brain matter. IHC ×400

7.1.3 Experimental Models

Of considerable interest are the results of quite numerous experimental studies devoted to the study of brain lesions with various strains of the influenza virus. C.N. Stuart-Harris already in 1939 showed that the influenza virus adapted to the brain of mice can multiply in it.

It was later shown that brain damage by influenza viruses depends on three main factors: the neurotropy of the strain, the age of the animals, and the amount of infection. Subsequently, this issue was studied in detail by a number of authors (for more details, see [1]). Intracerebral administration of a neurotropic strain of influenza A2 virus in newborn mice after 48 h virologically determined an increase in the amount of the virus by more than 100 times and morphologically noted necrosis of the ependyma and lymphocytic and polymorphocellular infiltration of the choroidal plexus, in the cells of which the influenza virus antigen was determined using IF microscopy. These changes were most pronounced 3–4 days after infection. After a few days, there were changes in most of the other parts of the brain, but less pronounced. Light microscopy was used to determine basophilic and oxyphilic inclusions in nerve cells and the proliferation of astrocytic glia. In EM, 24 h after infection, many filamentous viral particles were detected in the intercellular spaces of the hippocampus, and the "detaching" of viral particles from the surface of the neuron or its axon was determined. In addition, the cytoplasm of the "infected" neurons contained clusters of ribosomes associated with osmiophilic material of unknown nature, but absent in the control and located between numerous vacuoles, intracerebral infection of mice and ferrets with the influenza A virus caused acute incomplete infection of the ependymal cells of the cerebral ventricles and the choroidal plexus epithelium, in which a viral antigen is produced rather than a complete infectious virus. According to these authors, the number of ependymal cells infected with the influenza A virus is directly proportional to the amount of the virus injected. Ninety-three percent of suckers and 39% of adult ferrets infected with high doses of influenza A virus developed Sylvian aqueduct stenosis and hydrocephalus. Small doses caused a focal absence of ependyma in rodents of all ages. The infection did not manifest itself in any way, even in cases of clear lesions of ependymal cells with an acute inflammatory reaction.

Significant data on the pathogenesis of influenza-like brain lesions were also obtained in an experimental study performed on turkeys, with extensive use of histological, IF, and virological methods. Based on a comparative virological study of dynamics, it is shown that brain damage occurs against the background of the most pronounced viremia, which allowed the author to categorically speak in favor of hematogenic penetration of the pathogen. The choroidal plexuses are affected most early, followed by the spread of the virus through the soft meninges and ependyma of the cerebral ventricles, and in some cases, its penetration into the substance of the brain is possible. The main way of spreading the virus is liquor. Among the morphological changes, there were inflammatory changes at the sites of virus replication and perivascular leukomalacia in the brain substance, probably due to secondary mechanisms.

The most complete and comprehensive studies of brain lesions in white mice with intracerebral infection with eight different strains of influenza virus are given in the study of B.A. Osetrov et al. [for more details, see [1]]. They showed that the pathogenesis of brain damage is based on the reproduction of the virus in the cells of the ependyma and epithelium of the choriodal plexus of the cerebral ventricles, which led to dystrophic changes in these cells and reactive changes in the brain substance, designated by the author as acute primary viral influenza chorioependimatitis. The reproduction of the influenza virus in arachnoendothelium, nerve, and glial cells was rarely observed. The changes caused by the introduction of different strains of the influenza virus were fundamentally similar, although they differed in the severity of both structural changes and clinical manifestations. The inflammatory changes in the form of lymphocytic and plasmocytic infiltration, membrane fibrosis, and hydrocephalus detected by the authors 1–4 months after infection were regarded as an indirect sign of the formation of persistent influenza infection.

The study of pathological changes in the brain of mice with experimental influenza infection using virological, neurohistological, and EM methods was carried out by S.P. Semenov et al. [7]. This work once again confirmed the long-term circulation of the virus in the body with persistence in the brain and a number of internal organs. The vascular lesions identified by the authors, in particular the vascular plexus, are important, which creates prerequisites for a violation of BBB permeability.

Some authors conducted experimental studies on monkeys. In a *Cynocephalus babuin* monkey, C. Cateigne et al. [8] observed dyspnea and anorexia on day 6 after intracerebral administration of amniotic fluid containing a strain of influenza A1 virus and on day 7 photophobia, anisocoria, salivation, epileptic seizures, and hypothermia. The autopsy revealed macroscopically the phenomena of stagnation and fullness of blood in the vessels of the brain and membranes, as well as hemorrhages around several meningeal vessels. The microscopic examination revealed degenerative changes in most of the nerve cells of the cerebral cortex and, in smaller numbers, in other parts of the brain, except for the cerebellum and spinal cord.

G. Lussier et al. [9] reported experimental influenza encephalitis in monkeys following intracerebral and intranasal administration of the influenza A virus (strains A/Hong Kong/1/68 and A/PR-68). The pathomorphological examination revealed acute ependymatitis, choroiditis, and meningitis, which occurred with destructive desquamative changes in the ependyma. Infiltration of the choroidal plexus, ependyma of the lateral ventricles, and central canal of the spinal cord, as well as soft meninges were noted. The composition of the infiltrates was dominated by mononuclears. Perivascular infiltration was observed in the subependymal region. Hydrocephalus was observed in two animals. There were no changes in the brain parenchyma.

K. Miyoshi et al. [10] reported encephalitis caused by intracerebral administration of WSW and NWS strains of influenza virus in monkeys treated with immunosuppressants. Histologically, infiltration of the choroidal plexus, soft meninges, and subependimar structures by polymorphonuclear leukocytes was detected in the brain. Sometimes perivascular and parenchymal infiltrates in the gray matter of the brain were detected. Using IF microscopy, the viral antigen was detected in the subependimar regions, near the bottom of the fourth ventricle, in the area surrounding the central canal, as well as in glial cells.

We [1] conducted an experimental study in 2010. Influenza viruses A/WSN/33 (H1N1) and A/California/07/09 (H1N1) were obtained from the Influenza Research Institute virus collection. Before infection, the viruses were adapted to mice in three passages through the lung tissue of mice, followed by the passage through the allantoic cavity of 10–12-day-old chicken embryos for 48 hours at a temperature of 36 °C. We used inbred female mice weighing 18–20 g. Before the experiment, the animals were quarantined for 2 weeks. The experiment was planned in accordance with the principles of treatment of laboratory animals. The mouse-adapted virus was titrated to determine the lethal dose. For this purpose, mice (ten in each experimental group) were infected intranasally under anesthesia with 50 μL of serial dilutions (from 10–1 to 10–5) of lung homogenate from infected mice. The dose of the virus that causes the death of 50% of animals within 14 days after infection (LD50) was calculated according to the generally accepted method, which was later used for experiments. On day 3 after infection, five mice from each group infected with 1 LD50 of the virus were slaughtered; the chest was opened, and the lungs were extracted. The lungs were homogenized in a tenfold volume of sterile phosphate buffer. Serial dilutions (10-1–10-7) were prepared from each homogenate. MDCK cells were grown in 96-well plates, filled with 0.2 mL of each dilution of lung homogenate, and incubated at 36 °C for 48 h in an atmosphere of 5% CO2. After incubation, the culture fluid was collected and tested for the presence of influenza virus by mixing with an equal volume of 1% suspension of chicken red blood cells in saline solution. The maximum dilution that caused the hemagglutination reaction in the well was taken as the viral titer and expressed in log10EID50/20 mg of tissue. On days 3, 7, and 14 after infection, five mice from each group were slaughtered. For histological examination, the lungs, brain, and heart were taken. The organs were fixed in 10% formalin, passed through alcohols of ascending concentration, and poured into paraffin. The sections were stained with hematoxylin-eosin and partially PAS. To objectify the dynamics of inflammatory changes, slices were scanned and the area of airless foci was determined using Adobe Photoshop. As a control, we used intact mice and mice that were injected intranasally with saline solution in the same volume as the virus-containing suspension. Viruses effectively multiplied in the lung tissue of animals, reaching titers of 6.1–6.2 log10 EID50/20 mg of tissue on the third day after infection, depending on the strain used. Over time, the infectious activity of the virus decreased, and by the 11th day of the experiment, the A/WSN (H1N1) virus was practically not released from the lungs. The activity of another virus, A/

California/07/09 (H1N1), remained longer, but it also significantly decreased compared to the initial value (3 days). A histological examination of the control animals revealed no significant manifestations of spontaneous pathology. A histological examination of the experimental animals infected with both strains of the virus showed an increase in inflammatory infiltration in the lungs in the early stages, represented mainly by exudates consisting of neutrophils and macrophages in the lumen of the bronchi and around them. Later, there was a decline of individual alveoli with mainly mononuclear interstitial infiltration. The cells of the bronchial epithelium underwent pronounced degenerative changes, but in the case of the "swine" strain, they were practically not exfoliated. Some of the alveolar macrophages acquired enlarged light nuclei, which made them similar to the ones described by us in regard to the autopsy material. However, the cytoplasm of such cells was not always clearly traced. From the side of the brain in both studied groups, starting from day 3, the swelling of the endothelium of the blood vessels of the soft meninges and their fullness were naturally determined, as well as moderate mononuclear infiltration (Fig. 7.8). In the substance of the brain, along with dystrophic and necrobiotic changes in nerve cells, especially when infected with a neurotropic strain, small clusters of glial cells were determined in the substance of the brain (Figs. 7.9 and 7.10). In the myocardium of individual animals, vasculitis was noted. Signs typical of influenza lesions were also observed in plexus chorioideus (Figs. 7.11 and 7.12). During our previous studies, we succeeded to detect virus similar structures during EM in experimental influenza (Fig. 7.13). Thus, our experimental studies were able to confirm the generalization of influenza infection with brain damage, due not only to the classic neurotropic but also the current strain of influenza AH1N1 California/swine.

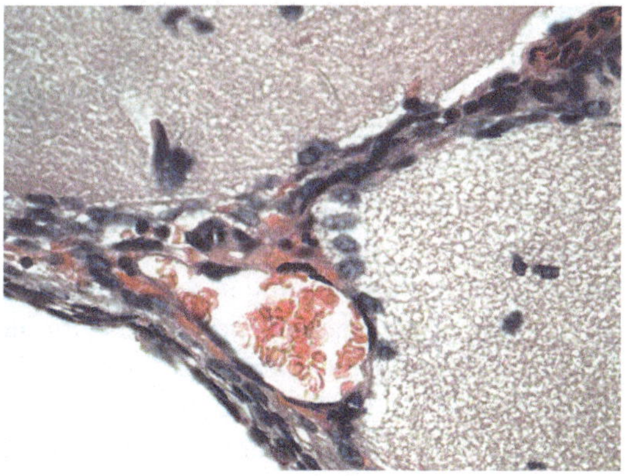

Fig. 7.8 Swelling of endothelium and perivascular infiltration in meninges of a mouse on the 14th day after intranasal challenge with influenza A/ H1N1/WSN. H-E ×400

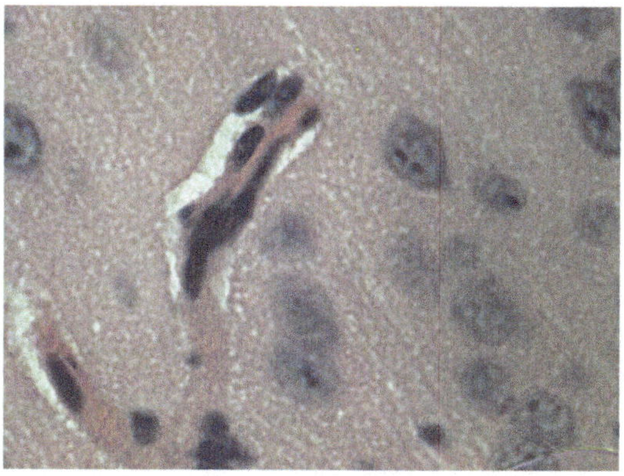

Fig. 7.9 Swelling of endothelium with moderate degenerative changes of adjacent cell in brain matter of mice on the third day after intranasal challenge with influenza A/ H1N1/WSN. H-E ×200

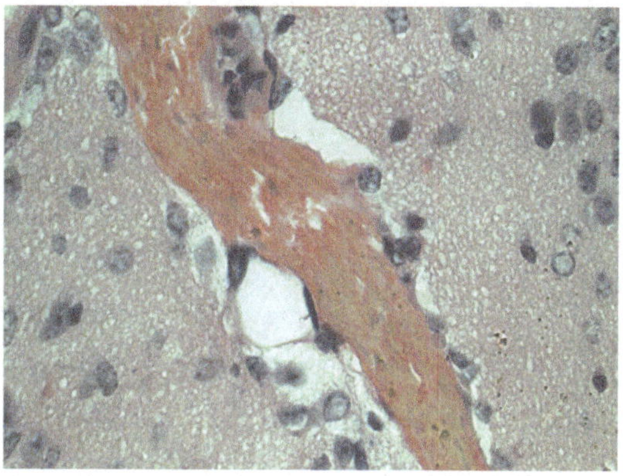

Fig. 7.10 Lesion of brain vessel in brain matter of mice on the 14th day after intranasal challenge with influenza A/ H1N1/WSN. H-E ×400

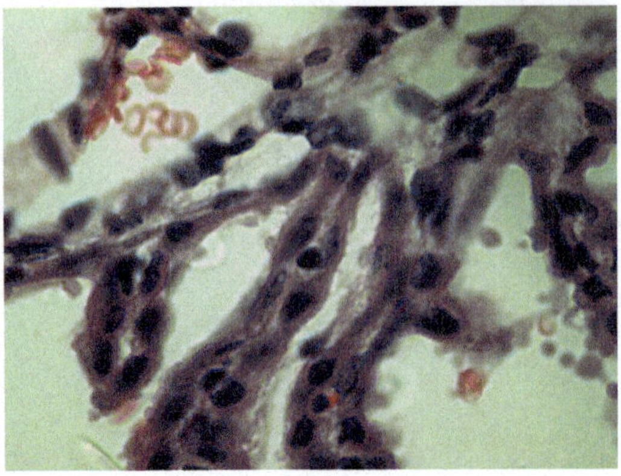

Fig. 7.11 Enlarged cells of plexus chorioideus with basophilic cytoplasm in experimental influenza. H-E ×600

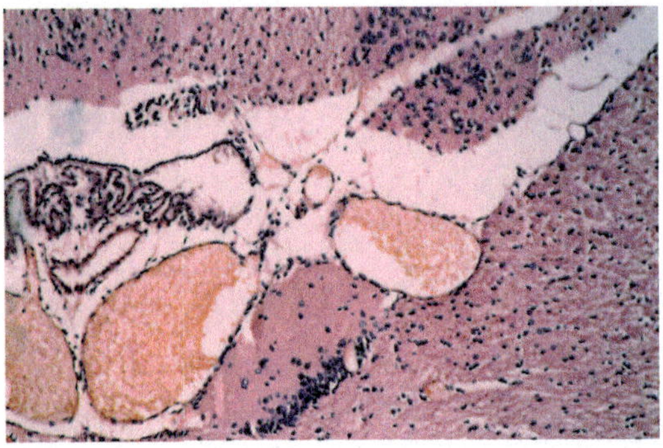

Fig. 7.12 Subependymal vessels, full blood, plexus chorioideus slightly enlarged in experimental influenza in mouse. H-E ×100

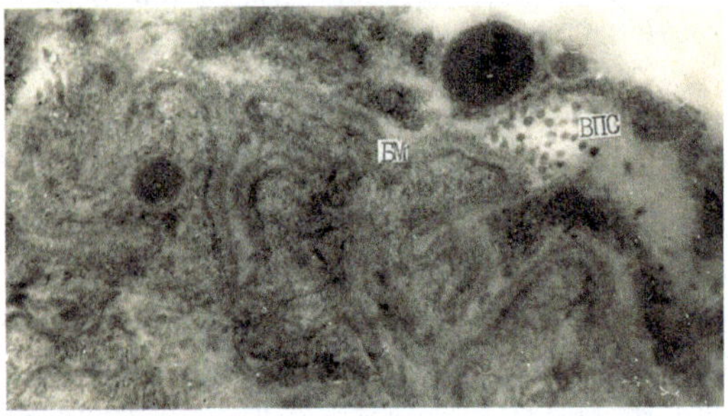

Fig. 7.13 Virus with similar structures near basal membrane in experimental influenza in mice. EM ×54,000

Thus, our experimental studies were able to confirm the generalization of influenza infection with brain damage due not only to the classic neurotropic but also to the current strain of influenza AH1N1 California/swine.

7.2 Other Respiratory Viral Infections

7.2.1 Brain Damage in Parainfluenza

Brain lesions with parainfluenza virus are described in the literature by a few authors. Clinical descriptions began to appear in 1953. There is practically no information about the frequency of such lesions in the literature.

The parainfluenza etiology of neurological lesions was established in patients mainly on the basis of a combination of clinical manifestations and the results of the serological examination of sera. Only in rare cases, the diagnosis was confirmed by isolation of the virus from the CSF or by serological examination of the CSF, investigators who summarized the most significant clinical materials, came to the conclusion that all 4 types of viruses can cause brain damage, however, in more than 80% of cases they are viruses of serotypes 2 and 3.

Clinical symptoms most often fit into the picture of serous meningitis or meningoencephalitis, as well as unstable meningeal or meningoencephalitic syndrome. In some cases, epileptic syndrome is described. It was noted that compared with the changes observed in influenza, the degree of intracranial hypertension is lesser, lymphocytic pleocytosis in the CSF is higher, there are no sharp vascular changes, and the focal symptoms are less pronounced.

There is practically no information about the morphological changes observed in rare cases of fatal outcomes in the literature.

Parainfluenza lesions of the brain in the experiment are devoted to quite a large number of literature in 1959–1980, mainly in connection with the discussion on the possible role of this virus in the etiology of subacute sclerosing panencephalitis. An overview of the literature of that time was done previously by us [1]. In modern literature, these issues were not discussed.

In our study [1], six observations of children who died from generalized parainfluenza at the age of 1 day to 6 years and 5 months (four boys and two girls) were analyzed. In five children, type 3 PI was diagnosed as a respiratory infection based on the results of IF, and in two cases, serological examination. In a girl who died 6 h after birth, PI was regarded as an intrauterine infection. Generalized PI developed in all children with an extremely unfavorable background: a boy, Mikhail A., 6 years and 2 months old, had a perinatal brain lesion caused by a conflict about the ABO system; a girl, Tatiana B., 10 months old, suffered from Down's disease. Two children (Mikhail S., 25 days old, and Yuri H., 8 months old) had signs of intrauterine infection (cytomegalic sialadenitis). Along with PI, most of the children had other diseases, although the severity of the associated lesions was relatively moderate at the time of death. In three children (Mikhail S., Mikhail A., Tatiana B.), there were residual changes of influenza in the respiratory organs (according to serological data in two cases A2 and one B); in Tatiana B., catarrhal enterocolitis caused by *Escherichia* O145 was also detected. In Pavel A., 1 year and 5 months old, with hyperplasia of the thymus gland and peripheral lymphoid tissue, the disease began a day after vaccination with smallpox. The girl T. was born in a state of intranatal asphyxia due to the entanglement of the umbilical cord around the neck and difficult delivery due to the narrowed pelvis of the mother.

Clinically, in four children, the disease was considered acute respiratory infection with neurotoxicosis with a duration of clinical manifestations from 2 to 17 days. In one child, the disease was regarded as intestinal toxicosis. In a girl who died in the first hours of life, asphyxia was considered as the cause of death.

A characteristic morphological picture of generalized PI [4] was detected in all cases in the lungs and kidneys and in three cases also in the liver and intestines.

Changes in the brain were characterized by moderate lymphomonocytic infiltration of the soft meninges and overgrowth of the epithelial cells of the choroidal plexus, of the ependymocytes of the lateral ventricles (Fig. 7.14), and of the endotheliocytes of small vessels with the formation of, in some cases, structures.

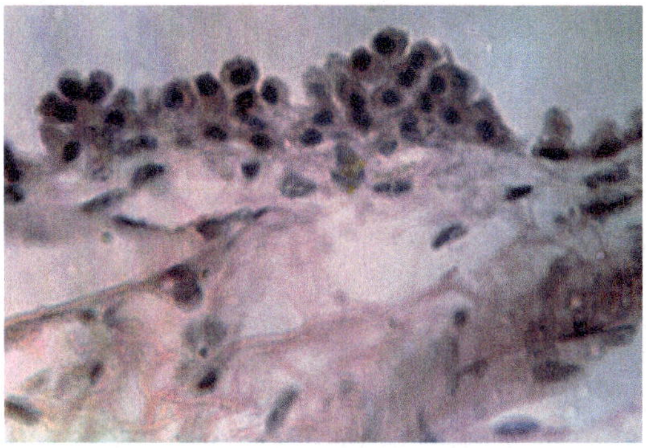

Fig. 7.14 Pillow-like overgrowths in plexus chorioideus of a child with parainfluenza brain lesions. H-E ×400

Shapes similar to "pillows" were detected in the respiratory organs. An example is the following observation.

Patient Yuri Kh., 8 months old, became acutely ill on June 6, with a rise in temperature, vomiting, and loose stools. The next day, an epileptic seizure was noted, after which the child was hospitalized in the Clinical Hospital of the Pediatric Institute. From that moment on, he was unconscious, almost constantly in an epileptic state. On June 8, the child died. Clinically, the disease was regarded as "intestinal toxicosis on the background of dysentery." The autopsy revealed the phenomena of laryngotracheobronchitis, focal bronchopneumonia, and catarrhal enteritis. The soft meninges are thin and transparent. The brain tissue is sharply swollen, flabby, of a jelly-like consistency. The convolutions of the brain are smoothed, and the furrows are flattened. On the incision, the ventricles are slit shaped, and their ependyma is smooth, shiny, and with moderately dilated and full-blooded vessels. In some areas, mainly in the frontal and occipital lobes, the border between the white and gray substances of the cortex, as well as the nodes of the base, is indistinct. In the IF study, the antigen of the PI-3 virus was detected in smears from the trachea, the lungs, of the intestine, as well as sections from various parts of the brain (cerebral cortex and basal nodes). The results of the IF study for other RV and mycoplasmas, as well as bacteriological studies, were negative. A detailed histological examination of the brain revealed fullness of the soft meninges, swelling of the endothelial nuclei of blood vessels, and pronounced perivascular and pericellular edema. There were dystrophic changes in nerve cells in the form of "acute swelling" or "severe lesions." In the soft medulla corresponding to the occipital lobe, pillow-like growths of vascular endotheliocytes were found, and similar growths of ependymocytes were found in the area of the lateral ventricle. Small glial nodules were found in the area of the basal nodes. The histological examination of the internal organs revealed changes typical of parainfluenza in the respiratory organs, kidneys, and intestines. In addition, signs of cytomegalovirus sialadenitis were found in the salivary glands. Thus, the boy of 8 months died due to parainfluenza 3 serotype with a distinct generalization, including in the brain, of the development of characteristic structural changes in the soft meninges and cerebral ventricles. In all other observations, the nature of the changes detected in the brain was similar to that described above. In addition, a child suffering from encephalopathy was found to have glial nodules in the area of the base nodes and a child suffering from IUI, moderate sclerosis of the soft meninges. In a child who died from intrauterine PG, there were also distinct signs of brain immaturity in the form of absence of clearly differentiated layers of the cortex, pronounced subperpendicular clusters of poorly differentiated glia, and a distinct external granular layer in the cerebellum. Thus, PI brain lesions in the studied children's sectional material were quite rare and were detected only in children with a very unfavorable premorbid background. Changes typical of PI were detected exclusively in the cells of the membranes, ependymocytes of the choroidal plexus and lateral ventricles, and vascular endothelium, along with nonspecific hemo- and cerebrospinal fluid changes in the brain substance. A clear clinical and morphological picture of acute parainfluenza encephalitis could not be identified. In subsequent years, deaths from generalized PI with brain damage on the autopsy material of Leningrad/In St. Petersburg, were absent. With the deceased adults in St. Petersburg, the diagnosis of generalized parainfluenza was never made; however, when studying microscopic changes in one of the deceased with a clinical diagnosis of "influenza" (without confirmation by any laboratory data), we [V.A. Zinserling] revealed changes typical of generalized PI.

7.2.2 Brain Damage in Respiratory Syncytial Infection

The clinical picture of pneumonia caused by the RS virus in young children describes the phenomenon of neurotoxicosis. We reviewed not so numerous old literature [1]. No recent publications were found.

Based on our material [1], we analyzed three observations of children who died from generalized RS infection at the age of 4.5 months to 1 year and 3 months. There were two girls and one boy among them. The diagnosis in all cases was made on the basis of an IF study; in one case, it was confirmed by the results of a serological study. In two children, generalized RS infection developed on a very unfavorable background. Stanislav S., 1 year and 3 months, had congenital tubulopathy and tubular acidosis, and Natalia S., 4.5 months, had residual changes in intrauterine cytomegaly. In the third child (Marianna A., 8 months), no distinct adverse background conditions were detected. Clinically, the disease in all cases was regarded as acute respiratory infection with neurotoxicosis, with a clinical manifestation duration of 2–6 days; acute leukemia could not be clinically excluded in one child. The characteristic morphological picture of generalized RS infection was detected, in addition to the brain, in the lungs, kidneys, liver, and intestines. Changes in the brain typical of RS infection were expressed relatively moderately, were similar to those described in parainfluenza, and consisted mainly in the overgrowth of the cells of the lining of the vascular plexus and the ependymocytes of the lateral ventricles, fundamentally similar to those detected in this infection in the respiratory organs [4]. As an example, the following observation can be presented. Natalia S., 4.5 months old, was born from the first normal pregnancy, urgent delivery, full term. In the neonatal period, she had prolonged jaundice. From 2 months, the child has had manifestations of exudative diathesis. She got sick for the first time on November 24. With the phenomenon of acute respiratory infection, the temperature was kept for 2 weeks at subfebrile figures (Fig. 7.14). From December 20, the girl became sluggish, her appetite worsened, and sleepiness appeared. After the appearance of repeated vomiting on December 24, the girl with suspected meningitis was hospitalized. At the time of admission, the condition was severe, the girl was conscious, her gaze was fixed. There was some agitation and general hyperesthesia. The large fontanelle is tense and bulging, and there was rigidity of the occipital muscles. There were no other meningeal symptoms. On the part of the internal organs, there were no distinct signs of pathology. After lumbar puncture (cytosis 1, 1×10^6/l, protein 0.165 g/l), the diagnosis of meningitis was declined. In the blood test, anemia and leucocytosis with a shift to the left were found. Despite intensive medical measures, including antibiotics and infusion preparations, the child's condition remained serious, and 19 h after admission to the clinic, the girl died. Clinically, the child's disease remained unclear, and a differential diagnosis was made between acute respiratory infection (pneumonia) and acute leukemia. At the autopsy on the parts of the respiratory organs, catarrhal laryngotracheobronchitis with focal viral pneumonia was detected in 1.2 segments of the lower lobe of the right lung. On the liver section, there were separate yellowish areas on a pale brown background. No significant changes were detected in other internal organs, including the spleen and bone marrow. The brain weighs 710 g (with an average age norm of 600 g), has a flabby consistency, but retains its shape on the table. The soft meninges are swollen, and their vessels are sharply expanded. On the incision, the border between the gray and white substances is blurred, and in both cases, single small-point hemorrhages are noted. The cerebral ventricles are slit shaped, and the vascular plexuses are reddish in color. Histological changes on the part of the brain were characterized by moderate lymphomonocytic infiltration of the soft meninges and overgrowth of the epithelial cells of the choroidal plexus, of the ependymocytes of the lateral ventricles, and of the endotheliocytes of small vessels with the formation in some cases of structures similar to "papilla" detected in the respiratory organs. Similar moderately pronounced changes were also observed on the part of the endothelium of small vessels and ependymocytes of the cerebral ventricles. Distinct signs of RS infection against the background of influenza were detected in the lungs. Signs of generalization of RS infection were also detected in the liver, kidneys, and intestines in the form of overgrowth of the epithelial cells of these organs. Focal lymphocytic infiltration with the participation of cells with enlarged hyperchromic nuclei and moderate interstitial sclerosis were found in the parotid glands, kidneys, and liver. Thus, the girl Natalia S., 4.5 months old, died from a mixed viral infection—influenza B and, later, RS infection, which occurred with pronounced generalization, including in the brain. Respiratory infections developed against the background of residual changes in generalized cytomegaly.

Thus, brain lesions caused by the RS virus were detected on the studied autopsy material quite rarely and mainly in children with an unfavorable premorbid background. The changes typical for RS infection were detected exclusively from the cells of the membranes, vascular endothelium, and ependyma and were identical to those described in parainfluenza. Encephalitis caused by the RS virus could not be detected. In the last decades, no deaths from generalized RS infection with brain damage have been diagnosed in children in St. Petersburg. There were no observations of RS virus brain damage in adults in our material as well.

7.2.3 Brain Damage in Adenovirus Infection

Brain lesions with adenoviruses (Ads) are among the relatively well-studied ones. The clinical manifestations of CNS lesions in Ad infection have been regularly described by many researchers since 1956. Information about the frequency of such lesions is uncertain. Ad etiology was established from 2.5% to 20.1% of the total number of deciphered CNS infections. The frequency of neurological complications in Ad infection ranges from 1.7% to 26% [1].

The etiology of these lesions was established in patients on the basis of a combination of clinical manifestations with the release of the virus from the CSF or at least the feces and respiratory tract, as well as on the basis of positive results of serological studies of sera. Even the presence of antibodies to this pathogen in the CSF is considered sufficient to detect the adenovirus etiology of the process.

Analyzing the features of the clinical course of brain lesions of Ad-etiology clinicians came to the conclusion that the primary lesion of the central nervous system in young children occur during two-wave fever. The main clinical manifestations are moderate hypertensive meningeal symptoms and pleiocytosis. The disease ends in most cases, safely leaving behind an asthenic syndrome of varying intensity and duration. Several cases of meningoencephalitis were described, the etiology of which was confirmed by the isolation of this pathogen from the CSF. They believe that for such a severe course of adenovirus infection, an unfavorable background is necessary. Ad-meningoencephalitis is described in children after surgery for astrocytoma and against the background of acute lymphoblastic leukemia and in an adult woman against the background of intoxication with "home-made whiskey," which is confirmed by biochemical studies.

A fairly complete description of morphological changes is given only in the article by S.M. Chou et al. [11]. They describe subacute focal adenovirus encephalitis in a man treated with immunosuppressive drugs for leukemia. Light microscopy revealed cells typical of this disease with intracranial basophilic inclusions, the specificity of which was confirmed by IF microscopy. In addition, astro- and microgliosis, petechial hemorrhage, perivascular lymphoid infiltrates, and necrosis in the white matter of the brain were determined. There were focal calcium deposits under the soft meninges. With EM, the authors were able to detect clusters of particles morphologically identified as adenoviruses in nerve cells. In the postmortem virological study, adenovirus 32 serotype was isolated from the brain tissue.

There are almost no works devoted to the study of Ad brain lesions in the experiment.

We studied 13 cases of acute generalized adenovirus infection with the development of specific brain lesions. The diagnosis of Ad infection in all cases was made on the basis of the results of IF and histological studies. In four cases, it was confirmed by the isolation of the virus (three times from the respiratory system and one time from the brain) and in seven cases serologically. Typical adenovirus lesions were naturally detected, in addition to the brain, in the respiratory organs, as well as in the intestines (in five people), in the kidneys (in eight children), and in a number of other internal organs.

The deceased children (six boys and seven girls) were aged 1.5 months to 1 year and 9 months. In most cases, the disease developed on an unfavorable background in the form of perinatal brain lesions (six observations), congenital heart defects (two observations), and multiple malformations and pylorostenosis (one observation). In five cases, the course of Ad infection was complicated by severe bacterial pneumonia caused by staphylococci, *Enterobacter*, and other pathogens. In most cases, the Ad infection developed against the background of other acute respiratory infections, more often influenza, however, without clear signs of generalization. Significant background pathology was absent only in two children.

Changes in the brain typical of Ad infection are characterized by changes in meningocytes, ependymocytes, endotheliocytes, nerve, and astro- and oligodendroglial cells. These changes are fundamentally similar to those detected in Ad infection in the lungs, as well as in a number of other internal organs [4], and consist in the appearance of large basophilic inclusions in the nuclei, sometimes clearly surrounded by zones of enlightenment.

The conducted clinical, laboratory, and morphological analysis showed the heterogeneity of this group. Two children aged 3 and 11 months died within the first 2 days of the onset of the disease. The clinical picture of their disease in vivo was regarded as neurotoxicosis. As an example of an acute course of generalized Ad infection, the following observation is given.

Lydia Sh., 3 months old, became very ill. Within a few hours after the onset of the disease, she was hospitalized in an extremely serious condition. The hospital was diagnosed with pneumonia and neurotoxicosis of the fourth degree. In addition, alcohol intoxication was noted (the mother who fed the girl with breast milk was an alcoholic). Despite intensive resuscitation measures, the girl died after 10 h. Clinically, was diagnosed ARI, complicated by bilateral small focal pneumonia, complicated by neurotoxicosis IV with thrombohemorrhagic syndrome on the background of hypotrophy.

Catarrhal laryngotracheobronchitis, focal pneumonia, catarrhal enterocolitis, and pylorostenosis were noted at the autopsy. There were no distinct changes in the brain and spinal cord.

During cytological examination, lung smears contain a lot of cytoplasmic fuchsinofilic inclusions. IF examination of smears from the respiratory organs, intestines, liver, kidneys, and brain revealed the antigen of adenoviruses. During bacteriological examination, a hemophilic bacillus was isolated from the lung, and no pathogenic microflora was found in other organs.

The histological examination of the central nervous system revealed distinct specific and nonspecific changes. The changes in the part of the nerve cells were of the greatest interest. Their nuclei were dramatically enlarged as a result of the appearance of large hyperchromic inclusions, clearly marked by hematoxylin, thionin, and azur. In parts of the cells, it was possible to see that they were separated from the little-modified part of the nucleus by a zone of illumination (Fig. 7.15). During the IF study, these inclusions were intensely lightening. On the part of a number of other nerve cells, the phenomena of lysis and pycnosis were noted. The endothelial cells of individual blood vessels were hypertrophied, and the nuclei of individual blood vessels were hyperchromic. Around such vessels, there was an accumulation of protein-rich fluid with an admixture of red blood cells. Sometimes there were also small clusters of lymphoid cells. Along with this, small, mostly perivascular, hemorrhages were detected throughout the brain, especially in the cerebellum. The soft meninges were sharply full blooded and edematous and contained loose lymphohistiocytic infiltrates. The nuclei of the ependymal cells of the cerebral ventricles had an irregular shape in places, which were hyperchromic and incorrectly located.

Similar changes, indicating the presence of Ad infection, were found in other organs. In particular, catarrhal laryngotracheobronchitis and focal

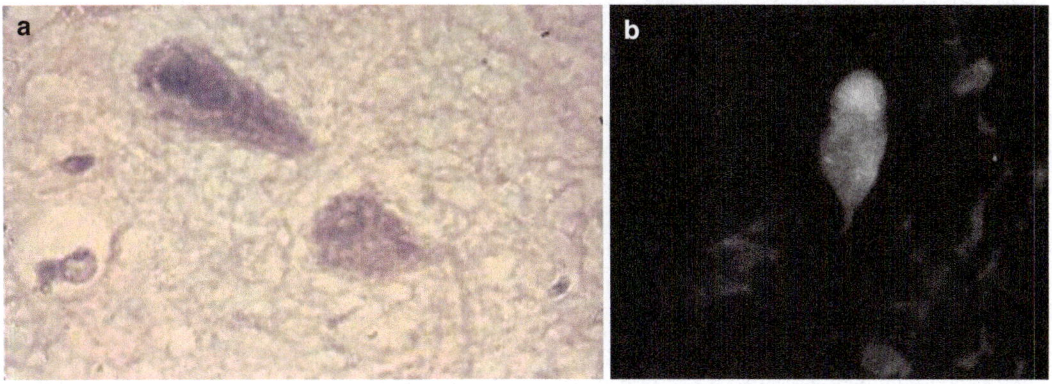

Fig. 7.15 Brain lesion in adenovirus infection in a girl, Sh., 11 mon. (**a**) Intranuclear basophilic inclusion in brain stem neuron H-E X600. (**b**) Antigen of adenovirus in the same child. IF ×1350

pneumonia with serous macrophage exudates were detected, which were mixed with a few neutrophilic leukocytes and red blood cells. Part of the cells of the ciliated and alveolar epithelium underwent a typical giant cell transformation for this disease. The intestine was sharply affected—many cells of the epithelium of the mucous membrane acquired the character of "adenovirus"; there were phenomena of fine-grained decay of these cells and moderate mononuclear infiltration. In the liver, pronounced dystrophic changes in hepatocytes were detected, the nuclei of some of which were hyperchromic. In the kidneys, there was swelling of the glomerular capillary loops, proliferation of mesangial cells, and dystrophic changes in the nephrothelium. The nuclei of individual cells were hyperchromic. The girl became acutely ill, and the Ad infection proceeded with a very early and pronounced generalization, which was probably associated with the development of the disease in the background of alcohol intoxication. Meningoencephalitis occurred along with other manifestations of generalization, among which enterocolitis was the most severe.

Similar changes were found in a boy of 1.5 months. However, the duration of clinical manifestations of "neurotoxicosis" was 11 days. During histological examination, along with changes similar to those described above, moderate gliosis was detected in the area of the basal nodes.

Increasing neurological symptoms within 2 weeks, which made it possible to clinically diagnose acute encephalitis, were detected in one child. Information about it is given in more detail.

The girl Julia K., 1 years 8 months before, the present disease developed according to age. She became acutely ill on April 25 with symptoms of acute respiratory infections and was treated on an outpatient basis. On day 3, the temperature was up to 39 °C, and there was lethargy, shortness of breath, and conjunctivitis; therefore, she was hospitalized with a diagnosis of adenovirus infection, right-sided bronchopneumonia. On May 5, clonic-tonic convulsions with loss of consciousness and impaired breathing rhythm were noted. At the same time, an increase in the blood level of transaminases was detected (ALT—18.7, AST—15). At puncture on 5/05-cytosis 2×10^6/l, protein 0.066 g/l. 12/05 in a serious condition, she was transferred to the clinic, where there was a lack of active movement, high deep reflexes D > S. During the puncture, no significant changes were detected on the part of the cerebrospinal fluid. On the EEG, pronounced changes in the organic type were noted and on the EchoEG, signs of increased intracranial pressure. The complex therapy was ineffective, and on 19/05 the girl died with the phenomenon of increasing edema of lungs and brain. The autopsy revealed the phenomena of catarrhal laryngotracheobronchitis and viral pneumonia. The brain is swollen, weighing 960 g (with an average age norm of 890 g). The vessels of the meninges and white matter are full blooded, and the lateral ventricles are dilated. The cytological examination revealed cells with enlarged hyperchromic nuclei in smears from the trachea, lung, and soft medulla. An IF study revealed the Ad antigen in smears from the lungs and soft meninges. During serological examination, antibodies to adenoviruses were detected in the blood at a titer of 1:160 and in the CSF of 1:40. During virological examination on the culture of L-41 cells and myeloid-derived suppressor cells (MDSCs), an adenovirus was isolated from the brain, which could not be typed. Interferon in the CSF was 2.2 lg (after warming up, 1.6 lg), in the brain tissue 2.6 lg (after warming up, 1.3 lg), in the choriodal plexus 1.8 lg (after warming up, 0.6), and in the lungs 1.9 lg (after warming up, 1.4 lg). On a histological examination, the soft meninges are swollen and full blooded and moderately infiltrated by lymphocytes. The endothelium of the small vessels of the membranes and the substance of the brain are swollen, often hyperchromic nuclei. Pronounced perivascular edema, often small hemorrhages, is noted, as well as lymphocytic infiltration around the part of the vessels. Occasionally, there is demyelination of nerve fibers in the white matter. Pronounced alterative and necrobiotic changes in nerve cells, up to small areas of their loss. Many of them have hyperchromic or "matte" cores. In the same area, there is some hyperplasia, as well as edema of astrocytic glia. Many oligodendroglia cells have enlarged hyperchromic nuclei. Ependymocytes of the cerebral ventricles are partially drained and regenerated, and some cells of the lining of the vascular plexus have enlarged hyperchromic nuclei. In the liver, kidneys, and lungs, changes typical of generalized Ad infection were also detected; in addition, "adenovirus cells" and fine-grained decay were also noted in the spleen and lymph nodes. Conclusion: thus, the results of a comparison of clinical, laboratory, and morphological data allowed us to regard the identified brain changes as adenovirus meningoencephalitis—the leading manifestation of the generalization of this infection.

In two children, the duration of Ad infection with brain damage was 1–5 weeks, according to clinical and laboratory data. However, due to the fact that the disease developed in them on the background of a pronounced perinatal brain lesion with hydrocephalus in one child, they did not have a clear clinical picture of acute encephalitis. A histological examination, along with the "adenovirus metamorphosis" of many nerve and glial cells, meningocytes, and ependymocytes, revealed focal clusters of glial cells mainly in the trunk area, with moderate perivascular calcium deposits. In one child (Valentina V., 1 year and 6 months), the morphological manifestations of a clinically diagnosed perinatal brain lesion with cystic adhesive arachnoiditis fit into the picture of sluggish meningoencephalitis. In the soft meninges, cysts with distinct lymphocytic infiltration of their walls, swelling, and proliferation of astrocytic and oligodendroglia cells forming small nodules in the caudate nucleus region were detected. In the area of the parietal lobe, there was a small calcification. The presence of a confirmed by IF (positive lightening in smears from the lungs and meninges) and serologically (antibodies in the blood and CSF) of a long-running generalized Ad infection in the girl allows us to presumably associate the detected changes with it, especially since the cells characteristics typical for Ad were also present in the area of lymphocytic and glial infiltrates.

In five children, the generalization of Ad infection occurred, according to laboratory and morphological data, a few days before death against the background of severe viral and bacterial RI, which occurred with the phenomenon of toxicosis. In this regard, only relatively moderate changes associated with adenoviruses were observed in the brain against the background of pronounced hemodynamic changes and vasculitis. They consisted mainly in the "adenovirus metamorphosis" of meningocytes, ependymocytes of the choriodal plexus, and, to a lesser extent, nerve and glial cells. Particular attention was drawn to the natural Ad damage of endotheliocytes of small blood vessels.

The clinical and morphological manifestations of the disease in Ekaterina S., 7 months old, differed significantly from those described above due to the fact that generalized Ad infection with brain damage was combined with ascending encephalomyelopolyradiculoneuritis. The duration of the main disease of the child, characterized by demyelination in the white matter of the spinal cord, trunk, and large hemispheres, swelling and lysis of oligodendrocytes, as well as severe dystrophic and necrobiotic changes in nerve cells and lymphocytic infiltration of the roots of the spinal nerves, was about a month. Clinical, laboratory, and morphological data suggest the existence of a generalized Ad infection with lung, brain, spleen, peripheral lymph node, and liver damage in the child at about the same time. The high titer (1:160) of antibodies to this pathogen in the cerebrospinal fluid and the detection of typical cells in the soft meninges and vascular plexus spoke in favor of brain damage with blood pressure. In addition, in the choriodal plexus, the substance of the brain, and the cerebrospinal fluid, fairly high content of interferon is found (2.3, 2.8, and 3.2 lg, respectively). A characteristic feature of this case was a sharp suppression of immunogenesis, which consisted in an expressed accidental involution of the thymus, with the appearance of secondary lymphoid follicles in the cortical layer and a sharp decrease in the number of lymphocytes in the spleen and peripheral lymph nodes. The high content of anticerebroside antibodies in the blood (1:256) as well as distinct vasculitis in the brain and liver, interstitial myocarditis, and glomerulitis in the kidneys allow us to document the autoimmune nature of the underlying disease. Given the long course of Ad infection, which caused damage to both the brain and the organs by immunogenesis, we can assume its possible significance in the pathogenesis of encephalomyelopolyradiculoneuritis.

These materials confirm the possibility of developing Ad lesions of the central nervous system. Such lesions are more likely to develop in children with an unfavorable premorbid background and can clinically both occur with a picture of neurotoxicosis or encephalitis and give relatively moderate manifestations on the background of preexisting lesions. In the morphological study, the most typical is the "adenovirus metamorphosis" of the nervous, glial, ependymal, endothelial (Fig. 7.16), and meningeal cells, which is fundamentally similar to that observed in this infection in the respiratory organs, kidneys, intestines, liver, adrenal glands, and pancreas. With a longer course of the inflammatory process in the brain, there is a distinct, although moderate, glial reaction and foci of perivascular demyelination. In recent years, very rarely is Ad infection diagnosed in children in St. Petersburg, both on clinical and autopsy material; deaths from generalized forms with brain damage were not noted. Generalized Ad infection with brain damage on adult autopsy material has not been diagnosed once over the years.

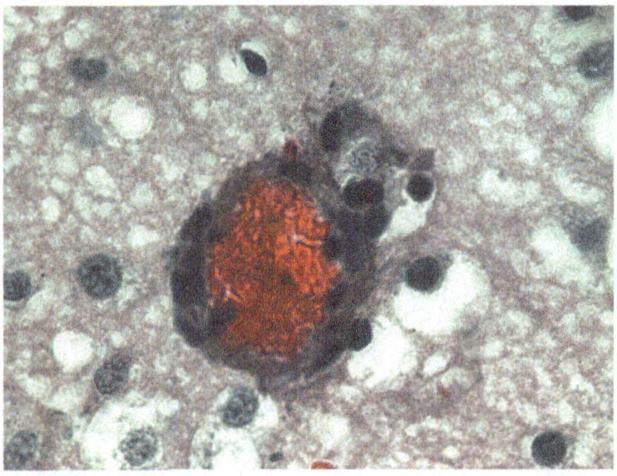

Fig. 7.16 Brain vascular lesion in a boy with generalized adenovirus infection. H-E ×400

7.3 Brain Damage in Respiratory Mycoplasmosis

Mycoplasmas were first described by Nokar, Roux, Borrel, and other outstanding microbiologists of the Pasteur school in 1893–1898 as the causative agent of contagious bovine pneumonia, currently called *Mycoplasma mycoides*. Initially, all similar pathogens of pneumonia were grouped into the group PPLO (pleuropneumoniae-like organisms). The general characteristics of the pathogens and the history of their study have been presented by us elsewhere [4].

The fundamental ability of mycoplasmas to penetrate the hemato-encephalic barrier has been proven. The clinical symptoms of nervous system lesions in respiratory mycoplasmosis are very diverse. Among the most common forms are meningitis and meningoencephalitis, the description of the symptoms of which on the background of the respiratory infectious clinic was first made in 1956 [1]. Subsequently, on the background of a diagnostic increase in antibodies to *Mycoplasma pneumoniae* (MP), meningitis was described in several hundred patients by numerous researchers. In most of the described observations, there were initial symptoms of respiratory tract damage. No correlation was found between the severity of its lesion and neurological manifestations. The disease was accompanied by headache and vomiting. Meningeal symptoms were observed in all patients, but the degree of their severity in many was insignificant. Cerebrospinal puncture showed an increase in CSF pressure and mainly lymphocytic (and sometimes polynuclear) pleiocytosis, ranging from 100 to 3000 cells per 1 μl with normal or slightly elevated protein content. The condition of such patients, as a rule, improved gradually, in a period of up to 7 days; there was a disappearance of clinical symptoms within 2–3 weeks. There was also a sanation of the cerebrospinal fluid. According to the literature, no deaths were observed in this form of the disease. The residual changes were not described by any of the authors.

In a number of cases, various authors describe the addition to the above-described clinical picture of both general cerebral symptoms and focal symptoms (pyramidal, subcortical hyperkinesis, oculomotor muscle paresis), which made it possible to diagnose meningoencephalitis. The cerebrospinal fluid picture in these cases, along with the changes described in meningitis, was characterized by an increase in the content of proteins in the cerebrospinal fluid. The course of the disease was sometimes more severe, and G. Sterner and G. Biberfeld [12], for the first time, give a description of a fatal observation. The residual changes observed in five of the 29 cases reviewed by H. W. Murray et al. [13] were persistent nystagmus, sensory aphasia, gait disorders, and focal changes in the EEG.

Some authors present encephalitis similar in its manifestations to those described above but not accompanied by meningeal syndrome. Among other, much rarer forms of nervous system lesions associated with *M. pneumoniae*, a number of cases of acute psychosis are described, most of which ended in recovery. Isolated cases of cerebellar ataxia are also described. The information available in the literature allows us to talk about the possibility of damage to this type of mycoplasma and also to the spinal cord, the nerve roots, and the spinal nerves themselves. The clinical picture of Guillain-Barre syndrome was quite characteristic of these cases. On the background of mycoplasma infection, transient hemiplegia is also described. When analyzing a large clinical material, it was concluded that the mycoplasmic etiology is related to 8% of all polyradiculoneurites, which can occur both with protein cell dissociation and with pleocytosis. No fatal cases have been described in this group of lesion.

From the very beginning of the clinical and serological study of nervous system lesions in respiratory mycoplasmosis, many authors have proposed a wide variety of mostly speculative considerations about their possible nature. Some authors assign a leading place in the pathogenesis of the brain lesions to intravascular coagulation, without paying serious attention to existing neuron lesions. Subsequent researchers mostly discussed other hypotheses: the influence of a hypothetical neurotoxin, damage of an immunological nature, and the presence of pathogens. However, only a few authors [12] provided incomplete descriptions of the pathological picture of single fatal cases of respiratory mycoplasmosis, which occurred with neurological complications. The etiology of the process in all cases was determined only in vivo on the basis of serological examination data. In all described observations, the brain was macroscopically unchanged, except for the moderate edema described in some cases. On a microscopic examination, the above authors observed, in most cases, perivascular edema and small hemorrhages, as well as blood clots in small vessels at various stages of development and, mainly, round-cell infiltration of the soft meninges. Some authors doubt the possibility of developing CNS lesions caused by *M. pneumoniae*. In the recent literature, the issues of mycoplasma brain lesions are not described.

To study the possibility of brain damage with the development of a distinct clinical picture in the generalization of respiratory mycoplasmosis, we conducted in 1977–1980 an in-depth study of 11 sectional observations of children over the age of 2 months who suffered from a generalized infection caused by *M. pneumoniae* confirmed in vivo or postmortem by serological or IF methods [1]. The conducted clinical and morphological analysis revealed the heterogeneity of this group. Only in three cases that the analysis of the clinical course of the disease made it possible to clearly identify the relationship between respiratory infection and the development of encephalitis, as well as to exclude the possibility of intrauterine infection. The following observation may be given as an example.

The girl Tatiana S., 11.5 months old, was born in time with a weight of 3300 from 3 pregnancy, which proceeded with toxicosis in the first half with a weight of 3300. She screamed immediately after birth, being attached to breast on day 3, as often regurgitated on the first day. On day 5, she was discharged from the maternity hospital. Early motor and mental development was slightly delayed. The disease began at the age of 9 months. With lethargy, refusal to eat, runny nose, and cough, which occurred at a normal temperature. ARI was diagnosed. On the fifth day of the disease, the girl lost consciousness, but there were convulsive seizures. A few hours later, she was taken to the intensive care unit. The condition at admission was extremely serious; consciousness was lost. Temperature was 37.3 °C. The skin was of the usual color; the lips were slightly cyanotic. Heart rate was 180 beats in 1 min. Blood pressure was 100/60 mmHg. Heart tones were rhythmic but muted. Breathing 20 per minute per minute, shallow wheezing was not heard. The abdomen was evenly swollen. The liver and spleen were not palpable. The pupils were narrow and uniform, and the reaction to light was sluggish. The fundus was normal. There were constant clonic convulsions in the left extremities. Deep reflexes were high—on the left lower than on the right. Abdominal and plantar reflexes were not triggered. No abnormal foot reflexes were detected. The meningeal symptoms were not pronounced. During lumbar puncture, there was an increased pressure of the cerebrospinal fluid. The cytosis was normal (8/3), and the protein content was 0.66%°. In the blood, leukocytosis was 14, 1×10^9 (E-1, P-2, S-74, L-18, M-5); ESR was 7 mm/h. On the seventh day of the illness, consciousness was restored, but the condition remained severe. The girl began to open her eyes, follow the objects, and react with tears to the examination. Active movement appeared in the right limb, and myoclonic hyperkinesis appeared in the left limb. The deep reflexes on the left are lower than on the right. This condition was present in the child until the 17th day of the disease. Further deterioration was noted due to the associated pneumonia, the appearance of propulsive epileptic seizures, and the generalization of hyperkinesis. Bilateral ptosis of the eyelids and converging strabismus began to be noted. The temperature became febrile. Propulsive seizures occurred in series. Consciousness was constantly lost. In the following days, heart and respiratory failure joined. The serological examination conducted on the eighth and 17th days of the disease showed an increase in the titer of antibodies to *M. pneumoniae* from 1:40 to 1:160. Despite treatment with antibiotics, anticonvulsants, and cardiac agents, the child died on the 52nd day of the disease. The clinical diagnosis was encephalitis, viral-mycoplasma infection, and interstitial pneumonia. The autopsy revealed catarrhal tracheobronchitis and small focal pneumonia. The brain and spinal cord were of the usual size and shape; it was possible to note only an uneven blood supply. In an IF study, the *M. pneumoniae* antigen was found in the lungs, brain, and kidneys. The histological examination revealed changes typical of mycoplasmosis in many organs. In particular, desquamative pneumonia was detected, the most typical feature of which was hypertrophy of alveolocytes with the appearance of mycoplasmas in their cytoplasm, surrounded by a zone of enlightenment [4]. Changes characteristic of mycoplasmosis were also found in the kidneys, mainly in the epithelium of the tubules, as well as in some other organs. In addition to these changes, cytomegalovirus sialadenitis was detected.

In the central nervous system, the maximum changes were detected on the part of nerve cells, especially in the right frontal lobe, in the area of the right central gyrus, and the nodes of the base on the right (Fig. 7.17). Small nerve cells have dark nuclei, enlarged in size and irregular in shape, and there was no change in the volume of the cytoplasm. A significant part of the large cells of the cortex and the nodes of the base are pale, enlarged in size, and the contours of some of them are erased. The cell nuclei are poor in chromatin, and the nucleoli are lightly swollen, sometimes irregular in shape. In the cytoplasm, as well as in the nuclei of such cells, there are a large number of small inclusions that are stained with thionine based on Nissl, azur, and PAS reaction. The inclusions are surrounded by small areas of lightening. The reaction to iron, based on Prussian blue, was negative. In addition, there were significantly pronounced changes in the walls of blood vessels in the form of proliferation and swelling of endothelial cells, in which there were focal clearances, in violation of the permeability of the vascular wall with the formation of small, often numerous hemorrhages. The vessels are overflowing with blood, often hemolyzed, and their endothelium is swollen. The meninges are thickened and full blooded with a moderate increase in the number of cellular elements. Vascular plexuses are full blooded and edema-

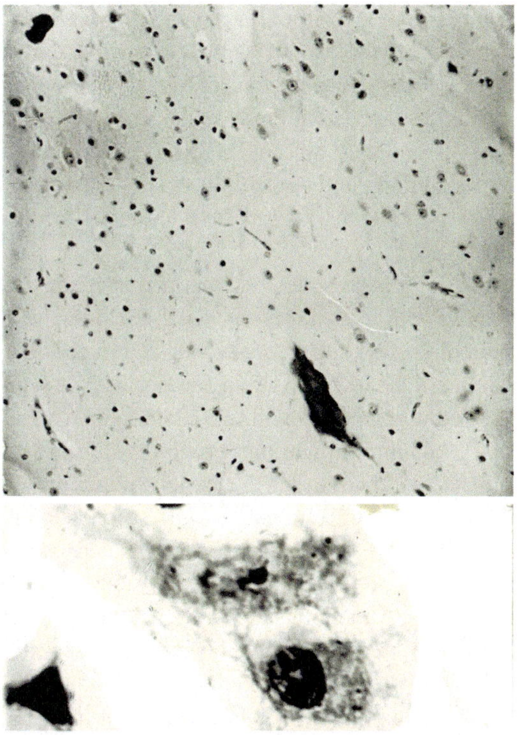

Fig. 7.17 Brain changes in encephalitis due to *Mycoplasma pneumoniae* in 11-month girl. (**a**) General overview. H-E. X100. (**b**) Neuron lesion in the same case. Note of small vacuolization of cytoplasm, containing small dot-like inclusions. Stained thionine by Nissl. ×1000

tous, many cells are enlarged in size, and focal clearances are visible in their cytoplasm. Ependymal cells are irregular in shape and of different sizes; the nuclei of most of them are dark, and others are much lighter than the rest. In EM of brain tissue obtained from the dewaxed block, artificial changes in ultrastructure were noted due to postmortem autolysis and the features of the methods used. In the better-preserved areas, it was possible to identify cell nuclei, mitochondria, tubules of the endoplasmic reticulum with ribosomes, and pinocytic vesicles. Special attention was paid to the oval bodies of 0.25–0.5 microns in size, bounded by a membrane and having a homogeneous electron-dense content of the layered structure. These formations were located in the nucleus, cytoplasm, mitochondria, and phagosomes. In some cases, the division of these bodies was observed, as well as their budding. They were similar to the mycoplasmas on the figures given by other authors. Clinical, laboratory, and morphological data made it possible to diagnose encephalitis caused by *M. pneumoniae* on the background of generalized respiratory mycoplasmosis.

Experimental studies of MP began in 1944 with the work of M.D. Eaton. The literature provides numerous data on the results of modeling respiratory mycoplasmosis in various animal species and mycoplasmas, especially intensively in the 1960–1970s of the twentieth century. The most commonly used model was infecting Syrian hamsters with MP. In these works, almost exclusive attention was paid to changes in the respiratory system. There is evidence of the possibility of brain damage in experimental infections in birds (*M. neuroliticum*), cattle (*M. bovirhinis*), and rats (*M. pulmonis*). Ependymatitis, periventricular encephalitis, and focal productive meningitis were described during experimental infection of calves, with the most pronounced changes located in the olfactory bulbs. Mycoplasmas were detected in the cells of the ependyma and epithelium of the choriodal plexus, causing changes in them similar to those described in the respiratory organs. In subsequent years, experimental work on experimental respiratory mycoplasmosis was carried out only to a very limited extent, and information about brain lesions is completely absent.

This leads us to cite the results of our experimental work. A study was conducted on 163 Syrian hamsters, 3 weeks old, which were infected with *M. pneumoniae* (strain No. 13) in four series of experiments. In the first series of experiments, 45 intact animals were used, which were intranasally treated with 0.1 suspension of mycoplasma at a concentration of 108 CFU/ml. Animals were slaughtered on days 1, 3, 5, 10, 15, 20, and 25 after infection, and the materials from all the most important organs were collected for a detailed histological examination using GE stains, azur-eosin, PAS, and tionin according to Nissl on paraffin sections prepared according to standard methods, as well as IF studies on cryostat sections. In parallel, quantitative isolation of mycoplasmas from the lungs was carried out on days 5, 10, 15, and 20 and determination of antibodies to them in the blood of animals in the neutralization reaction on days 5, 10, 15, 20, and 25. As a control, both intact animals and hamsters were used, which were injected into the nasal passages with a medium for growing mycoplasmas. In this series of experiments, it was possible to reproduce a generalized mycoplasma infection and trace its development. After hematogenic dissemination in the body, which was recorded histobacterioscopically as early as day 1, severe lesions of various internal organs developed later. The morphological pattern observed in the lungs, kidneys, and liver was similar to that described in mycoplasmosis. The results of a microbiological study of the lungs of infected animals showed that the intensity of mycoplasma reproduction increased with each day of infection, reaching a maximum by 15 days after infection, which correlated with the highest degree of morphological changes in the lungs. The results of the serological study were consistent with the microbiological data. The increase in the level of neutralizing antibodies occurred evenly following the increase in the titer of mycoplasmas in the lungs of infected animals. The maximum level of neutralizing antibodies (1:16) was detected on the 20th day of infection and remained during the subsequent development of the pathological process. Of particular interest was the analysis of the observed brain lesions. The absence of similar changes in the control animals; the dynamics of their development, which fits into the framework of the course of generalized mycoplasmosis throughout the body; the data of IF and histobacterioscopic studies leave no doubt about the mycoplasmic etiology of the observed process. It should probably be considered characteristic of the initial appearance of the pathogen in the areas adjacent to the BBB (vascular plexuses and soft meninges) with a rapid appearance of them, especially clearly in the last lymphohistiocytic infiltration (Fig. 7.18). In subsequent periods, the pathogen penetrates into the various parts of the brain substance (olfactory brain, cortex of the large hemispheres, and, less often, the nodes of the base Ammon horn), where it persists in the cytoplasm of large nerve cells, causing their changes in the form of an increase and vacuolation of the cytoplasm of such cells. In other cases, perivascularly located foci of lymphohistiocytic infiltration appear in these areas. Such foci contain a significant amount of mycoplasmas, both extracellularly and intracellularly. In the center of the largest lesions, foci of destruction and necrosis were observed.

In the second series of experiments conducted jointly with A.S. Kozlyuk with 35 animals, a radiobiological and IF study was conducted. The culture of the MP N13 strain was grown on a standard culture medium with the addition of 2 μk/ml of H3 thymidine. The first group of animals was infected intranasally at the same dose, as in the first series of experiments. In the second group, under the same conditions, an inactivated pathogen was introduced. In group 3, a live culture at the same dose was administered intraperitoneally. The animals were examined on the first, third, seventh, and 14th days after infection. For radiological examination, the lower lobe of the right lung, the cerebral cortex of one of the hemispheres, as well as the hypothalamic region with the medulla oblongata were taken. A hydrolysate was prepared from the pieces of tissue according to standard methods, to which a scintillation liquid was added, and the pulses were counted on a MARK-II counter. To obtain reliable results, the meter readings were correlated with 1/10 of the body weight. The obtained results were subjected to statistical processing (Table 7.1). The organs of uninfected animals served as controls. In parallel, histological and IF studies were conducted. The results of a comprehensive study of materials from animals of the first subgroup demonstrate a distinct reproduction of mycoplasmas in the lungs. However, in contrast to the first series of experiments, a large number of pathogens were not located intracellularly but lay freely or were adsorbed onto the surface of the bronchial and alveolar epithelium. In most animals, there were no pronounced structural changes associated with exposure to mycoplasmas, and only on day 14 did a number of animals show moderate histiocytic infiltration and small vessel thrombosis. Radiobiological, IF, and histological studies proved the ability of mycoplasmas in this experiment to disseminate to the brain,

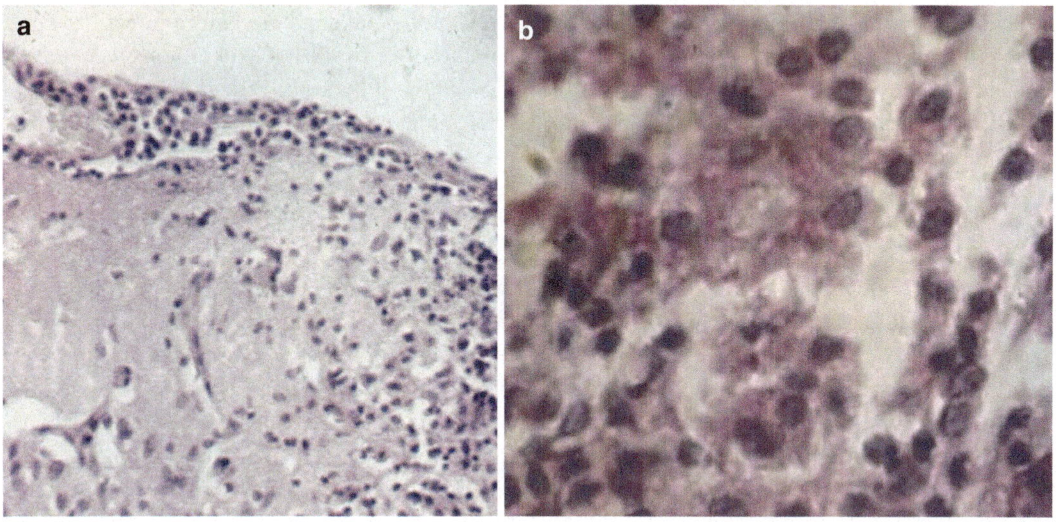

Fig. 7.18 Brain lesion in experimental *Mycoplasma pneumoniae* infection on the 7 th day after intranasal challenge with highly pathogenic strain. PAS reaction. (**a**) General view of meningoencephalitis. ×200. (**b**) Detail of the previous slide. Note expressed infiltration by macrophages containing numerous PAS-positive inclusions ×1000

Table 7.1 Results of radiobiologic investigation of Syrian hamsters (in impulses)

Group	Object of investigation	Days of experiment			
		1	3	7	14
Intranasal challenge with viable pathogen	Lungs	117.3 ± 37	20.1 ± 4.0	59.8 ± 6.6	47.8 ± 1.9
	Big hemispheres of brain	9.0 ± 2.0	2.5 ± 0.3	19.0 ± 7.0	14.2 ± 2.4
	Brain stem and medulla oblongata	2.3 ± 0.2	2.4 ± 0.3	13.9 ± 5.4	28.6 ± 11.0
Intranasal challenge with inactivated pathogen	Lungs	23.2 ± 3.1	9.4 ± 1.1	5.0 ± 0.8	3.9 ± 0.8
	Big hemispheres of brain	3.5 ± 0.6	1.8 ± 0.3	2.7 ± 0.5	3.0 ± 0.2
	Brain stem and medulla oblongata	2.4 ± 0.4	1.9 ± 0.5	1.2 ± 0.1	1.8 ± 0.1
Intraperitoneal challenge with viable pathogen	Lungs	4.4 ± 0.4	10.5 ± 3.5	36.5 ± 6.8	66.3 ± 17.0
	Big hemispheres of brain	3.1 ± 0.9	7.5 ± 0.9	18.4 ± 8.0	29.5 ± 4.0
	Brain stem and medulla oblongata	2.1 ± 0.4	5.5 ± 0.4	16.3 ± 5.8	24.8 ± 6.5
Control animals	Lungs	4.1 ± 0.4			
	Big hemispheres of brain	2.6 ± 0.4			
	Brain stem and medulla oblongata	2.4 ± 0.4			

where they were located mainly on the surface and, less often, in the cytoplasm of ependymocytes of the vascular plexus, as well as extracellularly in the perivascular spaces. The results of the study of the second group indicate that inactivated mycoplasmas do not penetrate into the animal's body beyond the lumen of the bronchi and lose their ability to adsorb onto the surface of the cells. The absence of mycoplasmas in the brain confirms that with intranasal infection, hematogenic dissemination of only viable pathogen is possible. The results of a comprehensive study of materials from animals of the third group indicate a significantly pronounced hematogenic dissemination of the pathogen during its intraperitoneal administration. It can be assumed that the transfer of mycoplasmas is facilitated by their ability to adsorb onto blood cells. Pronounced penetration of the pathogen into the lungs and brain occurred 3 days after infection and reached a maximum on day 14. Significant structural changes associated with mycoplasmosis in the lungs and brain could not be detected, perhaps due to insufficient follow-up.

In the third series of experiments (together with V.M. Soldatova), infection of 43 animals was carried out, as in the first series of experiments, but with a strain that underwent additional passages and lyophilization. Animals were sacrificed on days 3, 6, 9, 12, 15, 18, 21, 24, 27, and 30 after infection. Histologically and microbiologically (days 6 and 12), the lungs and brain were examined. The data obtained in the third series of experiments indicated that the *M. pneumoniae* strain used for infection had undergone significant changes in its properties during its one-and-a-half-year storage. A clear microbiological explanation for this phenomenon could not be given. In this series of experiments with morphological and microbiological studies, it was shown that the pathogen as a result of an intranasal infection in a fairly significant amount got into the lungs, where it multiplied and, despite partial elimination, continued to persist in moderate amounts even at the latest of the studied periods after infection (30 days). The localization of the pathogen was radically different from that described in the first series of experiments. Almost exclusively, the extracellular location of the pathogen was noted, mainly around the bronchi and blood vessels and in the lumen of the alveoli. The almost complete absence of brain damage, both according to morphological and microbiological data, suggests that the culture of the strain used in this study, along with the ability to penetrate cells and cause pronounced inflammatory changes in the lungs, has also lost the ability to penetrate blood vessels, as well as other organs, in particular the brain, and cause generalized infection.

In the fourth series of experiments, performed simultaneously with the first one, together with S.S. Avtushenko by a similar method, the animals were vaccinated once (for 3 weeks) or twice (for 4 and 3 weeks) intramuscularly with an inactivated ultrasound culture before infection. Forty animals of this series of experiments were examined on the fifth, 10th, 15th, 20th, and 25th days after infection using histological, morphometric, microbiological, and serological methods. In this series of experiments it was shown that although vaccination initially inhibits the reproduction of pathogens, later it increases, in parallel with which there was an enlargement of airless foci in the lung. At the same time, there is an increase in the area of perivascular lymphoplasmocytic infiltrates and the average thickness of the vascular wall, which can be considered as indirect signs of the development of immunopathological processes. Starting from the 10th day, were noted moderate, and from the 15th day distinct morphological signs of generalization of the process with damage to the kidneys, liver, and brain, the nature of the changes in which fundamentally corresponded to those described in the first series of experiments.

The data obtained in this experiment indicate that the course of respiratory mycoplasmosis, including the generalization of brain damage, depends not only on the severity of the inflammatory process and the level of specific antibodies. Immunopathological reactions are also of great importance among the morphological manifestations, of which we were able to evaluate peribronchial and peribronchial infiltrates in lymphoid cells, which the literature data allow us to associate with T-cell cytotoxicity. It should be mentioned that changes of this kind are considered characteristic of mycoplasmosis, which is characterized by the intracellular location of the pathogen. As a consequence of these processes, we can consider an increase in their permeability, which facilitates the dissemination of the pathogen. Thus, in our experimental studies, with the help of various methods, for the first time in the world, the ability of mycoplasmas to penetrate into the brain and cause pronounced structural changes was definitely proved. The dissemination of pathogens occurs only when cultures are used, the microorganisms of which are able to be adsorbed onto the cell surface. The penetration properties of mycoplasmas are clearly related to their ability to cause pronounced structural changes in both the lungs and other internal organs, including the brain. The development of extrapulmonary lesions is delayed in the presence of antibodies in animals, but they do not protect hamsters from more severe processes after a decrease in their titer. Sensitization of animals after their unsuccessful vaccination leads to the development of immunopathological processes in the lungs, probably by the type of delayed hypersensitivity and pathological immune complexes, and violation of its permeability, which contributes to the late generalization of the process.

7.4 Measles

The causative agent of measles is a virus belonging to the family *Paramyxoviridae* [14]. In addition to humans, monkeys are susceptible to measles, a disease that can be caused experimentally. Related viruses can cause similar diseases in dogs, sea lions, dolphins, cattle, goats, and sheep. Measles is one of the most common infections in all continents of the globe, and previous eras were characterized by very high morbidity and mortality of this disease. After the widespread introduction of the measles vaccination, the frequency of this infection in many countries has significantly decreased, and it is possible to talk about the prospects for its complete elimination. The source of infection is the patient. The main route of transmission is airborne, and only rarely are described observations with the transmission of the virus over placenta. People of all age groups are susceptible to measles; in previous years, there was a maximum incidence of children under 5 years old, and later, it moved toward an older age. A pathology of respiratory lesions has been described by us [4]. The frequency of lesions of the nervous system in children is 0.4–0.5% and in adolescents and adults 1.1–1.8%. The pathogenesis of measles encephalitis has not yet been fully elucidated. The most common theory is about the infectious allergic genesis of measles encephalitis. The main argument in favor of this point of view is the morphological changes described by a number of authors in previous years, according to which diffuse perivascular demyelination is described in the absence of "inflammatory changes." For many decades, a number of authors have expressed the existence of neurotropic strains of the virus, which can directly cause damage to the brain and its membranes. These views are supported by the possibility of isolating measles viruses from the brains of those who died from measles encephalitis, as well as the occurence of encephalitis before the rash. In addition, the possibility of developing a generalized infection with characteristic lesions of a number of internal organs in measles is known. Currently, it is common to distinguish three forms of CNS damage in measles: acute postinfectious measles encephalomyelitis (APME), "measles inclusion body encephalitis" (measles inclusion body encephalitis), and subacute sclerosing panencephalitis (SSPE) [15]. APME develops with a frequency of one case per 1000 cases of measles, usually within 2 weeks after the onset of rash. Neuropathological examination shows perivenous demyelination, but there are no inclusions. The measles virus cannot be isolated from brain tissue, and viral antigens and RNA are also not detected. Moreover, it does not determine the synthesis of antibodies to the measles virus outside the BBB. The time of onset of the disease suggests the role of immunopathological processes in the pathogenesis of APME. The detection of T lymphocytes specific to the main myelin protein supports the hypothesis of an autoimmune mechanism of the disease. There are also numerous analogies between APME and experimental allergic encephalomyelitis, which is widely used to study autoimmune processes in the central nervous system and is modeled in laboratory animals by injection of the mainmyelin protein, followed by the appearance of reactive T-lymphocytes. The mechanisms by which the own antigens lose their ability to immune tolerance are presumably (1) molecular mimicry, (2) damage to the cell surface with changes in its antigenic structure, (3) interaction with certain components of the immune system, and (4) disorders in the system of immunoregulatory molecules, such as antigens of the large histocompatibility complex. All of these events can lead to an imbalance in the immune system. Cellular autoimmune responses to brain antigens in the outcome of measles are likely to have significance in pathogenesis. The exact mechanisms leading to the distortion of the normal immune response under the influence of a viral infection are still unknown. Measles encephalitis and SSPE are formed in connection with persistent infection in the central nervous system. Measles encephalitis usually develops in patients with immunodeficiency weeks or months after the disease. In the absence of a characteristic measles rash, patients may also have giant cell measles pneumonia. SSPE is a chronic progressive inflammatory disease of the central nervous system, leading to a fatal outcome, which develops mainly in adolescents and young adults without visible disorders in the immune system. This classic slow viral infection has a very long incubation period: 7–10 years. A characteristic feature is the high titer of antibodies against all proteins of the measles virus in the blood, serum, and CSF. The oligoclonal nature of immunoglobulins supports the synthesis of immunoglobulins behind the barrier.

Both acute measles encephalitis and SSPE intracranial and intracytoplasmic inclusions are accompanied by pronounced inflammatory changes and demyelination to varying degrees. A prerequisite for the formation of persistent, rather than lytic, infection in the brain cells is a change in the function of viral genes, which may be due to certain factors on the part of the host. Molecular biological studies have shown that the persistence of the measles virus in the central nervous system is probably due to violations in the replication of viruses, which is associated with the genes encoding the virus envelope. In addition, mutations are detected in transcripts that cause translation delay. This allows the measles virus to survive inside the cells for a long incubation period while remaining inaccessible to the host's immune response. Despite the significant number of differences between the "wild" strain of the measles virus and the one isolated in SSPE, there is no reason to say that the latter is caused by a single variant of the pathogen. Mutations are likely to accumulate during the subclinical latency period. The expression of measles virus proteins in CNS cells in SSPE is absent or very low. This is due to the exceptionally low frequency of the corresponding messenger RNA (mRNA) and/or a change in the coding sequences within this reading frame, which leads to truncation or defective expression of proteins or complete termination of translation. The violation of the transcription of the measles virus was reproduced experimentally both in vivo and in vitro under the influence of neutralizing antibodies against H protein using nerve cell culture and experimental infection in rodents. The mechanisms of the occurrence and maintenance of the persistence of the measles virus remain unencrypted. A decrease in the cytolytic effect of the measles virus may be associated with the ability of individual viral isolates and vaccine strains to disrupt the expression of CD46 molecules on target cells. There is evidence that the measles virus does not directly cause the expression of class 1 antigens of the large histocompatibility complex, but it can be mediated by interferon γ. The morphological diagnosis of SSPE is based on five histological signs: (1) degenerative changes in neurons, (2) intracranial and intracytoplasmic eosinophilic inclusions in neurons and macroglia, (3) diffuse-focal proliferation of astro- and microglia, (4) widespread inflammatory mesenchymal-glial reaction, and (5) disintegration of myelin sheaths in the white matter. At the same time, the alternative process prevails in children, and the productive process prevails in adults. In addition to the above-described forms of CNS lesions in measles, the literature provides information about the possibility of developing other variants of complications. Thus, in children, symptoms of encephalitis are sometimes described before or in the first days after the appearance of the rash. In relatively rare cases, the development of serous meningitis is described. In young children, on the background of fever and intoxication, there may be general cerebral and rapidly disappearing focal symptoms, which are most likely associated with disorders of hemo- and cerebrospinal fluid dynamics. According to a number of authors, subclinical brain damage is observed in almost 50% of patients with measles. The degree of neurological disorders can be different—from mild subclinical forms to the most severe.

The clinical diagnosis of cortical lesions of the central nervous system is based on the assessment of the neurological status, epidemiological data, and the chronological relationship of neurological disorders with blood. For laboratory confirmation of measles, nasopharyngeal flushes, CSF, and blood taken during the first 3 days of the disease are examined. The infection of tissue cultures is carried out with the subsequent identification of viruses. The study of paired sera and CSF by serological methods is also very informative. Neurological disorders in young children in the initial period of the disease at the height of intoxication and fever usually pass without trace, although in previous years, there were isolated deaths. The prognosis of nervous system lesions of the type of acute postinfectious encephalomyelitis is relatively favorable. The worst prognosis is for measles encephalitis, which occurs in the prodromal period of measles. These forms are often followed by gross organic lesions. In general, according to various authors, the frequency of residual events in measles lesions of the nervous system is 20–40%. We studied several cases of death from measles with central nervous system damage in young adults, weakened by various causes.

As an example, we present one of the observations. Yu. A. A., 21 years old, had a history of cold, infertility, and acute adnexitis. On May 14, the child was acutely ill with pain in the lower abdomen, fever, frequent loose stools, and rashes on the skin. Since May 18, the pain has intensified, acquiring the character of sharp pain. Within a week, she was treated independently, but on May 21, with a diagnosis of measles, acute enteritis, and peritonitis, she was hospitalized in a serious condition. In connection with the suspected acute surgical pathology, she was urgently operated on in the evening of the same day. The operation revealed fibrinous purulent peritonitis; appendectomy and resection of the large omentum were fulfilled. After the operation, the condition remains bad, the fever of the wrong type persists, but the reverse development of peritonitis is noted. On the fifth day after the operation, the condition deteriorates sharply, the phenomenon of respiratory failure increases against the background of wet and dry wheezing in the lungs. Due to "endogenous intoxication," hemosorption was performed twice. On May 27, the child had a sudden cardiac arrest. Resuscitation measures were taken without effect. The clinical diagnosis was formulated as acute gangrenous perforated appendicitis, complicated by spilled purulent peritonitis. Measles was regarded as a concomitant disease. At the clinical autopsy, macroscopic data indicated the presence of fibrinous peritonitis in the stage of reverse development, bilateral bronchopneumonia, and polycystic ovaries (according to the type of Stein-Leventhal syndrome). The histological examination revealed a severe generalized viral infection with giant cell metamorphosis of epithelial cells with damage to the respiratory system, myocardium, kidneys, liver, appendix, and brain, which allowed us to consider measles as the main disease. Brain lesions were macroscopically uncharacteristic. Only edema of the soft meninges with uneven vascular fullness, paleness of the brain substance, narrowing of the cerebral ventricles, slight smoothness, and flatness of the convolutions were noted. On the lower surface of the cerebellum, there is an indistinct mark from a depression in the large occipital foramen. A microscopic examination of the brain tissue showed common signs of perivascular and pericellular edema, pronounced vasculitis with significant swelling of endothelial cells, and insignificant perivascular activation of glia (Figs. 7.19 and 7.20).

7.5 Chickenpox/Herpes Zoster

Among the most common infections is chickenpox. The frequency of lesions of the nervous system with it is 0.1–0.2%. Its causative agent is a virus from the family *Herpesviridae* (varicella-zoster, HV-3), which also acts as a causative agent of herpes zoster mainly in the elderly and senile. Like other viruses of this family, it has a certain neurotropism (see Chap. 5). A herpetic infection caused by the varicella-zoster virus

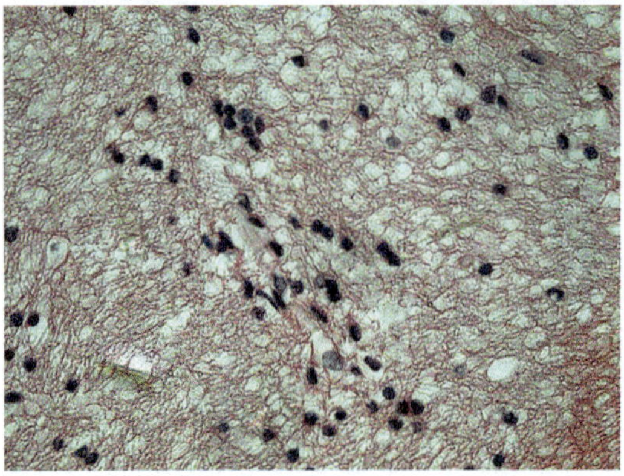

Fig. 7.19 Brain lesion in measles encephalitis. Note the formation of glial nodule. H-E ×100

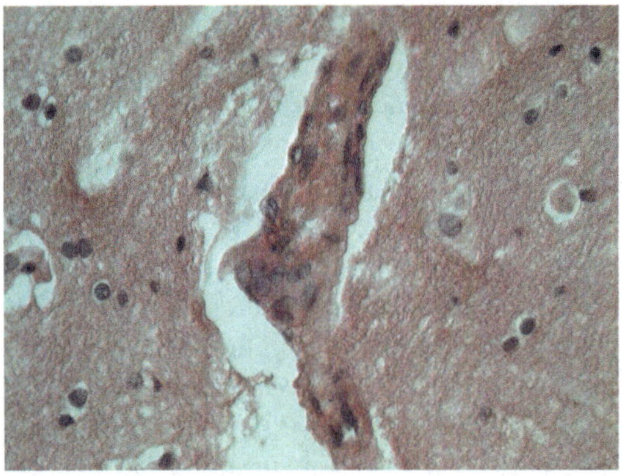

Fig. 7.20 Brain lesion in measles encephalitis. Note the swelling of endothelial cells. H-E ×200

leads to the development of chickenpox in childhood. Lesions of the nervous system in this disease occur mainly in children under the age of 2 years in the form of chickenpox encephalitis or encephalomyelitis. Herpes zoster, in 75% of cases, occurs in the elderly. In most cases, herpes zoster mainly affects thoracic dermatomas and areas of innervation of the trigeminal nerve. However, vesicular rashes in the area of innervation of the first branch of the trigeminal nerve are especially dangerous since they are often accompanied by the development of ocular herpes.

Neurological lesions in herpes zoster can manifest as follows: neuralgia, radiculoplexalgia, and neuropathy of the cranial and peripheral nerves. Usually, a few days or hours before the vesicular rash, burning and paroxysmal pains develop in the affected area, increasing at night. If such pain develops in the lumbar region, patients often associate them with the manifestation of osteochondrosis of the spine.

A rare clinical manifestation of herpes zoster is the development of acute inflammatory demyelinating polyradiculoneuropathy Guillain-Barre syndrome.

In chickenpox, lesions of the nervous system of various localizations are possible: encephalitis and encephalitic reactions, opticomyelitis and myelitis, polyradiculoneuritis, and serous meningitis; however, the highest specific weight is encephalitis, which makes up to 90% of their total number. There is no relationship between the severity of the course of chickenpox and the appearance and course of neurological complications—the latter can occur in both very severe and mild forms of the disease. Neurological disorders most often appear on days 3–8 of the rash but can develop simultaneously with the appearance of the rash or in a more distant period. In some cases, the symptoms of encephalitis precede the appearance of a rash—these forms are characterized by the most severe course. In young children, lesions of the nervous system sometimes occur as an encephalitic reaction; in these cases, there are general brain disorders (vomiting, generalized convulsions, disorders of consciousness), which usually pass quite quickly. Encephalitis, as a rule, occurs acutely on the background of high fever, but sometimes general cerebral symptoms develop gradually at normal or subfebrile temperature. In some children, the first manifestations are convulsions, disorders of consciousness, and brain damage in 18–20% of cases. Focal symptoms can be diverse; the most typical are cerebellar and vestibular disorders, which are relatively rare in children with encephalitis of other etiologies. There is shaking of the head, nystagmus, chanting speech, intentional tremor, and difficulty to perform coordination tests; symptoms are one or two sided. Some children develop static ataxia—patients can neither sit nor stand. Cerebellar syndrome may be the only manifestation of chickenpox encephalitis, but it can be combined with other focal symptoms: pyramidal signs, hemiparesis, and lesions of some cranial nerves. Possible forms of the disease with a predominance of disorders of consciousness, agitation, convulsions, hyperkinesis, chickenpox encephalitis with aphasia, and agnosia are described. Sometimes the spinal cord is involved in the process, and there are pathological signs, sensitivity disorders, and violation of the function of the pelvic organs. Meningeal syndrome is usually absent or moderately expressed; in the CSF, some patients have moderate lymphocytic cytosis and a slight increase in the amount of protein. The disease usually has an acute course with recovery after 3–6 weeks. Modern data on the pathogenesis and structural changes in chickenpox encephalitis are completely absent in the literature. When presenting this question, they are usually based on data from half a century ago: perivenous inflammatory infiltrates with micro- and macroglial reactions and demyelination, according to which the infectious allergic genesis of the lesions is postulated. There is also evidence of a possible direct etiological role of the virus. The histological picture usually indicates inflammatory perivenous changes and glial reaction and demyelination. Our own small experience concerning fatal observations in children and adults who developed chickenpox on the background of severe immunodeficiency, more often on the background of hemoblastosis, confirms the possibility of the development of both vasculitis and nerve and glial cells, including the formation of intracranial basophilic inclusions and hyperchromatosis. V.A. Zinserling et al. [1] studied the clinical and pathological data of ten people who died at the age of 60–90 years from a generalized form of herpes zoster. The duration of the disease ranged from 14 to 90 days. The disease began with general malaise, a rise in temperature to 39.5 °C, catarrhal phenomena, and characteristic herpetic rashes on the skin of the face, scalp, conjunctiva, and mucous membranes of the mouth; in the IV-V intercostal space of the chest; and on the extremities. Neurological symptoms appeared on the 5th–7th day of the disease: deafness, sopor, meningeal symptoms, in 6 cases – paresis of the facial nerve. The generalization of infection caused by herpes zoster led to the development of acute or subacute meningoencephalitis with focal serous meningitis, productive thrombovasculitis, small focal necrosis, followed by perifocal gliosis and petrification.

7.6 Brain Damage in Rubella

Rubella is also one of the most common human infections and can occur both as a congenital and acquired disease. Information about brain lesions in rubella embryos and fetopathy is given in Sect. 16.2. Lesions of the nervous system in acquired rubella are determined very rarely. Neurological disorders usually occur on days 3–4 of the rash but can develop on days 1–15 of the disease or precede the appearance of a rash on days 1–12. It is also possible to develop rubella encephalitis without a rash; the diagnosis in these cases is made on the basis of the results of a serological examination. Sometimes the appearance of neurological symptoms is accompanied by a secondary rash. All authors draw attention to the lack of a link between the severity of rubella and the development of neurological disorders. The disease usually begins acutely, with the appearance of headache, vomiting, and high fever; less often, the temperature is subfebrile. Almost all children have disorders of consciousness of varying degrees of severity. Hallucinations and delirium are possible. The most characteristic is the rapid onset of the disease with disorders of consciousness and generalized tonic-clonic convulsions. Motor disorders quickly develop in the form of hyperkinesis of various types, less often central paresis, as well as lesions of the cranial nerves; cerebellar, diencephalic, and bulbar disorders; ataxia; hyperthermia; central respiratory disorders; and cardiovascular activity. Myelitis and polyradiculoneuritis are described. In some cases, psychotic disorders develop up to the picture of acute psychosis. It is characterized by a very frequent involvement of the meninges in the pathological process. The CSF is characterized by moderate or significant cytosis with a predominance of lymphocytes and a slight increase in protein and sometimes sugar. In most cases, dehydration therapy leads to a rapid disappearance of symptoms. The catamnesis of children who have

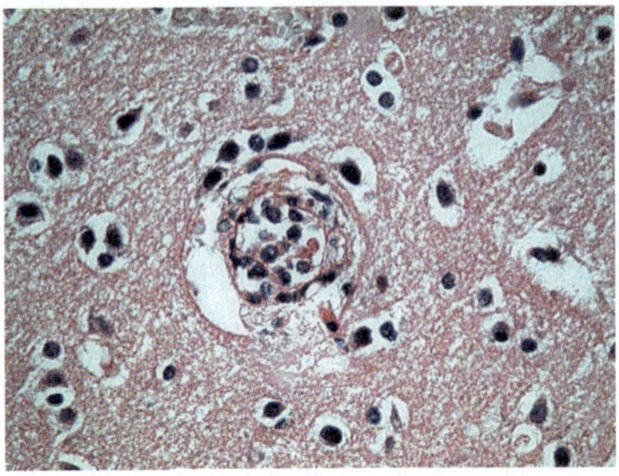

Fig. 7.21 Brain lesion in rubella. Vasculitis and perivascular edema. H-E ×300

suffered from rubella encephalitis is quite successful. The pathogenesis of postnatal rubella encephalitis has not yet been definitively elucidated. There are opinions about the direct etiological role of the rubella virus, "toxic vascular damage," allergic mechanisms, and the activation of the previously latent neurotropic virus in the body by rubella. Due to the absence of fatal outcomes from rubella encephalitis in recent decades, there are no complete descriptions of structural changes in the literature, and the existing ones in previous years are fragmentary. When reviewing archival observations of clinically documented cases of fatal outcomes from rubella encephalitis, we [1] showed that the pathological picture in an extremely severe course of the disease with the development of cerebral coma can be reduced to the phenomenon of moderate vasculitis with pronounced disorders of hemo- and cerebrovascular dynamics, manifested in the form of significant perivascular and pericellular edema (Fig. 7.21).

7.7 Brain Lesions in COVID-19

During the last two years, COVID-19 infection became one of the most important and widely discussed issues. Everyone accepts that nearby respiratory tract other organs and systems are involved during COVID-19 infection. Lesions of central and peripheral nervous system can be considered as frequent and important from clinical point of view. The pathogenesis of various neurological and psychiatric complications remains unclear and probably includes direct virus lesions and those modulated through immunopathology reactions. Unfortunately, there are till now no studies with detailed clinico-neuropathological comparisons. We, as other investigators, can state that the most typical changes can be referred to vasculitis of brain vessels (Fig. 7.22), sometimes with surrounding infiltration with the cells of macrophage lineage (Fig. 7.23) and detection of SARS-CoV-2 antigen by IHC (Fig. 7.24). Without a doubt further studies are urgently necessary.

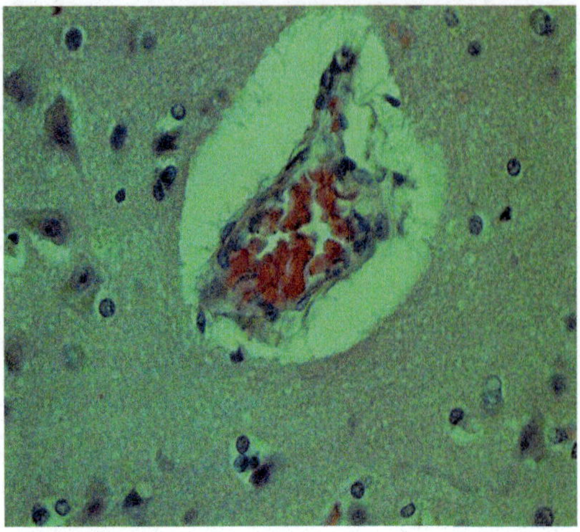

Fig. 7.22 Brain vascular lesion In COVID-19 infection. Note the swelling of endothelium. H-E ×200

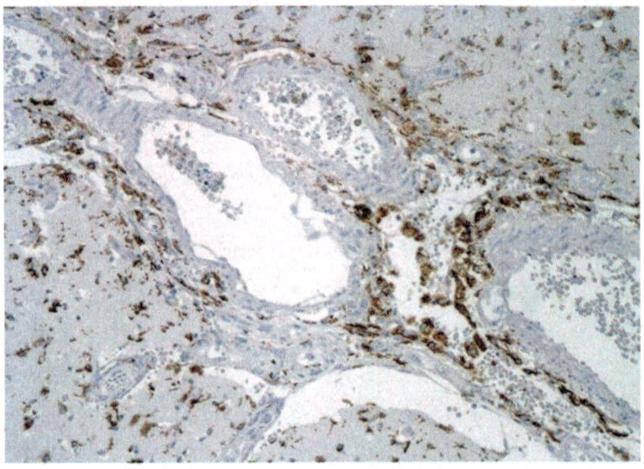

Fig. 7.23 Brain lesion in Covid-19. Accumulation of $CD68^+$ cells around the vessel. IHC ×200

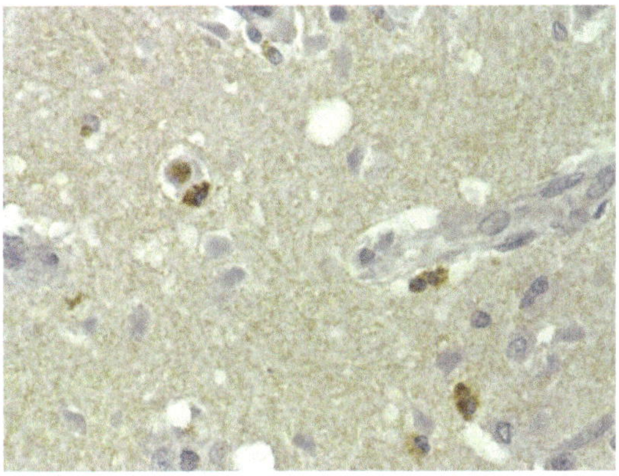

Fig. 7.24 N protein of SARS-CoV2 in brain matter. IHC ×200

References

1. Zinserling VA, Chukhlovina ML. Infectious lesions of nervous system. Issues of etiology, pathogenesis and diagnostics. Saint-Petersburg: ElbiSPb; 2011. p. 583. (In Russian)
2. Liang C-Y, Yang C-H, Lin J-N. Focal encephalitis, meningitis, and acute respiratory distress syndrome associated with influenza A infection. Med Princ Pract. 2018;27(2):193–6.
3. Sejvar JJ, Uyeki TN. Neurologic complications of 2009 influenza A(H1N1). Neurology. 2010;74(13):1020.
4. Zinserling VA. Infectious pathology of the respiratory tract. Springer International Publishing; 2021. https://doi.org/10.1007/978-3-030-66325-4. ISBN 978-3—030-66324-7
5. Takahashi M, Yamada T, Nakashita Y, Saikusa H, Deguchi M, Kida H, Tashiro M, Toyoda T. Influenza virus-induced encephalopathy: clinicopathologic study of an autopsied case. Pediatr Int. 2000;42(2):204–14. https://doi.org/10.1046/j.1442-200x2000.01203x.
6. Isakov VA, Chepik EB, Shamanova MG, Zhukova AO, Parsagashvili EZ, Ivannikov IG. Mortality and lethality of influenza and acute respiratory diseases. Vest Ross Akad Med Nauk. 1994;6:61–4. (in Russian)
7. Semenov SP, Konovalov GV, Taros LI, Kudriavtseva VK. The pathomorphological changes in brain and internal organs in experimental influenza infection in mice. Arkh Patol. 1990;52(5):50–5. (in Russian)
8. Cateigne G, Brygoo P, Fauconnier B. Experimental demonstration in the monkey of the neuropic properties of influenza virus CR Hebd seances. Acad Sci. 1951;232(16):1511–3. (In French)
9. Lussier G, Boudreault A, Pavilanis V, Fi-Franco DE. Lesions of the central nervous system induced in nonhuman primates by life influenza viruses. Can J Comp Med. 1974;38(4):398–405.
10. Miyoshi K, Gamboa ET, Harter DH, Wof A, Hsu KC. Influenza virus encephalitis in squirrel monkeys receiving immunosuppressive therapy. J Immunol. 1971;106(4):119–21.
11. Chou SM, Roos R, Burrel R, Gutman L, Harley JB. Subacute focal adenovirus encephalitis. J Neoropathol Exp Neurol. 1973;32(1):34–50. https://doi.org/10.1097/00005072-197301000-00003.
12. Sterner G, Biberfeld G. Central nervous system complications of mycoplasma pneumoniae infection. Scand J Infect Dis. 1969;8(2):71–3.
13. Murray HW, Masur H, Senterfit LB, Roberts RB. The protean manifestations of Mycoplasma pneumoniae infection in adults. Am J Med. 1975;58(2):229–42. https://doi.org/10.1016/0002-934(75)90574-4.
14. Lasono BM, de Vries RD, McQuaid S, Duprex WP, de Swart RL. Measles virus host invasion and pathogenesis. Viruses. 2016;8(8):210. https://doi.org/10.3390/v8080210.
15. Liebert UG. Measles virus infections of the central nervous system. Intervirology. 1997;40(21–3):176–84. https://doi.org/10.1159/000150544.

8 Brain Lesion Due to HIV and its Complications

Infection due to human immunodeficient virus (HIV) remains one of the most frequent in the world. Despite the tremendous success in treatment strategies allowing majority of patient to lead a normal lifestyle, full recovery with virus elimination is still a rare exception and lethal outcomes are not rare. Among the issues only rarely discussed in the literature, the histopathology of changes directly caused by the virus has to be noted [1]. Neurological symptoms and signs of cognitive impairment in HIV infection are observed in at least 80% of patients, among whom 10% have severe symptoms [2]. The range of causes of their occurrence is quite wide: these include brain tumors (lymphomas, metastases from other tumors), infections (meningitis, encephalitis, brain abscesses), peripheral nerve changes, and dementia [2]. Additionally, there are lesions of the nervous system that are not conditionally associated with HIV infection, but are caused by the toxic effects of narcotic substances, alcohol, and the presence of somatic pathology. In these cases, the absence of an inflammatory component in the clinical picture of neurological deficits and psychotic disorders is considered as evidence of the toxic effect of these substances on the cells of the central nervous system. There is no complete morphological description of such lesions in the literature. In pathology practice, more than 50% of those who die from HIV infection have an indication of neurocognitive disorders in the structure of the diagnosis. According to our experience, morphological studies in almost all cases reveal various brain changes expressed to varying degrees [3, 4]. Exact correlations between cognitive disorders and the nature of structural changes have not been established. The damage to the nervous system in HIV infection can be primary, directly related to the cytopathic effect of the virus, secondary, due to opportunistic infections that develop in AIDS patients in conditions of immunodeficiency, or combined, due to both opportunistic infections and continuing effect of HIV itself. In this chapter, we try to distinguish the lesions directly connected with HIV and by other courses.

8.1 Neurology and Neuropathology of HIV Infection

In HIV infection, the human immunodeficiency virus enters the brain at an early stage, where it can persist and develop, causing chronic progressive encephalitis [1], which, according to our data, has characteristic morphological features [3–5]. Brain macrophages and microglia are the key cell types in which the virus develops, and they are likely to mediate the neurodegeneration seen in dementia patients. Virus replication in these cells occurs at a low rate, and the infection is latent, but the exact pathogenesis of this neurodegeneration is still unclear.

V. Zinserling, *Infectious Lesions of the Central Nervous System*,
https://doi.org/10.1007/978-3-030-96260-9_8

Certain role in pathogenesis of brain lesions in HIV infection may play also toll-like receptor (TLRs).

Primary HIV neuropathologies can affect all levels of nervous system in all stages of the disease. HIV encephalitis, HIV myelitis and diffuse infiltrative lymphocytosis of peripheral nerve are considered to develop due to productive viral infection. While vacuolar meyelopathy, distal symmetric polyneuropathy, and central and peripheral nervous system demyelination, are not clearly related to regional viral replication, and reflect more complex cascades of disregulated host immunity and metabolic dysfunction. In pediatric patients, the spectrum of neuropathology is altered by the impacts of HIV on the developing nervous system with microcephaly, abundant brain mineralization, and corticospinal tract degeneration [6].

Microglia are the main target of HIV-1 infection in the brain [7]. There are viral particles in the infected microglia, suggesting that they may be a potential virus reservoir [8]. The main features of HIV-1 encephalitis are considered to be the formation of multinucleated giant cells, microglia nodules, and macrophage infiltration into the central nervous system [9]. The formation of multinucleated giant cells reflects the infection of HIV-1 microglia in vitro. Active infection of microglia is ultimately associated with astrogliosis, myelin pallor, and neuronal loss. Although there are ample pieces of evidence that activated microglia have neuropathic effects in HIV-1 encephalitis, there a data suggesting that microglia may have some neuroprotective effects in the early stages of the disease [10].

In the field of brain lesions in HIV infection is assumed that astroglial disfunction- mediated neuronal stress is a major factor contributing to HIV-1 neuropathogenesis. There are numerous evidence that astrocytes harbor HIV-1 and serve as "safe haven" for the dormant virus in the brain, the indirect pathway of neuronal damage in its contribution to neuropathogenesis of this infection [11]. In the modern literature, there are no hints about virus location in neurons and their direct lesions as it was not excluded before. Disruption of blood-brain barrier is explained by action of HIV-envelope protein gp120 [12].

Detection of p24 in tissues by IHC is rarely used in diagnostics, although there are data proving that it can be informative while studying different organs, including brain [13].

Our own observation generally coincides with above cited with only exclusion; till approx. 2015 we did not observe giant cell formation, later they appeared (Figs. 8.1, 8.2, 8.3).

8.2 Brain Complications of HIV Infections

Exposure to opportunistic infections is associated with the amount of CD4. Thus, multifocal leukoencephalopathy usually occurs in patients with a CD4 count of less than 200 cl / mcl, toxoplasmosis, and cryptococcosis develop with a cell count of less than 100, mycobacterial and cytomegalovirus encephalitis with a CD4 count of less than 50. It should be noted that a significant proportion of patients with HIV infection receiving therapy still have neurological disorders, which affects the predicted long-term survival. However, according to our data, there is no strict relationship between the immune status and the etiology of brain lesions. I.

We can divide the complications according to their etiology into infectious and noninfectious (tumor). It is notable that the frequency of the complications due to unclear courses varies on our material in different periods of observation.

8.2.1 Infectious Complications

Toxoplasma meningoencephalitis is considered to be the most common pathology of the central nervous system in HIV (see Chap. 14), and in some rare cases it occurs as a generalized process involving the lungs and heart. A pathological feature is the presence of multiple destructive foci in all brain structures with the presence of a large number of parasites on the periphery of brain tissue necrosis. The second place in the frequency of CNS pathology is occupied by *tuberculous meningoencephalitis*, often as a manifestation of a generalized process with lung damage. In HIV-

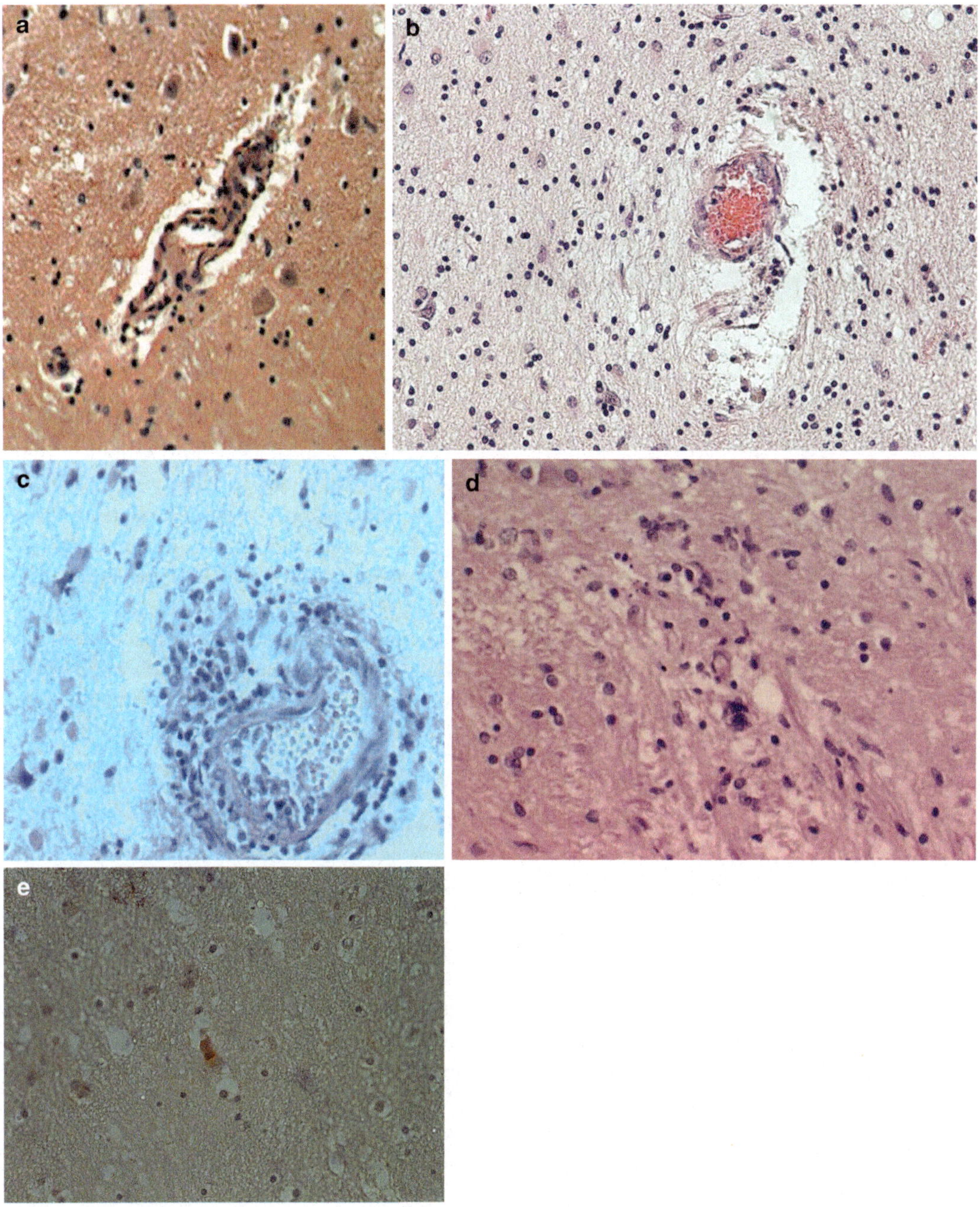

Fig. 8.1 Different patterns of brain vasculitis in HIV infection without giant-cell reaction H-E, **a**, **b** ×200, **c**, **d** ×400; **e** IHC detecting p24 antigen X400

infected patients, there is an extremely rapid progression of the pathological process and a sharp predominance of the alternative component of inflammation over the productive one, and microscopy shows a weak expression of giant cell transformation, which is a characteristic feature of the course of mycobacterial infection in HIV infection (see Chap. 13).

Progressive multifocal leukoencephalopathy (PML) is caused by the JS virus and is character-

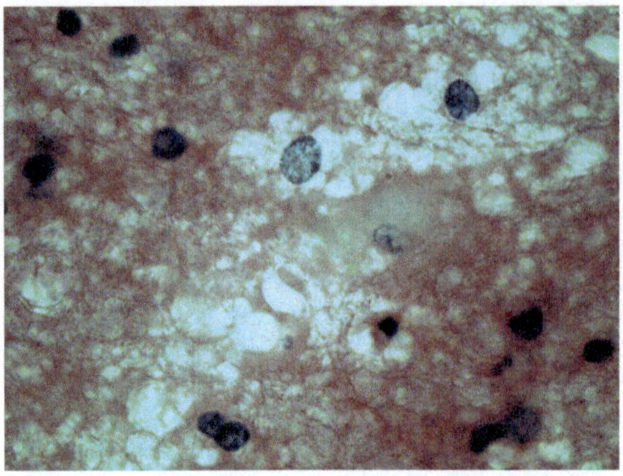

Fig. 8.2 Focal demyelization of white matter and hyperplasia of astrocytes. H-E ×400

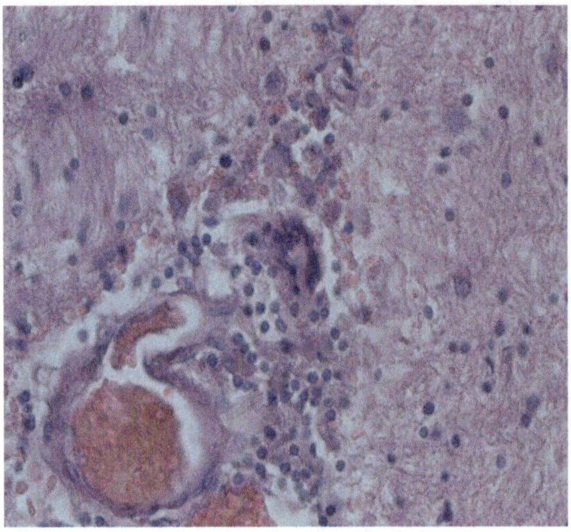

Fig. 8.3 Giant cell reaction in HIV vasculitis H-E ×400

ized by multifocal necrosis of various brain structures caused by demyelination of nerve fibers, on our material these lesions appeared only the middle of the tenth of this century. Macroscopically, the foci of necrosis in the brain are determined from 0.2 cm to the merging foci that occupy most of the hemisphere (Fig. 8.4). The diagnostic sign of PML is karyomegaly and intracranial inclusions in oligodendrocytes and granular neurons of the cerebellum (Fig. 8.5). There is a tendency to increase the number of deaths due to the lack of etiotropic therapy of the JC virus (Figs. 8.5 and 8.6).

Among the most important viral lesions, *cytomegaly* must be mentioned. Previously known as intrauterine infection (see Chap. 16), this pathogen became the course one of the most frequent secondary diseases in HIV although significantly varying in frequency in different decades. CMV is able to damage all brain structures with appearance of very typical "owl-eye-like" intranuclear basophilic inclusions. To detect all cell containing virus antigen it is advisable to perform IHC study (Figs. 8.7, 8.8, 8.9, 8.10). Lesions due to Herpes simplex viruses seem to develop relative rare due to unclear reasons (see Chap. 5).

Recently, clinical and morphological data have appeared on the possibility of developing encephalitis caused by the *Epstein-Barr virus* (Fig. 8.11), but there is no complete pathogenetic, epidemiological, clinical, and morphological characteristics of such lesions yet.

Among mycotic infections of the brain, the leading place is occupied by *cryptococcosis.* In hospital settings, the mortality rate from cryptococcal meningitis, which occurs in up to 6% of cases of brain damage in HIV, continues to be high, varying from 30% to 50%, even with antifungal therapy (see Chap. 13).

Among less famous lesions, those due to chlamydia should be mentioned.

It is assumed that C. pneumoniae is involved in the progression of AIDS-dement complex) [14]. It was identified in the central nervous system with the help of modern technologies in 17.4% (4/23) of patients with AIDS-dement complex. In two life-time examined patients with HIV in the AIDS stage, Chlamydia spp. was detected (culturally) in the cerebrospinal fluid, while antibodies were detected in the cerebrospinal fluid. In several observations we succeeded to prove the presence of Chlamydia with the help of PAS-staining and immunofluorescent microscopy (Fig. 8.12).

In many observations, a mixed etiology of the process is noted. It is possible that some of the infectious lesions for various reasons are currently not diagnosed.

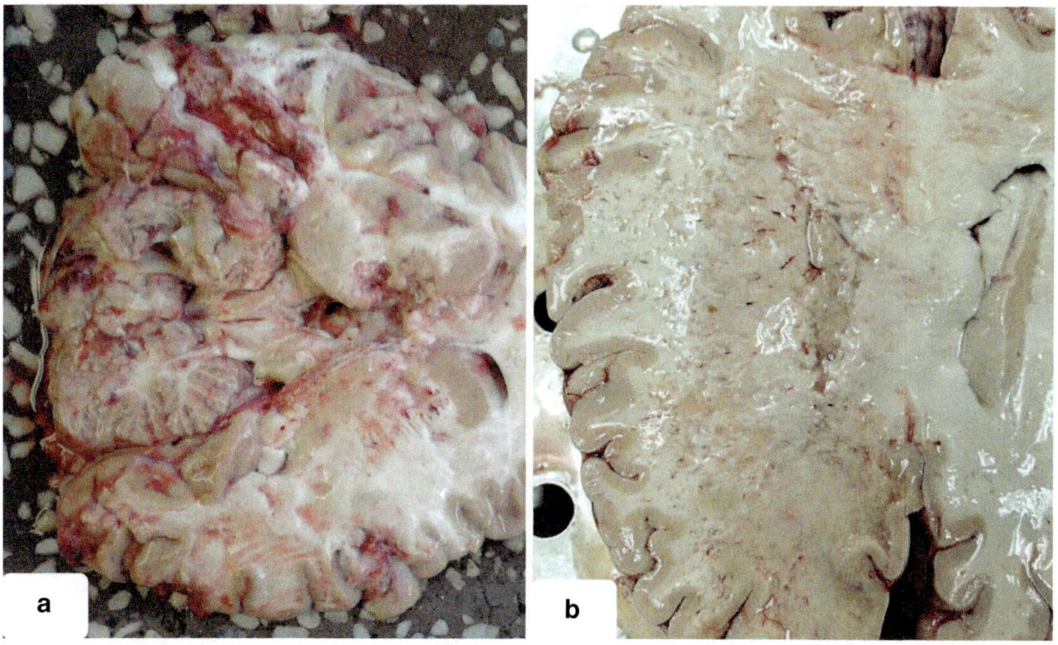

Fig. 8.4 Different patterns of PML. Unfixed macropreparations. (**a**) Necrotic changes in deep parts of the brain; (**b**) Subtotal lesion of hemisphere

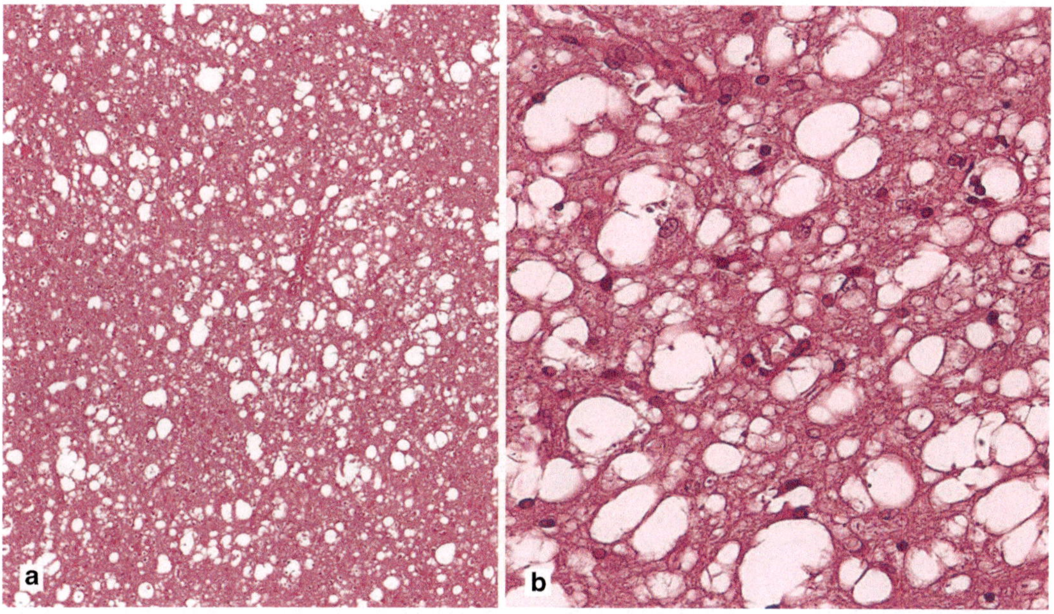

Fig. 8.5 HIV-associated multifocal progressive leukoencephalopathy. (**a**) A focus of gliosis in the substance of the brain (indicated by a round frame); (**b**) Dystrophic changes in the spongiosely altered substance of the brain with the formation of axonal balls (blue starch or amyloid corpuscles), some of the balls (corpuscles) are indicated by arrows. H-E. **a** – ×100; **b** – ×200. (Courtesy of Y.R. Zyuzya)

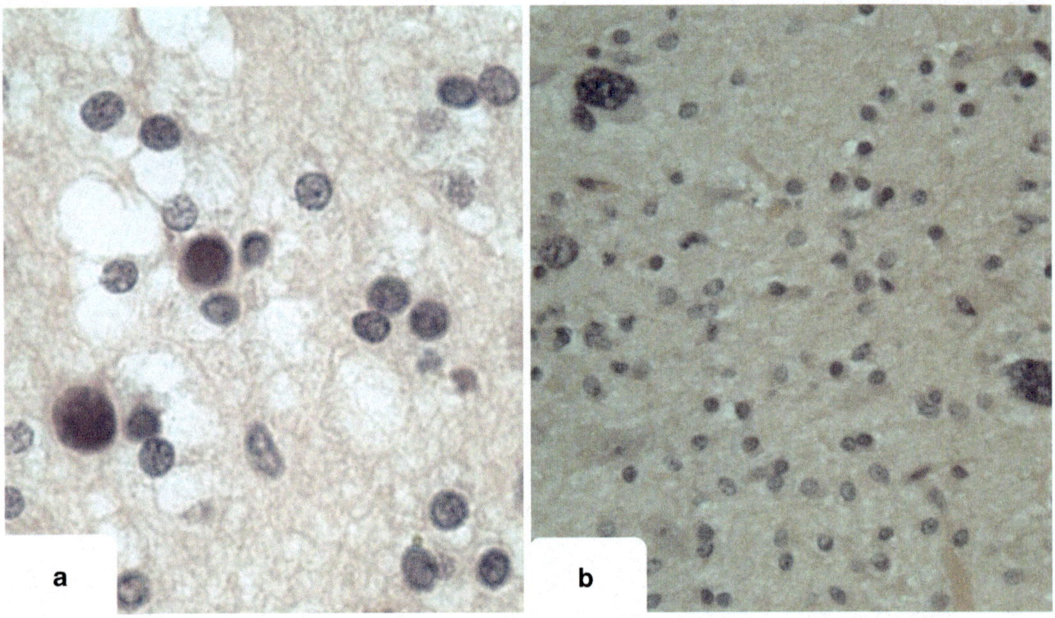

Fig. 8.6 Cell changes in HIV-associated leukoencephalopathy. H-E. (**a**) Diffuse hyperchromatosis of nuclei at early stage of the lesion. ×400; (**b**) Hyperchromatosis of small dots at later stage of the lesion ×200

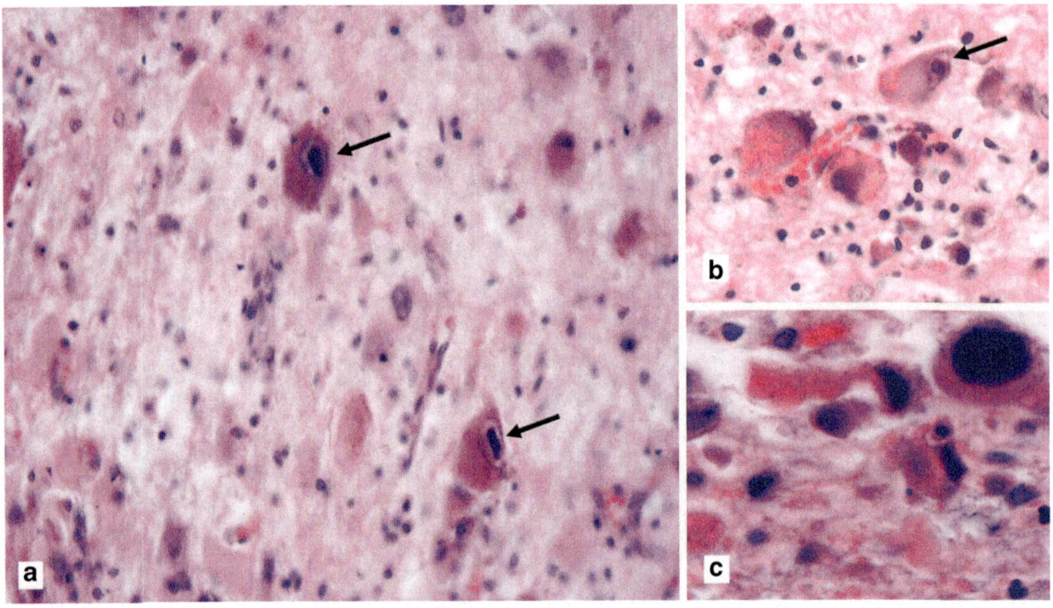

Fig. 8.7 Cytomegalovirus encephalitis. Cells with cytomegalic transformation in the brain substance. The cells of the "owl's eye" are indicated by arrows. **a**, **b** ×400, **c** ×800. (Courtesy of Y.R. Zyuzya)

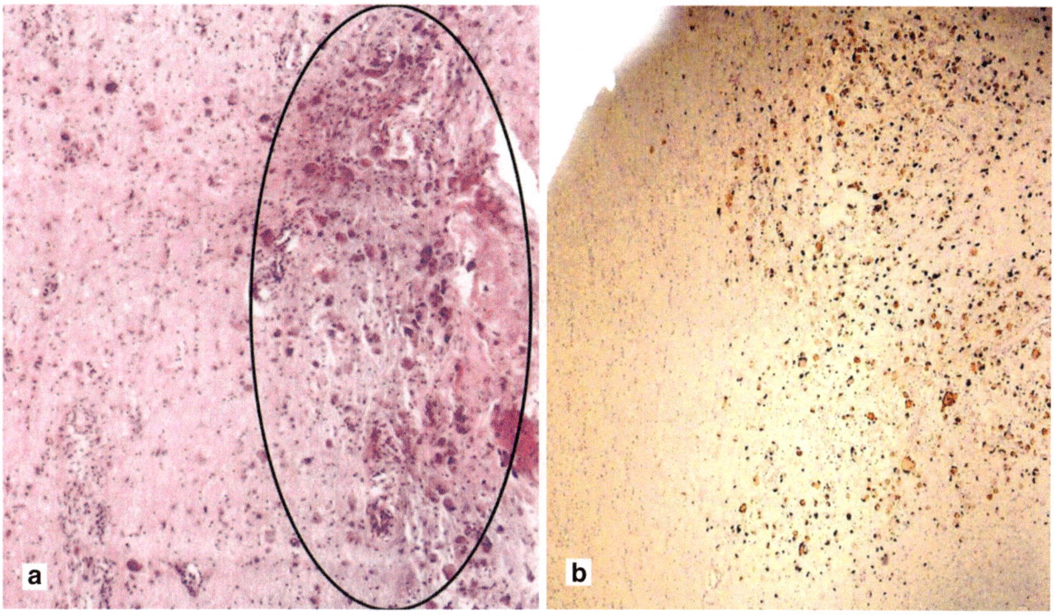

Fig. 8.8 Cytomegalovirus encephalitis. (**a**) Cluster of cells with cytomegalic metamorphosis in the brain substance (circled by an oval frame); (**b**) Positive expression of cytomegalovirus antibodies in the affected area of the brain. **a** – staining with hematoxylin and eosin. ×100; **b** – immunohistochemical reaction with cytomegalovirus antibodies. ×400. (Courtesy of Y.R. Zyuzya)

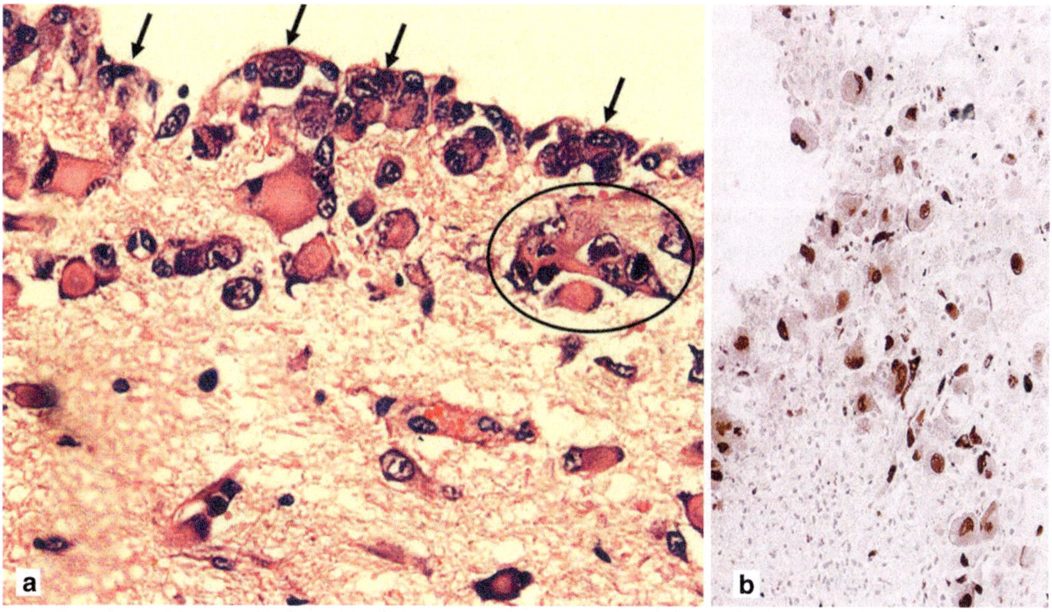

Fig. 8.9 Cytomegalovirus encephalitis (cytomegalovirus ventriculitis). (**a**) Cytomegalovirus lesion of ependymal cells of the lateral ventricle of the brain (ependyma is indicated by arrows); in the substance of the brain under the ependyma there are also multiple cells with cytomegalic transformation, the cells of the "owl's eye" are encircled by a round frame; (**b**) expression of antibodies to cytomegalovirus in the cells of the wall of the lateral ventricle of the brain. (**a**) H-E. ×400; (**b**) Immunohistochemical reaction with cytomegalovirus antibodies. ×100. (Courtesy of Y.R. Zyuzya)

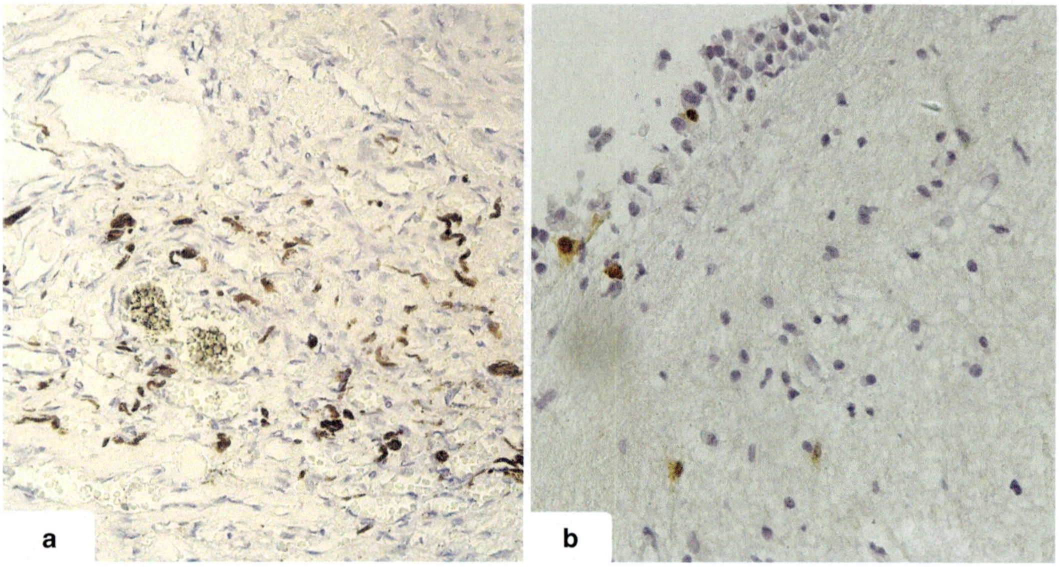

Fig. 8.10 Cytomegalovirus leptomeningitis. Cells of arachnoendothelium and endothelium of individual capillaries with cytomegalic transformation and expression of cytomegalovirus antibodies (colored brown) IHC with cytomegalovirus antibodies. (**a**) Part of the affected cells with clear expression of CMV antibodies without signs of cytomegaly (positive reaction before the development of cytomegalic metamorphosis of cells). ×100. (Courtesy of Y.R. Zyuzya). (**b**) Positive reaction in ependyma ×400

8.2.2 Tumor Complication

Tumor lesions of the nervous system are represented by the following neoplasms: primary lymphoma of the central nervous system, systemic lymphoma with cerebral metastasis, less often—Kaposi's sarcoma. Brain lymphoma in AIDS patients is an extra-nodular lymphomatous infiltration (B-cell lymphoma) with a high degree of malignancy. Currently, there is a tendency to increase the incidence rate. Clinical picture of focal brain damage (most often—frontal, temporal, parietal areas; cerebellum) has no specific symptoms, as a result of which differential diagnosis is carried out with a wide range of AIDS-associated opportunistic infections. Most researchers associate the formation of brain lymphomas with the action of the Epstein-Barr virus (EBV).

Primary malignant brain lymphomas (PMBL) account for less than 2% of all tumors of this localization. However, in AIDS patients, such lymphomas develop much more often: their frequency in these cases is 3.6×10^3–7.8×10^3 higher than in the general population. It is believed that their development is characteristic of the transition of HIV infection to the stage of AIDS. PMBL almost always have a B-cell immunophenotype. Unlike lymphomas developing in immunocompetent patients, in AIDS patients they are often biclonal. An exceptionally high detection rate of EBV (up to 100%) in tumor cells has been established using various modern methods.

We, together with E.E. Leenman and K.M. Pozharissky [15], specially studied six cases of primary malignant non-Hodgkin's lymphomas of the brain in SP. Botkin Infectious Hospital. Among the deceased were five men and one woman aged from 27 to 47 years. In most patients, HIV infection occurred sexually, and in three cases homosexual. The duration of HIV infection is from months to 7 years. The diagnosis of lymphoma in three cases was made in vivo based on the results of neurological examination, computed tomography, in the remaining three was postmortem. Along with detailed macro- and microscopic examination, tumor tissue was studied using a wide range of antibodies (LCA, CD20, CD3, CD30, EMA, anti-kappa, anti-lambda, CD68 bcl-2 p53 Ki-67, LMP-1 ZEBRA), which allowed phenotyping of tumor cells, evaluation

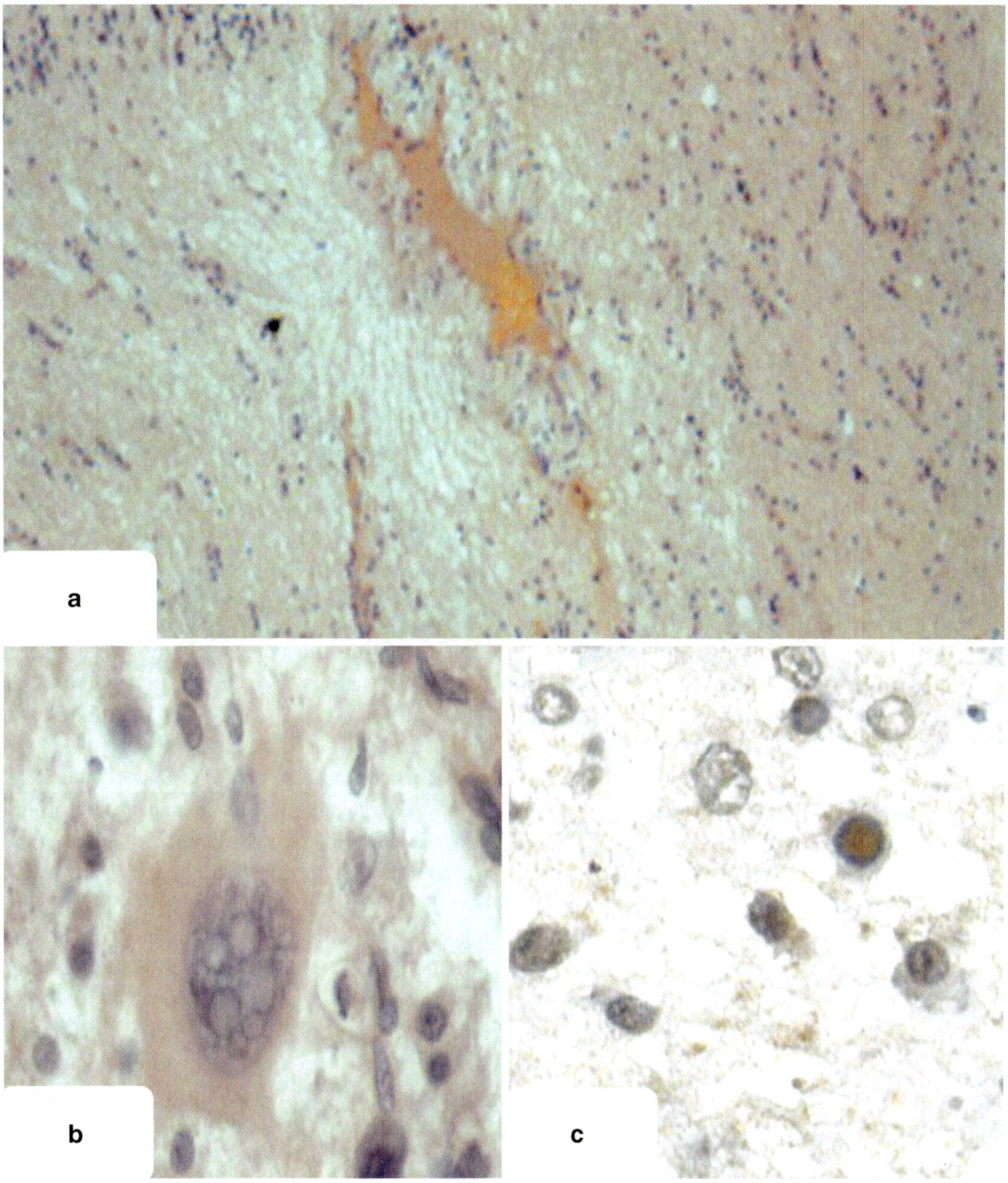

Fig. 8.11 Brain changes related to EBV. (**a**) General view of the lesion. H-E X50; (**b**) Peculiar lesion of individual cell H-E X 1000; (**c**) Positive IHC reaction with serum against EBV ×400

of their proliferative activity, apoptosis, as well as latent and lytic forms of EBV. In addition, in situ hybridization was performed to evaluate EBV with the detection of RNA - EBER-1,2 and EA-R (lytic cycle).

All the deceased posthumously showed signs of HIV encephalitis (including 3 significantly pronounced) and numerous opportunistic infections (most often cryptococcosis), which proceeded generically, including with brain damage.

Tumor lesions in all cases were of a multiple nature, foci were usually localized supratentorially, mainly in the hemispheres of the brain

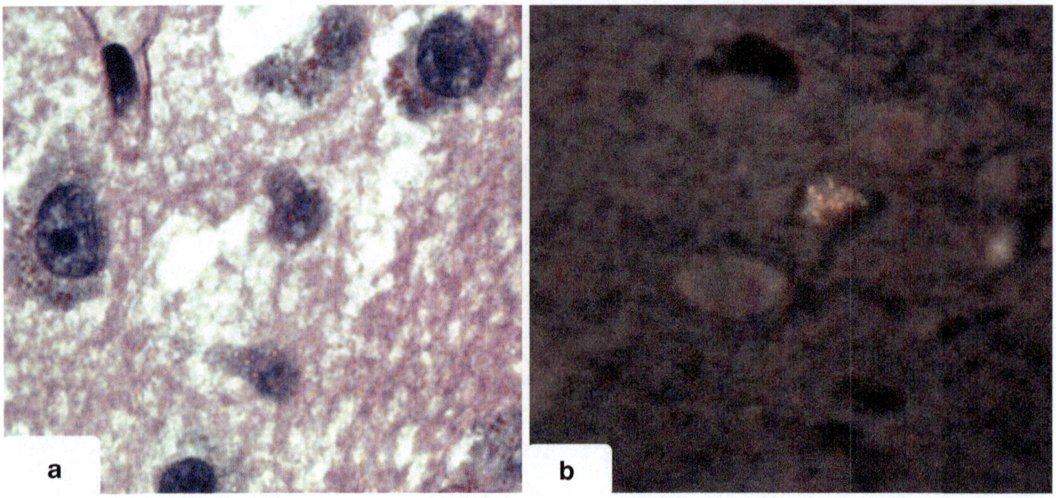

Fig. 8.12 Probable lesions related to Chlamydia. (**a**) Small intracytoplasmic inclusions. PAS-reaction X400; (**b**) Lightening of nervous cells in luminescent microscopy with serum against Chlamydia. Luminescent microscopy X 1000

(Fig. 8.13). The soft meninges were infiltrated by the tumor in only one patient. The tumor tissue had a gray-pink color with a yellowish swelling, the size of the foci ranged from 9.5 to 9 cm, in three observations their boundaries were clear and in 3—blurred. Necrosis was noted in all the deceased, and in 5—focal hemorrhages in the tumor growth zone.

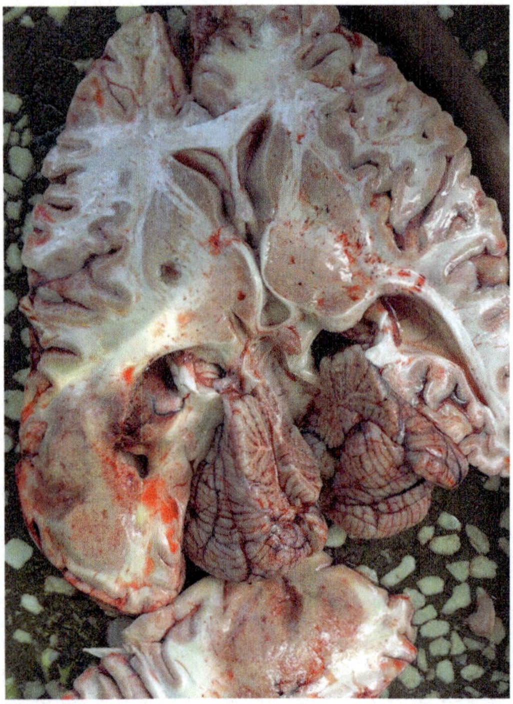

Fig. 8.13 Brain lymphoma. Unfixed macropreparation

Microscopically, the tumor had a polymorphic appearance with a predominance of large cells. Based on histological criteria in accordance with the Kiel classification, 3 lymphomas were regarded as immunoblastic with plasmocytic differentiation, 2 as centroblastic polymorphic lymphoma and 1 as large-cell anaplastic. Diffuse and perivascular types of tumor cell proliferation with high cell content in both components were noted in all observations. During the IHC analysis, it was found that in all the studied observations, tumor lymphocytes had a B-cell origin based on the strong membrane expression of the pan-B-cell antigen CD20. Thus, according to the International Histological Classification, all cases were regarded as diffuse large-cell B-cell lymphomas. Only in one observation monoclonality along the kappa chain was noted, in the remaining cases there were both kappa and lambda-positive cells. Moderate expression of activation antigen CD30 was detected in two observations, no other activation antigen EMA was detected (Fig. 8.13).

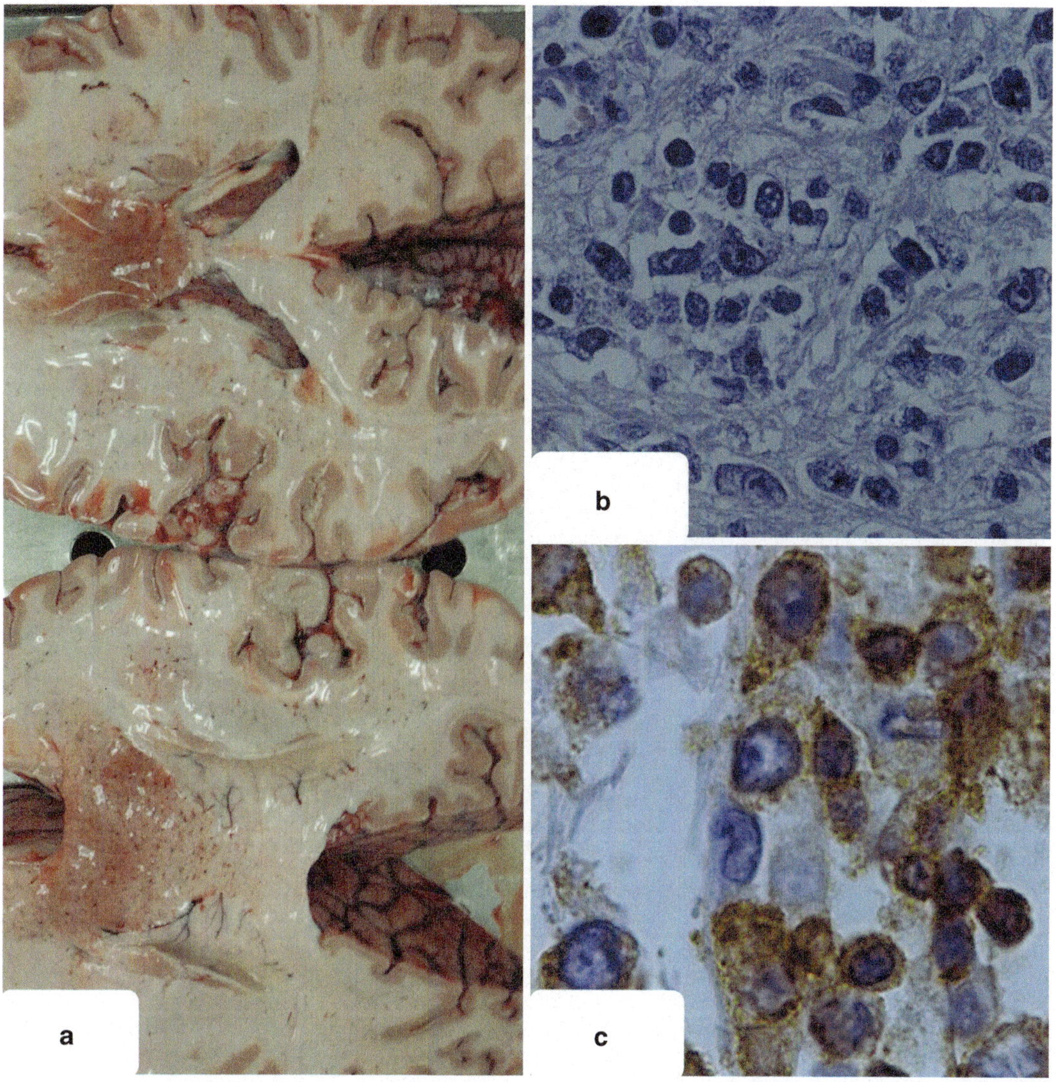

Fig. 8.14 Atypical case of brain lymphoma. (**a**) Unfixed macropreparation (Courtesy of N.A. Lugovskaya); (**b**) Cell content H-E X400; (**c**) Positive IHC reaction with $CD45^{+}$ cells

The apoptosis antagonist protein bcl-2 was detected in 5, and the suppressor protein p53 in two observations. Proliferative antigen Ki-67 was detected in four observations. T-lymphocytes and macrophages were also identified as part of the tumor infiltrate. EBV was detected in all patients. The expression of latent membrane protein LMP-1 was noted in 100% of observations, but in part of tumor cells (from 28 to 60%). The ZEBRA lytic protein was detected in a small amount in only 1 observation. During in situ hybridization, EB-encoded EBER-1,2 RNAs were detected in almost all tumor cells. The EA-R lytic cycle RNA was noted only in the same observation where the ZEBRA protein was expressed. It should be noted that both in IHC reactions and in situ hybridization, EBV was detected exclusively in tumor lymphocytes. Analyzing the data presented, it can be noted that for the first time, data correspond to the characteristics available in the literature. Later, we have met the case in which macroscopic picture presented certain difficulties in differential diagnostics with focal encephalitis (Fig. 8.14).

We have not observed other tumors in the central nervous system with HIV infection.

References

1. Zinserling AV, Zinserling VA. Modern infections: pathological anatomy and questions of pathogenesis Guide. 2nd ed. "Sotis", 2002 2002, 346 p. (in Russian).
2. Spudich S, Gonzalez-Scarano F. HIV-1-related central nervous system disease: current issues in pathogenesis, diagnosis, and treatment. Cold Spring Harb Perspect Med. 2012;2(6):a007120. https://doi.org/10.1101/cshper4spect.a007120.
3. Tsinzerling VA, Komarova DV, Vasil'eva MV, Karev VE. Pathological anatomy of HIV infection according to data in saint-Petersburg. Arkh Patol. 2003;65(1):42–5.
4. Tsinzerling VA, Komarova DV, Rakhmanova AG, Yakovlev AA, Leonova ON. Actual problems of morphological diagnostics and pathomorphosis of HIV infection. Arkh Patol. 2010;67(2):26–30. (in Russian)
5. Zinserling VA, Chukhlovina ML. Infectious lesions of nervous system. Issues of etiology, pathogenesis and diagnostics. Saint-Petersburg: ElbiSPb; 2011. p. 583. (in Russian)
6. Morgello S. HIV neuropathology. Handb Clin Neurol. 2018;152:3–19. https://doi.org/10.1016/B978-0-444-63849-6.00002-5.
7. Cosenza MA, Zhao ML, Si Q, Lee SC. Humas brain parenchymal microglia express CD14 and CD45 and are productively infected by HIV-1 in HIV-1 encephalitis. Brain Pathol. 2002;12:442–55. https://doi.org/10.1111/j.1750-3639.2002.tb00461.x.
8. Williams KC, Hickeyu WF. Central nervous system damage, monocytes and macrophages, and neurological disorders in AIDS Ann. Rev Neurosci. 2002;25:537–62.
9. Persidsky Y, Gendelman HE. Mononuclear phagocyte immunity and the neuropathogenesis of HIV-1 infection. J Leukoc Biol. 2003;74:691–701.
10. Gras GF, Chretien AV, Vallat-Dedcouvellaere G, et al. Regulated expression of sodium-dependent glutamate transporters and synthetaser: a neuroprotective role for activated microglia and macrophages in HIV infection? Brain Pathol. 2003;13:211–22. https://doi.org/10.1111/j.1750-3639.2003.tb00020.x.
11. Pandey HS, Seth P. Friends turn foe-astrocytes contribute to neduronal damage in NeuroAIDS. J Mol Neurosci. 2019;69:286–97. https://doi.org/10.1007/s12031-019-0113357-1.
12. Louboutin J-P, Strayer DS. Blood-brain barrier abnormalities caused by HIV-1 gp120:mechanistic and therapeutic implications. ScientificWorldJournal. 2012;2012:482575. https://doi.org/10.1100/2012/482575.
13. MoonimMT AL, Freeman J, Mahadeva U, van der Walt JD, Lucas SB. Identifying HIV infection in diagnostic histopathology tissue samples—the role of HIV-1 P24 immunohistochemistry in identifying clinically unsuspected HIV infection: a 3-year analysis. Histopathology. 2010;56(4):530–41. https://doi.org/10.1111/j.1365-2559.2010.03513x.
14. Contini C, Seraceni S, Cultera R, Castellazzi M, Granieri E, Fainardi E. Chlamydophila pneumoniae infection and its role in neurological disorders. Interdiscip Perspect Infect Dis. 2010;2010:273573. https://doi.org/10.1155/2010/273573.
15. Leenman EE, Tsinzerling VA, Pozharisskiĭ KM. Morphological and immunohistochemical characteristics of primary brain lymphomas in AIDS patients. Arkh Patol. 2002;64(1):25–9. (in Russian)

9 Meningococcal Infection

Neisseria meningitidis is gram-negative diplococcus considered as the most frequent course of acute neuroinfections all over the world. Historically, the main clinical form was called epidemical cerebrospinal meningitis with very high lethality. Recent update of pathogens properties can be found in several reviews [1, 2]. Nowadays, most frequent in clinical practice are serotypes A, B, C, W135, and Y. The immunization against N. meningitidis serotypes A and C has resulted in a significant decrease in meningococcal disease. Choroid plexuses are considered as the main site of meningococcus entry in the central nervous system. N. meningitidis can bind to human brain microvascular endothelial cells via the 37/67-kDa laminin receptor, as the ligands are considered type IV pili, PilQ, PorA and Opc. The pathogen is thought to invade endothelial cells primarily by paracellular mechanisms. Following initial bacterial attachment, the meningococcal minor pilin protein, PilV, triggers a cellular response during which endothelial cells form protrusions around the pathogen. These cellular projections further protect the bacterial microcolony from mechanical damage due to high velocity blood flow. The further steps of pathogen-host interactions have been studied in detail in vitro without direct extrapolation to different clinical forms of meningococcal infection. Animal models of infection have also highlighted the possibility of bacteria to invade the olfactory bulb within the brain from the nasal mucosa [3, 4]. Main clinical forms are meningitis, meningococcemia and mixed.

9.1 Meningococcemia

Among the most important clinical forms of meningococcal infection, which provides maximum mortality, is meningococcemia. From a formal point of view, we are talking about acute meningococcal sepsis. It can be stated that this example makes obvious the need to revise the traditional view about the independence of sepsis manifestations from the causative agent. Based on many years of experience, it can be stated that the most important clinical and morphological manifestations of this disease are strictly specific for meningococcemia, and we do not know cases in which it would be possible to associate a similar clinical and morphological picture with another pathogen. In cases with no seeding of meningococcus, more often in connection with the initiated treatment with antibiotics, it is quite often possible to sow a variety of microflora, but its significance in the etiology of the disease, as a rule, remains unproven. In those cases, in which meningococcemia is combined with meningitis, it is customary to talk about a mixed form of meningococcal infection. It should be noted that the distinction between these two forms is often very conditional, since in many observations with typical clinical and morphological

V. Zinserling, *Infectious Lesions of the Central Nervous System*,
https://doi.org/10.1007/978-3-030-96260-9_9

manifestations of meningococcemia, minimal inflammatory changes in the soft meninges are determined, and bean-shaped diplococci with cytological or histobacterioscopic studies are naturally detected already in deceased at the earliest stages of the disease. The pathogenesis of meningococcemia is usually considered in connection with bacteremia, accompanied by the release of significant amounts of endotoxin, which causes the development of severe disseminated intravascular coagulation (DIC) syndrome, the most significant in the diagnosis of this becomes a hemorrhagic rash, in combination with meningeal symptoms, and in the hemorrhages (hemorrhagic necrosis) of the adrenal glands, the last play the leading role in thanatogenesis. Despite the absolute value of such views, they do not allow us to answer all questions that arise in the study of meningococcal infection. Thus, it remains unclear why, even in cases without treatment, the number of diplococci detected in microvessels, similar to meningococcus, varies so much. No one has ever tried to explain the greater clinical effectiveness in the treatment of meningococcemia of a bactericidal drug (penicillin family) compared to a bacteriostatic drug (levomycetinum family for example), although theoretically penicillin should exacerbate the development of endotoxin shock. Many other issues related to the characteristics of immune responses and the identification of the pathogen remain unclear. In principle, meningococcemia can occur at any age. However, it is much more common (and for reasons that are not entirely clear) to develop in children. According to the literature, the clinical course of meningococcemia in children is characterized by an acute onset with a rise in temperature to 38–39 °C [5–7]. Characteristic is the appearance on the skin a few hours after the onset of the disease of a hemorrhagic rash of various sizes and shapes from small-point petechial to extensive hemorrhage: the most typical hemorrhagic rash is in the form of irregular stars, dense to the touch, protruding above the skin level (Fig. 9.1). The number of elements of the rash is very different—from single ones to covering the entire surface of the body. Often, a hemorrhagic rash is combined with roseolous or roseolous-papular elements. The latter may precede the appearance of hemorrhage. Since the rash does not occur at the same time, the different elements of the rash in the same patient have different colors. Most often, the rash is localized on the buttocks, back of the thighs and shins, eyelids, and sclera, less often on the face. The reverse development of the rash depends on its nature and the extent of the skin lesion. Roseolous and roseolous-papular rashes quickly disappear, leaving no traces. Significant hemorrhages in the skin often give necrosis (Fig. 9.2), followed by rejection of necrotic areas; after rejection, scars may remain. In 3–5% of patients with meningococcemia, joint damage is noted, most often fingers, but the ankle, wrist, knee, and hip joints can also be affected. The intensity of their damage is different—from a barely noticeable swelling to purulent inflammation with redness of the skin, edema, fluctuation, and exudates in the cavity. With recovery, the function of the joints is fully restored. Occasionally, iridocyclitis is observed, in which

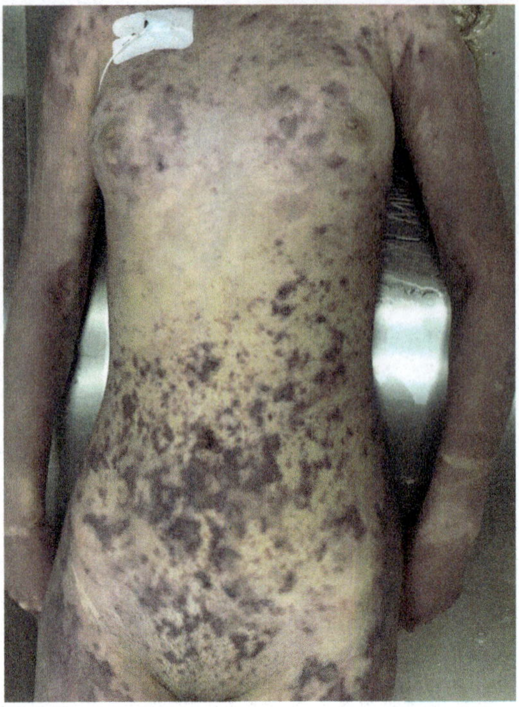

Fig. 9.1 Typical hemorrhagic rash in the deceased due to meningococcemia. Courtesy of A.N. Isakov

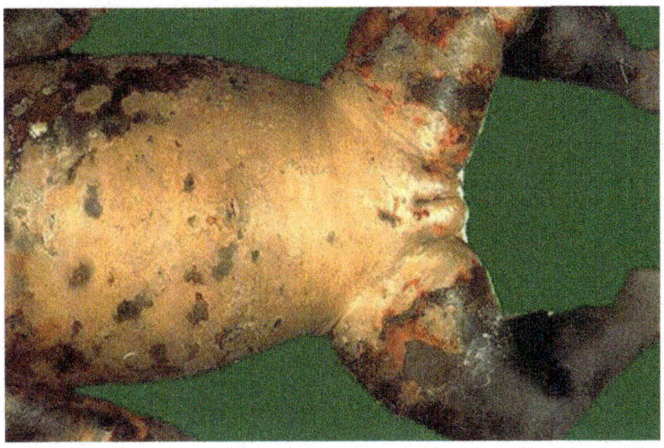

Fig. 9.2 Hemorrhagic rash and skin necrosis in child died on the 7 day of meningococcemia

the color of the iris often acquires a rusty hue, as well as conjunctivitis. The temperature in meningococcemia is most often intermittent. During 1–2 days of illness, the temperature is usually high (39–41 °C). Attention is drawn to pronounced intoxication, tachycardia, less often mild cyanosis, and a decrease in blood pressure. Often there is shortness of breath, dry skin, overlaid tongue, increased thirst, lack of appetite. Possible urinary retention, older children have constipation. Infants may have loose stools. In some cases, hepatolienal syndrome is detected, and the liver and spleen remain soft, and therefore are not always well palpated. With a severe course of the disease, the appearance of proteinuria, microhematuria, leukocyturia, a decrease in glomerular filtration, indicating the development of glomerulonephritis, is possible. Among the metabolic changes, meningococcemia is most characterized by metabolic acidosis, arterial hypoxemia, venous hyperoxia, and hypocapnia. Most patients in the acute period of the disease have a decrease in the level of potassium in the plasma. The hemogram is usually characterized by high leukocytosis (20–40 × 10^9/l), neutrophils shift to young, and sometimes to myelocytes, aneosinophilia, and an increase in ESR. A decrease in white blood cell count is a poor prognostic sign. Meningitis can develop simultaneously with meningococcemia, but more often on the 2–3 days of the disease. With a severe course of the disease, disorders of consciousness, convulsions, or focal symptoms of the nervous system are detected. There are different approaches to classifying meningococcemia. We agree to base the classification on the degree of shock: no shock, shock of I, II, III, and IV degrees.

We analyzed the clinical course of the most severe forms of meningococcemia, which ended fatally in 108 children [8]. The children were admitted to the intensive care unit in an extremely serious and terminal condition with a rapid increase in intoxication and rash. Thus, the time from the rise in body temperature to admission to the hospital ranged from four to 12 hours (an average of 10 h), the time from the appearance of a rash to admission to the hospital—from two to 10 h, more often 4–6 h. Forty-nine patients stayed in the hospital from 10 min to 6 h. The duration of the disease in them was about a day. Eighteen patients stayed in the hospital for 12–24 h, 21 children for more than a day. In children, there was a rapid development of manifestations of toxicosis. The condition was regarded as extremely serious. The skin is sharply pale, pronounced cyanosis, a large hemorrhagic rash spreading throughout the body with the formation of extensive purplish cyanotic areas on the upper and lower extremities, venous stasis of the "cadaverous spots" on the posterior surface of the trunk. All patients had severe symptoms of toxicosis, a decrease in blood pressure to 40% of normal or to zero values, tachycardia of more than 200% with a violation of the heart rhythm, tachypnea of more than 170% with a violation of the respiratory rhythm, which required the use of resuscitation aids and artificial ventilation. In the intensive care unit, patients were given large doses of hormones and dopamine. Some of the children received several sessions of hemosorbtion during their stay in the hospital, antimeningococcal plasma was transfused, and ultraviolet irradiation of the blood was performed. All children showed signs of DIC-syndrome, the leading manifestation of which was hemorrhagic necrosis of the adrenal glands, detected in 94.7% of the deceased. Structural changes in this most severe form of meningococcal infection consist of moderately pronounced inflammatory changes and sharply prevailing in the clinical and morphological manifestations of circulatory disorders, primarily caused by thrombo-hemorrhagic syndrome (THC).

Microscopically, it is typical to detect small clusters of meningococci in the tissues of various organs, surrounded by a very moderate loose neutrophil-lymphocytic infiltration. Most naturally (in 46% of cases, based on our material), they are observed in the soft meninges, less often in the heart, liver, kidneys, skin, and occasionally in the thymus and lungs. Certain patterns in the timing of development and the degree of severity of lesions of various organs cannot be identified. A distinct predominantly neutrophilic infiltration of the soft meninges in isolated cases is observed already on the first day from the onset of the disease, along with this, it may be absent in the death of children on 3–5 days. It is also necessary to mention the possibility of a discrepancy between a certain cytosis in the cerebrospinal fluid (460 x 10^6/l) in vivo (a few hours before death) and the complete absence of inflammatory infiltration of the soft meninges during post-mortem histological examination. It should be noted that in terms of observations, quite significant clusters of microbes can be detected without a significant reaction to them. Such findings are most frequent in smears from the tracheal mucosa, less often in the lumen of the renal tubules and occasionally in the lungs. Macroscopically, inflammatory changes except for moderate thickening and turbidity of the soft meninges are not determined. A mandatory component in meningococcemia is the manifestation of THS. In typical cases, the most important diagnostic value is the rash. With a minimal degree of severity (roseolous rash), a histological examination reveals a stagnant fullness of small venules with swelling of the vascular endothelium and minor serous edema. With a greater severity of the process (petechial rash), in addition, small extravasates and very moderate lymphocytic infiltration of mainly the walls of blood vessels are detected. Occasionally, blood clots are detected in the lumen of small vessels. There are dystrophic changes in the multilayer squamous epithelium. Meningococci in the lumen of the vessels or in the perivascular space are detected intermittently and often in small quantities. Microbial microthrombs described in the literature are detected extremely rarely. In the case of a spilled rash, in addition, diffuse blood penetration of all layers of the skin and areas of necrosis are determined. Macroscopically, small elements are initially noted in the skin, which have the character of roseolous and roseolous papular. Subsequently, there is an increase in the size of the hemorrhagic rash, which often takes on a stellate shape. In the center of large drain elements, yellowish areas of necrosis may be noted. The most unfavorable in prognostic terms are spilled elements in the extremities. Depending on the age of the rash, the elements can be bright red, reddish-bluish, or brownish. The most typical localization of the rash is on the buttocks, the back of the thighs, and shins. With a severe course of the disease, the rash is located on the entire surface of the body. It should be noted that in the first hours after death, the rash may slightly change its appearance, while becoming more clearly delineated from the surrounding tissues. Another major manifestation of THS, developing, according to our data, in parallel with the development of the rash, is the defeat of the adrenal glands. In most cases, total or subtotal hemorrhages are detected, followed by necrosis of both the cortical and medullary matter. In some cases, changes of this kind are focal in nature and only occasionally in the adrenal glands, only pronounced fullness with small perivascular hemorrhages is determined (Fig. 9.3a,b). Some of the small vessels are thrombosed, and a moderate amount of diplococci can be found in them. Cortical cells outside the hemorrhage zone are rich in lipids and nucleic acids. Other characteristic locations of hemorrhage in meningococcal infections include the mucous membranes of the digestive tract, trachea, and bladder, as well as, although less frequently, the soft meninges, lungs, endo - and pericardium, thymus, spleen, and other organs. It is not possible to identify patterns in the degree of damage to various organs. Hemorrhages are more often pinpointed and are arranged in groups. Histological examination in these areas often determines the swelling of all layers of the vascular wall, rounding and increase in the size of the endothelial nuclei. Microthrombosis and significant concentrations of diplococci in these areas are relatively rare. Thrombosis of small vessels in the capillaries of

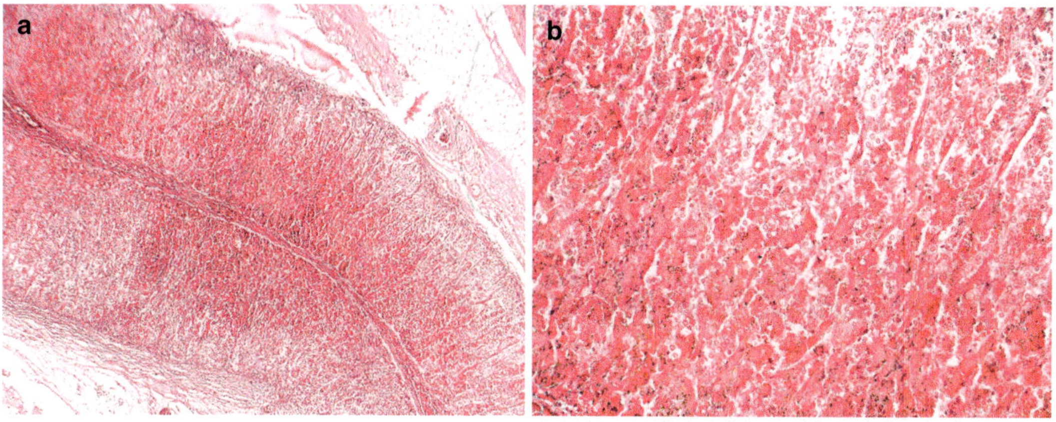

Fig. 9.3 Hemorrhages in adrenals in meningococcemia in a child. Stained H.-E. (**a**)- × 250; (**b**) × 400

the renal glomeruli, choroidal plexuses, as well as the lungs and spleen, is more natural. Often identified kidney lesions can be associated with THS. Pronounced alterative changes in the epithelium of the convoluted tubules are detected in almost all observations, and in some of them, especially in clinically pronounced renal insufficiency, there is a clear picture of coagulation necrosis of the epithelium of the convoluted tubules. We also studied the dynamics of thrombosis depending on the duration of meningococcemia using colors according to Mallory, and orange-red-blue on a limited material (Fig. 9.4a,b,c). The results of the study showed that in the first hours of meningococcemia, damage to the platelet and vascular components of hemostasis prevails. During histological examination, the appearance of platelet aggregates was typical. With an increase in the duration of the disease, the phenomena of thrombocytopenia, generalized thrombosis of small vessels, consumption, coagulation, and activation of fibrinolysis increase, which leads to the development of common hemorrhages. In histological examination at the end of the second day, the presence of hyaline blood clots in the capillaries is typical. The nature of hemostatic disorders depends little on the volume and nature of resuscitation measures in the terminal period. Meningococcemia often occurs on the background of violations of the immune system. In histological examination, the changes detected in the organs of the immune system are heterogeneous. In some cases, there is a gradual development of accidental transformation of the thymus, accompanied by a significant loss of lymphocytes from the peripheral immune organs. In other observations, there are pronounced changes in the peripheral lymph nodes and spleen, up to karyorrhexis and fibrinoid necrosis in the light centers, developing against the background of seemingly relatively moderate changes in the thymus. Finally, in part of the observations, it is possible to identify the initial, and sometimes clearly expressed follicle-like structures in the thymus, indicating the appearance of B-dependent zones in it. In a few cases, there is a distinct hyperplasia of the light centers of the spleen, tonsils, and lymph nodes, which are rich in plasma and blast cells. There is no direct natural dependence of these structural changes on the time elapsed from the onset of the disease.

In the recent time on the stage appeared the new serotype of N. meningitides W-135 [9]. Which leads to the most severe course is in older children and adults; subacute appearance of hemorrhagic exanthema from 6 h to 3 days from the onset of the disease; severe lymphopenia and a higher level of CRP; more pronounced exudative cellular character of organ lesions in meningococcemia; involvement of the cortical hemispheres (meningoencephalitis); formation of foci of necrobiosis and necrosis of brain substance (including with intracerebral hemorrhages) (Fig. 9.5). Recent publications show that clinical course and pathological picture remain similar [10].

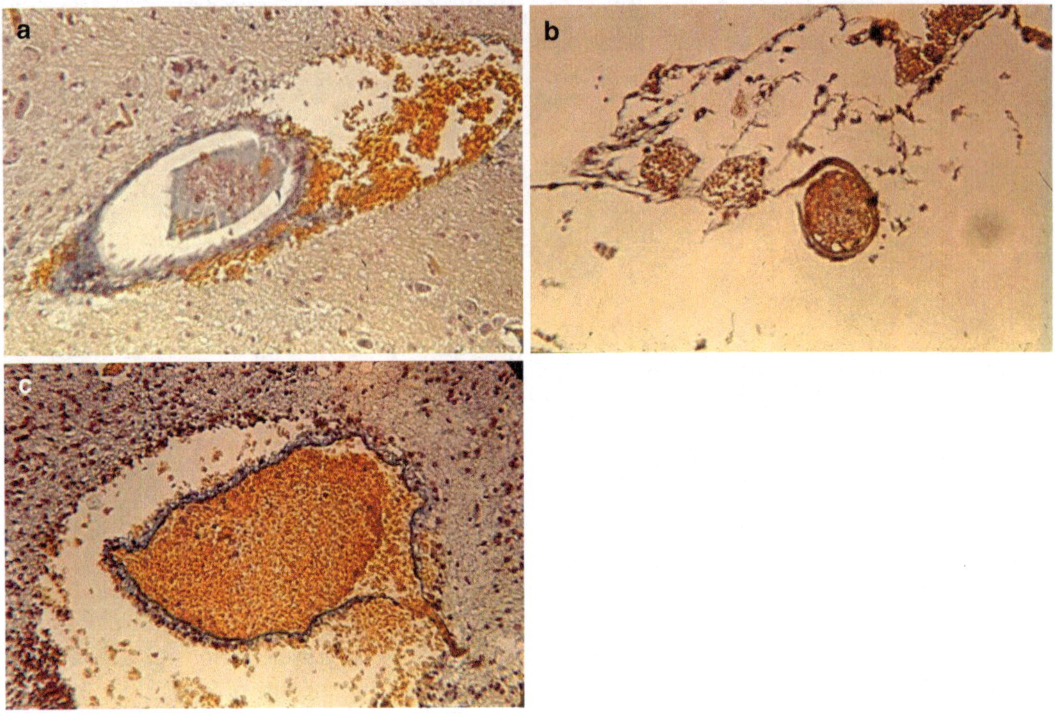

Fig. 9.4 Formation of thrombi in the brain of a child died from meningococcemia. Stained by Martius Scarlet Blue. (**a**) Formation of fibrin thrombus and perivascular hemorrhage. x100; (**b**) Development of predominantly thrombocytic thrombus, ×100; (**c**) Formation of erythrocytic thrombus, ×200

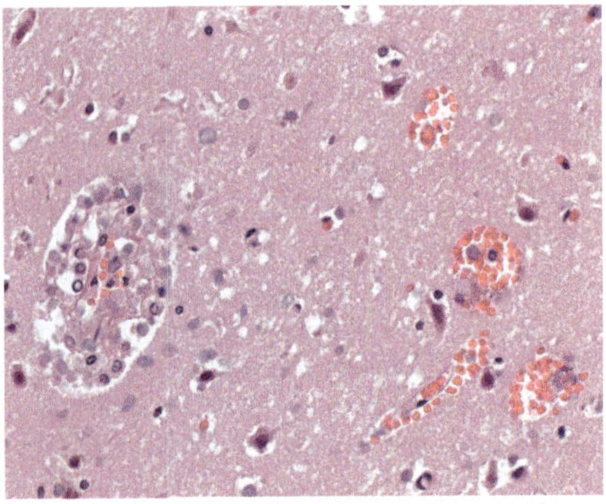

Fig. 9.5 Encephalitis due N.menigitidis W-135. Stained by H.E. ×100 Courtesy of V.E. Karev

9.2 Meningococcal Meningitis in Children

Clinical manifestations of this disease in children are characterized by an acute onset with the appearance of typical cerebral and meningeal symptoms. On our material [8], the presence of single petechiae was noted in 2/3 of the patients. Convulsive seizures at the prehospital stage were observed in 1/5 of patients. Epileptic status developed only in isolated children. Compared with other forms of purulent meningitis, consciousness was more often preserved or stunned (26.3%). Less than 30% of patients were admitted in a state of constipation and coma. Indicators of the extreme severity of the condition are disorders of the frequency and rhythm of breathing (less than 20%), with the appearance of which about half of the patients die. Neurological symptoms are characterized by "flickering" of focal symptoms, anisoreflexia and hyperreflexia are detected in the vast majority of patients. Pronounced hemiparesis was detected in nine patients (15.0%), which recovered by the end of the acute period. Almost half of the children had cranial nerve lesions. One- or two-sided ptosis, pupil constriction, anisocoria, floating movements of the eyeballs, converging and diverging strabismus were more often detected, which in 15 patients was combined with respiratory disorders.

Disorders on the part of other cranial nerves were unstable and passed during the first or second week of the disease. Paresis of the facial muscles of the central type, vestibular ataxia were also revealed. Four patients developed hearing loss.

The analysis of neurological symptoms showed that in meningococcal meningitis, the main manifestations of the disease were pronounced cerebral and meningeal symptoms caused by intracranial hypertension. With EchoEG, the expansion of the M-echo to 10–12 mm, an increase in the index of the cerebral and ventricles of the brain, the appearance of additional pulsations were determined. Pronounced diffuse disturbances of bioelectric activity with a predominance of slow-wave activity were noted on the EEG. Pronounced cerebrospinal hypertension was also detected during lumbar puncture: the cerebrospinal pressure increased to 30–34 mmHg. (300–400 mm of water), averaging 29.4 ± 1.3 mmHg; perfusion pressure was more often within the normal range or decreased slightly and amounted to 60.7 ± 3.2 mmHg. In children admitted on the first day of the disease, cytosis was 330.5 × 10^6/l ± 31.3, there was an increase in cytosis within 12–48 hours after the start of therapy, the maximum index was 2493 ± 620 × 10^6/l in half of cases, up to 6720 ± 130 × 10^6/l in a third of cases, 10,000 × 10^6/l in 10 patients, which indicated high BBB permeability.

In cases of uncomplicated purulent meningitis, CT and MRI scans are usually little changed. The images obtained with the help of FLAIR IP may show a moderately hyperintensive signal from the cerebrospinal fluid in the subshell space, compared with the cerebrospinal fluid in the ventricles of the brain or other parts of the unchanged subarachnoid space. Exudate accumulation is usually localized primarily in the projection of the frontal lobes and along the interhemispheric fissure. At the same time, sometimes there is a slight smoothness of the convolutions. The most reliable sign of the inflammatory process is a selective increase in the intensity of the signal from the brain membranes in postcontrast images.

During cytological examination of CSF at the beginning of the disease, a neutrophil reaction with pronounced destruction of cells was noted, which is why accurate counting of cellular elements was sometimes impossible. Single monocytes and lymphoid cells (0.5–1%) were present in clusters of neutrophils. A large number of bean-shaped diplococci were located inside and extracellularly, the percentage of phagocytosis was 43–50%. In 1/3 of cases, the early appearance of macrophages, which make up 2–3% of cells, was noted.

Unlike other purulent meningitis, the cytogram of the cerebrospinal fluid in meningococcal meningitis changes rapidly, due to its sanitation, which is evidenced by the disappearance of bacteria, the typical forms of which are not determined bacterioscopically already on the third-fourth day of the disease. At the same time, there is a 2–three-fold decrease in cytosis, there is a distinct tendency to increase the number of mononuclears. The content of small, medium and large lymphocytes increases to 7–15%, monocytes—up to 6–10%, plasmocytes—up to 0.2–0.5%. On the 5th–sixth day, the lymphoid-monocyte type of reaction becomes the main one and indicates recovery. The exception was five patients, in whose cerebrospinal fluid smears meningococci were detected until the 5th–7th day of the disease, the rehabilitation of their cerebrospinal fluid was delayed until the 12th–14th day of the disease. In four cases complicated by subdural effusion, CSF sanitation occurred only at the third week of the disease.

Changes in peripheral blood were characterized by leukocytosis up to 10–20 × 109/l with a shift of the formula to the left: up to 4–20 rod-shaped in half of the patients, in 10 patients—up to young cells and up to myelocytes—in three children. During treatment, the onset of cerebrospinal fluid sanitation was accompanied by normalization of the leukocyte formula in most children, except for 13 patients whose course of the disease was complicated by acute respiratory viral infections and pneumonia.

During the pathological study, in all five lethally terminated observations, there was a

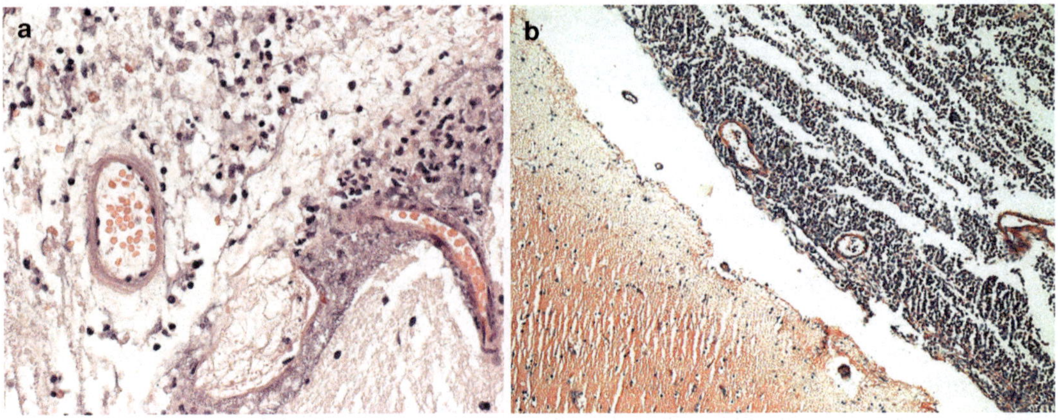

Fig. 9.6 Menigococcal meningitis in a child. Stained by azur-eosine. (**a**) Mixed infiltration of the meninges at the early stage of the disease, several free lying and phagocytized cocci. ×650; (**b**) Dense neutrophilic infiltration of the meninges. ×100

characteristic morphological picture of purulent meningoencephalitis.

In thanatogenesis, only in two cases we can talk about the significance of meningoencephalitis, which led to a sharp swelling of the brain and dislocation of the trunk. Meningoencephalitis was diagnosed in vivo, the child received appropriate dehydration therapy, which proved ineffective due to the development of anuria (in the section—necrosis of the cortical layer of the kidneys). In the second case, a child who was admitted in a terminal state was found to have purulent meningitis of the brain and spinal cord and local encephalitis of the trunk, which was obviously the cause of sudden respiratory arrest and ineffectiveness of the resuscitation aid.

Of the 60 patients, 51 recovered completely; five died in the acute period, four had moderately pronounced hemiparesis, two had deafness.

Morphological changes in the case of currently very rare deaths from this form of meningococcal infection almost completely correspond to detailed classical descriptions.

Microscopic examination reveals a gradually increasing infiltration of the soft meninges, represented mainly by neutrophilic leukocytes with an admixture of lymphocytes, monocytes and a small number of eosinophils (Fig. 9.6a,b). Maximally dense infiltrates with a large participation of lymphoid cells are formed around blood vessels and in their walls. Clusters of neutrophilic leukocytes and small blood clots are usually detected in the lumen of the vessels. Similar, though much less pronounced changes are observed in the wall of the cerebral ventricles. In the substance of the brain, inflammatory changes are usually determined in the form of purulent vasculitis, capturing mainly the vessels adjacent to the soft meninges and ventricles of the brain. In addition, there are pronounced degenerative and ischemic changes in nerve and glial cells. In the late stages of the development of the process (starting from 5 to 6 days from the onset of the disease), along with predominantly decaying neutrophilic leukocytes, the number of monocytes, lymphocytes and macrophages increases significantly, moderate fibrin deposits are noted. Exudate resorption occurs. Later, fibroblasts also appear, and the production of a few collagen fibers begins. Mainly around the ventricles there is a proliferation of glia. Perivascular lymphoplasmacytic infiltrates also appear.

Macroscopically, the inflammatory process developing in the meninges is initially serous-purulent in nature. From 2 to 3 days, the exudate becomes purulent and accumulates mainly in the form of yellowish-gray masses in the furrows around the veins. Purulent infiltration can initially be located both on the basal, particularly around the intersection of the optic nerves, and on the convexital surface. In some cases, the entire brain may be covered with a continuous layer of yellowish-green purulent masses. The exudate that performs the subarachnoid spaces and impregnates the soft shell in the first days of the disease is liquid, subsequently it turns into a soft elastic purulent fibrinous mass. From the medulla oblongata, the inflammatory process can directly pass to the membranes of the cranial and spinal nerves. Changes in the spinal cord, at least according to the data of children's and adult autopsies of St. Petersburg, are unstable and usually expressed relatively moderately.

Convalescents of purulent meningitis have had thickening and whitishness of the soft meninges for at least several weeks.

Among the complications of meningococcal meningitis in previous years, internal hydrocephalus was most often described, leading to atrophy of the brain substance. This complication, as well as other, rarer and earlier processes (neuritis, subdural abscesses), are currently practically not found at the autopsy. Recently appeared new data concerning the mechanisms of overcoming of BBB by meningococci [11].

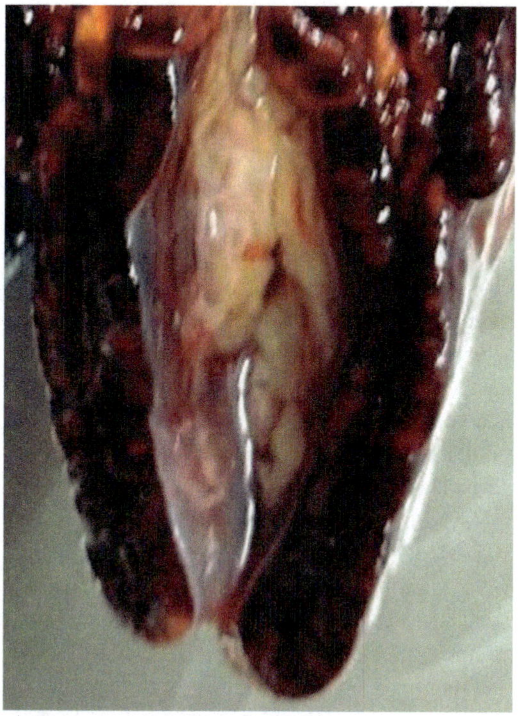

Fig. 9.7 Subtotal hemorrhage in adrenals in an adult. Courtesy of A.N. Isakov

9.3 Meningococcal Infection in Adults

Based on the material of pathology department of SP Botkin infectious hospital in the period from 2001 to 2020, 69 cases of meningococcal infection in adults aged 18–86 years were analyzed. It is possible to note some fluctuations in its frequency on the autopsy material. In most cases, the development of meningococcemia was noted, in about half of the observations in combination with incipient purulent meningitis. The clinical picture of the disease was typical with the development of a characteristic hemorrhagic rash in the first 12 hours of the disease (see Fig. 9.1). In three people with a missing spleen, it was less pronounced. All persons over 30 years of age have a diverse comorbid pathology. The most common direct death cause was hemorrhages in the adrenal glands (Fig. 9.7), within the framework of the Waterhouse-Frederichsen syndrome, which was considered as a manifestation of infectious-toxic shock along with other signs of DIC. In isolated cases of isolated meningitis (mainly in elderly people), edema-swelling of the brain was considered as the direct cause of death. In the literature as a very seldom form empyema is described [12].

9.4 Experimental Models of Meningococcal Infection

In the literature of various years, it is shown that meningococcal infection in animals is practically not modeled [13]. In our study [8], performed jointly with bacteriologist N. A. Korzhuyeva, and virologists O. A. Aksenov and E. A. Murina, it was also shown that intranasal infection of mongrel white mice with various strains of Meningococcus resulted only in short-term (up to 1 day) neutrophil infiltration in the lungs and their edema. Microbes, according to both bacteriological and histobacterioscopic studies, did not multiply and did not cause generalized infection. In the case of mixed influenza-meningococcal infection (see also Chap. 18), it was possible to show a significant severe process in comparison with monoinfections. At the same time, despite the negative results of bacteriological cultures (conducted according to the standard scheme for diagnosing meningococcal infection in patients), a number of data allowed us to talk about the development of an infectious process caused by meningococcus in these mice. Positive effect of treatment of mice with mixed infection with penicillin was shown. According to our data, small diplococci were detected in the lungs and brain during histobacterioscopic examination, which were absent in all control and comparison groups. In some animals, the histological picture of bacterial lung damage and meninges was also determined. Bacterial-like structures were found in the brain and in EM. We postulated the presence of a mixed infectious process in mice infected with various influenza viruses and meningococci.

References

1. Hollingshead S, Tang CM. An overview of Neisseria meningitidis. Methods Mol Biol. 2019;1969(1):1–16. https://doi.org/10.1007/978-1-4939-9202-7_1.
2. Read RC. *Neisseria meningitidis* and meningococcal disease: recent discoveries and innovations. Curr Opin Infect Dis. 2019;32:601–8.
3. Sjölinder H, Jonson AB. Olfactory nerve—a novel invasion route of *Neisseria meningitidis* to reach the meninges. PLoS One. 2010;5:e14034.
4. Dando SA, Mackay-Sim A, Norton R, et al. Pathogens penetrating the central nervous system: infection pathways and the cellular and molecular mechanisms of invasion. Clin Microbiol Rev. 2014;27(4):691–726.
5. Campbell H, Borrow R, Arrumugan C, et al. Invasive meningococcal disease as a cause of sudden and unexpected death in a teenager: the public health importance of confirming the diagnosis. J Infect. 2019;78:323–37.
6. Beebeejaun K, Parikh SR, Campbell H, et al. Invasive meningococcal disease: timing and cause of death in England, 2008–2015. J Infect. 2020;80:286–90.
7. Wang B, Santoreneos R, Giles L, et al. Case fatality rates of invasive meningococcal disease by serogroup and age: a systematic review and meta-analysis. Vaccine. 2019;37:2768–82.
8. Zinserling VA, Chukhlovina ML. Infectious lesions of the nervous system. Issues of etiology, pathogenesis, and diagnostics. Saint-Petersburg: ElbiSPb; 2011. p. 583. (In Russian)
9. Krone M, Gray S, Abad R, et al. Increase of invasive meningococcal serogroup W disease in Europe, 2013–2017. Euro Surveill. 2019;24(14):1–9.
10. Brady RC. Meningococcal infection in children and adolescents: update and prevention. Adv Pediatr Infect Dis. 2020;67:29–46. https://doi.org/10.1016/yapd.2020.03.007.
11. Jamil Al-Obaidi MM, Mohd Desa MN. Mechanisms of blood brain barrier disruption by different types of bacteria, and bacterial-host interactions facilitate the bacterial pathogen invading the brain. Cell Mol Neurobiol. 2018;38:1349–68.
12. Bajaj D, Agraval A, Gandhi D et al. (2018), Intraventricular empyema caused by Neisseria meningitides ID Cases, 15:1–4 https://doi.org/10.1016/j.idcr2019.e00503.
13. Orihuella CJ, Machdavi J, Thornton J, et al. Laminin receptor initiates bacterial contact with the blood-brain barrier in experimental meningitides model. J Clin Invest. 2009;119:1638–46. https://doi.org/10.1172/JCI36759.

Purulent Meningitis and Meningoencephalitis

10

Purulent meningitis stays an important death threating disease able also to lead to invalidity. Strictly we usually deal with leptomeningitis, simultaneously involving in purulent inflammation pia mater and tunica arachnoidea. Inflammation in dura mater is called pachymeningitis and usually develops as result of brain trauma. Diagnosing purulent meningoencephalitis, we postulate brain matter involvement as vasculitis and/or choroiditis and epididymitis. It is important to note that structural changes in viral and bacterial encephalitis are quite different. According to localization of inflammation can be distinguished basal and cerebrospinal meningitis. Due to clinical history primary and secondary (as complication of otitis, sinusitis and pneumonia) are discriminated. Etiology of purulent meningitis includes waste spectrum of microorganisms, but in practice we usually meet *meningococcus, pneumococcus, haemophilus influenzae*. But we have to note that even in specialized departments exact etiology may not be established. (Figs. 10.1, 10.2, 10.3, 10.4, 10.5). Certain aspects of pathogenesis have been discussed before in Chap. 2.

10.1 Pneumococcal Meningoencephalitis

One of the most common pathogens of meningoencephalitis is pneumococci (*Streptococcus pneumoniae*) of various serotypes, having a lanceolate shape, arranged in pairs, Gram-positive and sometimes having a mucous capsule. Pneumococcus was discovered in 1886, and its historical name is diplococcus Weichselbaum-Fränkel, after the name of the authors who identified it in pure culture. Until now, not all microbiologists share the validity of including Pneumococcus in the genus Streptococcus for a number of phenotypic features. P. are widely distributed among the population. Detailed modern data related to the pathogen have been reviewed [1–3]. Histopathology of pneumococcal lung lesions was updated by us [4].

In terms of frequency, pneumococcal meningoencephalitis (PME) occupies the second or third place in patients older than 1 year, accounting for 10–15% of the total number of purulent meningoencephalitis. The mortality rate in pneumococcal meningoencephalitis even in conditions of complex therapy with the appointment of massive doses of antibiotics reaches 30–50%, which significantly exceeds the corresponding indicators in purulent meningoencephalitis of other etiologies. In recent years, there has been evidence of the existence of particularly virulent neurotropic clones of *Pneumococcus,* and receptors for it have been identified on the surface of endothelial cells in the central nervous system [5]. In addition, it was shown that in the subarachnoid space, there is no purification of the cerebrospinal fluid from pneumococci, as it is carried out in the bloodstream by the spleen, and

V. Zinserling, *Infectious Lesions of the Central Nervous System*,
https://doi.org/10.1007/978-3-030-96260-9_10

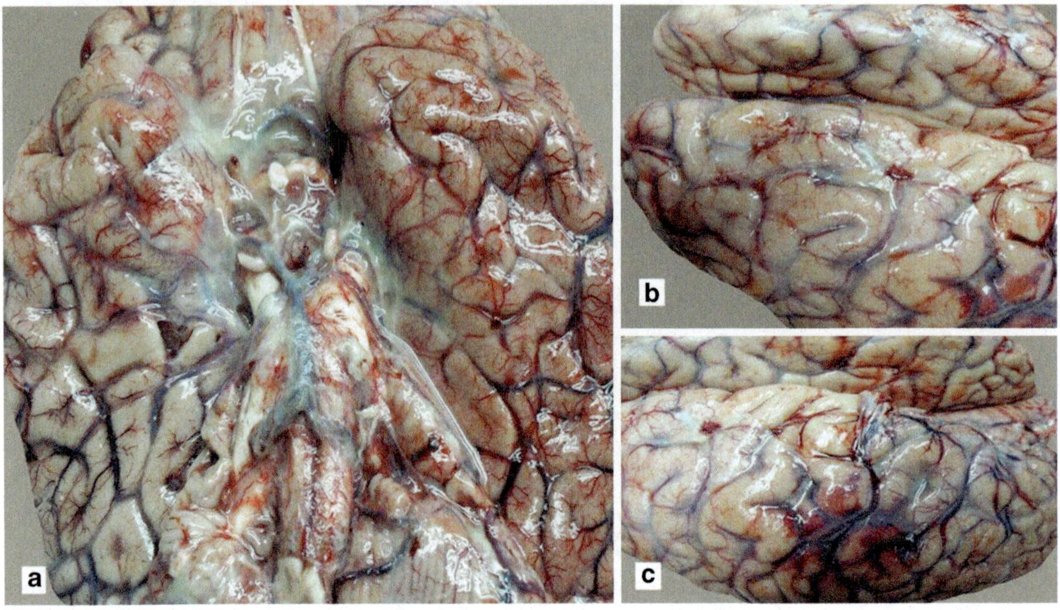

Fig. 10.1 Purulent leptomeningitis in adult of unknown etiology. Pronounced fullness and purulent impregnation of the soft meninges. (**a**) The soft meninges of the base of the brain, inflammation is spread throughout the basal surface of the brain; (**b**, **c**) Lesions of the soft meninges of the convexital surfaces of the brain. Unfixed macropreparations (courtesy of Y.R. Zyuzya)

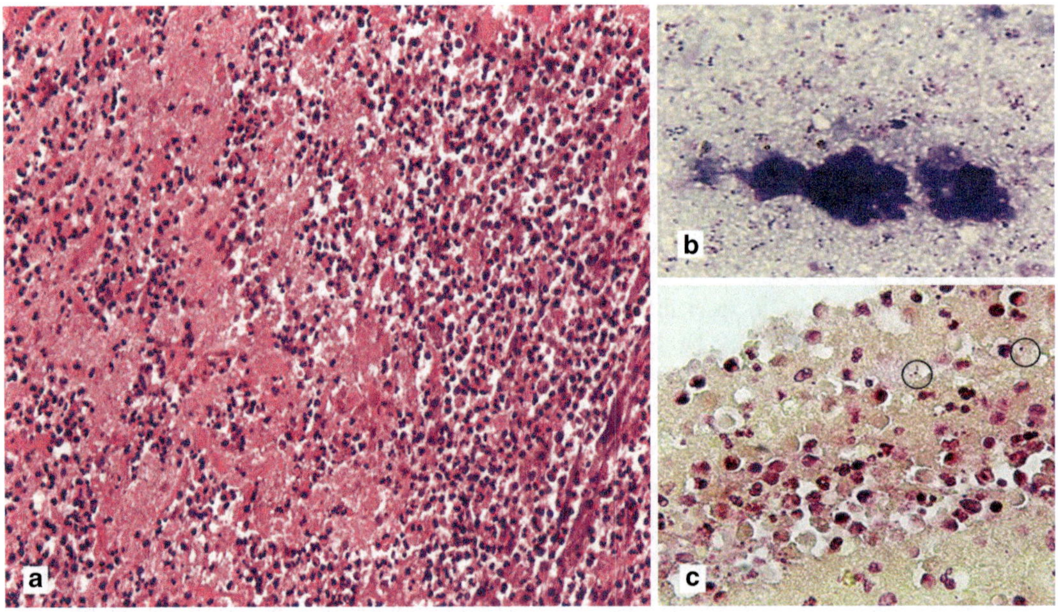

Fig. 10.2 Purulent encephalitis in adult of unknown etiology. (**a**) Pronounced leukocyte infiltration of the brain substance; (**b**) In the smear-imprint of the focus of purulent inflammation, leukocytes and an abundance of coccal microflora; (**c**) Gram-positive coccal microflora in the area of purulent inflammation (circled with round frames). (**a**) H-E. X100; (**b**) methylene blue staining. ×1000 (cytological preparation); (**b**) – Brown-Hopps staining. ×1000 (courtesy of Y.R. Zyuzya)

neutrophilic leukocytes in the cerebrospinal fluid do not have bactericidal properties [6].

Ideas about the pathogenesis and pathological picture of mainly secondary pneumococcal meningitis developed in the 20–30s of the twentieth century. At the same time, all researchers emphasized the identity of changes in purulent meningitis of various etiologies. Subsequently, the original publications devoted to this problem were practically absent in the literature, and only brief summary morphological descriptions of purulent meningoencephalitis of various etiologies were given in the relevant sections of the generalized manual. At the same time, the presence of a number of clinical features of pneumococcal meningoencephalitis was constantly pointed out.

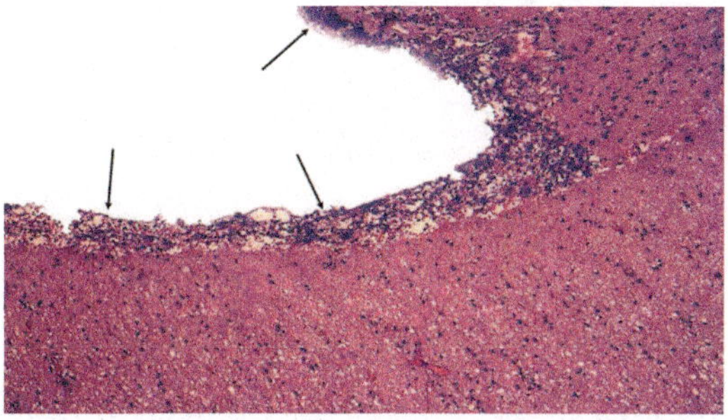

Fig. 10.3 Purulent ventriculitis in adult of unknown etiology. H-E. ×100 (courtesy of Y.R. Zyuzya)

Clinical manifestations of the disease in children are characterized, according to our data [6], by acute development, a rapid increase in toxicosis. Only half of the patients report about the presence of a primary focus of infection (otitis, sinusitis, pneumonia), in other cases, meningitis developed as a primary infection of the central nervous system. In all cases, children had a rapid rise in temperature to 39-40 °C. Evidence of neurotoxicosis was the persistence of hyperthermia, or sharp fluctuations in body temperature from 40 to 35 °C for several hours, which were accompanied by pronounced vegetative symptoms—pallor, hyperemia, hyperhidrosis of the head, change of tachy and bradycardia, indicating early lesions of the hypothalamic structures of the brain. In infants, there was lethargy, anxiety, refusal to eat, in older children severe headache, repeated vomiting. In 1/3 of cases, focal symptoms appeared: strabismus, ptosis, paresis of the extremities, local and general convulsive seizures. The children were admitted in an extremely serious con-

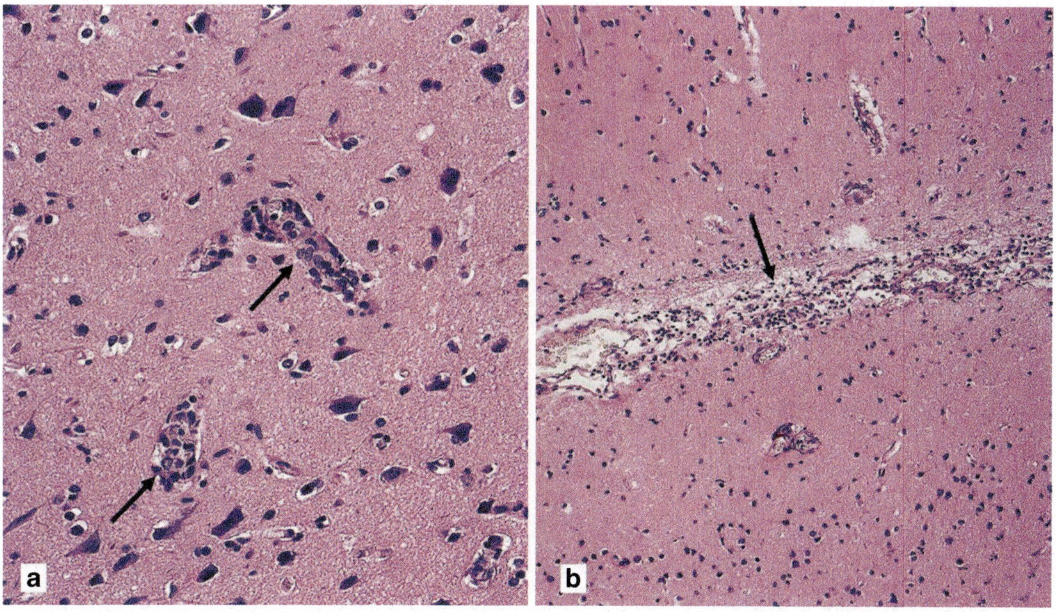

Fig. 10.4 Purulent meningoencephalitis in adult of unknown etiology. (**a**) Productive reactive capillaritis; (**b**) Productive perivasculitis. H-E (**a**) – ×400; (**b**) – ×100 (courtesy of Y.R. Zyuzya)

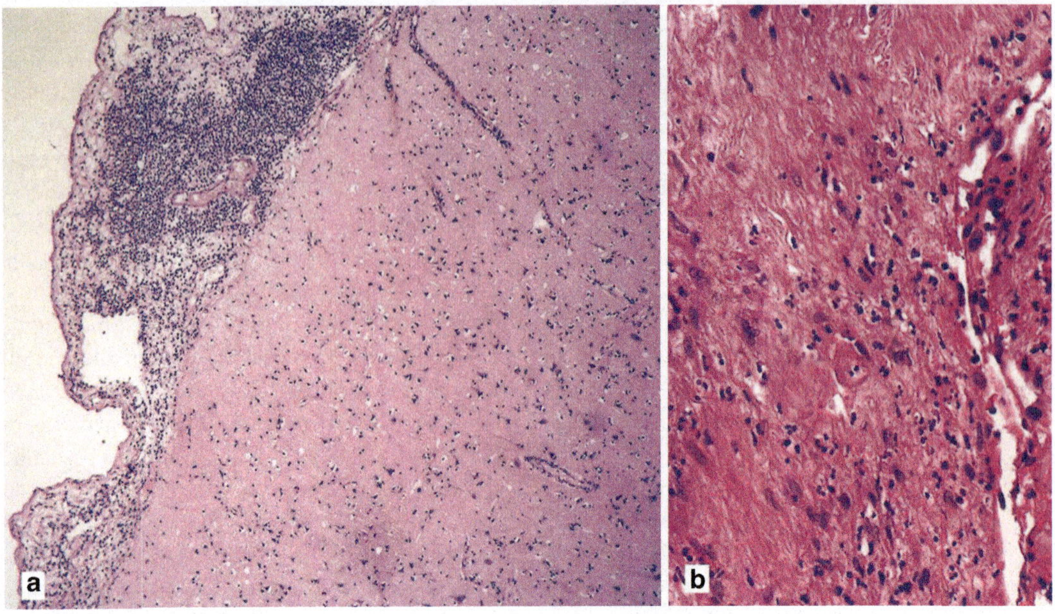

Fig. 10.5 Purulent leptomeningitis in adult of unknown etiology. Edema, fullness of blood, leukocyte infiltration of the soft meninges. H-E **a** – ×100; **b** – ×400 (courtesy of Y.R. Zyuzya)

dition with severe hypertension hydrocephalus syndrome. In young children, divergence of the cranial sutures, bulging and tension of the large fontanelle, hydrocephalic sound during cranial percussion, and signs of hypertension were determined according to EchoEG data. However, in four cases, the fontanelle was sunken, and on autopsy in one of these observations, the absence of cerebrospinal fluid in the ventricles of the brain and the subarachnoid space was found, which indicated a violation of the secretion of cerebrospinal fluid and pronounced swelling of the brain. A sharp deterioration of the condition on the 2–4 days of the disease was also characteristic, when meningeal symptoms appeared against the background of toxicosis, disorders of consciousness progressed to sopor and coma, convulsions occurred, and half of the patients developed a convulsive comatose syndrome typical of pneumococcal meningoencephalitis. When patients were admitted to the intensive care unit, meningeal symptoms were detected in 72.5%, there was rigidity of the occipital muscles with less severity, and even the absence of other meningeal symptoms. Generalized and partial seizures, epileptic status, lasting from 2 to 20 h (survival with minimal consequences) or lasting up to 7–12 days. Thus, the convulsive syndrome occurred in 72.5% of cases. Disorders of consciousness were equally severe in children: relative rare of the type of stun, and in more than half of the cases—sopor and coma. They were accompanied by significant respiratory disorders of the central type, up to apnea. Lethality was 43%. The death occurred with the initial respiratory arrest followed by the cessation of cardiovascular activity, in some cases—on the 10th–12th day of the patients stay on the ventilator. Analysis of individual focal symptoms shows that among the deceased, more than half were in a state of decerebration and decortication at the time of death, among the survivors, this pathology was in 36.9% of children. Hemiparesis, developed in half of the patients (54.9%), was often accompanied by Jackson's seizures, was characterized by persistence, slow recovery, and in some of the survivors were observed in the period of late convalescence. A third of the patients had extrapyramidal muscle tone disorders, tremor, myoclonic hyperkinesis, astasia phenomena abasia, ataxia; in children under 1 year a violation of the installation reflexes, which, even with a favorable course, was restored only within 4–6 days. Sensorineural hearing loss was detected in some patients in the period of early convalescence. Symptoms of cranial nerve damage in the form of oculomotor disorders (73.6%), which indicated a predominantly diencephalic-mesencephalic (46.6%) or stem (53.2%) level of damage. The majority of patients (62.0%) initially had a decrease in plasma osmolarity (265 (50.5 mosm/l).

In nine cases with an hyperacute course, the duration of the disease was 12–49 h. All patients were taken to the intensive care unit in a terminal condition. In the clinical picture, attention was drawn to the acute development of toxicosis hyperthermia, lethargy, refusal to eat, tachycardia, shortness of breath, and after 7–20 h—the development of convulsive comatose syndrome with impaired breathing and cardiac activity. Children were admitted with signs of irreversible brain dislocation in the large occipital foramen, and all died in the next few hours while on a ventilator. Five patients had symptoms of DIC syndrome with the presence of a single or widespread spot hemorrhagic rash. In all patients with a hyperacute course, the cerebrospinal fluid during lumbar puncture was changed by the type of protein cell dissociation, neutrophil cytosis was 6–31 × 10^6/l, protein-2.4–3.3 g/l. With lumbar puncture (with patency of the cerebrospinal fluid pathway) or with fontanelle ventricular puncture, high intracerebral pressure was determined, except for few cases with hypotensive syndrome. The values of the liquor pressure were 15–45 mmHg (200–600 mmHg), on average—32.0 ± 4.5 mmHg. Brain perfusion pressure was usually reduced in cases with a fatal outcome—up to 7 mm Hg; the average values were 42.5 ± 13.4 mm Hg and indicated a pronounced violation of cerebral blood flow, which in itself determines the development of cerebral edema. When studying the cerebrospinal fluid in children admitted on the 2–3 days of the disease, cytosis was more often determined from 700 to 5–6 thousand cells in 1 μl, which increases with 10–50 thousand cells in 1 μl in the next 1–2 days. Characteristic of the cytological examination of the cerebrospinal fluid for the most severe course of pneumococcal meningitis (meningoencephalitis) is the mass of bacteria (diplococci in the form of a candle flame) in the field of view, and the number of neutrophils does not correspond to the microbial mass. Usually, bacteria are detected in neutrophils, the cells are destructively changed, sometimes they are differentiated only by the nature of the nuclear substance. Usually, all neutrophils are connected by fibrin filaments in conglomerates. With the predominance of neutrophilic leukocytes, a significant number of choriodic, ependymal, and arachnoendothelial cells were determined, while monocytes and lymphocytes are isolated. Until the 4th–fifth day, the nature of cytosis is monotonous. On the 6-ninth day, and sometimes later, the lympho-monocytic cell reaction begins, small, medium, and large lymphocytes appear, the number of which increases, in contrast to meningococcal meningitis, gradually. By days 9–11, the number of lymphoid cells is 20%, monocytes-10%. At the second week of the disease, macrophages appear, in which bacteria can be detected, and the content of ependymal and arachnoendothelial cells increases. Sanation (the number of cells—up to 30x106/l) occurs with a favorable course by the 14th–17th day, and in complicated cases at the third week of the disease. We observed two patients in whom significant cytosis (800–12,000 in 1 μl) was observed for 6–8 weeks, both children died, and pneumococcus was postmortem isolated from the brain in both cases, which indicates the possibility of a chronically progressive course of pneumococcal meningitis.

V. A. Zinserling et al. [7] conducted a detailed study of 31 children who died from PME. During the first half of life, six children died, nine children died in the second half of life, eight children aged from 1 to 3 years, six children aged from 3 to 7 years, and two children aged over 7 years. Most of the children had a favorable history, only one child had Down's disease and three had perinatal brain damage. Previous severe bacterial pneumonia was not diagnosed in any child, catarrhal or purulent otitis media was observed in only seven children. Several variants of the course of this disease were identified, including: (a) hypertoxic course and duration of the disease to death only 12–48 h (six observations); (b) acute course and death on 3–7 days (20 observations); and c) with an acute course with a transition to chronic progredient and death after 10 days–1.5 months from the beginning of the disease (five observa-

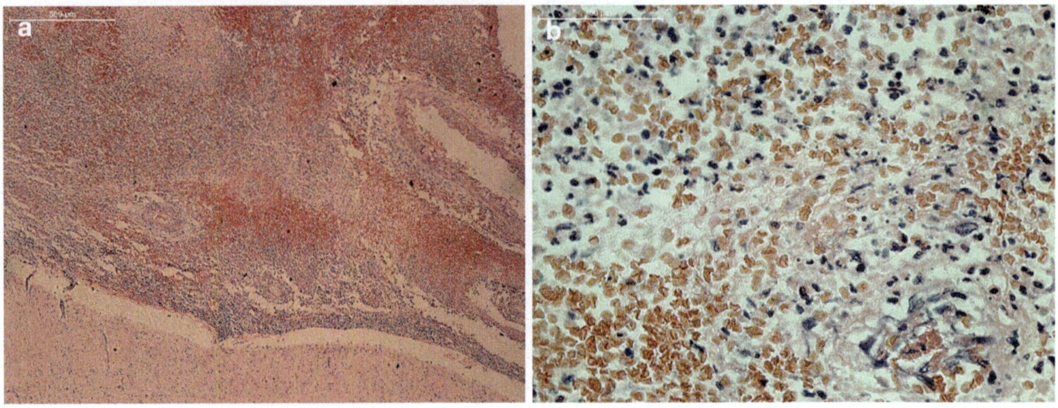

Fig. 10.6 Purulent meningitis due to *S. pneumoniae* in a child. Stained by azur-eosin. (**a**) General view ×100; (**b**) Detail. Note numerous Cocci. ×1000

tions). The hypertoxic course was characterized by the most acute symptoms of neurotoxicosis—persistent hyperthermia, progressive impaired consciousness, shortness of breath, tachycardia, pallor, and after 7–20 h—convulsive comatose and meningeal syndrome with respiratory and cardiovascular disorders. Five patients had a petechial hemorrhagic rash. Lumbar puncture was performed in five patients, in three of them purulent CSF was obtained in two opalescent with changes in the type of protein-cell dissociation. The acute course of PME was characterized by the fact that even in the presence of previous respiratory viral infection, there was a sharp deterioration in the condition in the form of an increase in general cerebral symptoms, autonomic disorders, central hyperthermia, and on the 3–4 days, as a rule, a comatose-convulsive syndrome with pronounced meningeal symptoms developed. Upon admission to the clinic, diencephalic mesencephalic coma was diagnosed in 15 patients, lower-stem coma in 12. Lumbar puncture was performed in 16 patients, 10 of them had purulent cerebrospinal fluid, and six had changes characteristic of protein cell dissociation. A chronically progredient course was observed in five patients with a long stay on artificial lung ventilation. Already 5–7 days after the onset of the disease, symptoms of decortication and decerebration occurred, and neurotrophic disorders progressed. Pneumoencephalography revealed internal and external hydrocephalus, the phenomenon of cystic arachnoiditis. The etiological diagnosis was made based on in vivo and postmortem bacteriological studies. It was possible to type the pathogen in nine cases. Five strains belonged to serotype 1, two to serotype 2, one to serotypes 1 and 19.

Microscopic examination (cytological and histological) in both first groups shows focal clusters of partially phagocytized pneumococci and little-changed neutrophilic leukocytes. Starting from day 2, there is a more intense infiltration of the meninges, which becomes leukocyte-macrophage. Due to these changes and edema, the soft meninges thicken significantly. Along with this, fibrin thrombi in the vessels are detected, and later purulent vasculitis in all parts of the brain (Fig. 10.6a, b). Perivascular hemorrhages are often detected in the hypertoxic course of the disease. Sometimes there is a transition of purulent inflammation from the meninges to the substance of the brain itself. The ependyma of the cerebral ventricles with pronounced dystrophic changes, its cells are partially drained. Often there are leukocyte infiltrates near the ependyma. Infiltration of choroidal plexuses was also detected in almost all children. Changes in the spinal cord are usually minimal, purulent infiltration in the membranes of the spinal cord was noted only in one observation.

Macroscopic changes consist in thickening and turbidity of the soft meninges mainly on the convexital (especially in the frontal, parietal and temporal lobes), less often basal (especially in the posterior cranial fossa) surfaces. In the depth of the furrows, greenish masses are determined, unlike purulent meningitis of another etiology, in which they are yellowish. The brain is compacted, with smoothed convolutions, its mass exceeded the age norm by 13.9%. Spot hemorrhages are determined on the incision. The cerebral ventricles are more often somewhat dilated, less often slit-shaped. The ependyma lining them is cloudy and rough. There are usually pus-like overlays on the choroidal plexuses. The cerebrospinal fluid in the early stages of the disease is yellowish, later greenish, it was absent in three observations.

With a chronic progressive course of the disease, internal and external hydrocephalus, the phenomena of cystic arachnoiditis are detected. There are also more pronounced focal alterative changes. In the soft meninges and choriodal plexuses, the proliferation of collagen fibers is determined, among which foci of purulent inflammation and microbes are detected during histobacterioscopic examination, which in a number of observations corresponded to pneumococcal seeding during postmortem bacteriological examination. In joint studies with M.O. Volkova [7] it was shown that these strains, when assessing their virulence in mice, had less pronounced pathogenic properties compared to the original strains isolated from the same patient at the beginning of the disease.

Acute viral respiratory infections of various etiologies were naturally diagnosed, with some of them there was brain damage as one of the manifestations of their generalization.

In subsequent years, is observed wave-like fluctuations in the frequency of pneumococcal meningoencephalitis on children's autopsy material.

10.1.1 Pneumococcal Meningoencephalitis in Adult

Clinical manifestations of PME are characterized by fever, intense headache, generalized convulsive seizures, disorder of consciousness, and the development of meningeal symptoms. The occurrence of PM is often preceded by pneumonia, otitis media, sinusitis, and infectious endocarditis, although the primary development of the disease is possible. Pneumococcal infection is more often detected in people suffering from diabetes, alcohol abusers.

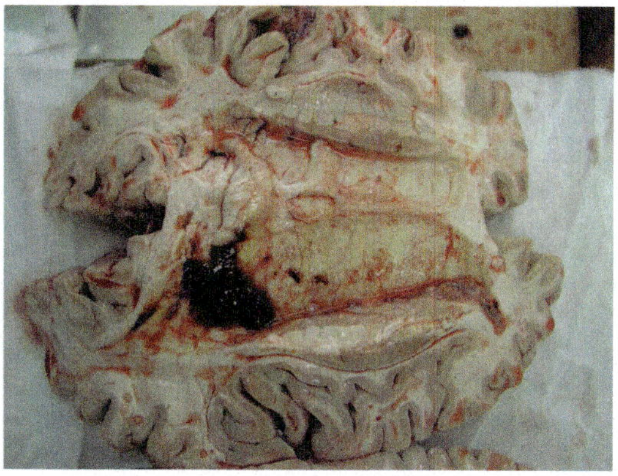

Fig. 10.7 Secondary purulent ventriculitis as complication of pneumococcal lobar croupose) pneumonia. Fresh macroprepation. Courtesy of V.V. Svistunov

Together with V. V. Svistunov et al., we analyzed 152 deaths from pneumococcal pneumonia in Irkutsk [8]. Damage to the meninges was noted in 17 cases (11.2%), of which meningoencephalitis occurred in nine cases, which was accompanied by ventriculitis in five cases. In case one, ventriculitis was complicated by hemorrhage in the vascular plexus. The soft medulla, in cases of meningitis and meningoencephalitis, was sharply edematous, cloudy, green-yellow in color with a gray tinge. Microscopically, there was pronounced edema, circulatory disorders in the form of full blood, infiltration of the shell by white blood cells, fibrin in the form of threads, films, infiltrated by white blood cells was visible on the outer surface of the shell. In case of meningoencephalitis, vascular damage was noted (Figs. 10.7, 10.8, 10.9). When stained with azur-eosin, lanceolate diplococcus was determined. In smears-prints—Gr + diplococcus. In seven cases with meningitis, pneumococcus was sown on culture media.

According the data of pathology department of SP Botkin infectious Hospital among 269 deceased from croupose (lobar) pneumonia purulent meningitis and meningoencephalitis were diagnosed 68 times, which was 25.3%.

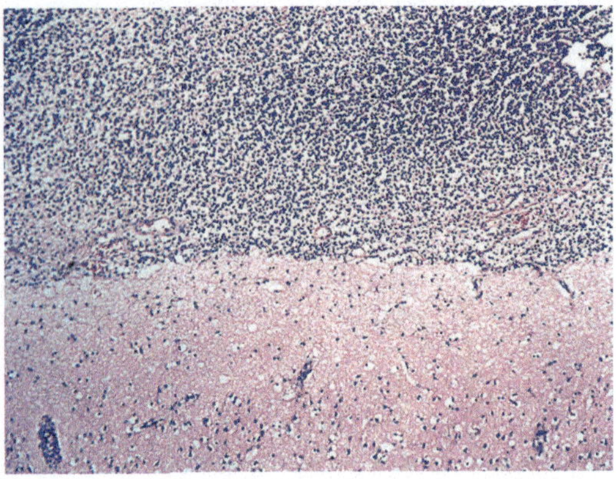

Fig. 10.8 Secondary meningoencephalitis as complication of pneumococcal lobar croupose) pneumonia. H-E. ×100 Courtesy of V.V. Svistunov

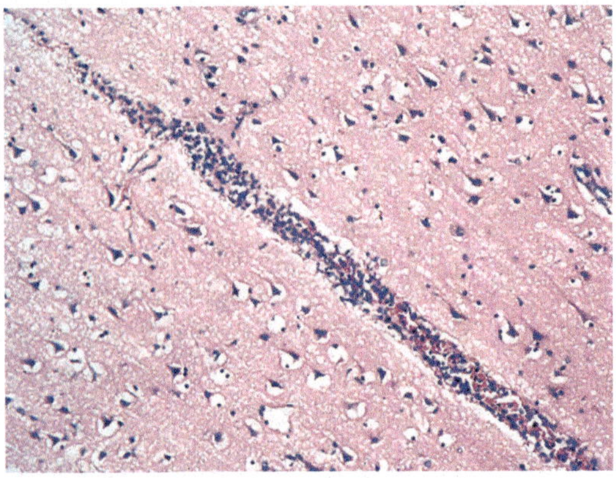

Fig. 10.9 Purulent inflammation of brain vascular walls as complication of pneumococcal lobar croupose) pneumonia. H-E. ×200 Courtesy of V.V. Svistunov

During the same period of time, 44 patients with secondary purulent meningitis with other primary foci, including 13 polysinusitis and 3 otitis media, were examined at the SP Botkin infectious hospital. Despite the lack of direct bacteriological data in some cases, it can be confidently assumed that pneumococcus was the causative agent in the vast majority of these observations. Almost all patients were middle-aged and elderly with a slight predominance of men. Morphologically significant differences from the primary meningoencephalitis were not revealed, they were naturally accompanied by the phenomena of ventriculitis and vasculitis of the cerebral vessels. Pneumococcal purulent meningitis may be complicated by subdural empyema.

10.1.2 Experimental Models of Pneumococcal Meningoencephalitis

- Experimental pneumococcal meningoencephalitis is traditionally reproduced in suboccipital infection of rabbits. The development of experimental models of PME was carried out in the 20–30 years of the twentieth century. A very detailed study of the pathomorphology and pathogenesis of the disease was one of the first conducted by L. S. Bibinova [1936]. To study some aspects of the pathogenesis of PME, we [7] conducted an experimental study on 18 rabbits. Infection was carried out suboccipitally at a dose of 1 × 105–2 × 105 microbial cells per animal. Three strains of Pneumococcus were used for infection: a serotype 1 strain isolated from the brain of a girl who died from PME within a day from the onset of the disease; a serotype 27 strain isolated from the cerebrospinal fluid of a boy who had a moderate form of the same disease; an atypical one isolated from the ear of a patient without a clinical picture of otitis media. All animals infected with Pneumococcus serotypes 1 and 27 developed meningoencephalitis on day 1, characterized by an increase in body temperature, loss of appetite, and convulsive twitching of the limbs. By the end of 2 days, all nine animals infected with serotype 1 pneumococcus had died. Six animals infected with Pneumococcus serotype 27 fell by the end of 3 days, one rabbit after 4 days. Morphological examination of all animals revealed massive, mainly granulocytic, infiltration of the soft meninges. However, the changes caused by Pneumococcus serotype 1 were significantly more pronounced: in these animals, a large number of microbes were detected histobacterioscopically in the soft meninges, and there was a clearly pronounced hemorrhagic syndrome, both in the soft meninges and in the brain substance. Granulocytic infiltration was naturally determined around the vessels in the brain substance, in the villi of the choriodal plexus, and subependimar, including in the area of the ammonian horn. When animals were infected with an untyped strain of Pneumococcus, even in very significant doses (1×10^9 microbial bodies per animal), their condition did not significantly worsen. At the control slaughter of two animals on the tenth day, they had only a rather loose lymphoplasmacytic infiltration of the soft meninges. Effective complex treatment, including penicillin (to which the studied strains were sensitive) and transfusion of liquor, was accompanied by the appearance of focal perivascular lymphoplasmacytic infiltration in the soft meninges.

10.2 Hemophilic Meningoencephalitis

Haemophilus influenzae (HiB) was previously called Afanasyev-Pfeiffer's rod. It is a Gram-negative, facultative anaerobic, and pathogenic bacterium belonging to the Pasteurellaceae family [9]. Among the pathogens of purulent meningitis possesses the third, and according to some authors, the second place with a frequency of about 10% is characterized by a pronounced polymorphism during bacterio—and histobacterioscopic examination—along with thin, delicate sticks, small coccoid forms can also be determined. In practical work, it is also necessary to remember that the high demands of the pathogen from the nutrient media, as well as the suppression of its growth by the accompanying microflora, significantly complicate its isolation.

Purulent meningitis caused by this pathogen is most common in the age group from 3 months to 3 years but can develop in adult as well. The mortality rate from hemophilic meningitis, according to various authors, ranges from 5% to 10%.

The main portals that let HiB enter the CNS are laminin receptor (LR) and platelet-activating factor receptor (PAFR). Similarly, H. influenzae OmpP2 can target the common carboxy-terminal domain of LR to start initial interaction with brain endothelium. It was stated that Haemophilus species pili probably interact with PAFR on brain endothelial cells [10].

In the clinic, it is more often acute. According to our data [6] less than 30% of children had previous acute respiratory viral infection and otitis media. The severity of meningitis was due to toxicosis, more often to hyperthermia up to 390C, lethargy, pallor, but meningeal symptoms usually increased only by the third–fourth day of the disease. Therefore, when patients were admitted, the diagnosis often remained uncertain and was established only after a lumbar puncture. In 1/3 of cases, the fontanelle does not bulge, the pulsation is reduced. In most children, a typical hypertension syndrome is determined by a bulging fontanelle, a divergence of the sutures of the skull. Usually, with hemophilic meningitis, the phenomenon of normochromic anemia occurs early. There were disorders of consciousness in the form of stun (31.2%), less often—sopor (15.6%) and coma (9.3%). Convulsive syndrome was manifested in the form of generalized clonic tonic seizures (19.4%) and epileptic status (6.2%). The initial signs of the disease were muscle hypotension, tremor of the fingers when moving the hands. At the same time, there was a decrease in oral and installation reflexes. In all patients, violations of the reflex sphere were detected in the form of hyper- or anisoreflexia, more often (12.6%) than in other purulent meningoencephalitis, hyporeflexia with a decrease in deep and superficial reflexes was encountered. A severe consequence was deafness in four patients. The course of meningitis was characterized by a wave-like deterioration and improvement of the condition, which correlated with a decrease and increase in inflammatory phenomena in the cerebrospinal fluid, the rehabilitation of which was delayed up to 3–6 weeks. The cerebrospinal fluid pressure was increased to 200–400 mm Hg, averaging 23.0 ± 3.4 mm Hg. IVD was more often reduced, its average values were 55.0 ± 4.9 mm Hg. In the study of CSF in the first days of the disease, neutrophilic pleocytosis was noted (from 355 to $15,000 \times 10^6$/l) with pronounced destruction of neutrophils, which was accompanied by the presence of lymphocytes (about 1%) and monocytes (36) in the cytogram, in one case, pronounced eosinophilia (up to 10%) was noted. In high pleocytosis, the cell compound was usually mixed with a predominance of neutrophils. Pronounced manifestations of intracranial hyper-

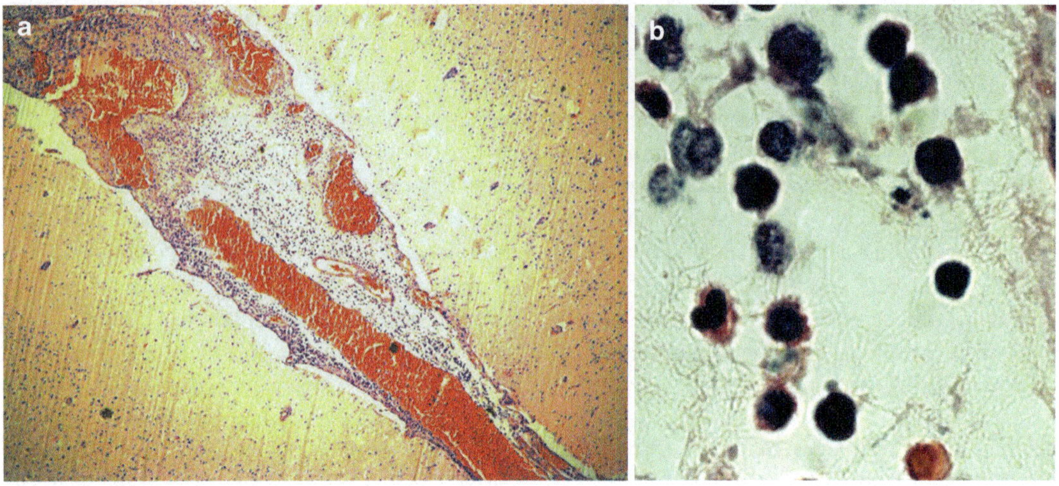

Fig. 10.10 Brain lesions due to *Haemophilus influenzae*. Stained by azur-eosin. (**a**) General view. ×40; (**b**) Detail note cocci-like microorganisms. ×1000

tension, convulsive seizures, and disorders of consciousness were observed in 23 patients (71.3%) with plasma hypoosmolarity, the average values of which were 260 (1.8 mosm/l. Oculomotor disorders in combination with respiratory disorders, hemi and tetraparesis were the basis for the diagnosis of wedging syndrome in 12 patients (43.9%), and in nine cases of them (26.1%), the dislocation syndrome was caused by the development of subdural effusion, which was detected during puncture of the subdural space and subsequently drained. At the same time, six children recovered, and one died in the phenomenon of transtentorial insertion of the brain stem. In two other fatal cases, there was an hyperacute course of the disease lasting 24 and 36 hours. With acute development of toxicosis, severe intracranial hypertension (repeated vomiting, impaired consciousness, convulsive seizures.

Children with meningitis caused by Hemophilus coli often develop a sterile subdural effusion. In such cases, CT or MRI images in the frontal parietal region visualize a sickle-shaped zone of the pathological signal, the characteristics of which correspond to the parameters of the unchanged cerebrospinal fluid. The lesion is always bilateral, regressing within a few days. Intravenous contrast is usually not effective. Sometimes, post-contrast images show a local increase in the adjacent surface of the brain substance, indicating the presence of an acute pathological process, such as inflammation or ischemia. This radiation pattern suggests the presence of meningoencephalitis.

As an example, we can present a child Sh. 1, five-year-old who was admitted with a respiratory disorder, blood pressure = 0, violation of microcirculation. In LP: cytosis 1024 × 10^6/l, protein-0.62 g/L, LP-20 mmHg, brain perfusion pressure negative-20 mmHg, which corresponds to a Glasgow scale of 3 points (brain death). On autopsy: on the soft meninges of the superimposition of light green pus, the convolutions are flattened, the furrows are smoothed, the ventricles are slit-shaped. There are a lot of rods and slightly modified neutrophils in the smears from the soft medulla. Degenerative changes of nerve cells are expressed.

In another case, the child E., 11 months old, was admitted in a convulsive comatose state and died six hours later. A feature of the disease was hemorrhage in the right hemisphere in the presence of pronounced inflammatory changes in the soft meninges, perivascular infiltrates in the brain substance, indicating widespread vasculitis, which was surely the cause of cerebral hemorrhage (Fig. 10.10a, b).

The nature of the macro- and microscopic changes caused by this pathogen in the brain, according to the literature data and the results of our own research, is very similar to those detected in meningococcal purulent meningitis. We did, however, diagnose individual cases with a more pronounced thrombohemorrhagic syndrome, which required a differential diagnosis with meningococcemia in combination with meningoencephalitis.

Hemophilic meningitis was not diagnosed on the adult autopsy material of S. P. Botkin Infectious Hospital. This may be due to some objective difficulties in isolating and identifying hemophilic bacilli from autopsy material. It should be noted that among both primary and secondary meningitis, there were a quite a significant number of observations in which bacteriological cultures did not allow to make an etiological diagnosis. In quite numerous experimental studies, hemophilic meningitis is usually reproduced in suboccipital infection of rabbits. This model is used to study both the pathogenesis of purulent meningoencephalitis and to develop therapeutic tactics.

10.3 Meningitis Due to Streptococcus Pyogenes

Streptococcus pyogenes (previously S. hemolyticus group A) is one of the most frequent human pathogens able to course wide spectrum of lesions of all localizations [11]. In collaboration with K.G. Ioakimova we studied the lethal outcomes due to this pathogen, including with the brain lesions. This group consisted of four children of different ages (from 2 months to 15 years). Clinically, the disease was considered: in one child as meningitis, in one as a generalized viral infection. In two children, no clinical diagnosis could be formulated. Three children did not receive antibiotic therapy, all of them received only antipyretics. Inadequate antibacterial therapy was provided to only one child. The children were born full-term. Three children grew and developed according to their age. One child had myelomeningocele of the lumbar region with rupture of the hernia membranes with their subsequent infection, and liquorrhea a week before the present disease. Two children were considered healthy before the present disease. In one child had previously osteomyelitis, streptoderma, catarrhal otitis, frequent. In three children, the disease began acutely with rapidly increasing symptoms of intoxication: lethargy, weakness, anorexia, and sleep disorders, then after 2–4 h, the temperature rose to high numbers (39–40 °C), which was accompanied by the appearance of a sharp pallor of the skin. In 1 of them, repeated vomiting, delirium, headache, weakness, and paresthesia, convulsive twitching in the left arm in two children were observed meningeal symptoms, primarily rigidity of the occipital muscles. Duration of streptococcal infection: 13 h in one child, 1.5 days—in two, and one—sudden death.

At the autopsy dura mater of the children looked smooth, shiny, gray-pink the soft meninges on the convexital surface of the large hemispheres of the brain were swollen, not transparent, gray-red, in 3-with a yellow-green, cloudy, moderate amount of liquid content with sharply expanded full-blooded vessels. In two children, the upper surface of the pia mater of the cerebellum had the same appearance. The soft meninges at the base of the brain were swollen with sharply dilated, overflowing blood vessels. In all observations, flattening of the convolutions and smoothness of the furrows of the brain were noted. In one child, numerous pinpoint dark-red hemorrhages were visible on the surface of hemispheres. The brain tissue at the incision were sharply full-blooded, homogeneous, in three children with a clear division into gray and white matter, and in one at the age of 1 month, the border between gray and white matter was erased. Brain tissue in two children was of the usual consistency, in two—flabbier. In one child with spinal hernia, atrophy of the brain substance was determined, and its width was 2.0 cm. The lateral ventricles of three children were sharply narrowed, slit-shaped, and a child with spinal hernia had a sharp expansion of all ventricles of the brain, containing about 500 ml of opalescent fluid. Vascular plexuses were dark red, edematous. The spinal cord tissue in four children was gray-pink with the preservation of the "butterfly" pattern, in one of them it was detected only in the cervical and thoracic spine. The cerebrospinal fluid in all children

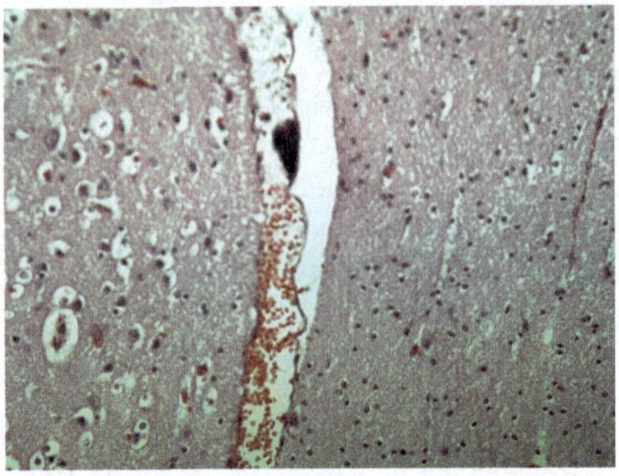

Fig. 10.11 Brain lesion in Streptococcus pyogenic infection. Note accumulation of pathogens in blood vessel. H-E × 100

was opalescent. In other internal organs, except for fullness and moderate edema, no significant changes were found. The results of the bacteriological study. In four children, β – hemolytic streptococcus was isolated from brain tissue, soft meninges, and cerebrospinal fluid. With a lower frequency, it was found in other organs.

During the histological investigation soft meninges in all children were sharply edematous, their vessels are paretically expanded with aggregation of erythrocytes, the endothelium is swollen, partially drained. The subarachnoid space is expanded, it contains exudate, represented by whole and decaying neutrophilic leucocytes with single macrophages and an abundance of free-lying and phagocytized gram-positive cocci, in one child they also form clusters around blood vessels, including in areas of the brain adjacent to the membranes. The substance of the brain is full-blooded, two children had small, multiple hemorrhages and microbial embols in the surface layers of the cortex (Fig. 10.11). Pronounced perivascular and pericellular edema, dystrophic changes of individual neurons are detected in the brain tissue. In two children, moderate dystrophic changes of the ependyma are detected, in one child they are more pronounced: ependymocytes with pycnotic nuclei, small clusters of glial cells in sub-perpendicular zones. In the vascular plexuses of the brain, the vessels are paretically expanded with aggregation of erythrocytes in them, their endothelium is swollen, partially desquamated, small LL infiltrates are observed in one child.

10.4 Purulent Meningoencephalitis of Other Etiology in Older Children and Adults

The literature indicates the fundamental ability of many pathogens to cause purulent meningoencephalitis.

In most cases described in the literature, the causative agent is Staphylococcus aureus and only rarely epidermal (S. epidermidis). Primary staphylococcal meningitis is diagnosed with a frequency of 0.2–2% of the total number of purulent meningitis. More often, the staphylococcal etiology of the process is determined by secondary meningitis and brain abscesses against the background of otitis media, mastoiditis, sinusitis, injuries and sepsis. Relatively often, this pathogen is detected in spinal epidural abscesses and neurological complications of infectious endocarditis (more often in the form of infected emboli); in the latter case, purulent pleocytosis is characteristic of the cerebrospinal fluid [12]. Macro- and microscopic changes in staphylococcal meningitis are not given in the literature. According to the own data of the analysis of several children's sectional observations, the formation of small abscesses is the most characteristic of staphylococcal meningoencephalitis.

In the outbreak of hospital klebsiella infection studied by the author in children of different ages, against the background of various neuroinfections, there was a severe lesion of both the membranes and the substance of the brain. At the same time, histobacterioscopically, against the background of a minimally pronounced cellular reaction, very significant clusters of rods were detected in the soft meninges and brain matter (mainly near blood vessels) (Fig. 10.12).

In recent years, a number of reports on the possible role of various anaerobic pathogens in the etiology of purulent meningitis has increased in the literature. As the causative agents of

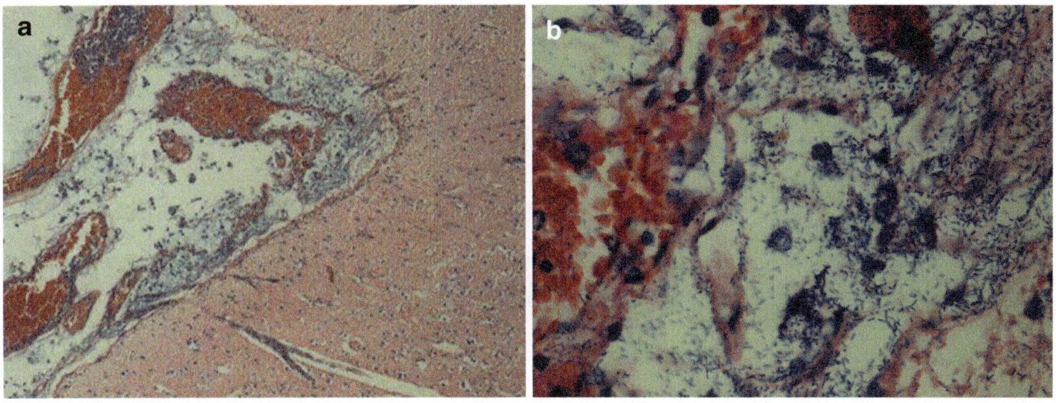

Fig. 10.12 Brain lesions in a probable nosocomial sepsis due to *Klebsiella pneumonia* in a child. Note numerous rods. Stained by azur-eosin. (**a**) General view ×50; (**b**) Detail ×640

meningitis, most often, especially in postoperative and posttraumatic patients, consider bacteroids (especially Bacteroides fragilis) and propionobacteria (especially Propionobacterium acnes) [13]. The pathogens can also influence upon the brain indirectly through toxins and metabolites [14]. Unfortunately, due to the difficulties in isolating and identifying these pathogens, the true frequency of the lesions caused by them remains unknown, and the features of the structural changes caused by them are not described in the literature. We do not have our own observations of purulent meningitis with a proven anaerobic etiology of the process. In the research devoted to "hidden" encephalitis (Chap. 17) bacteroids detected in brain appeared to play a significant but not fully understood role.

10.5 Purulent Meningoencephalitis of Other Etiology in the Newborns

Most often, brain lesions are diagnosed in newborns on the background of a generalized infection caused by group B streptococcus [15]. We have only a small number of such observations. Infection in these cases is usually considered as intranatal and associated with frequent colonization of the vagina by this pathogen. The mortality rate in such forms of damage reaches 40–100%.

As pathogens of bacterial lesions of the brain, often, especially in newborns, many Gram-negative rods can act: Escherichia, Klebsiella, Pseudomonas (Pseudomonas aeruginosa), Acinetobacter, serratii, Enterobacter, providence, Moraxella. According to the literature data, summarized by V. I. Kocherovets et al. [12], bacteroids and propionibacteria can also act as pathogens of purulent meningitis in newborns. Clinically, such lesions are usually extremely difficult, and their diagnosis is often difficult. Information about the features of morphological changes caused by individual Gram-negative pathogens is practically absent in the literature. There are only indications that in the diseases caused by many of them, the development of ventriculitis and pyocephaly is typical. S. D. Popov and E. D. Popova [14] analyzed the results of morphological and bacteriological studies of 143 autopsies of children who died of sepsis in the period 1994–2000 in two large children's hospitals in St. Petersburg. Among monoinfections, the most common pathogens were fungi of the genus Candida (33), Klebsiella (29), Escherichia (13), serratia (11), enterococci (9), Pseudomonas aeruginosa (7), Staphylococcus aureus (3). In 13 children, the disease was caused by bacterial-bacterial and bacterial-fungal associations in 10. Most of the children (95) suffered from various severe neonatal pathologies, were in the intensive care unit for newborns, and died from sepsis at the age of 17 h to 3 months. Among septic foci characterized by purulent inflammation and necrosis, brain lesions occupied one of the most prominent places they were found in 52 cases, second only to the gastrointestinal tract (63) and lungs (56) in frequency.

In previous years, the specific weight of Pseudomonas aeruginosa sepsis was significantly higher. Thus, in the period from 1977 to 1982 in Leningrad, 195 children died and 29 recovered from Pseudomonas aeruginosa infection, of which 14 died before the age of 28 days and two died before the age of 1 year, one older than a year with purulent meningitis, most often against the background of pseudomonas aeruginosa sepsis. Pseudomonas aeruginosa meningitis ended in recovery only in one child over a year old. The most frequent symptoms of purulent meningitis in newborns, there were a decrease in physiological reflexes, a change in body temperature (in seven people, it increased to 37.5–38 °C, four children developed hypothermia), adynamia (10), convulsive seizures (8). Neutrophilic pleocytosis was detected in the CSF: in newborns, on average, 345.8 ± 67.8 × 106/l, as well as an increased total protein content of 4.1 ± 0.7 g/l. Foci of purulent inflammation of the meninges with the accumulation of gram-negative rods in them and alterative changes in exudate cells were detected. An in-depth bacteriological study of Pseudomonas aeruginosa strains allowed V. F. Tsinzerling to prove their hospital origin based on intraspecific typing (with the determination of immuno-, phago-, and pyocinotypes), and to study their pathogenic properties both in vitro (plasma coagulase, hemolysin, DNase, lipase, protease, and lecithinase) and in vivo (with intratracheal infection of white rats) it was possible to prove a significantly greater pathogenicity of hospital strains compared to "wild" ones. The result of the complex study [16] was the implementation of anti-epidemic measures, which led to a sharp decrease in the frequency of all forms of Pseudomonas aeruginosa infection in this hospital.

E. D. Popova and S. D. Popov [17] were the first to analyze in more detail 35 autopsy observations of infection caused by Serratia marcescens in 1994–2000. Most of the children (28) were born prematurely. Monoinfection with serrations was observed in 21 cases, and in 14 cases it was combined with other pathogens. Twelve children were diagnosed with sepsis. Among the organ lesions, along with the gastrointestinal tract (11 observations), central nervous system lesions were most often noted (nine observations). Macroscopically, these lesions were characterized by gray-red or pink foci of softening. Microscopic examination of necrotic foci naturally determined hemorrhage, in the zone of which a substantial number of bacteria was determined. Neutrophil infiltration was determined only in part of the observations. Manifestations of DIC syndrome were also typical.

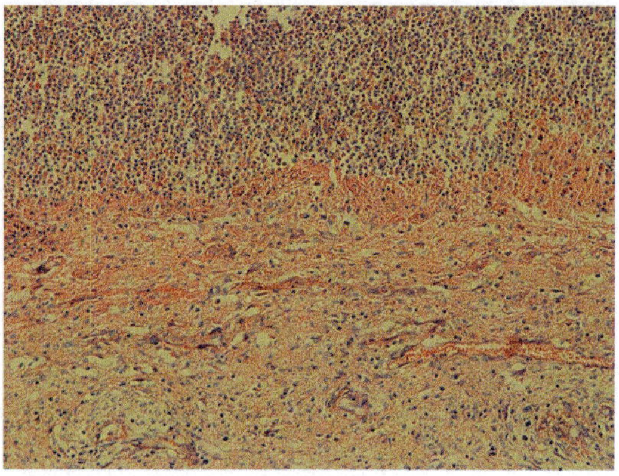

Fig. 10.13 Wall of the brain ventricle in course of long-term purulent lesion in a one-month-old girl. H-E × 200

On their own material, they managed to establish some interesting facts. Thus, in a one-month-old girl, as a result of a comparison of microbiological and morphological, including experimental data [6], it was possible to talk about purulent ventriculitis caused by E. coli O4 (Fig. 10.13). The long-term existence of this microorganism within the brain led to a greater expression of K-antigen and a significant increase in pathogenic properties in the test on an isolated rabbit loop compared to the original strain from the intestine.

References

1. Weiser JN, Ferreira DM, Paton JC. Streptococcus pneumonie: transmission, colonization and invasion. Nat Rev Microbiol. 2018;16(6):355–67. https://doi.org/10.1038/s41579-018-0001-8.

2. Loughran AJ, Orihuela CJ, Tuomanen EI. Streptococcus pneumoniaer: invasion and inflammation. Microbiol Spectr. 2019;7(2):10.1128. https://doi.org/10.1128/microbiolspec.GPP3-0004-2018.
3. Dion CF, Ashurst JV. Streptococcus pneumoniae. In: StatPearls[internet]. Tresure Island (FL): StatPeartls Publishing; 2021.
4. Zinserling VA (2021) Infectious Pathology of the respiratory tract Springer International Publishing DOI https://doi.org/10.1007/978-3-030-66325-4. ISBN 978-3—030-66324-7.
5. Dando SA, Mackay-Sim A, Norton R, et al. Pathogens penetrating the central nervous system: infection pathways and the cellular and molecular mechanisms of invasion. Clin Microbiol Rev. 2014;27(4):691–726.
6. Zinserling VA, Chukhlovina ML. Infectious lesions of nervous system. Issues of etiology, pathogenesis and diagnostics. Saint-Petersburg, ElbiSPb; 2011. p. 583. (In Russian)
7. Tsinzerling VA, Sorokina MN, Volkova MO, Bass RL, Zaitsev VS. Pathological anatomy and problems of the pathogenesios of pneumococcal meningoencephalitis in children. Arkjh Patol. 1987;49(4):38–45.
8. Zinserling VA, Svistunov VV, Botvinkin AD, Stepanenko LA, Makarova AE (2021) Lobar (croupose) pneumonia: old and new data Infection Sep1:1–8 doi:https://doi.org/10.10007/s15010-021-01689-4.
9. Khattak ZE, Anjum F. Haemophilus Infuenzae. In: StatPearls [internet]. Treasure Island, FL: StatPearls Publishing; 2021. PMID: 32965847.
10. Jamil Al-Obaidi MM, Mohd Desa MN. Mechanisms of blood brain barrier disruption by different types of bacteria, and bacterial-host interactions facilitate the bacterial pathogen invading the brain. Cell Mol Neurobiol. 2018;38:1349–68.
11. Ijaz M, Ameen F, Alfopteih YA, et al. Dissecting streptococcus pyogenes interaction with human. Arch Microbiol. 2020;202(8):2023–32. https://doi.org/10.1007/s00203-020-01932-w.
12. AguilaR J, Urdayt-Cornejo V, Donabedian S, et al. Staphylococcus aureus menongitis: case series and literature review. Medicine (Baltimore). 2010;89(2):117–25.
13. Kocherovets VI, Usanov EI, Matveev NV (1988) Nonclostridial anaerobic infections of the central nervous system Zh VoprNeirokhir im NN Burdenko (6):42–45 (in Russian).
14. Jang NI, Chiu IM. Bacterial signaling to the nervous system through toxins and metabolites. J Mol Biol. 2017;429(5):587–605. https://doi.org/10.1016/j.mb.2016.12.023.
15. Tazi A, Bellais S, Tardieux I, et al. Group B streptococcus surface proteins as major determinants for meningeal tropism. Curr Opin Microbiol. 2012;15(1):44–9. https://doi.org/10.1016/j.mib.2011.12.002.
16. Krasnogorski IN, Indikova MG, Tsinzerling VF, Boikov SG. Pathologic anatomy of Pseudomonas aeruginosa infections in children. Arkh pastol. 1983;45(1–0):9–14.
17. Popov SD, Popova ED (2001) [cited by 6].

11 Brain Abscesses

A brain abscess is a focal infection of the brain that begins as a localized area of inflammation and develops into a collection of pus surrounded by a well-vasculated capsule [1, 2].

Among intracranial volume formations, brain abscesses make up 2–8%. The incidence has been estimated as 0.3–0.9 per 100,000 inhabitants in developed countries, with a male-to-female sex ratio of 2:1 to 3:1, and a median age of 30–40 years. Brain abscess was a fatal disease with mortality between 30% and 60% until the late 1970s with a prognosis dramatically improved due to advances in brain imaging, minimally invasive neurosurgery and use of more efficient antibacterial agents. Nowadays the rate of cure should be >90% [2].

According to the mechanism of occurrence, it is customary to distinguish between brain abscesses that have developed through contact (more often with nasopharyngeal pathology, otogenic), posttraumatic, metastatic, and post-encephalitic. In approximately 10–20% of cases, the mechanism of abscess development remains unknown. Metastatic brain abscesses of pulmonary origin are the most common in clinical practice. It is shown that up to 33.3% of brain abscesses are located in the frontal lobe, up to 24% in the parietal lobe, up to 13.6% in the temporal lobe, and up to 7.6% in the occipital lobe. A study from Finland suggested that the proportion of brain abscesses due to dental infections might be on rise [3]. Brain abscess was encountered in only 0.5% of patients with bacterial meningitis in the nationwide prospective cohort from the Netherlands [4].

During experimental study on dogs R.H. Britt et al. (1981) determined following stages of formation of streptococcal brain abscess: early cerebritis (days 1–3), late cerebritis (days 4–9), early capsule formation (days 10–13), and late capsule formation (14 days and older). In lesions that were well encapsulated five distinct histological zones were apparent: (a) well-formed necrotic center; (b) peripheral zone of inflammatory cells, macrophages and fibroblasts; (c) the dense collagenous capsule; (d) a layer of neovascularization associated with continuing cerebritis; and (e) astrogliosis, and cerebral oedema external to the capsule [5]. According to our experience in men brain abscess has similar structure (Figs. 11.1, 11.2, 11.3). In clinical practice, it usually takes 4–6 weeks for the abscess capsule to form.

It should be emphasized that often for a long time the brain abscess has no clinical manifestations, the patient's well-being remains satisfactory. There is an initial stage of the disease, including the first reaction to infection, and a latent stage, during which the abscess is separated from the brain tissue and the capsule is formed. At the neurological examination during this period, focal symptoms and meningeal symptoms are not observed. The deterioration of the patient's condition occurs sharply within a few hours or days: intense head-

V. Zinserling, *Infectious Lesions of the Central Nervous System*,
https://doi.org/10.1007/978-3-030-96260-9_11

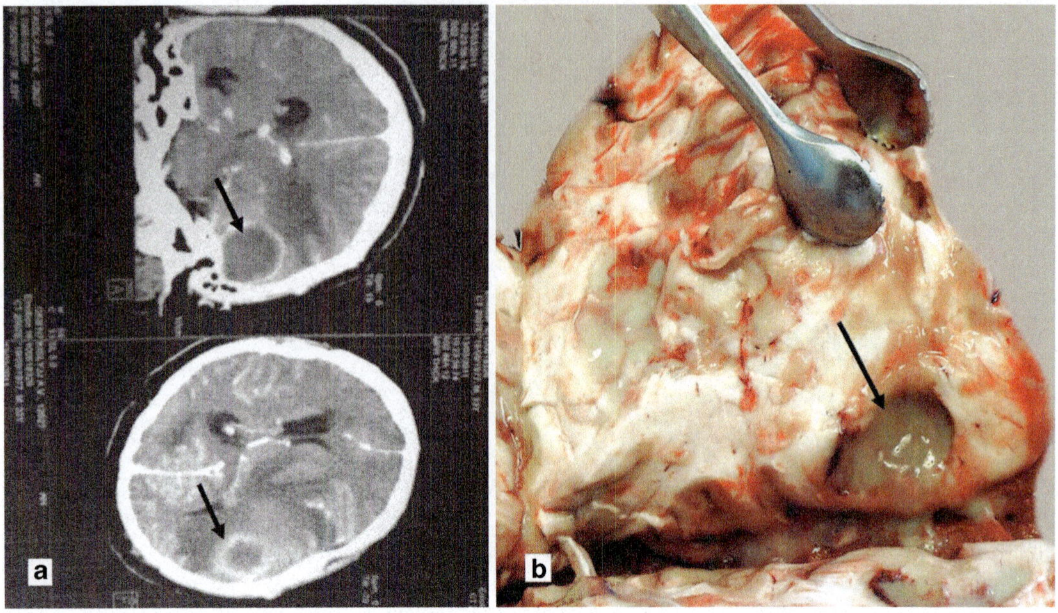

Fig. 11.1 Brain abscess (indicated by arrows). (**a**) Computed tomography; (**b**) Not a fixed specimen. (Courtesy of Y.R. Zyuzya)

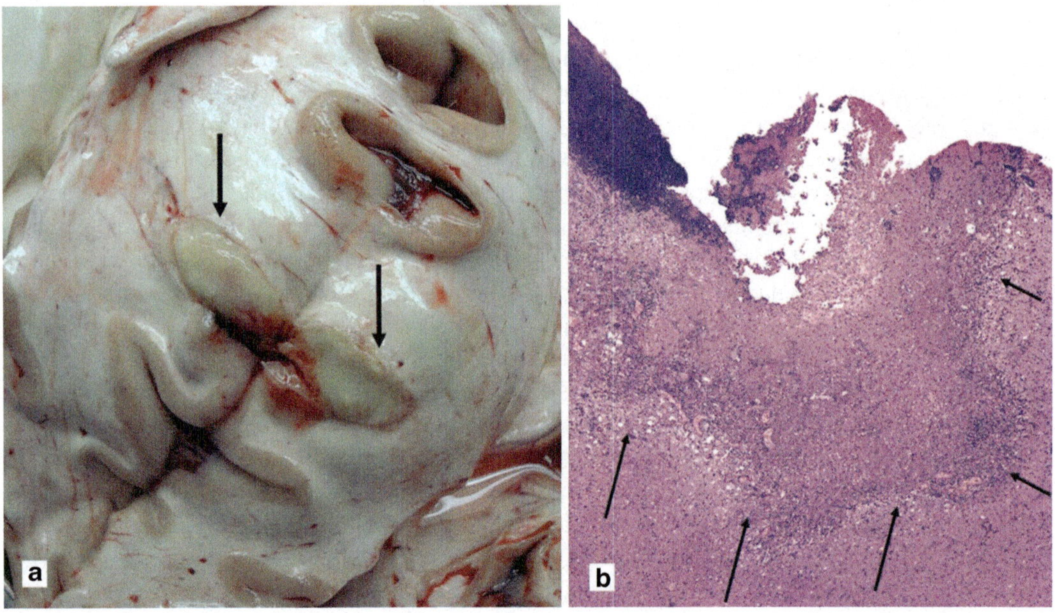

Fig. 11.2 Brain abscess (indicated by arrows). (**a**) Not a fixed specimen; (**b**) The wall of the brain abscess; staining H-E. ×100. (Courtesy of Y.R. Zyuzya)

aches, nausea, vomiting, bradycardia, and fever develop. The clinical picture in the manifest stage is caused by hypertension hydrocephalus syndrome, irritation or compression of the adjacent structures of the brain, it is represented by a combination of general cerebral and focal symptoms, meningeal syndrome, and there may be generalized convulsive seizures. During this period, the

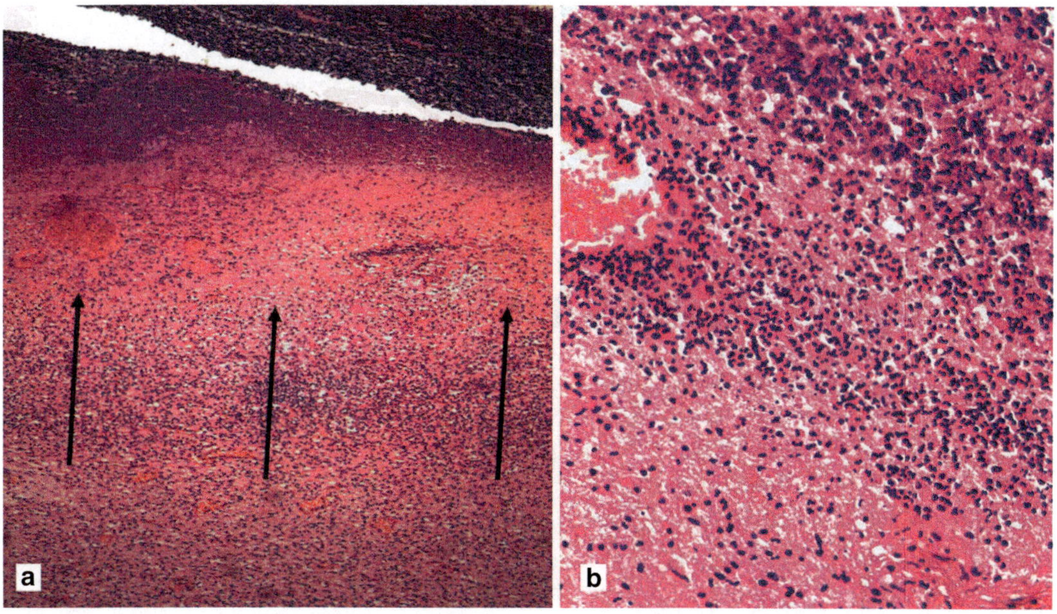

Fig. 11.3 Brain abscess. (**a**) The wall of the abscess (indicated by arrows); (**b**) Fragment of the wall of an acute abscess of the brain with an abundance of neutrophilic leukocytes, edema in the adjacent substance of the brain, vascular fullness and microhemorrhages. Stained with H-E. **a** – ×100; **b** – ×200. (Courtesy of Y.R. Zyuzya)

blood test may show leukocytosis with a shift of the formula to the left, in the cerebrospinal fluid neutrophil pleocytosis with an increase in protein content. With late admission to the hospital, the ineffectiveness of the therapy often comes after the stage of decompensation of the disease with symptoms of brain dislocation, pronounced meningeal signs associated with the rupture of the abscess capsule. Diagnosis of an abscess in the initial and latent stages is quite difficult, and sometimes at the prehospital stage is almost impossible. Thus, M.L. Chukhlovina [6] described a case when an abscess of the deep part of the right parietal lobe was not diagnosed before admission to the hospital due to objective reasons. A 40-year-old patient went to the clinic for fever, runny nose, cough. For 3 weeks, she was observed by a polyclinic therapist with a diagnosis of acute tracheobronchitis, and received antibacterial therapy. According to the records in the outpatient card, the patient did not complain of headache, there was no nausea, and vomiting. There were no grounds for consulting a neurologist. However, after 3 weeks at home, there was an intense headache with nausea, vomiting, the patient was hospitalized in the infectious department by ambulance, where meningeal symptoms were detected and pleocytosis with a predominance of neutrophils and an increase in protein content were found in the cerebrospinal fluid. After performing a CT scan of the brain, a diagnosis was made—a brain abscess and the patient was transferred to the neurosurgical department for further treatment. It should be noted that the asymptomatic course of the brain abscess in the patient was also associated with the peculiarities of the localization of the pathological focus—the abscess was located in the deep part of the right parietal lobe. Such localization may not manifest itself clinically for a long time, since focal symptoms and increased intracranial pressure occur in the late stages of the disease.

Radiation semiotics of the abscess, does not depend on the type of pathogen. The duration of abscess maturation from 2 weeks to several months, patients are usually treated at the stage of late cerebritis. Early manifestations of cerebritis—encephalitic stage (3–5 days): poorly defined areas of softening of the substance with inclusions of necrosis, edema, petechial hemorrhage and perivascular infiltration. CT scans show areas of abnormal density in the subcortical parts of the white matter, mass effect, and moderate central accumulation of the contrast agent. In MRI, poorly defined hypo- and isointensive areas are visualized on T1VI, and a hyperintensive zone is visualized on T2VI, and the destruction site is practically not differentiated from edema. The accumulation of the contrast agent is expressed slightly, heterogeneously. In the early stage of abscess formation, DWI is more specific than CT and MRI with contrast. A change (decrease in the high) DWI signal and a decrease in the lesion volume is a criterion for the effectiveness of treatment, especially in neurosurgical interventions. Radiation picture of the abscess in the period from 4–5 days to 2 weeks: a round-shaped pathological formation with a thin-walled capsule. On CT, a zone of reduced density is determined, surrounded by perifocal edema with signs of mass effect, moderate peripheral amplification in the form of a thin ring, traced in fragments. In MRI, on T1VI, the capsule appears to be hyperintensive, compared to the cerebrospinal fluid; the center of the abscess is characterized by a hyperintensive signal. On T2 VI, the hypointensive ring corresponds to a capsule surrounded by perifocal edema. The hypointensity of the capsule is due to collagen, hemorrhage products, and free radicals. With successful treatment, this phenomenon disappears, while the reaction to the contrast agent still remains. The contents of the abscess are heterogeneous. The capsule thickness of an acute abscess is 5–8 mm, while that of a chronic abscess is thicker. The inner contour may be smooth, but in 20–30%—bumpy. The time of capsule formation varies depending on the immune status of the patient, the pathogenic properties of the pathogen, etc. the less pronounced the formation of the capsule, the worse the prognosis of the disease. Abscess formation in children differs from the formation of abscesses in adults by large size and rapid growth, periventricular localization, and poor capsule formation.

Before the introduction of brain CT into clinical practice, the diagnosis of abscesses was usually late, the mortality rate reached 30–60%; after the use of modern neuroimaging methods, this indicator decreased to 10% [2].

In bacterial abscesses of the brain, strictly anaerobes (most often bacteroids, fusobacteria, anaerobic streptococci) can be isolated in 81.4% of cases. In 31.4%, it is possible to establish the otogenic origin of the abscess [7]. Introduction in clinical practice of metagenomics allowed to detect much more pathogens, such as Staphylococcus aureus, Streptococcus pneumoniae, piogenes, anginosus, constellatus, intermedius; *Clostridium sp, Prevotella sp., Bacteroides sp, Actinomices sp. Fusobaterium sp., Haemophilus aspp, Aggregatibacter spp, Cardiobacterium spp, Eikenella corrodens, Kingella spp.* and others. Total number of detected pathogen species is more than 100 [8]. Brain abscesses due to *Mycobacteria tuberculosis* are presented in Chap. **13**. The most unfavorable are considered to be mixed etiology with dominant role of gram-negative bacteria [9]. However, the clinical significance of these large number of bacteria (as many as 16 distinct species in a single brain abscess), identified only through metagenomic analysis, but not by conventional cultures, remains to be proven.

We analyzed four cases in which brain abscesses were considered as a primary disease in S. P. Botkin Infectious Hospital. In all cases, they were men aged 25, 26, 43, and 70 years. The duration of their hospitalization ranged from 5 to 29 days.

Recently, we have come across an observation of a chronic brain abscess (surgical material) caused by Streptomyces. At the same time, the morphology of pathogens that were clearly determined in the neutrophil infiltration zone in its center when stained according to the Romanovsky method fully corresponded to the microbes isolated and identified during bacteriological research (Fig. 11.4). The factors contributing to the development of the disease of such a rare etiology remain unclear.

In children, brain abscesses account for about 1.4% of all diseases of the central nervous system, 4.4% of neurosurgical pathology. The most common pathogens of the disease are Staphylococcus

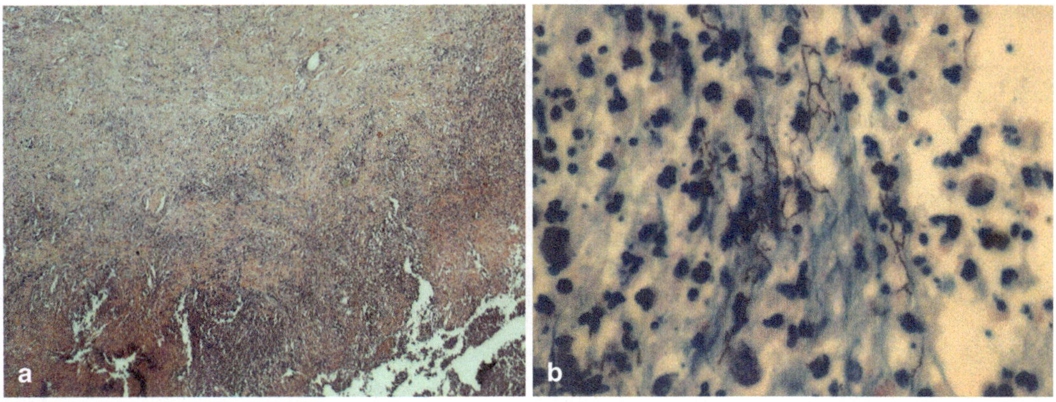

Fig. 11.4 Brain abscess due to Streptomyces in surgical material. (**a**) General view. Stained H-E, ×25; (**b**) Stained by Romanovsky, ×640

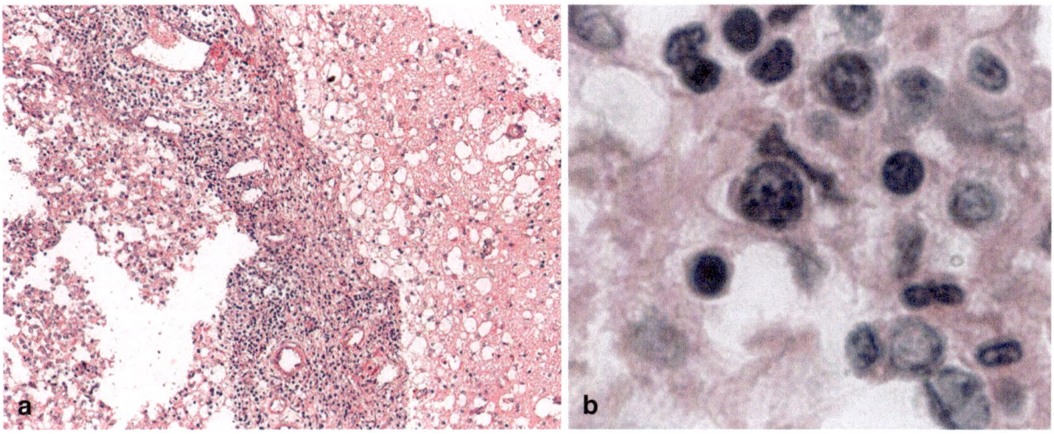

Fig. 11.5 Wall of chronic brain abscess in an eight-year-old girl. (**a**) General view. Stained H-E, ×100; (**b**) Detail of the same picture. Note intranuclear basophilic inclusions. ×1000

aureus and white staphylococcus, streptococcus. Localization is predominantly supratentorial. Children with brain abscesses are less likely than adults to develop bradycardia, congestive discs of the optic nerves to the fundus. Brain abscesses as an independent nosological form were not observed in the children's autopsy material of St. Petersburg. In one of our former observations related to an eight-year-old girl deceased due to chronic abscess, we diagnosed basing upon comparative serological study of blood and liquor adenoviral brain lesion with appearance in capsule of cells with typical for this infection nuclear inclusions (Fig. 11.5).

References

1. Brouwer MC, Tunkel AR, McKhan GM 2nd, van de Beek D. Brain abscess. N Engl J Med. 2014;371:447–56.
2. Sonneville R, Ruimy R, Benzonana N, et al. An update on bacterial brain abscess in immunocompetent patients. Clin Microbiol Infect. 2017;23:614–20. https://doi.org/10.1016/j.cmi.2017.05.004.
3. Laulajainen-Hongisto A, Lempinen I, Farkkila E, et al. Intracranial abscesses over the last four decades: changes in aetiology, diagnostics, treatment and outcome. Infect Dis (Lond). 2016;48:310–6.
4. Jim KK, Brower MC, van der Ende A, van de Bek D. Cerebral abscesses in patients with bacterial meningitis. J Infect. 2012;64:236–8.

5. Britt RH, Enzmann DR, Yeager AS. Neuropathological and computerized tomographic findings in experimental brain abscess. J Neurosurg. 1981;55:590–603.
6. Zinserling VA, Chukhlovina ML. Infectious lesions of nervous system. Issues of etiology, pathogenesis and diagnostics. Saint-Petersburg: ELBI-SPb; 2011. p. 584. (in Russian)
7. Prasad KN, Mishra AM, Gupta D, et al. Analysis of microbial etiology and mortality in patients with brain abscess. J Infect. 2006;53:221–7.
8. Mishra AK, Dufour H, Roche PH, et al. Molecular revolution in the diagnosis of microbial brain abscess. Eur J Clin Microbiol Infect Dis. 2014;33:2083–93.
9. Al Masalma M, Lonjon M, Richet H, et al. Metagenomic analysis of brain abscesses identifies specific bacterial associations. Clin Infect Dis. 2012;54:202–10.

Brain Lesions in Generalized Bacterial Infections

12

Brain can be involved practically in all generalized bacterial infections. In present chapter will be discussed those we have certain own experience. Mechanisms of the lesions differ and can be either associated with exotoxin influence or dissemination of the pathogen itself.

12.1 Damage to the Nervous System in Diphtheria

At the beginning of the nineteenth century, there were publications devoted to the clinical manifestations and treatment of diphtheria. The name of the disease itself comes from the Greek word dipthera, which means a piece of skin film, and was given in 1821 by the French scientist Pierre Bretonneau. It was he who first pointed out the possible connection between diphtheria and the development of paralysis. In 1851. Trousseau described diphtheria paralysis. Later, J. Charcot and A. Vulpian gave a detailed description of the paralysis of the soft palate in diphtheria. In 1898, I. A. Klimov, one of the first to study changes in the vegetative nodes involved in the innervation of the heart in diphtheria.

The causative agent of diphtheria, Corynebacterium diphtheriae, was discovered in sections of diphtheria films by Klebs in 1883. A year later, Leffler was able to isolate it and infect experimental animals. It was found that C. diphtheriae, a thin Gram-positive rod (1–8 microns long) with club-shaped thickening at the ends, produces an exotoxin with a strong toxigenic effect. According to the cultural and biochemical properties, there are three types of C. diphtheriae: gravis, mitis, intermedius, as well as varieties—toxigenic and non-toxigenic, a number of serological types and phagotypes. On the territory of Russia, all three types circulate, with the most common types being gravis and mitis. It is proved that non-toxigenic corynebacteria can turn into toxigenic ones under the influence of a phage. It is shown that toxigenic strains, unlike non-toxigenic ones, have a profag in their chromosome—the genome of a moderate phage beta, of which the diphtheria toxin gene (tox gene) is a component. Expression of the tox gene leads to the formation of diphtheria toxin. The causative agent of diphtheria is highly resistant to environmental factors: on films removed from the tonsils of patients, it remains active for up to 3–5 months, in dust up to 2 months, on food—up to 18 days [1].

In Russia, as a result of the creation of a high level of anti-diphtheria immunity in children in the 60–70s, the incidence of diphtheria was sporadic. Diphtheria infection was mainly manifested by bacterial transmission and rare cases of manifest disease: there were reasons to believe that it would soon be eradicated. However, in the 80–90 years, the frequency of diphtheria cases increased sharply, and the rise in the incidence was for the first time due to the predominant

V. Zinserling, *Infectious Lesions of the Central Nervous System*,
https://doi.org/10.1007/978-3-030-96260-9_12

disease of adults. The pathogen also changed: the cultural and biochemical type of C. diphtheriae gravis was replaced in the 90s by the mitis type; the carrier of toxigenic strains increased to 5%, and non-toxigenic—to 22%. In recent years, the causative agent of diphtheria gravis has been frequently detected again. The source of diphtheria is a person, both a patient and a bacterial carrier, and the infection is transmitted by airborne droplets. In the early 90s, it turned out that the number of nonimmune persons among the adult population reaches 70–75%. The latter is explained by the fact that the creation of a high immune layer among children in 1960–1980 reduced the number of patients with diphtheria, reducing the level of bacterial transmission of toxigenic corynebacteria of diphtheria. As a result, there was a decrease in the natural immunization of the adult population, at the same time, who lost post-vaccination immunity over the years. In Russia, during the epidemic of diphtheria in 1993–1996, the number of patients with this serious disease increased dramatically, and 5000 deaths were noted. In 1994 alone, 40,000 cases of diphtheria were registered. Based on the material of the pathology department of the SP Botkin Infectious Hospital, we (V. A. Zinserling, S. N. Kadyrova) observed about 130 deaths in adults from diphtheria, including those complicated by polyneuritis. Due to the increased incidence of diphtheria in 1992–1996, the frequency of lesions of the nervous system in this pathology also increased. However, cases of diphtheria in children and adults continue to be reported.

It was found that diphtheria toxin has neurotropicity and a complex structure [1]. It is a single polypeptide chain that is easily divided into A-and B-fragments by the action of trypsin or other proteolytic enzymes. The B-fragment binds the toxin to the cell surface receptors and facilitates the transfer of the A-fragment to the cytosol. At the same time, the A-fragment is an ADP-riboxylating agent that alters and inactivates the elongating factor-II and disrupts protein synthesis. Diphtheria toxin binds to the receptors rather slowly. There are two stages in this process. The first stage is reversible, lasts about 30 minutes, during which time the toxin is fixed on the surface of the cytoplasmic membrane, and can be neutralized with antitoxic serum. The second irreversible stage lasts 30–60 minutes; it ends with the formation of a transport system for the A-fragment and its entry into the cytosol, where the latter is inaccessible to antitoxic serum. Diphtheria toxin penetrates the cells of the host by adsorption endocytosis and pinocytosis. Enzymes that are produced by diphtheria bacilli, such as neuraminidase, facilitate the passage of the toxin into the cell. It should be emphasized that after the addition of diphtheria toxin to tissue cultures, metabolic disorders are detected after 2–3 h, morphological after 5 hours. The latter is due to the complexity, multi-stage pathogenetic mechanisms that provide the cytopathogenic effect of diphtheria toxin. It was found that when diphtheria toxin was administered to experimental animals, the synthesis of the main protein myelin was suppressed by 75% and proteolipid by 50%. At the same time, the compactness of myelin changes, which leads to an increase in the process of lipid peroxidation and proteolysis. This explains the fact that demyelination is the pathophysiological basis of diphtheria polyneuropathy. Pathologically, diphtheria lesions have the form of periaxial Wallerian degeneration of the nerves and anterior roots. The revealed segmental demyelination of the Schwann sheath decreases the speed of nerve conduction, and the absence of residual phenomena in most cases. When studying the morphological features of modern diphtheria, V. A. Zinserling, together with S. N. Kadyrova and D. V. Komarova [2], established the following. In adults who died of diphtheria, polyradiculoneuropathy was detected in 18.5% of cases, mainly in forms that occurred with the development of toxic neck edema of II-III degree. If patients died on the 1st–20th days of the disease, degenerative ischemic changes in nerve cells and fibers were detected, more pronounced in the peripheral nervous system. In the nerve trunks, against the background of different degrees of edema of the peri- and epineurium, foci of neurolysis were found in their myelin sheath, when stained according to Nissl, focal vacuolization, granular disintegration and disappearance of myelin were constant. In diphtheria, accompanied by edema of the neck of the II-III degree, there was swelling and focal loosening of the axial cylinders. In patients with diphtheria who died on the 25–50 days of the disease, small focal proliferation of oligodendroglia cells in the brain tissue was detected, and intermittently in the anterior horns of the spinal cord, focal proliferation of lemmocytes in the peripheral nerve trunks. Histological changes detected in various parts of the nervous system after 55–60 days of illness were most pronounced in the nerve trunks. Thickening of endoneural connective tissue, focal fibrosis of nerve fibers and nerve ganglia, as well as activation of perineural fibroblasts and uneven growth of perineural connective tissue were noted. It is now recognized that damage to the nervous system in diphtheria can occur when the diphtheria toxin penetrates through the nerve tissue in the case of early paralysis (particularly soft palate paralysis) and through the blood in late paralysis. The severity of diphtheria is largely determined by the biological properties of the pathogen. In patients with toxic forms of diphtheria, strains with high activity of superoxide dismutase, catalase, and protease were isolated. In localized forms of the disease, C. diphtheriae strains with lower activity of DNase, phosphatase, and protease are detected.

12.2 Damage to the Nervous System in Botulism

Since the beginning of the eighteenth century, descriptions of the clinical manifestations of poisoning with "sausage poison" began to appear in the scientific literature. Later it was noticed that a similar clinical picture of the disease can develop when eating dried fish. The great Russian surgeon N. I. Pirogov described the results of the autopsy of patients who died due to poisoning with "fish poison." Lesions of the nervous system in these poisonings were most often manifested in the form of bulbar paralysis with the development of dysphagia, dysphonia, and dysarthria. Belgian scientist Emil Ermengen in 1894, isolated the causative agent of the disease from the spleen and intestines of the deceased person, as well as from the ham that he ate. Working with an experimental model of botulism in monkeys, the Romanian neurologist G. Marinescu revealed significant lesions of neurons and neuroglia of the brain.

The causative of the disease is Clostridium botulinum (from lat. Botulus sausage), depending on the antigenic structure, can be of the following serological types: A, B, C, D, E, F, G [3]. This strict anaerobe, a mobile gram-positive rod (length 4–9 microns, width-0.6–0.9 microns), forms spores and secretes an exotoxin. The latter is the strongest natural poison. The vegetative forms of microbes die at a temperature of 80 ° C for 10–15 min, and the spores endure boiling for 5 h. In canned food, botulinum toxins can persist for several years without changing the organoleptic properties of food. The disease occurs when botulism bacteria are poisoned by toxins and is accompanied by severe damage to the central nervous system. The natural reservoir of botulism is domestic herbivores in the intestines of which Clostridium botulini lives. When water bodies are infected with livestock secretions, fish become carriers of the pathogen of botulism. The spread of botulism can also be associated with birds. The disease develops after eating foods infected with botulism bacillus and its toxins. This can be various kinds of canned food (zucchini caviar, canned fish, compotes), as well as meat products, sausages, ham, salted, and dried fish. Currently, there is a classic form of botulism associated with eating foods contaminated with toxins, wound botulism caused by infection with spores of the pathogen, infantile, caused by colonization of the pathogen in the gastrointestinal tract of infants who received mixtures infected with botulism. There are also observations of an adult form of infantile botulism, when the disease occurs in persons suffering from achlorhydria, Crohn's disease, as a result of the multiplication of toxin-producing bacteria in the gastrointestinal tract. In recent years, isolated cases of botulism have been described in individuals treated with botulinum toxin for the treatment of spastic torticollis and other dystonic syndromes. In addition, there are known cases of botulism infection in orthopedics during musculoskeletal tissue transplantation. Botulism occurs as isolated or familial outbreaks worldwide. In the United States, cases of botulism are mainly associated with the consumption of canned vegetables in Germany—with sausages, ham, in Russia—with fish cooked at home without observing the necessary sanitary and hygienic requirements, with mushrooms. When using modern tactics of management, the mortality rate of this severe infection reduces to 1.02% [3].

It is believed that the disease is caused by botulinum toxin, which enters the body along with infected food or is produced as a result of the vital activity of microbes living in the gastrointestinal tract, as well as penetrating through the damaged skin. Through the lymph and blood, botulinum toxin spreads throughout the body. It has neurotropism. It is shown that botulinum toxin binds to the receptors of the presynaptic membrane and prevents the release of acetylcholine into the synaptic cleft, as a result, the synaptic transmission of the impulse in the cholinergic system is disrupted. The innervation of the muscles responsible for the movements of the eyeballs, the muscles of the pharynx, larynx, and respiratory muscles mainly suffers. In addition, the autonomic innervation is disturbed, which leads to disorders of the secretion of the digestive glands. Pathological changes in botulism are most pronounced in the medulla oblongata, in the nuclei of the oculomotor and abductor nerves, are alternative and infiltrative, are noted in the cortex, subcortical nuclei, in the motor neurons of the anterior horns of the spinal cord. In ganglion cells, vacuolization of the cytoplasm, disintegration of nuclei, and destruction of processes are observed.

The incubation period ranges from 2 h to 10 days, but most often about a day. Often, within a few hours after poisoning, nausea, vomiting, abdominal pain, and sometimes stool disorders occur. Unlike other acute infections with botulism, there is no increase in temperature, and therefore patients do not immediately consult a doctor. The first symptoms of botulism are caused by intoxication and are expressed by headaches, dry mouth, decreased lacrimation, shaky gait and gastrointestinal disorders, and a decrease in the frequency of urination. Patients with botulism have general weakness, fatigue, fever, dizziness. Symptoms associated with the lesion of the oculomotor nerve quickly join: double vision, ptosis of the upper eyelid, divergent strabismus, paralysis of convergence, and accommodation. There is a picture of toxicoinfection with repeated vomiting, unpleasant sensations in the abdomen, and there is usually no stool. In this regard, such patients are often hospitalized with a diagnosis of intestinal obstruction. It is possible to develop a symptom of a "hanging" head when the patient has to hold it with his hands. As a result of damage to the neuromuscular synapses of the respiratory muscles and diaphragm aspiration due to swallowing disorders, pronounced respiratory disorders occur, usually requiring the patient to be connected to a ventilator. A diffuse toxic lesion of the heart can be detected. Consciousness in adults is usually preserved in children its violation is possible. Deep reflexes decrease or disappear. Sensitivity is preserved. In particularly severe clinical variants of the course of botulism, all four described syndromes can be combined and sometimes quickly lead to death. In a typical course, a detailed picture of botulism occurs by 3–4 days. It is important to emphasize that the CSF always remains normal. The high virulence of the pathogen is indicated by data on mortality in botulism. It reaches 70% in the absence of adequate therapy, in this regard, the outcome of the disease depends on the early diagnosis of botulism and timely treatment, which consists in the introduction of polyvalent anti-botulinum serum. After establishing the type of pathogen, the appropriate serum is administered, and subcutaneous administration of anatoxin is used to develop active immunity, along with the serum. The diagnosis of botulism is confirmed by the detection of botulinum toxin in the blood, food residues, vomit, and stool. A biological test on animals were used: a neutralization reaction on white mice.

Unfortunately, cases of botulism, especially with delayed hospitalization in an infectious disease hospital, often end fatally.

As an example, we give one of our observations from previous years.

Alexander D, 67 years old, artist. In the past, chronic bronchitis, contusion. On the eve of the disease, he ate homemade salted whitefish. On the night of 19/VIII at 2 a.m., dry mouth, continuous severe vomiting, weakness appeared. Initially, he sought help in a multidisciplinary hospital from where he was redirected to the SP Botkin Infectious Hospital with a diagnosis of food poisoning. Upon receipt (at 23.45 min. The same day) the condition is severe shivering; the pulse was 80 per minute. The heart tones are muffled, the tongue is dry, the abdomen is sensitive in the right iliac region, hypochondrium. Liver and spleen under the costal arch. Hoarseness of voice. In the blood test, HB-162 g/l, leukocytes – 10.5 × 10^9/l, neutrophils 49%, bilirubin 30 mg/l, ALT-0.68. He was taken to the intensive care unit in extremely serious condition. There is difficulty breathing, a feeling of lack of air, bilateral ptosis and mydriasis. Blood pressure 100/70 mm Hg. At 2 h. 20/VIII, an anti-botulinum serum was administered. The patient's condition rapidly progressively worsened. Respiratory and cardiac muscle damage was noted. Despite the ventilator and resuscitation measures 20/VIII at 6 o'clock PM, death was pronounced.

The clinical diagnosis is formulated as a severe form of botulism complicated by acute respiratory failure, acute myocarditis and acute cardiovascular insufficiency. The diagnosis of botulism was confirmed by a biological test on mice.

At the clinical autopsy the corpse of a man of large build, above average height, normosthenic constitution was found. The dura mater is noticeably not tense, gray-bluish shiny, liquid blood in its sinuses. The soft meninges are thin transparent, shiny full-blooded. The convolutions of the large hemispheres are relief, the furrows normally expressed. The brain tissue is slightly flabby, full-blooded with the correct distribution of white and gray matter, a clear boundary between them. The ventricles of the brain are not dilated, their inner surface is smooth, shiny. At the bottom of the fourth ventricle, there is a slight variegation of tissue. Vascular plexuses are soft, full-blooded, bluish-red, shiny.

During macroscopic examination of internal organs, moderate manifestations of atherosclerosis of the aorta and arteries of the heart attracted attention. Hyperplasia of the spleen (weight 215 g). Uneven acute venous fullness of internal organs, small focal hemorrhages in the lungs and the mucous membrane of the small intestine. Parenchymal liver degeneration, lung dystelectasis.

Under microscopic examination in the brain, unevenly pronounced acute fullness. In the stem sections, small focal perivascular hemorrhages and small foci of softening. Necrobiotic and necrotic changes of nerve cells. Moderate activation of glia, rare and small perivascular infiltrates. Perivascular and pericellular edema. Swelling and fullness of the soft meninges. Microscopic examination of the internal organs revealed only moderately pronounced signs of background pathology and acute circulatory disorders. The results of postmortem bacteriological studies are negative. Comparison of characteristic anamnestic, clinical and laboratory data with scant morphological findings allowed to confirm the clinical diagnosis of botulism.

To prevent cases of botulism, strict compliance with the sanitary rules of harvesting, storage of vegetable, fish, meat semi-finished products, as well as the preservation regime of products is necessary.

12.3 Tick-Borne Borreliosis

In recent years, the special attention of doctors has been attracted by ixodic tick-borne borreliosis—a natural focal infection, a multisystem, inflammatory disease that is caused by borrelias and tends to chronic and recurrent courses [4]. In 1910, Arvid Afzelius first described skin manifestations and suggested the role of ticks in the occurrence of the disease. The peculiarities of the course of the developing skin syndrome gave rise to such names of the disease as Afcelius erythema, chronic migrating ring-shaped erythema. Further studies have shown that this disease can develop symptoms of infectious toxicosis, damage to the skin, heart, joints, central, and peripheral nervous system. In 1975, after cases of mass disease with a picture of juvenile rheumatoid polyarthritis in the American city of Lyme, an intensive search for the pathogen began. In 1982, Burgdorfer established that an epidemic outbreak in the city of Lyme was caused by a special type of spirochete, which was called borrelia Burgdorfer, and the disease was Lyme disease.

Currently, the causative agent of tick-borne systemic borreliosis is spirochaeta, which belongs to the family Spirochaetaceae, the genus Borrelia. The following species of Borrelia are distinguished: Borrelia burgdorferi, Borrelia garinii, Borrelia afzelii, etc. The disease is transmitted by ixodic ticks. When bitten, the pathogen enters the blood with saliva, infection is possible if the tick's feces get on the damaged skin. The source of infection is small rodents, dogs, horses, deer, and birds. Tick-borne borreliosis is widespread in the forest zones of the Northern Hemisphere. It is believed that the strains circulating in America belong to B. Burgdorferi, and in Europe and Asia, all three main types of pathogens are found. Tick-borne borreliosis is characterized by seasonality associated with the period of tick activation (April–October), it is in the spring-summer period that most cases of the disease are registered. Currently, tick-borne borreliosis is one of the most common vector-borne infections in our country. Within 1 year, 5000–7000 cases of tick-borne borreliosis are detected on the territory of Russia. At the same time, official statistics on the incidence of ixodic tick-borne borreliosis in Russia in most cases are based on the detection of an early stage, a significant part of non-erythemic forms are not detected at all. Tick-borne borreliosis significantly outstrips tick-borne encephalitis. However, to date, the clinical manifestations and pathogenesis of tick-borne borreliosis remain insufficiently studied. Radiation semiotics of disseminated encephalitis caused by B. burgdorferi In Lyme disease, in all cases, changes in the substance of the brain are multifocal in nature. The foci have a rounded, oval, and irregular shape with a tendency to merge and form demyelination zones. Some large foci / zones are surrounded by perifocal edema. They are characterized by a hyperintensive signal on T2 VI and FLAIR IP. Single foci with the most pronounced changes in the brain substance are traced from T1 VI. It is possible for the process to follow the type of leukoencephalitis with the presence of extensive zones of altered MR signals, extending from the subcortical to subependymal parts of the white matter and occupying several lobes of the brain. The volume effect is expressed slightly and does not correspond to the volume of the lesion. In the vast majority of cases, focal changes are localized in the white matter of the hemispheres of the brain. A characteristic feature of the borrelious etiology of the process is also the involvement of the brain stem, the corpus callosum. Damage to the structure of the posterior cranial fossa occurs in half of the observations, while it is necessary to note a much greater interest in the pedunculi of the cerebellum compared to the rest part. Localization of focal changes in the projection of the basal ganglia is not typical. There are no changes in the gray matter of the cerebral cortex. Intravenous administration of a paramagnet in more than half of cases leads to a change in the signal intensity at T1 VI. In this case, the central model of accumulation of the contrast agent is mainly observed in a smaller percentage of cases - the peripheral model. In dynamics, the following variants of the process flow are possible: - complete elimination of focal changes in the period from 20 days to 5 months; – multiphase course of the process with dissemination of focal changes in the time of appearance and localization in the brain substance, while the radiation pattern becomes similar to that in multiple sclerosis—the appearance of foci in the sub-perpendicular parts of the white matter, the corpus callosum, stem structures, as well as the characteristic transverse orientation of the sub-perpendicular foci with respect to the anterior-posterior axis; – gradual reverse development of focal changes with a decrease in their number and volume of the lesion. Atrophic changes in the brain substance in neuroborreliosis are characterized by moderate diffuse atrophy and are observed in less than half of cases.

Currently, it is assumed both the direct effect of the causative agent of tick-borne borreliosis on the nervous tissue, and its role as a trigger of the autoimmune demyelinating process in the central and peripheral nervous system. The study of the mechanisms of neuroborreliosis development is complicated by the fact that such experimental animals as mice, rabbits, and dogs do not suffer from this form. Experiments conducted on monkeys showed the following. Three months after infection with tick-borne borreliosis, the experimental animals developed polyneuritis. Biopsy of the affected nerves revealed cellular infiltrates with a large number of macrophages and B-lymphocytes, demyelination, and axonal phagocytosis. Immunohistochemically, pathogen or its antigen was detected in macrophages 46 months after infection, a biopsy of the nerve trunk revealed regenerative changes, stimulation of cytokine synthesis, and activation of nitric oxide production.

Currently, according to the classification of tick-borne borreliosis, there are typical and atypical forms (non-erythema—erythema is absent, a general infectious syndrome, regional lymphadenitis is detected, latent-asymptomatic, only the detection of a titer of 1:40 and higher to the causative agent of borreliosis is detected). By severity, there are light, moderate, and severe forms; by duration: acute—up to 3 months, prolonged up to 3–6, and chronic more than 6 months. Light and severe course of the disease is possible. The incubation period ranges from 3 to 32 days (an average of seven to 10 days). The disease often begins with a migrating erythema—a ring-shaped, increasing erythematous spot with a clearing in the center at the site of a tick bite, fever, and headache. There are three stages of tick-borne borreliosis: early stages I and II are the stages of localized infection and dissemination; late stage III are the stages of persistent infection.

Deaths from borreliosis have not been described. In this regard, there are descriptions of structural changes in the skin during biopsy. There is no data on the nature of changes in the central nervous system. In the examination of patients with Lyme disease, hyperactivity of the T-cell link of immunity was revealed: CD3+ CD4+ T-lymphocytes predominate in the early stages, and CD3+ CD8 + T - lymphocytes predominate in the late stages. In addition, at an early stage of tick-borne borreliosis, autoantibodies against platelets, lymphocytes, and neutrophils are detected, indicating a pronounced autoimmune component of the pathogenesis. At the same time, the leading role of the direct effect of the pathogen on the development of the pathological process is confirmed by the positive results of the use of the vaccine to prevent the occurrence of tick-borne borreliosis.

12.4 Generalized Listeriosis in Adults

The principal possibility of brain damage by Listeria (the most studied in this respect is the only species of L. monocytogenes) has been known for a long time. However, relatively complete information concerning this disease is provided only in relation to intrauterine infections [[5], see also Chap. 16]. Many authors briefly indicate the possibility of the development of serous meningitis of listeriosis etiology in adults. Detailed information about the pathogenesis of such lesions and the nature of the structural changes that occur in them is not available in the literature. In the last decade, there has been a significant increase in the frequency of listeriosis in the elderly on the background of concomitant pathology or when using immunosuppressive drugs [6, 7]. The molecular mechanism enabling Listeria to cross the blood-brain barrier may be associated with either or both of Listeria surface proteins In1A and In1B. These proteins mediate species-specific interactions with their host receptor, E cadherin, and by mesenchymal-epithelial transition across the microvascular endothelium and choroid plexus at the epithelial level. Additionally, expression of P- and E-selectin, intercellular adhesion molecular 1, vascular cell adhesion 1 and inflammatory factors (interleukin 6 and 8, monocyte chemoattractant protein 1) contribute to disruption of BBB [8]. It is shown that in patients with HIV infection, listeriosis is detected 150–300 times more often than in the general population. It is established that in adults listeriosis infection occurs mainly in the form of sepsis, meningitis, encephalitis. Listeriosis meningitis is usually characterized by

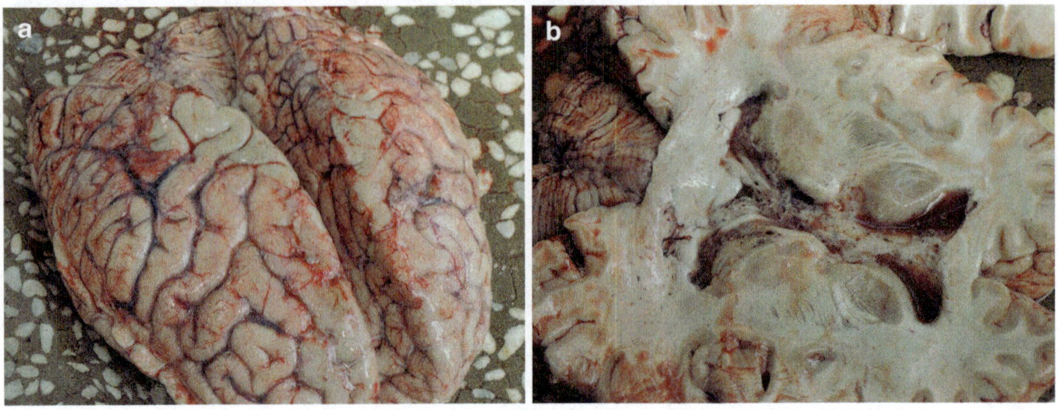

Fig. 12.1 Brain in listeriosis meningitis. Unfixed macropreparation. (**a**) General view; (**b**) Cut surface

an extremely severe course. It should be emphasized that during autopsy, listeria was detected in the brain stem not only in patients with clinical manifestations of stem encephalitis, but also in the absence of neurological deficits.

We present one of our rather rare autopsy observations. Patient L. S., 60 years old, retired. In anamnesis, joint pain was noted for a long time. The disease began abruptly on 23/01 with a rise in temperature, joint pain, cough, runny nose. Initial diagnosis: systemic connective tissue disease. She was admitted to the SP Botkin Infectious Hospital, where she stayed for 9 days. From 1/03 sopor, psychomotor agitation, cytosis 80 cl/ml, protein 5.5 g/l. A differential diagnosis was made between tuberculous and lupus meningoencephalitis, a brain abscess. From 6/03, L. monocytogenes was seeded into the CSF, during its study on the same day - protein 2.9 g/l, glucose 1.6, cytosis 5232/3, neutrophils 90%, during cytological examination, the similarity of fuchsinophilic rods is determined. 11/03 the patient died. Final clinical diagnosis: Listeriosis, septic form. Complications of the underlying disease: Purulent meningoencephalitis, ventriculitis, edema swelling of the brain. Dislocation syndrome from 8/03, ventilator from 9/03, bilateral bronchopneumonia, nephritis, and acute cardiovascular failure. Concomitant disease: systemic lupus erythematosus with damage to the joints, heart, and central nervous system. Common atherosclerosis. CHD. Hypertension II. Tuberculosis of the lymph nodes?

Extract from the protocol of clinical autopsy. Macroscopically: The bones of the skull and the dura mater are intact. The soft medulla is thickened, edematous, with greenish tinting, in the area of projection of the furrows in the parietal area—dull. On the base between the hemispheres of the cerebellum, in the area of the lower surface of the trunk, the chiasm is a cluster of gray-greenish dense pus-like masses. In the area of the arteries of the Vilisian circle, there are single rounded whitish foci up to 1 mm in diameter. The convolutions of the brain are flattened, the tissue is wet on the incision, it sticks to the knife. The pattern of the brain is preserved, the border between gray and white substances is clear. There is some variegation of gray and fullness of white matter (Fig. 12.1). The cerebral ventricles are dilated, which contain cloudy cerebrospinal fluid. The vascular plexuses are pale pink in color, with many small cysts. The ependyma is dull with an accentuated vascular pattern. In the cavity of the main sinus, there is a thick gray pus-like content.

Microscopically in the soft meninges, there is a significant leukocyte-macrophage infiltration (Fig. 12.2). Both fresh and decaying neutrophil granulocytes are detected. A distinct admixture of fibrin, which has an eosinophilic hue. In the area of fibrinous purulent exudate - basophilic shade. Focal perivascular hemorrhage in the cortex of the large hemisphere. Lymphocytic infiltration of the walls of blood vessels in the substance of the brain. Small granulomas of large

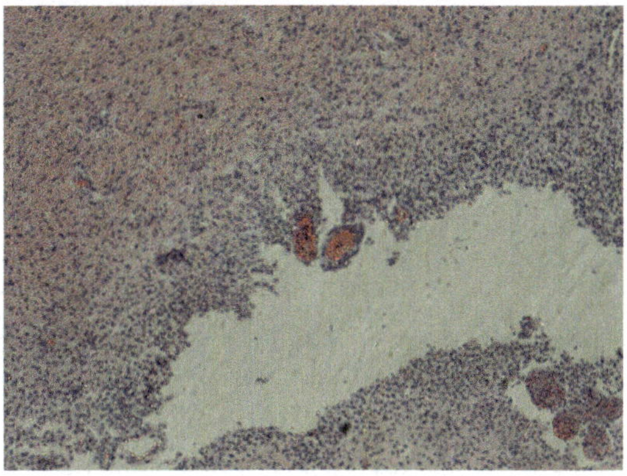

Fig. 12.2 Subependymal inflammation in listeriosis meningoencephalitis in adult H-E × 100

oval cells, closely adjacent to each other, surrounding small areas of necrosis. Ventricular ependyma with focal proliferation, "juicy," and its surface is a cluster of dystrophic altered white blood cells. Vascular plexuses are full-blooded with focal small calcifications, lymph-leukocyte infiltration. In the subependymal part, lymphocytic perivasculitis, small perivascular granulomas, areas of brain tissue dilution with lymphohistiocytic infiltration with an admixture of a few neutrophilic leukocytes. Pronounced alternative changes in nerve cells up to their necrobiosis. Perivascular and pericellular edema. In a postmortem bacteriological study, *L. monocytogenes* was isolated from the soft meninges and cerebral ventricles. In other crops (blood, main sinus, spleen, small intestine, esophagus), various representatives of conditionally pathogenic bacterial microflora and Candida fungi. In the serological study, antibodies to influenza A1 in titer 1:320, influenza A2–1: 40. Final pathological diagnosis: Listeriosis (in vivo seeding of L. monocytogenes from the cerebrospinal fluid, postmortem - from the soft meninges and ventricles of the brain): hyperplasia of the paraaortic and periportal lymph nodes, hyperplasia of the spleen, diffuse purulent leptomeningitis (with a predominant lesion of the basal parts of the brain) with the onset of organization, purulent ventriculitis, granulomatous encephalitis with the primary lesion of the cortical and subependymal parts of the brain. Left-sided lower lobe focal pneumonia. Systemic lupus erythematosus: focal myocarditis, focal nephritis. Fibrotic-focal tuberculosis of the upper lobe of the left lung without signs of exacerbation. Fibrosis, calcinosis, and anthracosis of bifurcation lymph nodes. Synechiae between the pleural leaflets. Pronounced atherosclerosis of the aorta, arteries of the heart and brain. Influenza A1 in the stage of residual events. Post-traumatic common purulent-necrotic tracheobronchitis. Parietal purulent-necrotic thrombophlebitis of the superior vena cava during cava catheterization. Large serous cyst of the right ovary.

This observation demonstrates the exceptional complexity of the correct clinical and pathological interpretation of the course of the disease in many patients, often suffering from many diseases at the same time. In this case, the elderly woman at the time of death had seven (7!) quite severe diseases and two resuscitation complications. At the same time, the complex of clinical, morphological, and bacteriological data allows us to assign a leading role in thanatogenesis to generalized listeriosis with a predominant brain lesion. Attention is drawn to the peculiar purulent productive nature of the inflammatory reaction, which can be considered characteristic of listeriosis. Schematically, the development of the disease in this patient can be represented as follows. An elderly woman with severe background pathology: atherosclerosis, focal tuberculosis, systemic lupus erythematosus got ill with influenza. Against the background of reduced resistance, there is probably an alimentary infection with listeriosis with primary damage to the periportal and then paraaortic lymph nodes, followed by hematogenic generalization of the infection with severe lesions of the meninges and ventricles, white and gray matter. Predominantly basal localization of the process significantly complicated the clinical diagnosis. During the disease, the addition of focal pneumonia was noted, possibly associated with purulent necrotic tracheobronchitis - a complication of intubation with mechanical ventilation. Purulent-necrotic thrombophlebitis of the superior vena cava, which is a complication of cava catheterization, could also be potentially life-threatening.

Here is a summary of another indicative observation of listeriosis in an adult. Patient T., 59 years old, with a history of alcohol abuse. Taken to the SP Botkin Infectious Hospital from the somatic hospital, where purulent leptomeningitis was detected. Since the admission is noncontact, the condition is extremely serious, the consciousness is confused. Blood pressure 80/60 mmHg, pulse 130 beats in min, marbled skin, meningeal symptoms are sharply positive, pathological foot reflexes on both sides. Despite active resuscitation therapy, the condition continued to deteriorate and on the fifth day of hospitalization (7–8 days of illness), without regaining consciousness, the patient died. In the blood test: Hb 173 g / l, e-5.4, L-18.7, ESR-6 mm/h. In the cerebrospinal fluid cytosis 2300/3, lymphocytes 48%. Seeding with liquor and blood - L. monocytogenes. At the clinical autopsy brain meninges were indistinctly thickened, grayish translucent, cloudy with the injection of small vessels. The surface of the brain is raised, the tissue is flabby elastic with a clear border between gray and white substances. The ventricles of the brain are dilated, their contents are grayish cloudy, their walls are dull, grayish-red. In the trunk area, a blurry area of grayish-red color. Microscopic examination revealed a picture of meningitis, ependymatitis with mixed infiltration, and pronounced leukocyte rexis. In some places, there are small granulomas in the brain substance. Posthumously, L. monocytogenes was isolated from the cerebral ventricles and membranes.

12.5 Typhoid Fever

Typhoid fever (TF) is a common, in some cases, a severe disease that leads to significant economic and social damage in many countries of the world. In the second half of the twentieth century, there was a significant decrease in the incidence of disease in developed countries as a result of targeted sanitary and anti-epidemic and therapeutic and preventive measures, but the disease remains a serious health problem in developing countries [9]. According to current estimates, 16–21 million new cases of TF and 200,000 to 600,000 cases of BT are registered annually in the world deaths associated with this disease. Before the use of antibacterial drugs, complications of typhoid fever were determined by 74–90% of deaths, in other cases, patients died from severe general intoxication caused by the disease. Among the complications that led to the death of patients with typhoid fever, perforation of typhoid ulcers with the development of peritonitis dominated (11–32%), ulcerative bleeding was less common—in 2–11% of the dead, pneumonia was detected in 32.5–74.4%. Often developed purulent complications (arthritis, periostitis, spondylitis, otitis), as well as sepsis, meningoencephalitis, ulcerative necrotic laryngitis, vasculitis, thrombophlebitis, damage to the hepatobiliary system and kidneys. Hemorrhagic forms of this infection are described. Changes in the nervous system are characterized by acute serous, purulent meningitis and acute encephalitis. In serous meningitis, typhoid bacilli are sometimes found in the membranes of the brain. However, it can also be of toxic origin. Acute purulent meningitis is rare, more often in children. Changes are localized mainly on the basis of the brain. Acute encephalitis is characterized by round-cell infiltrates around small blood vessels, thrombosis, and hemorrhage. On the material of the pathology department of the SP Botkin in a retrospective analysis of 122 sectional observations of typhoid fever in 1948–2003, we (V. A. Zinserling, A. N. Kovalenko) also managed to identify only two cases in which meningoencephalitis was probably caused by S. typhi abdominalis (Fig. 12.3).

12.6 Salmonellosis

Currently, several hundred serotypes of S. enteritidis are known to cause acute intestinal infection, which can be associated with both alimentary factors and hospital infection. The most often diagnosed are gastrointestinal, erased, atypical forms, much less often typhoid and septic. In the latter, hematogenic dissemination of the pathogen, especially in young children, can lead to damage to various organs, including the development of meningitis, which is documented by seeding Salmonella into the CSF. Focal brain

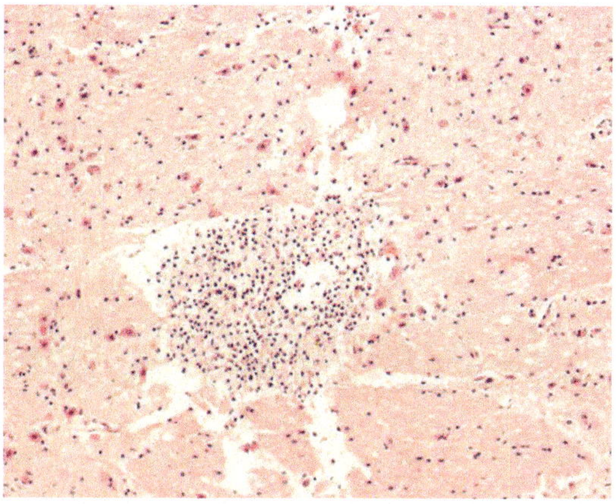

Fig. 12.3 Brain granuloma in typhoid fever H-E × 100

lesions caused by Salmonella are uncommon in adults. In the literature, we were able to find only references to such observations, mainly in the clinical literature of previous years. Modern guidelines on microbiology and infectiology do not provide data on this issue. However, traumatic brain injury, especially in combination with an immunodeficiency condition, predisposes to the development of this infection. In a retrospective analysis of long-term autopsy material of pathology department of SP Botkin Infectious Hospital, we were surprised to find no observations of generalized (septic) salmonellosis with brain lesions. The only exception was the observation of S. Ch., 26 years old, suffering from chronic alcoholism, who on the 4th–5th day of the disease dies from generalized salmonellosis of group C1 infants with catarrhal hemorrhagic, sometimes erosive gastritis, common catarrhal, sometimes catarrhal-erosive enteritis with hyperplasia of Peyer's plaques and mesenteric lymph nodes, catarrhal hemorrhagic colitis, focal ascending hepatitis, small-focal myocarditis and meningitis. Salmonella was shown in vivo and postmortem from the blood, intestinal contents, mesenteric lymph nodes, and liver. Changes on the part of the brain did not play a significant role in thanatogenesis (it was mainly determined by hemo - and liquorodynamic changes in the meninges unevenly expressed mononuclear infiltration, it was not possible to accurately determine the morphogenesis of which.

12.7 Infectious Endocarditis

Infectious endocarditis (formerly commonly referred to as septic endocarditis) is a very relevant worldwide disease that can develop on various heart valves, both altered (more often against the background of rheumatism) and unchanged, both in drug addicts and those leading a normal lifestyle. Without being able to analyze in detail the extremely complex and controversial problem of sepsis, in this work, we consider it necessary to note that a number of characteristic features of infectious endocarditis allow us to confidently distinguish them from the general group of "septic processes," which certainly need a more precise categorization. Numerous bacterial, fungal, and chlamydial pathogens are described as pathogens of infectious endocarditis. Many questions of their pathogenesis remain unclear. Clinical symptoms are often extremely severe, but it is not always possible to make a correct diagnosis without using instrumental methods (primarily ultrasound diagnostics), which in practice leads to a large number of erroneous diagnoses. General problems of infectious endocarditis are quite fully described in a number of modern reviews [10], note that among their complications, embolic lesions of the brain and its membranes are quite common. In clinical morphological comparisons were conducted jointly with V. I. Ulanova, it was found that the hospital mortality rate for infectious endocarditis in patients with drug dependence was 30%, and without it—42%. In the literature, there are few data on the features of brain lesions in the development of infectious endocarditis on the background of HIV infection. In such patients, morphological signs characteristic of HIV infection were detected in the brain tissue. In the majority of deceased HIV-infected patients with IE, signs of HIV encephalitis with the presence of multinucleated cells, phenomena of perivascular infiltration and endothelial proliferation, as well as fullness and infiltration of lymphocytes of the meninges as a manifestation of meningitis caused by HIV infection were determine. At the same time, according to the data of the pathological study of deceased patients with IE, the presence of HIV infection in the early stages did not significantly affect the nature of complications and the outcome of the underlying disease. In our material of pathology department of the SP Botkin Infectious Hospital, 46 fatal cases of infectious endocarditis were analyzed. Of these observations, 32 cases (67.4%) were diagnosed with embolic meningoencephalitis (17), encephalitis (12), or meningitis (3). In seven observations (21.9%), the underlying disease was not clinically recognized, most often due to the short duration of the patient's stay in the hospital and other objective reasons. In terms of observations, the attending physicians had difficulty in determining the embolic nature of brain lesions. In 21 cases, brain damage was the direct cause of death, most often diagnosed with a brain coma. In nine cases, neurological disorders developed on the background of infectious endocarditis with aortic valve damage in 12 – mitral, in 2 – mitral+aortic, in 3 – tricuspid, in 2 – tricuspid+mitral, in 4 – tricuspid+aortic. In 30 cases, infectious endocarditis developed against the background of unchanged valves, as well as in one case with congenital heart disease and rheumatism. There are data on drug abuse in 17 people, chronic alcoholism in six people. In addition, in 15 cases, drug addicts were found to have different forms of chronic viral hepatitis in terms of etiology and severity, and in seven cases the initial stages of HIV infection. Efforts were made to establish the etiology of the process. In 19 observations (mainly in drug addicts), based on in vivo and postmortem bacteriological studies, it was possible to talk about the staphylococcal etiology of the process, partly in combination with gram-negative rod microflora, in two cases there were grounds to consider pneumococcus and hemolytic streptococcus as the causative agent. In the remaining nine observations, despite the presence of a variety of seedings, it was not possible to determine the etiology of the process with certainty, although in some cases the seeding of Klebsiella and Acinetobacter attracted attention. In the morphological study, the diagnosis of embolic lesions is based on the detection of infected blood clots in small and medium-sized vessels, surrounded by foci of purulent inflammation, hemorrhage and necrosis, which allows in most cases to make the correct diagnosis already macroscopically. Microscopic examination in some cases reveals additional embolic lesions (Fig. 12.4).

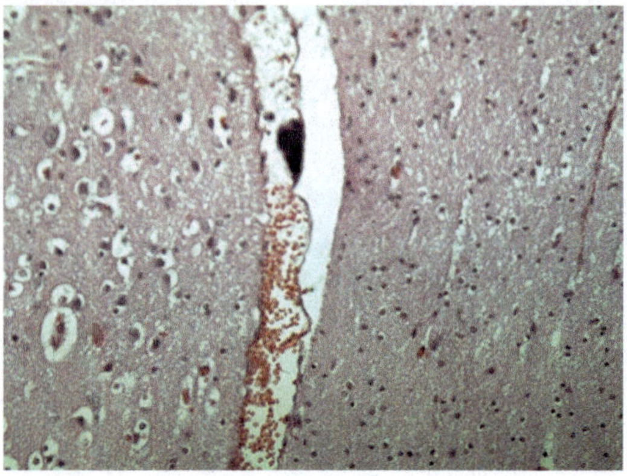

Fig. 12.4 Bacterial embolus in brain vessel in infectious endocarditis H-E × 200

12.8 Brain Lesions in Sepsis

Sepsis is one of the most important pathological processes in humans, the views on which have changed significantly over time and differ among specialists of different profiles and scientific schools. From the most accepted clinical positions, sepsis is a pathological process based on the reaction of the body in the form of systemic inflammation to an infection of various nature. However, some experts consider it possible to talk about antimicrobial sepsis. From the standpoint of pathology, sepsis is usually called a generalized bacterial or fungal infection with a predominantly hematogenic spread of the pathogen. The possibility of developing viral sepsis is not recognized by most researchers. It is necessary to differentiate sepsis from the clinical syndrome of "systemic inflammatory reaction (septic)" and bacteremia. Due to tradition, the term sepsis is not used for typhoid and typhoid fever, malaria, plague, anthrax, in which severe clinical symptoms are associated with the presence of pathogens in the blood.

Sepsis most often develops in weakened people: newborns, especially premature babies, burn patients, postoperative patients, etc. Although there is a widespread point of view that the etiological factor does not significantly affect the occurrence and manifestation of the disease, ideas about the exceptional importance of identifying the pathogen primarily for optimizing treatment dominate. The difficulties lie in the fact that when using standard nutrient media, the aerobic microbiota from the blood of septic patients is often not seeded. Modern technologies are not always used in the routine work of intensive care units. The most common pathogens of sepsis are staphylococci, Pseudomonas aeruginosa, klebsiella, enterococci, various gram-negative pathogens, including as part of a mixed infection. Pneumococcal sepsis develops almost exclusively in people without a spleen, more often associated with trauma. In addition to the activation of autoflora and the translocation of microbes from the intestine, exogenous infection with hospital strains of pathogens is also of great epidemiological importance. In some cases, a particularly high virulence of the pathogen is shown. The etiology of sepsis does not always significantly affect the clinical manifestations of the disease, but sometimes it can be assumed. Among the etiological forms of sepsis, meningococcemia stands out, having the brightest clinical and morphological features (see Chap. 9).

The main entrance gates for sepsis are the umbilical ring, large veins (during their catheterization), intestines, lungs, skin, endometrium (in the postpartum period), kidneys, tonsils, which is the basis of clinical and morphological classification. In some cases, it is not possible to identify the entrance gate for sepsis, and it is designated as cryptogenic.

Depending on the state of reactivity of the body, sepsis can occur with varying degrees of severity of clinical symptoms and exudative inflammatory reactions.

The main generally recognized variant of sepsis is septicopyemia, which is morphologically characterized by the presence of a primary focus of purulent inflammation, secondary hematogenous (metastatic) foci and signs of infectious and toxic shock with DIC syndrome.

The views on the second form of sepsis—septicemia, expressed by various specialists are ambiguous. The most common point of view is that septicemia is bacteremia without the formation of pyemic foci, in most cases it is a manifestation of infectious and toxic shock and precedes septicopyemia.

The pathological anatomy of sepsis consists of purulent (pyemic) foci, represented mainly by neutrophil infiltration, tending to blood vessels, vasculitis, often with the phenomena of microthrombosis and disseminated intravascular coagulation. The size of such foci can vary significantly, often they can be determined only by microscopic examination. The most important component of the morphological study is the detection of pathogens in septic foci using histobacterioscopic methods. The most important, although difficult to verify in an autopsy study, are alterative changes in parenchymal cells, with which it is customary to associate multiple organ failure.

Septic changes in the brain are usually differentiated from secondary purulent meningoencephalitis, most often of pneumococcal etiology, developing as complications of pneumonia, otitis, sinusitis (see Chap. 10).

Septic lesions of the brain have a fundamentally similar character to those observed in other organs (Figs. 12.5, 12.6, 12.7, 12.8, 12.9) and are detected in many observations. It should only be noted only the features of perivascular changes, represented by reactions from astrocytes in the form of swelling and proliferation of microglia, focal demyelination is possible.

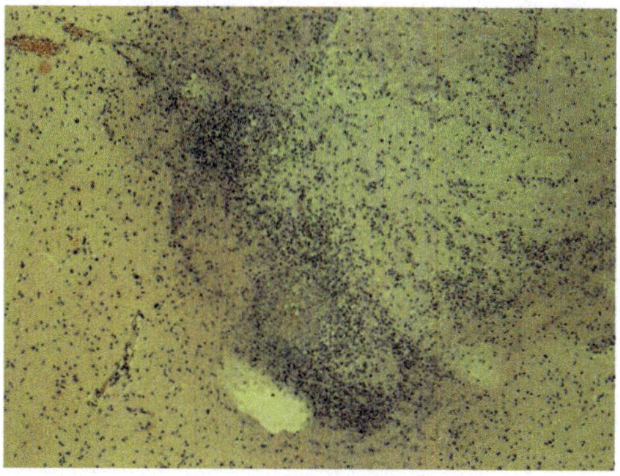

Fig. 12.5 Granuloma in brain matter in listeria meningoencephalitis in adult. H-E X600. (Courtesy of Y.R. Zyuzya)

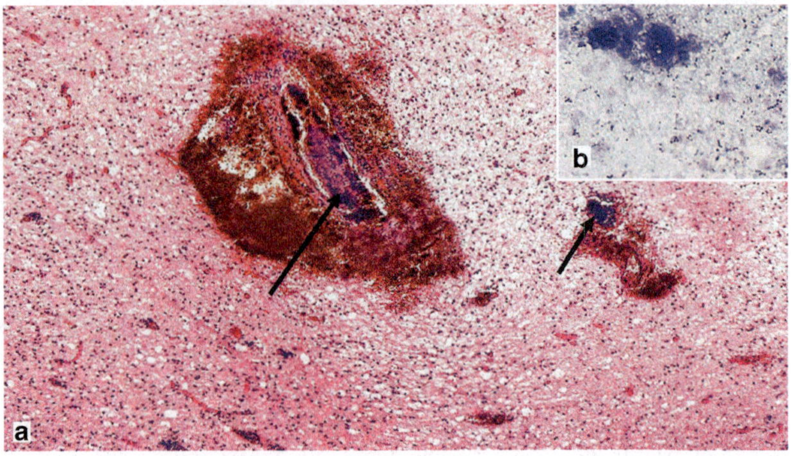

Fig. 12.6 Sepsis. (**a**) Microbial emboli in the vessels of the brain in sepsis (indicated by arrows); (**b**) Coccal microflora. **a** – H-E. ×100; **b** – methylene blue coloring. ×1000 (cytological preparation, smear imprint). (Courtesy of Y.R. Zyuzya)

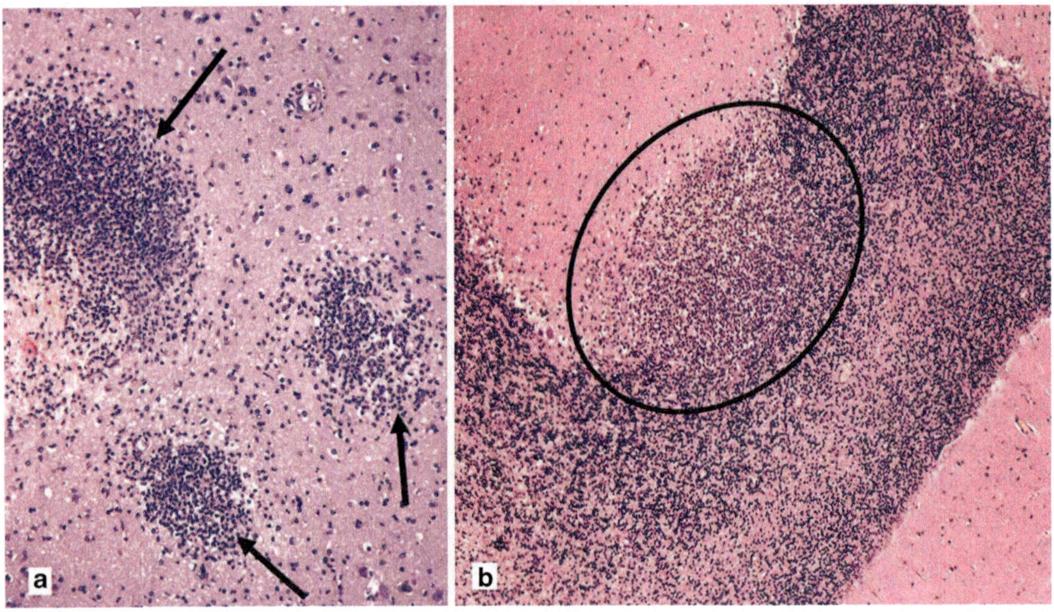

Fig. 12.7 Sepsis. (**a**) Pyemic foci in the substance of the brain (indicated by arrows); (**b**) Pyemic foci in the cerebellum (circled by a round frame). H-E **a** – ×100; **b** – ×40. (Courtesy of Y.R. Zyuzya)

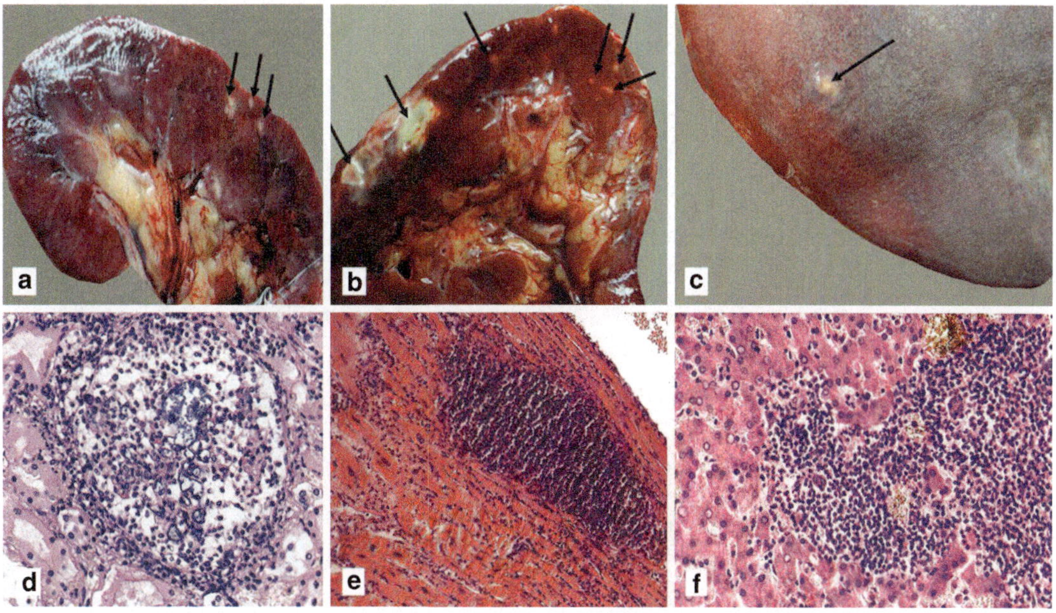

Fig. 12.8 Pyemic foci in various organs. (**a**) Pyemic foci in the cortical substance of the kidney (indicated by arrows); (**b**) Pyemic foci and kidney abscesses (indicated by arrows); (**c**) Pyemic focus in the liver (indicated by arrow); (**d**) Pyemic focus in the kidney, in the center of the accumulation of bacillary microflora; (**e**) Pyemic focus in the myocardium; (**f**) Pyemic focus in the liver. **a**, **b**, **c** – unfixed macropreparations; (**d**, **e**, **f**) H-E. (**d**, **f**) – ×200; (**e**) – ×100. (Courtesy of Y.R. Zyuzya)

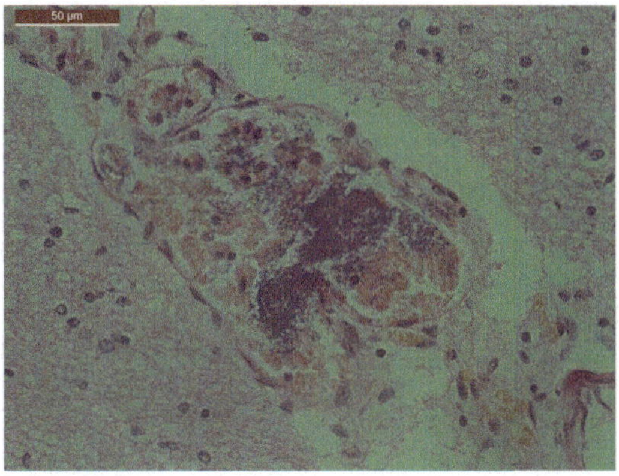

Fig. 12.9 Accumulation of cocci in meningeal blood vessel at the early stage of sepsis. Stained H-E, ×950

References

1. Chaudhary A, Panday S. Corynebacterium diphtheriae StatPearls [internet]. Treasure Island, FL: StatPearlsPublishing; 2021.
2. Zinserling VA, Chukhlovina M. Pathogenesis and immune response. Clin Lab Med. 35(4):745–64. https://doi.org/10.1016/j.cll.2015.07.004.
3. Tiwari A, Nagali S. Clostridium botulinum. In: Diphteriae StatPearls [internet]. Treasure Island, FL: StatPearlsPublishing; 2021.
4. Petzke M, Schwartz I. Borrelia burgdorferi pathogenesis and the immune response. Clin Lab Med. 2015;35(4):745–64. https://doi.org/10.1016/j.cll2015.07.004.
5. Zinserling VA, Melnikova VF. Perinatal Infections: issues of pathogenesis, morphological diagnostic and clinic-pathological correlations. Manual for doctors "Elbi-SPb", 351 p (in Russian) 2002.
6. Choi MH, Park YJ, Kim M, et al. Increasing incidence of listeriosis and infection-associated clinical outcomes. Ann Lab Med. 2018;38:102–9. https://doi.org/10.3343/alm.2018.38.2.1202.
7. De Noordhout CM, Devleesschauwer B, Angulo FJ, et al. The global burden of listeriosis: a systemic review and metaanalysis. Lancet Infect Dis. 2014;14:1073–82. https://doi.org/10.1016/S1473-3099(14)70870-9.
8. AlObaidi MMJ, Deasa MNM. Mechanisms of blood brain barrier disruption by different types of bacteria, and bacterial-host interactions facilitate the bacterial pathogen invading the brain. Cell Mol Neurobiol. 2018;38:1349–68. https://doi.org/10.1007/s10571-018-0609-12.
9. Bhutta ZA, GaffeyMF CJA, et al. Typhoid fever:way forward. Am J Trop Med Hyg. 2018;99(3_Suppl):89–96. https://doi.org/10.4269/ajtmh.18-0111.
10. Hubers SA, DeSimone DC, Gersh BJ, Anavekar NS. Infective endocarditis: a Contemporary review. Mayo Clin Proc. 2020;95(5):982–97. https://doi.org/10.1016/j.mayocp.2019.12.008.

13 Neurotuberculosis and Neurosyphilis (in Collaboration with Y.R. Zyuzya)

13.1 Tuberculosis of the Central Nervous System

The causative agent of tuberculosis (Mycobacterium tuberculosis) was discovered by the German bacteriologist R. Koch in 1882. Currently, the properties of this pathogen are studied in detail. Advances in molecular genetics made it possible to complete the decoding of its genome, which contains more than 4000 genes, by 1998 [1]. According to the World Health Organization (WHO), in 2016, the 10 most common causes of death are ischemic heart disease, stroke, chronic obstructive pulmonary disease, pneumonia, Alzheimer's disease and other dementias, respiratory cancers, diabetes mellitus, road accidents, intestinal infections, and tuberculosis [2].

It should be emphasized that the AIDS epidemic has led to an increase in cases of active tuberculosis, which has become the leading cause of death among HIV-1-infected patients in developing countries. HIV infection weakens the immune system, which leads to reactivation of latent tuberculosis infection and rapid progression of the disease in individuals infected with Mycobacterium tuberculosis. A complete morphological description of respiratory tuberculosis was given earlier [3].

13.1.1 Clinical Features

Tuberculosis meningitis has been described in many publications of the past years, information about its clinical and pathological features has been included in textbooks around the world on neurology, infectious diseases, phthisiology pediatrics, therapy, and pathological anatomy all over the world [4–7]. There is mainly a basal localization of the process, a kind of yellowish infiltrate, in which fuchsinophilic rods are determined when stained according to Ziehl-Nielsen (Z-N), a mixed neutrophil-mononuclear nature of the infiltration, a high protein content and low glucose in the CSF, which significantly distinguishes it from other nosological forms. All this, it seemed, would contribute to its successful clinical and morphological diagnosis. At the same time, the experience of pathological diagnosis of tuberculous meningitis in both adults and children indicates frequent significant difficulties. There are no modern works with a detailed description of structural changes in tuberculosis of the central nervous system in the world literature.

In the International Classification of 10—revision (ICD-10), there is a category of tuberculosis of the nervous system, including tuberculous meningitis, meningeal tuberculosis,

V. Zinserling, *Infectious Lesions of the Central Nervous System*,
https://doi.org/10.1007/978-3-030-96260-9_13

tuberculosis of the nervous system of other localizations, tuberculosis of the nervous system, unspecified; tuberculosis of the spine is considered separately. The classification of tuberculosis used in the Russian Federation separately distinguishes tuberculosis of the meninges and central nervous system; tuberculosis of bones and joints.

Special attention should be paid to the working classification of neurological complications in tuberculosis, which takes into account the variety of clinical manifestations of lesions of the nervous system in this pathology [5]. According to this classification, neurological complications in tuberculosis are divided into four large groups: I. Tuberculosis of the nervous system II. Nonspecific lesions of the nervous system III. Residual effects after tuberculosis of the nervous system IV. Lesions of the nervous system under the influence of anti-tuberculosis treatment. In the first group, lesions of the central nervous system (meningitis, meningoencephalitis, meningoencephalomyelitis, tuberculoma of the brain), peripheral nervous system (mononeuropathy, polyneuropathy) and spinal cord roots in tuberculous spondylitis are considered separately. In the second group, acute toxic encephalopathy and encephalomyelopolineuropathy are distinguished. The third group includes cerebral basal arachnoiditis (after meningitis, meningoencephalitis), lesions of the optic nerves and chiasm, and residual effects of damage to the spinal cord and roots after tuberculous spondylitis. The fourth group includes mono—and polyneuropathies, lesions of the optic nerve, and lesions of the vestibulocochlear nerve. It seems that this approach allows us to give an in-depth description of neurological complications in tuberculosis, to clarify the formulation of the diagnosis.

In clinical practice, among the lesions of the nervous system in tuberculosis, tuberculous meningitis is more common. It is shown that the age structure among patients with tuberculous meningitis is dominated by children under 2 years and young people from 18 to 24 years. In most cases, these patients can detect the primary focus of tuberculosis in the lungs. Symptoms of tuberculosis are usually divided into systemic and organ-specific. The first include subfebrile temperature, sweating, especially at night, decreased appetite, body weight, and general weakness. The second—with tuberculosis of the lungs include cough, pleural pain, hemoptysis. Tuberculosis meningitis in children can develop suddenly, in adolescents and adults more often gradually after prodromal phenomena. Along with general malaise, increased fatigue, irritability, headaches occur, the frequency and intensity of which increase, nausea and vomiting appear.

After 1–3 weeks, the prodromal period is replaced by the development of meningeal phenomena, the temperature rises to 38–39 °C. At this time, the patient is most concerned about constant severe headaches with nausea and vomiting, and the development of a convulsive syndrome is possible. There is drowsiness, lethargy, forced posture—eyes closed, head thrown back, legs bent at the knee and hip joints, pressed against the retracted abdomen, its muscles tense. Palpation of the eyeballs and skin becomes painful. In small children, a large fontanel bulges out. Meningeal symptoms are detected: rigidity of the occipital muscles, Kernig's symptoms, Brudzinsky's symptoms, often upper and lower. At the same time, meningeal symptoms are often not clearly expressed, their dissociation is noted: the presence of rigidity of the occipital muscles in the absence of symptoms of Kernig and Brudzinsky. Deep reflexes and superficial abdominal ones are reduced, quickly depleted. Periodically, episodes of motor arousal may occur, sometimes accompanied by delirium. Gradually, tachycardia is replaced by bradycardia, with a severe course, a comatose state develops. Due to the predominant lesion of the meninges of the base of the brain, the cranial nerves are often involved in the tuberculous process. Characteristics of the defeat of VI, III, and VII pairs of cranial nerves can be observed. A tuberculous lesion of the optic nerve is described. When the brain substance is involved in the pathological process, development of tuberculous meningoencephalitis is possible with the appearance of central paresis, paralysis. It should be emphasized that the classic course of tuberculous meningitis in children has changed in recent years, and the number of erased cases has increased.

When performing a lumbar puncture, a clear, colorless, sometimes xanthochromic cerebrospinal fluid flows out under pressure, pleocytosis is small—up to 120–300 cells in 1 mcl, of a mixed nature with a predominance of lymphocytes. The protein content can increase to 1–3 g/l, the glucose level is significantly reduced (to 0.8–1.5 mmol/l) with a slight decrease in the amount of chloride. If you put a few drops of liquor on the glass, a fibrin film is often formed within 12 h, in which in some cases Koch's rods can be detected.

Currently, highly sensitive tests are widely used to detect the Mycobacterium tuberculosis antigen in the cerebrospinal fluid using PCR. In the peripheral blood leukopenia with lymphopenia, a shift of the leukocyte formula to the left is detected.

It is proved that the correct recognition of the nature of the process is facilitated by indications of tuberculosis in the anamnesis, prolonged contact with tuberculosis patients, the presence of tuberculosis lesions of other organs, combined with the picture of intracranial neoplasm, acute infectious diseases, respiratory tract diseases and the appearance of the first symptoms of brain damage after these infections. The presence of the prodromal period of the disease, subfebrile temperature, children's and youth age of patients, subtentorial localization of the process, the presence of symptoms of multifocal brain damage, positive tuberculin reactions, increased protein and pleocytosis, mainly lymphocytic in the cerebrospinal fluid, are important. Prior to the introduction of modern methods of neuroimaging into clinical practice, in vivo recognition of brain tuberculosis occurred in 17.6% of cases.

Currently, tuberculomas of the brain in adults, which represent the maximum difficulties in differential diagnosis for neurosurgeons, occur in 0.87–8.8% in pulmonary tuberculosis and in 12.2% in tuberculous lesions of the central nervous system. Solitary tuberculomas are most often detected in the cerebellum, brain stem, and meninges, and are less often found in the large hemispheres. Patients with tuberculomas of the brain are admitted to neurological or neurosurgical departments with directional diagnoses: intracranial hypertension, volume formation of the brain, acute circulatory disorders of the brain. According to the clinical course, tuberculomas of the brain are similar to gliomas, meningiomas, and tumors of the posterior cranial fossa. During the 25 years in the neurosurgical department of the Mariinsky Hospital of St. Petersburg, among 2000 patients operated on for tumors of the central nervous system, brain tuberculoma was detected in four cases [8].

Among the lesions of the peripheral nervous system in tuberculosis, polyneuropathy is more common, manifested by numbness, pain in the toes, and fatigue when walking. In patients with osteoarticular tuberculosis, tuberculosis spondylitis is detected in 45–82% of cases. It should be emphasized that in patients with tuberculous spondylitis in the presence of a pronounced pain syndrome for 1.5–2 months, changes on radiographs are often not detected. Clinical observations indicate that in 90% of patients, contact destruction of two or three vertebrae is detected, and infiltration of paravertebral soft tissues is noted. In the diagnosis of tuberculous spondylitis, complicated by neurological disorders, along with radiography, computer tomography is successfully used. Using this method, it is possible to detect infiltrative changes in the epidural tissue. It is shown that the main cause of damage to the nervous system in tuberculosis spondylitis is the narrowing of the spinal canal due to infiltration and compression of the spinal cord and its roots. The presence of a reserve space in the spinal canal is also important. Thus, the most severe neurological disorders develop when the lower cervical and mid-thoracic parts of the spine are affected, where such spaces are not expressed. It is believed that tuberculosis of the spine (Pott's disease) develops as a result of hematogenous dissemination or when mycobacteria spread through the lymphatic vessels from the pleural cavity to the paravertebral lymph nodes. The progression of tuberculous spondylitis can lead to curvature of the spine and the appearance of cold abscesses. Diagnostic difficulties often arise in tuberculosis of flat bones and pelvic joints. Such patients may develop sacroiliitis with intense pain in the sacroiliac joint. During a neurological examination, more than half of the patients show pain during palpation of the paravertebral points, along the sciatic nerve, and sometimes the femoral nerve; there may be a decrease in the Achilles, knee reflexes, symptoms of tension of the nerve trunks (Laseg, Mackiewicz, Wasserman). Pathognomonic for sacroiliitis are the following symptoms: Gate -occurrence of pain in the area of the iliosacral joint with forced hip flexion in the hip joint with the knee joint bent in the supine position; Bonnet - pain in the same area when turning to the inner femoral surface of the leg, bent at the knee joint. Changes in radiographs in sacroiliitis usually develop much later than the onset of pain, which makes early diagnosis difficult. Provoking factors for the development of tuberculous sacroiliitis can be overcooling, trauma, and the postpartum period.

As noted, patients with tuberculosis may develop nonspecific lesions of the nervous system. The latter can be in the form of acute tuberculous encephalopathy, developing acutely with a violation of consciousness from stunning to coma, often with a convulsive syndrome, headache. In contrast to tuberculous meningitis, headache is usually moderate, vomiting is infrequent from meningeal symptoms, Kernig's symptoms can be detected, there are no symptoms of cranial nerve damage, the cerebrospinal fluid is not changed.

13.1.2 Pathology of Tuberculosis of the Central Nervous System without HIV Infection in Adults

Tuberculosis of the central nervous system includes lesions of the brain, spinal cord, and their membranes.

There are two main mechanisms of pathogenesis with leading role in pathogen's spreading through blood and cerebrospinal fluid [6].

Hematogenic phase of infection is considered as a link in the general chain of generalization of tuberculosis: initial reactive changes in the intima of the vessels of the meninges and vascular plexuses of the ventricles of the brain, the development of vasculitis with increased permeability of the vascular wall, thrombosis, violation of the vascular barrier (blood-brain barrier). Mycobacterium tuberculosis penetrates through the altered vascular walls, specific vasculitis develops, infection of the cerebrospinal fluid (cerebrospinal fluid phase) and the soft meninges.

Ya. L. Rapoport in 1936 established three conditions for the development of tuberculosis meningitis: general, local sensitization and tuberculosis bacteremia, which are considered relevant till present.

According to the lymphogenic theory, mycobacteria penetrate from the affected intra-thoracic mesenteric lymph nodes to the cervical ones, then to the base of the brain along the lymphatic pathways accompanying the large arterial trunks.

Some authors also suggest a contact pathway in the process of developing a tuberculous lesion of the central nervous system. According to this theory, there is an introduction of mycobacteria to the spine, skull, bones, ear cavities, nose, eye, orbit, tonsils. It is also considered possible for pathogens to enter the soft meninges and the cerebrospinal fluid space from tuberculous foci of the membranes and brain matter ("Rich's focus," including when the caseous focus of the brain breaks into the subarachnoid space), the bones of the skull.

Some authors distinguish four ways of infection of the meninges in tuberculosis—hematogenic, lymphogenic, cerebrospinal fluid, perineural.

Based on the pathogenetic principle, there are usually distinguished:

1. tuberculous meningitis with primary tuberculosis and early large focal generalization,
2. tuberculous meningitis in late (miliary) generalization,
3. tuberculous meningitis in hematogenic tuberculosis.

Items 1 and 2 are characteristic of primary ("child") tuberculosis and can also occur in elderly and senile people with the course of tuberculosis typical for primary tuberculosis in children.

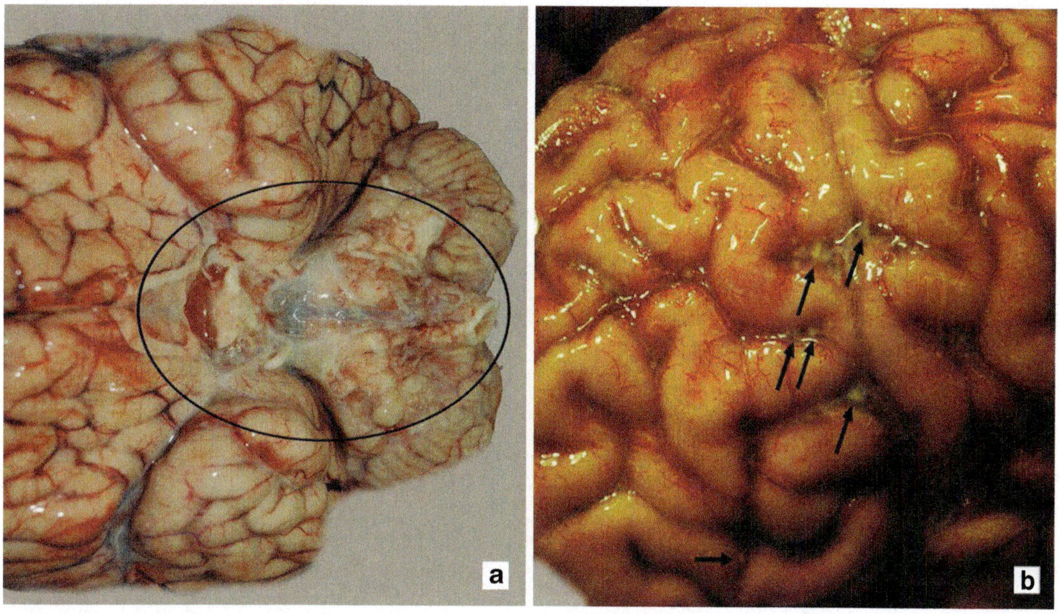

Fig. 13.1 (**a**) Basal tuberculous meningitis. The soft medulla of the base of the brain is jelly-like, translucent, slightly whitish, swollen (circled by a round frame); (**b**) Miliary rash in the soft medulla along the course of the blood vessels (indicated by arrows). Unfixed macropreparations

A number of authors believe that primary tuberculous meningitis can occur in the absence of visible tuberculous changes in the lungs or other organs—"isolated" primary meningitis, and secondary tuberculous meningitis occurs as a hematogenous generalization with damage to the meninges against the background of active pulmonary tuberculosis in children or in the presence of extrapulmonary tuberculosis.

Regarding "isolated" tuberculosis meningitis, many phthisiologists believe that it is necessary to search for an extracerebral focus of tuberculosis infection, including a small or even healed one, which can explain development of brain damage.

There are distinguished serous tuberculous meningitis, basilar tuberculous meningitis (the most common), meningoencephalitic (meningovascular) form and spinal (cerebrospinal) form. There are also tuberculomas of the brain and tuberculomas of the meninges, which are a lumpy focus of cord necrosis in the subcortical parts of the brain tissue or in the meninges.

According to the nature of the course, tuberculous meningitis is classified as acute, subacute, chronic, and recurrent.

Taking into account the nature of the exudate, serous, serous-fibrinous, purulent, and hemorrhagic meningitis are distinguished.

The most characteristic localization of tuberculous inflammation of the soft meninges is the area of the base of the brain. Macroscopic examination shows that the shells here are swollen, can reach a thickness of several millimeters, jelly-like, translucent, whitish, yellowish, or greenish-yellowish in color. On the surface, mostly along the course of the vessels, there are grayish-whitish miliary tubercles with a diameter of 1–2 mm (Fig. 13.1). Localization of specific lesions in tuberculosis meningitis in the soft meninges of the base of the brain from the intersection of the visual pathways to the medulla oblongata. The process can pass to the lateral surfaces of the hemispheres of the brain, usually during the Sylvian furrows, in this case, basilar convexital meningitis develops.

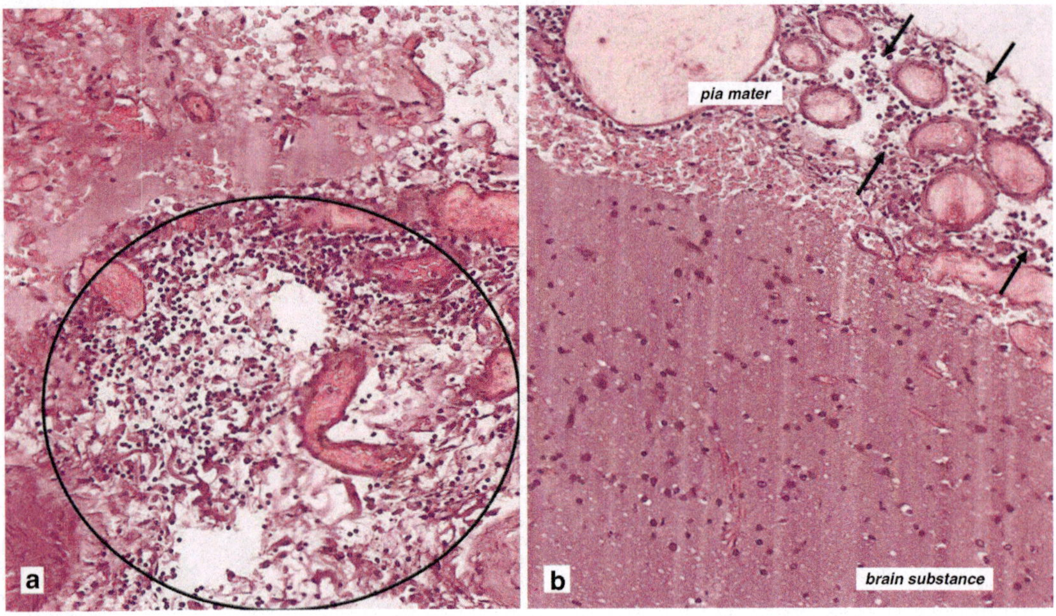

Fig. 13.2 Productive tuberculous leptomeningitis. In the soft medulla, there is moderate edema, fullness, and lymphoid reaction. (**a**) The inflammatory lymphoid infiltrate is circled by a round frame; (**b**) Areas of lymphoid infiltration are indicated by arrows. H-E; ×100

In macroscopic examination during autopsy, the cerebrospinal fluid in the lateral ventricles of the brain is usually transparent or cloudy. The ventricles of the brain can be dilated.

Microscopically, in the initial period of the disease, the inflammation has a "nonspecific" character, which is manifested by fullness, edema, and lymphoid infiltration. Macrophages and white blood cells may be present in the inflammatory infiltrate (Fig. 13.2). Later, after about 10 days, signs of "specific" inflammation are detected. Microscopic examination, in addition to edema, fibrosis, and diffuse focal, mainly lymphoid infiltration of the membranes, shows the formation of single and draining epithelioid giant cell granulomas, including those with caseous necrosis in the center (Figs. 13.3, 13.4, 13.5, 13.6).

When staining histological sections according to Z-N, acid-resistant bacteria are detected, especially in caseous necrotic foci, in areas with leukocyte infiltration, as well as in macrophages (Fig. 13.7a). Histobacterioscopy according to Z-N is usually effective approximately in 40%, but in cases of acute progressive process, in particular, in HIV-associated tuberculosis, the effectiveness can reach 80% [9]. Histobacterioscopy according to Z-N allows us to determine whether the microorganisms belong to the family of "acid- and alcohol-resistant bacteria." An IHC study using antibodies against M. tuberculosis clarifies the generic affiliation of acid-resistant bacteria to mycobacteria (Fig. 13.7b).

Exact identification of pathogens was carried out using bacteriological method - seeding of autopsy material (for example, CSF, brain matter, brain membranes) on special nutrient media. Currently, the polymerase chain reaction is used to detect the DNA of M. tuberculosis. It is advisable to take CSF from the lateral ventricles during autopsy for bacteriological research, including molecular genetic testing to detect the DNA of Mycobacterium tuberculosis. In the absence of native material, the material from the paraffin block can be examined by PCR.

Moreover, to establish the tuberculosis etiology of the process, a cytological study is valuable, for example, the study of a cytological preparation of a smear an imprint of the brain

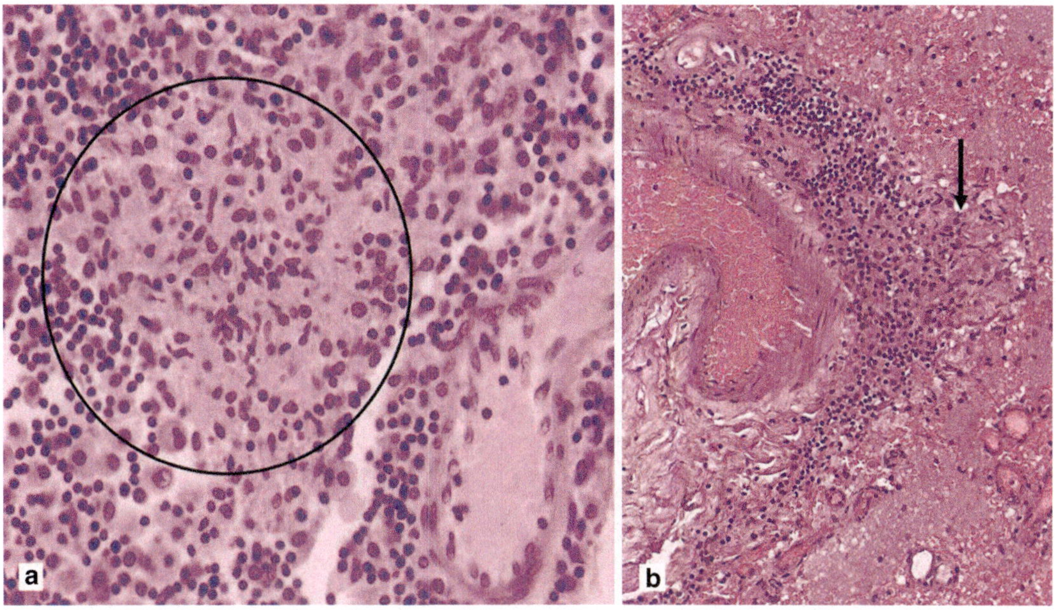

Fig. 13.3 Tuberculosis leptomeningitis. Forming perivascular macrophage epithelioid granulomas. (**a**) The granuloma is surrounded by a round frame; (**b**) The granuloma is indicated by an arrow. H-E; (**a**) × 200; (**b**) 100

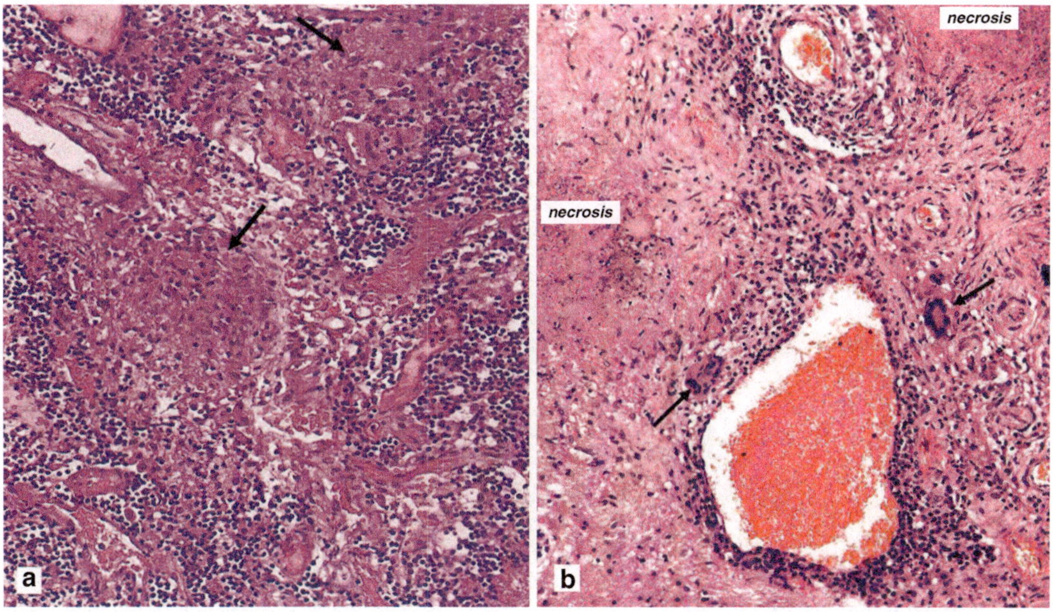

Fig. 13.4 Tuberculosis leptomeningitis. (**a**) Small macrophage-epithelioid granuloma (indicated by arrows), lymphoid infiltration; (**b**) Vascular fullness, uneven perivascular lymphoid infiltration and single giant multinucleated cells (indicated by arrows), areas of caseous necrosis with white blood cells and indistinct epithelioid cell reaction along the edge. H-E; (**a**) ×100; (**b**) × 200

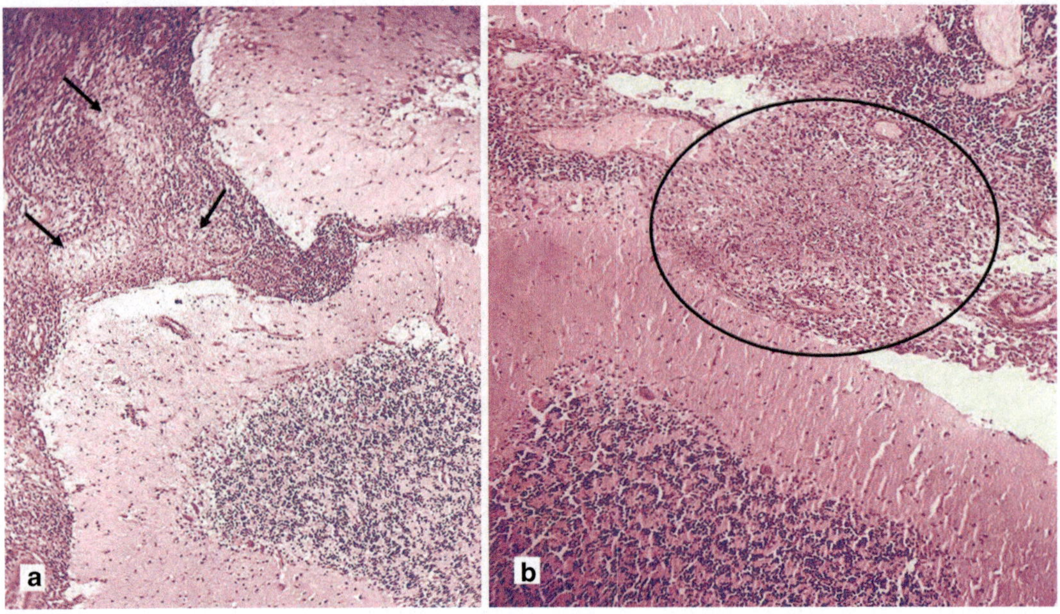

Fig. 13.5 Basal tuberculous meningitis (cerebellum, soft medulla). In the soft medulla, there is a dense lymphoid infiltrate, a fullness of blood vessels, and granulomas formed (Fig. "**a**" granulomas are indicated by arrows; in Fig. "**b**" - circled with a round border). H-E; ×100

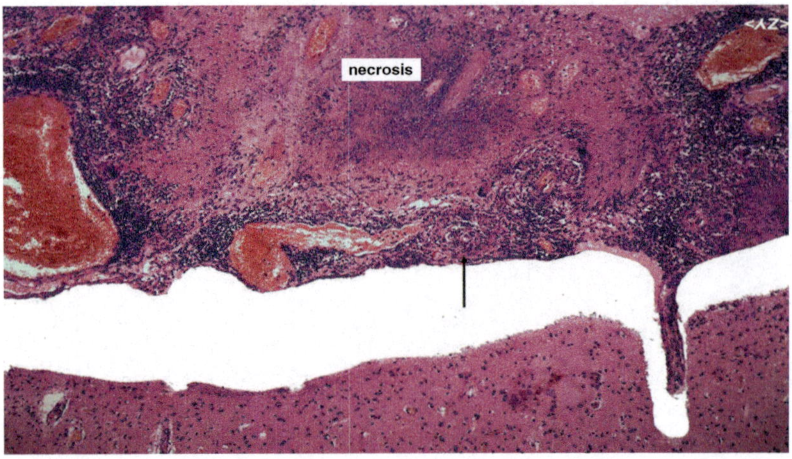

Fig. 13.6 Tuberculosis leptomeningitis. In the soft medulla, there is pronounced lymphoid infiltration, small granulomas (granuloma is indicated by an arrow), foci of caseous necrosis with leukocyte infiltration, epithelioid giant cell reaction at the periphery. H-E; ×100

membrane. This study allows us to identify elements of granulomatous inflammation, and when staining a cytological preparation according to Z-N or with luminescent microscopy with auramine-rhodamine staining, acid-resistant bacteria (Fig. 13.8).

Tuberculous meningitis is characterized by damage to blood vessels, mainly veins, as well as small and medium-sized arteries. The walls of blood vessels with signs of acute, subacute and productive vasculitis and thrombovasculitis (depending on the degree of activity of the tuberculosis process), which is manifested by neutrophilic, lymphoid-leukocyte, lymphoid infiltration of the vascular wall, edema, signs of increased vascular permeability (Fig. 13.9). Peri- and endo-

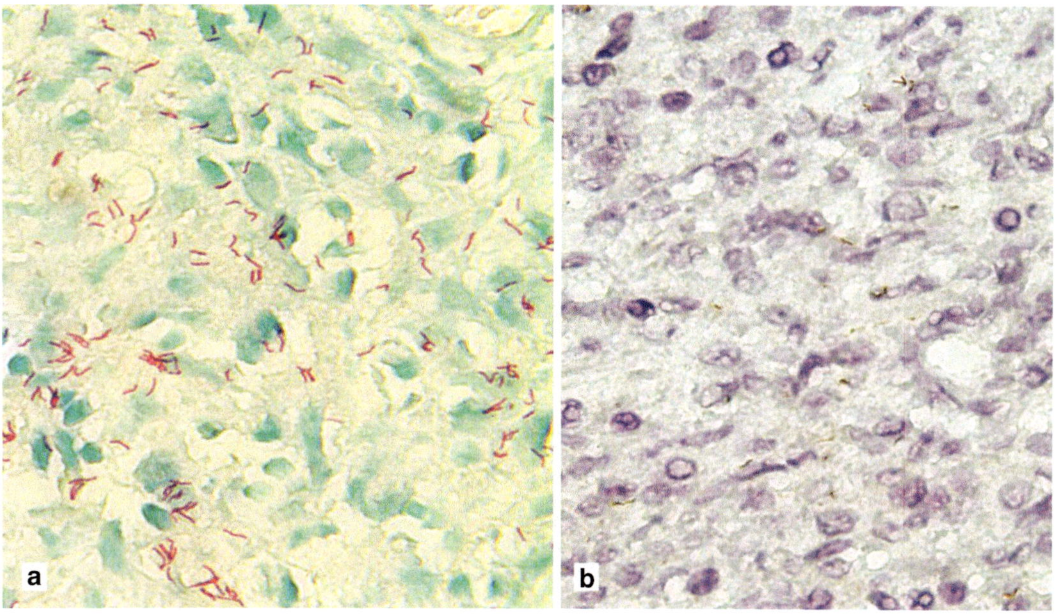

Fig. 13.7 (**a**) Acid-resistant bacteria (colored red); Z-N staining. ×1000; (**b**) Mycobacteria (colored brown); IHC study with tuberculosis antibodies. ×1000

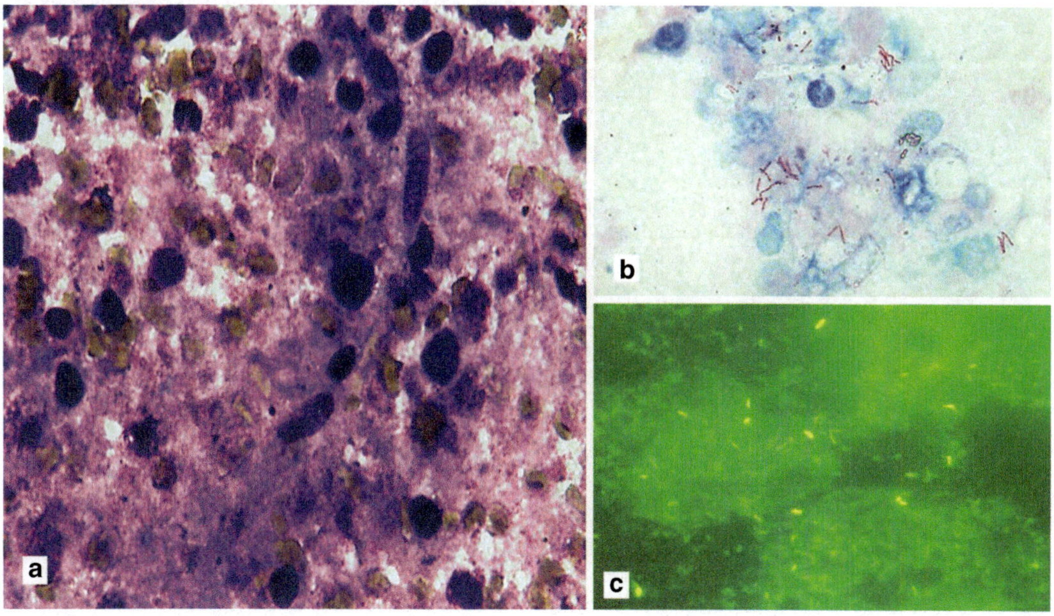

Fig. 13.8 Cytological preparations. (**a**) In the smear print, lymphocytes and epithelioid cells; (**b**) Acid-resistant bacteria (colored red); (**c**) Acid-resistant bacteria (colored golden yellow). Stainings: (**a**) according to Romanovsky-Giemsa. ×1000; (**b**) according to Zil-Nielsen. ×400; (**c**) immunofluorescence study with auramine-rhodamine staining. ×400

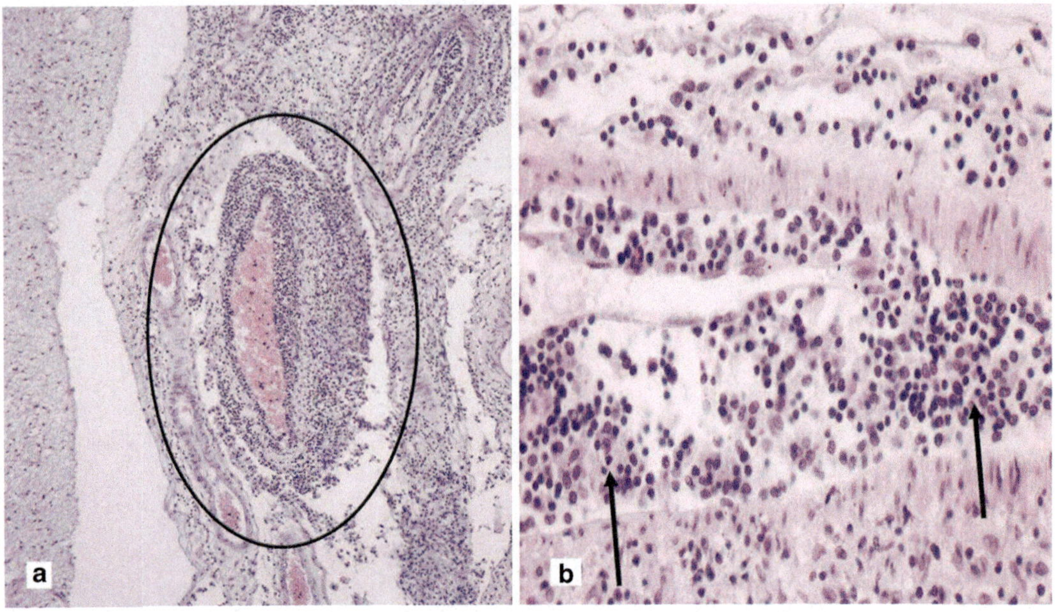

Fig. 13.9 Tuberculosis leptomeningitis. Productive vasculitis. (**a**) The vessel is surrounded by an oval frame; (**b**) The inflammatory infiltrate cells in the vessel wall are indicated by arrows. H-E; **a** – ×100; **b** – ×400

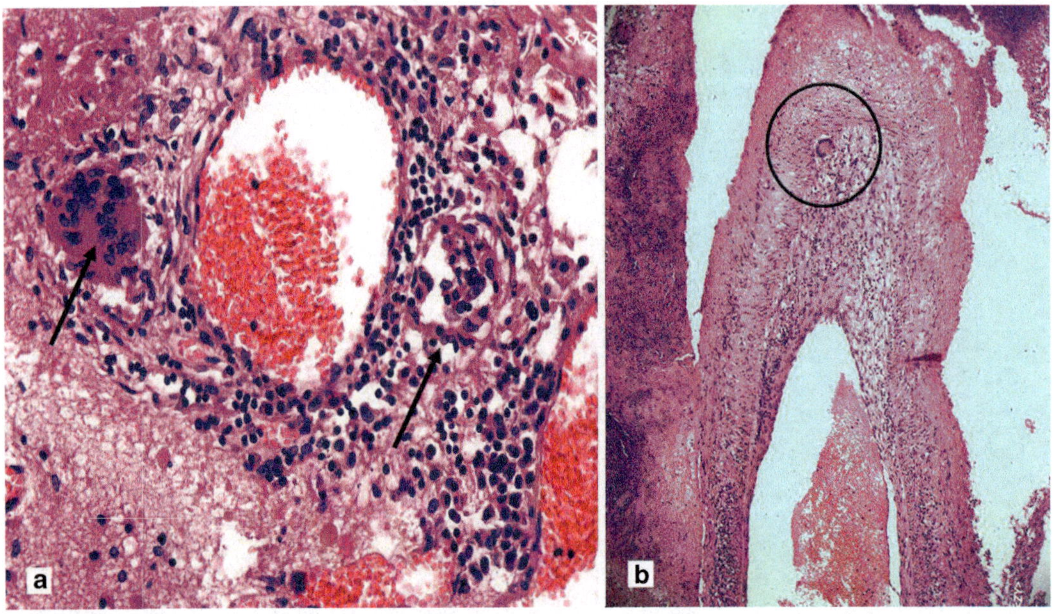

Fig. 13.10 Tuberculosis leptomeningitis. Tuberculous granulomatous vasculitis. H-E; **a** – X200; **b** – X100

vasculitis with proliferation of endotheliocytes and narrowing of the vessel lumen is detected. In addition to reactive vasculitis, tuberculous vasculitis develops with the formation of granulomas and necrotic changes in the vessel wall. Tuberculous vasculitis and perivasculitis occur in the form of a lymphoid infiltrate with the presence of epithelioid and giant multinucleated cells, without formation of distinct granulomas (Figs. 13.10 and 13.11).

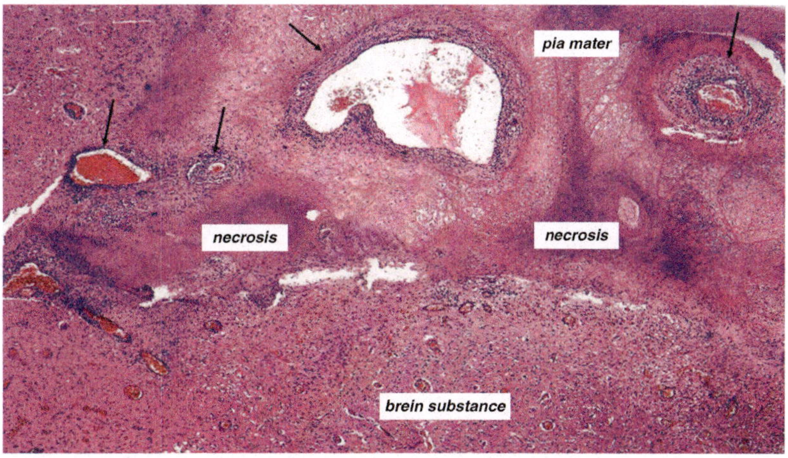

Fig. 13.11 Tuberculosis leptomeningitis. In the soft medulla, edema, areas of necrosis with leukocyte infiltration, vessels with signs of productive and granulomatous vasculitis (vessels are indicated by arrows)

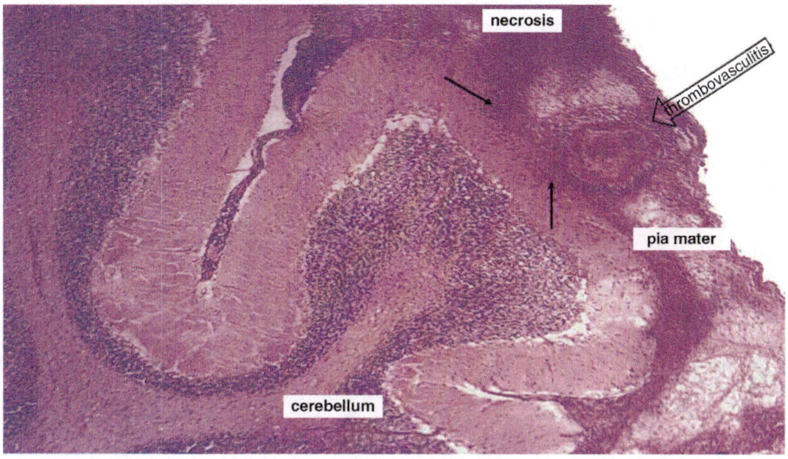

Fig. 13.12 Tuberculous meningoencephalitis (lesion of the basal parts of the brain). The inflammation spreads from the soft medulla to the cerebellum (indicated by the black arrows). H-E; ×40

The spread of inflammation to the adjacent substance of the brain leads to the appearance of foci of tuberculous lesions in the brain (Figs. 13.12, 13.13, 13.14). The development of "specific" or reactive productive and destructive vasculitis and thrombovasculitis in the membranes and substance of the brain contributes to this process and provokes the development of secondary ischemic infarction or infarcts, which increases the volume of brain damage and aggravates the severity of the patient's condition (Fig. 13.15). Occasionally there are also hemorrhagic brain lesions, such as extensive subarachnoid hemorrhages and hemorrhagic cerebral infarcts.

Morphological manifestations of tuberculous encephalitis are granulomas, often located perivascular (Figs. 13.16 and 13.17); miliary perivascular foci, often of necrotic type (necrotic tubercles) (Fig. 13.18), as well as tuberculous abscess of the brain (Fig. 13.19) and focal lesions—tuberculomas of the brain, which are a lumped focus of curd necrosis, usually located in the subcortical parts of the substance brain (Figs. 13.20 and 13.21).

In the wall of the tuberculous abscess there are elements of tuberculous inflammation—epithelioid and giant multinucleated cells (see Fig. 13.19b), granulomas; the inner purulent-necrotic layer is represented by caseous masses with leukocyte infiltration.

Changes of a "nonspecific," reactive nature are also found in the brain substance — edema of the brain substance (Fig. 13.22a), venous plethora, capillary plethora, fibrin-erythrocyte thrombi in small vessels with DIC syndrome (Fig. 13.22b), neuron degeneration, neuronophagy, focal

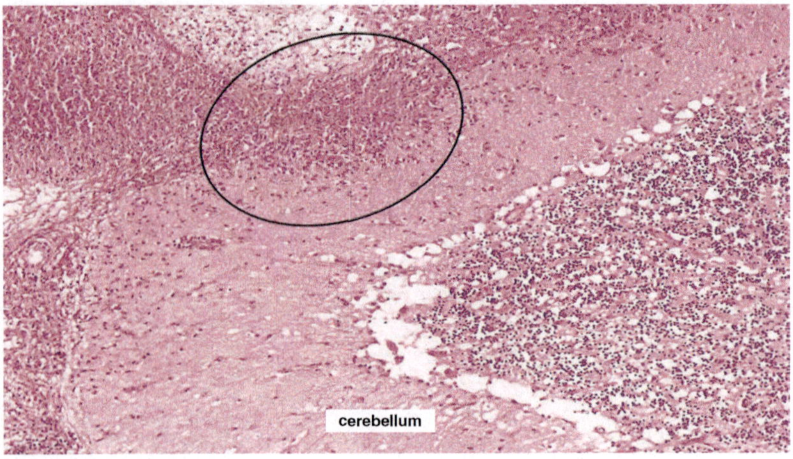

Fig. 13.13 Tuberculous meningoencephalitis (lesion of the basal parts of the brain). The spread of inflammation from the soft medulla to the cerebellum (indicated by a round frame). H-E; ×200

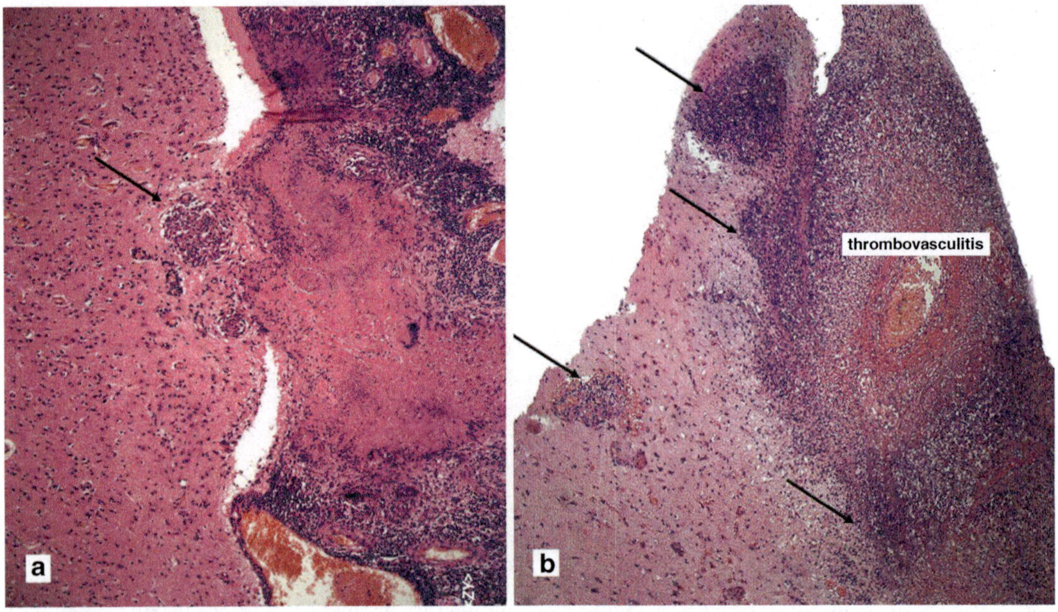

Fig. 13.14 Tuberculous meningoencephalitis. The spread of inflammation from the soft meninges to the underlying areas of the brain. (**a**) On the right the soft medulla with full blood, dense diffuse lymphoid infiltrate, the focus of caseous necrosis; on the left the underlying area of the brain with forming granulomas (indicated by the arrow); (**b**) In the soft medulla, thrombovasculitis, forming foci of tuberculous inflammation in the adjacent areas of the brain (indicated by the arrows). H-E; ×100

gliosis, perivascular muff-like lymphoid infiltration (Fig.13.22c).

To establish the mycobacterial etiology of the process allows histobacterioscopic examination with staining of sections according to Z-N and IHC with tuberculosis antibodies, as mentioned above. Cytological examination of smears-prints of the affected areas of the brain substance, stained according to Z-N, will also help to obtain data in favor of tuberculosis when acid-resistant bacteria are detected in smears.

If possible, it is advisable to take material from an abscess or a closed focus, suspicious of brain tuberculosis, for bacteriological (molecular biological) examination during an autopsy. With a tuberculous abscess or with tuberculoma of the

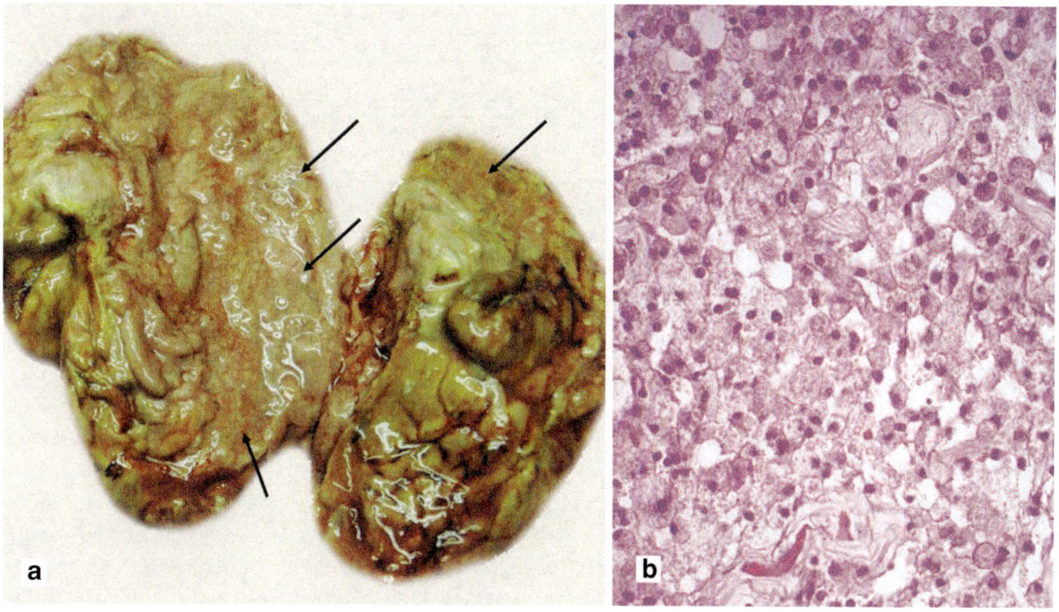

Fig. 13.15 Secondary ischemic brain infarction in tuberculous meningoencephalitis. (**a**) Extensive cerebral infarction (areas of destruction are indicated by arrows); (**b**) Cells of "granular balls" in the infarcted area of the brain. An unfixed macropreparation; (**b**) – H-E; ×400

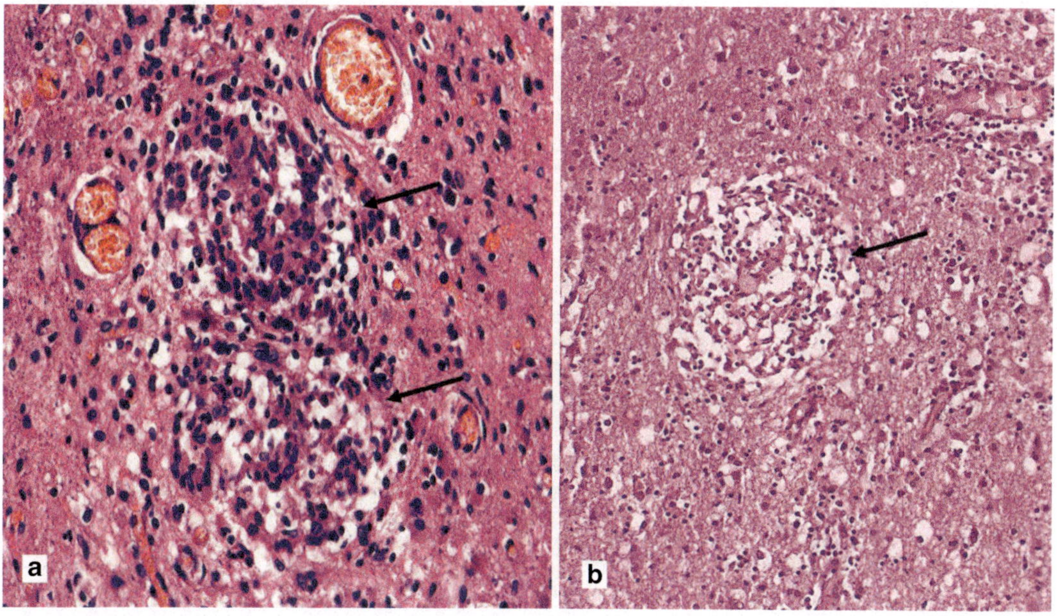

Fig. 13.16 Granulomas in the substance of the brain (indicated by arrows). H-E; **a** ×200; **b** ×100

brain (i.e., with delimited foci in the substance of the brain), Mycobacterium tuberculosis is often not found in the cerebrospinal fluid. It should be remembered that it is not typical for tuberculosis to detect "nonspecific" and pyogenic microflora in the lesions, except in cases of combined lesions, which is observed in immunosuppressive conditions. In tuberculous meningoencephalitis,

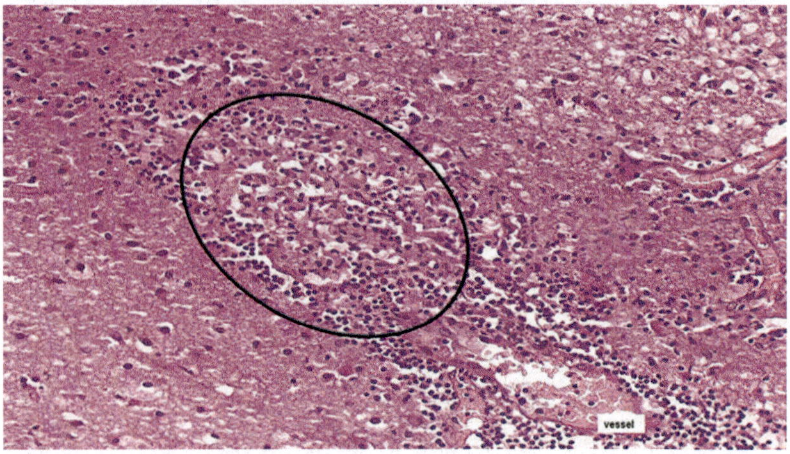

Fig. 13.17 Forming perivascular granulomas in the substance of the brain (circled by a round frame). H-E; ×200

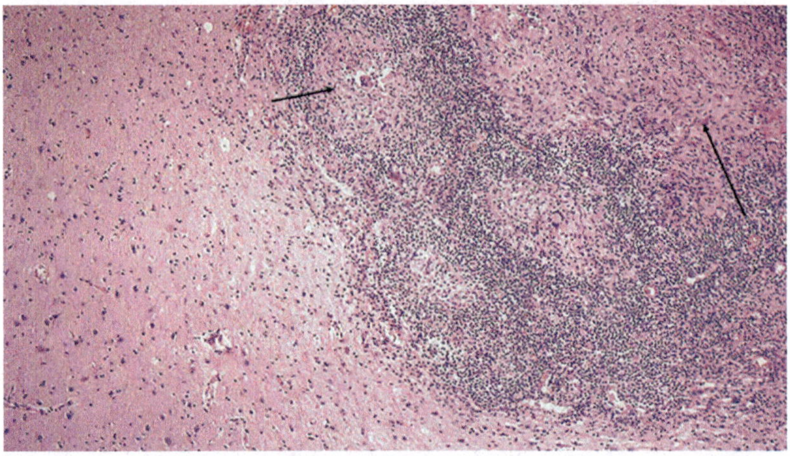

Fig. 13.18 Tuberculous "bumps" in the substance of the brain (indicated by arrows). H-E; ×200

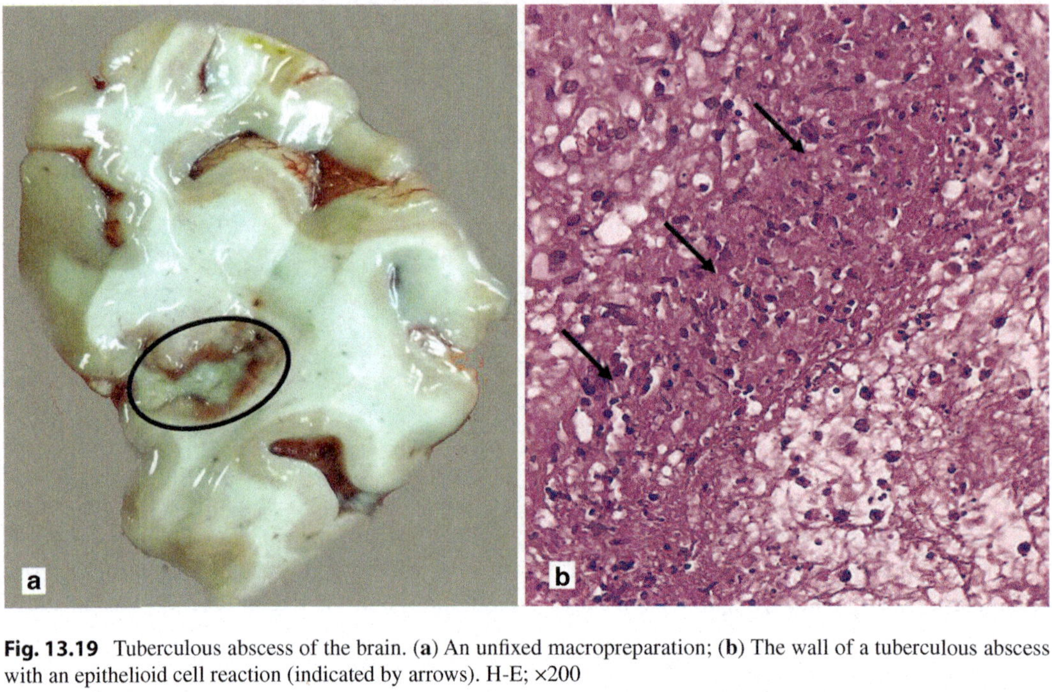

Fig. 13.19 Tuberculous abscess of the brain. (**a**) An unfixed macropreparation; (**b**) The wall of a tuberculous abscess with an epithelioid cell reaction (indicated by arrows). H-E; ×200

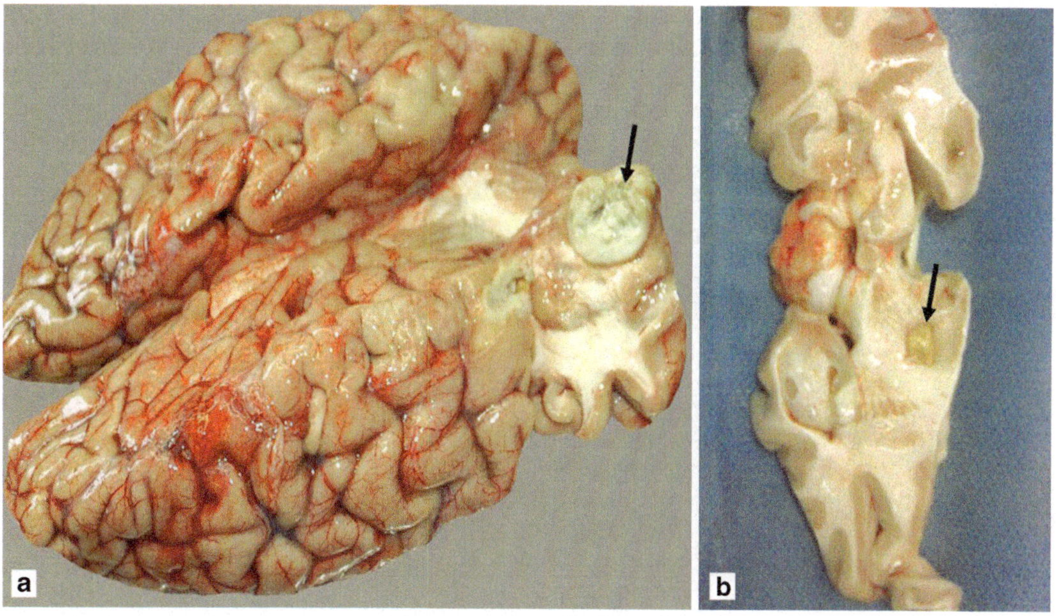

Fig. 13.20 Tuberculomas of the brain (indicated by arrows) **a**, **b** Unfixed macropreparation

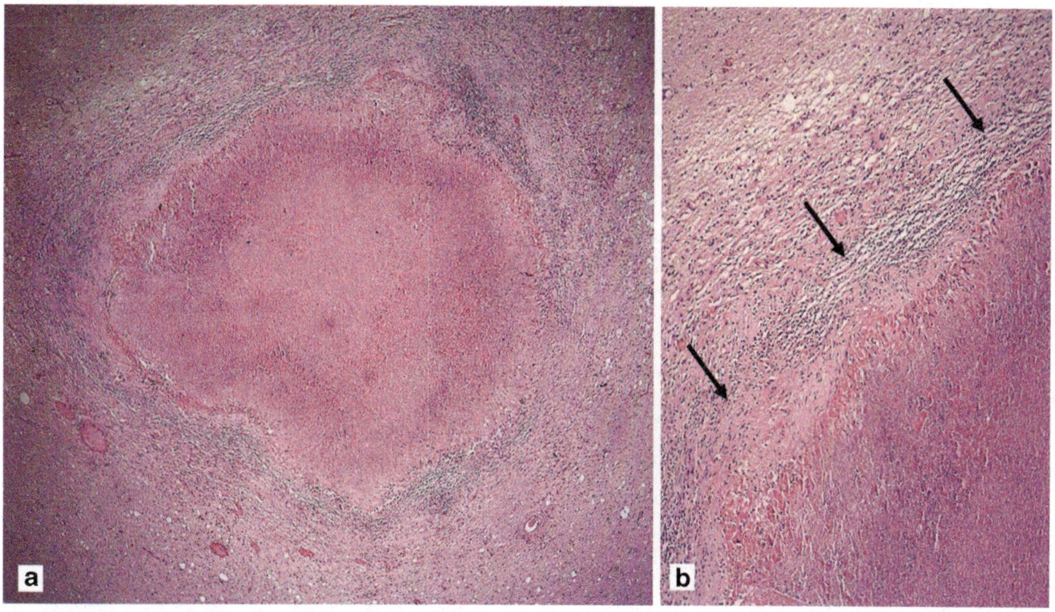

Fig. 13.21 (**a**) Tuberculoma of the brain; (**b**) A fragment of Fig. "**a**" - the edge of the encysted focus of caseous necrosis. H-E; **a** – ×40; **b** – 100

bacterial "nonspecific" and pyogenic flora growth is not observed in the contents of the abscess or tuberculoma.

Clinical manifestations of tuberculous lesions of the brain substance depend on the localization zone, the size of the lesions and the activity of the tuberculosis process.

In rare cases, tuberculous inflammation is found in the vascular plexuses of the ventricles of the brain—tuberculous ventriculitis

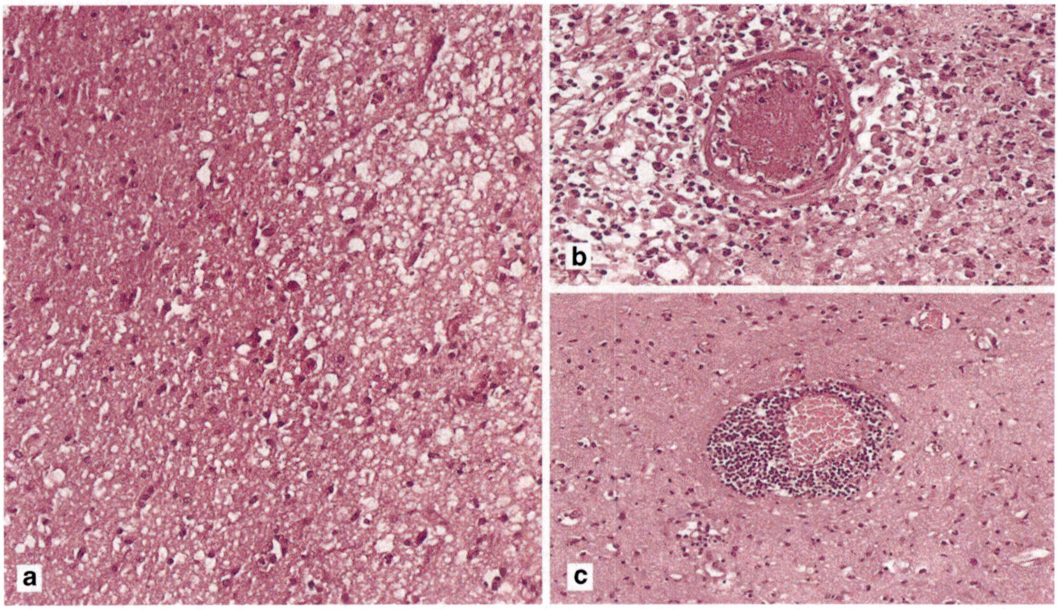

Fig. 13.22 Reactive changes in the brain in tuberculous meningoencephalitis: (**a**) Cerebral edema; (**b**) Fibrin thrombus in the brain microvessel in DIC syndrome; (**c**) Perivascular muff-like lymphoid infiltration. H-E; **a**, **b** – ×200; **c** – ×100

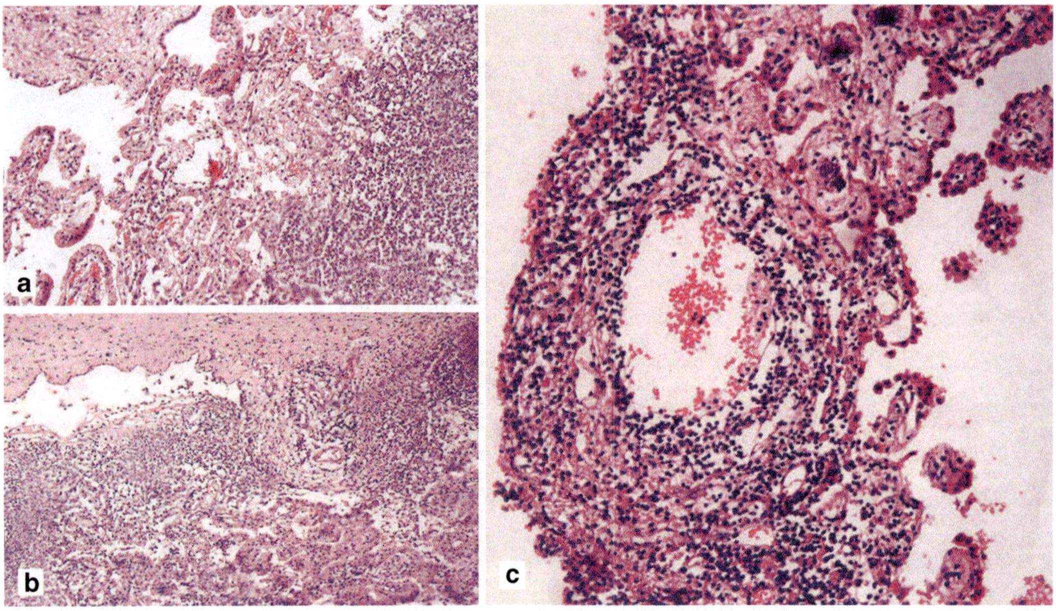

Fig. 13.23 Inflammation in the vascular plexuses of the lateral ventricles of the brain in tuberculous meningoencephalitis. H-E; **a**, **b** – ×40, **c** – ×100

(Fig. 13.23), as well as in the pituitary gland (Figs. 13.24 and 13.25), the cerebellum.

The cerebrospinal form is the most severe. The membranes of the spinal cord are affected (leptomeningitis, leptopachymeningitis), myelitis, tuberculosis of the spinal cord may develop, which is clinically manifested by peripheral paralysis or paresis mainly of the lower

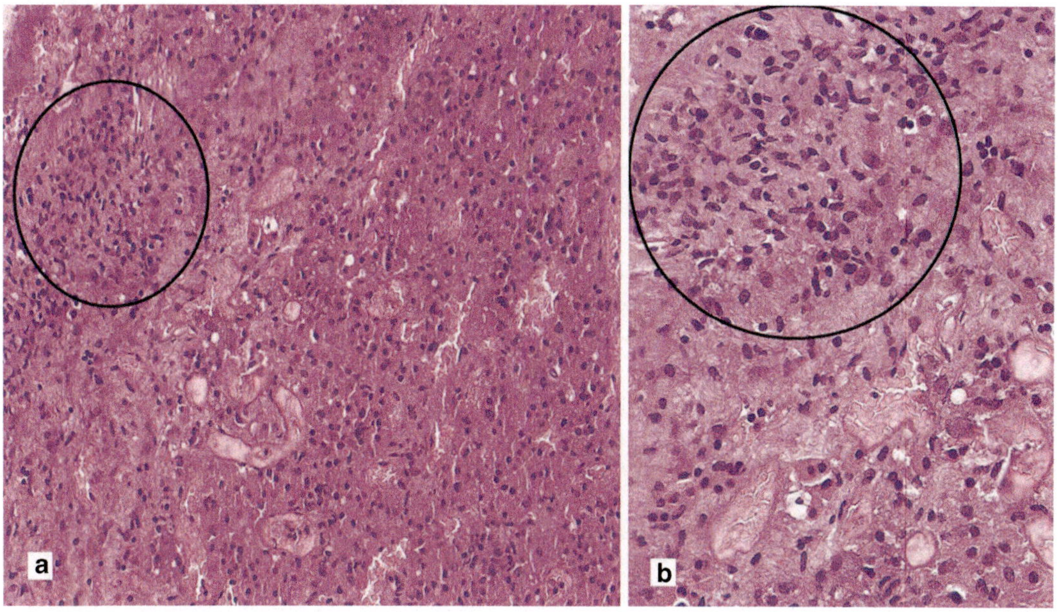

Fig. 13.24 Tuberculous lesion of the pituitary gland. Forming granuloma in the pituitary gland (circled by a round frame). H-E; **a** – X100; **b** – ×200 ("**b**" – fragment of Figure "**a**")

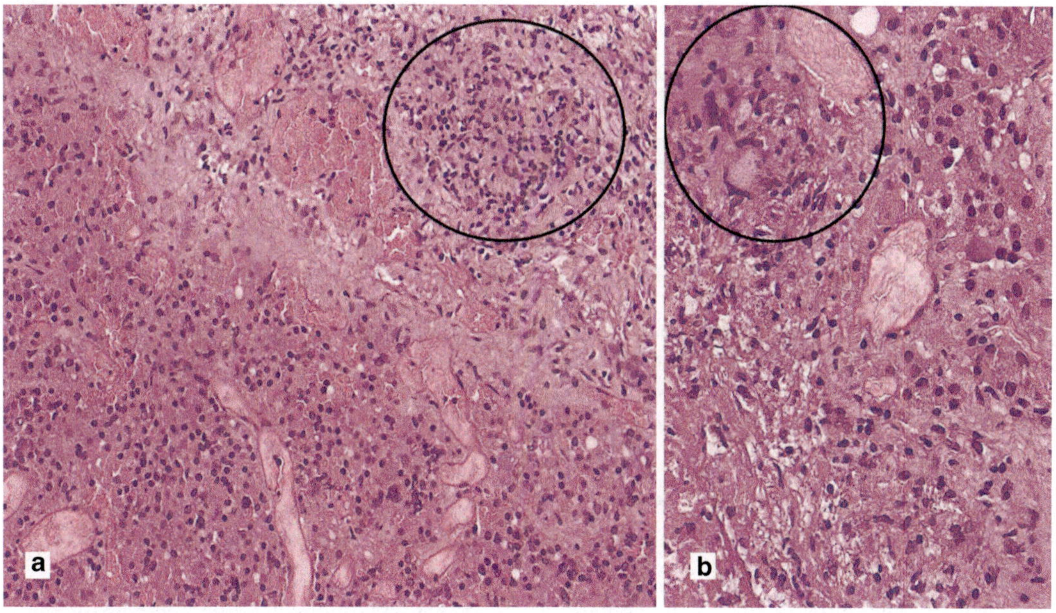

Fig. 13.25 Tuberculous lesion of the pituitary gland. Forming granulomas in the pituitary gland (circled by a round frame). H-E. **a** – ×100; **b** – ×200

extremities, disorders of the pelvic organs. When the process spreads to the root segment of the sensitive spinal nerves, pain of a shingling nature appears in the spine, chest, abdomen, very intense, sometimes not amenable to relief even with narcotic analgesics.

Microscopically, areas of productive inflammation, granulomatous inflammation, as well as

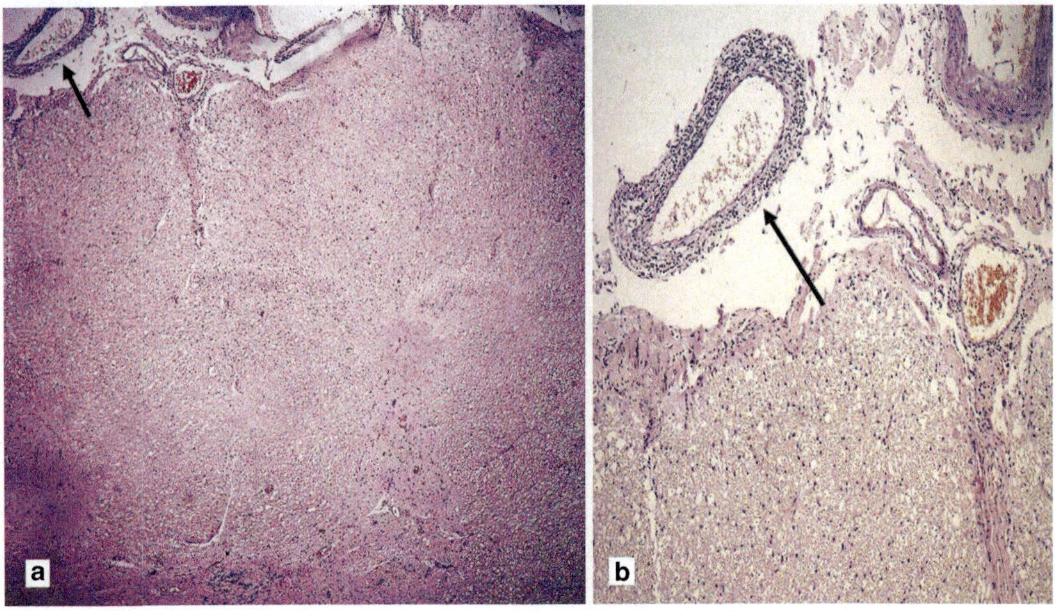

Fig. 13.26 Tuberculous lesion of the spinal cord (productive leptomeningitis, indicated by an arrow). H-E; **a** – ×40; **b** – ×200 (fragment of figure "**a**")

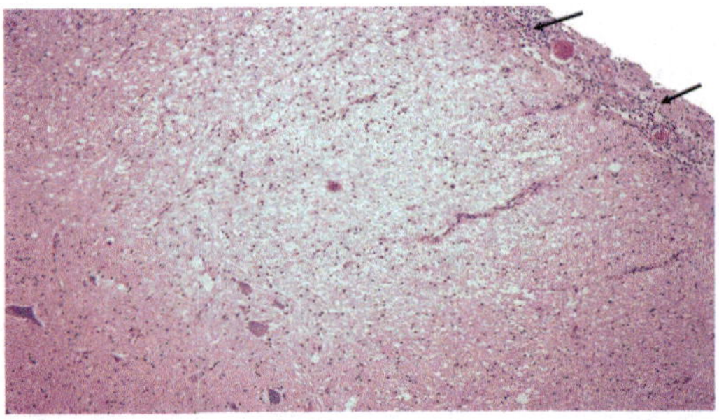

Fig. 13.27 Tuberculous lesion of the spinal cord (productive leptomeningitis, indicated by an arrow), edema. H-E × 40

edema of the brain substance, neuron dystrophy are detected (Figs. 13.26, 13.27, 13.28).

Complications and outcomes of tuberculous brain damage depend on the timing of diagnosis and the beginning of treatment. Complications of tuberculous meningitis include hydrocephalus, cranial nerve damage, paresis and limb paralysis, hyperkinesis, intracranial hypertension, decerebral rigidity, optic nerve atrophy, deafness, epilepsy, spinal arachnoiditis.

Tuberculosis meningitis is fatal in 16–55% of cases. The outcome of meningitis may be a cure with pronounced residual changes (decreased intelligence, motor disorder syndrome, hydrocephalus, epilepsy). In young children with tuberculous meningitis, hydrocephalus can develop very quickly, with irreversible consequences in the form of a decrease in intelligence (up to idiocy), persistent motor disorders, and blindness. After the treatment of tuberculous inflammation of the meninges, sclerotic changes, adhesions, and small calcifications can be detected. When organizing the tuberculoma of the brain in necrotic masses, the deposition of calcium salts can be observed, a wide capsule is formed around it (Fig. 13.29). A postinfarction cyst is a consequence of a secondary brain infarction. Endocrine-vegetative disorders, such as obesity, early puberty, and hypertrichosis, are described.

A favorable outcome of tuberculous meningitis is a cure without residual changes in the outcome of the disease, complete resorption of the exudate with complete tissue restoration can occur.

In some cases, it is necessary to conduct a differential diagnosis of tuberculous brain damage with another pathology. Thus, the differential

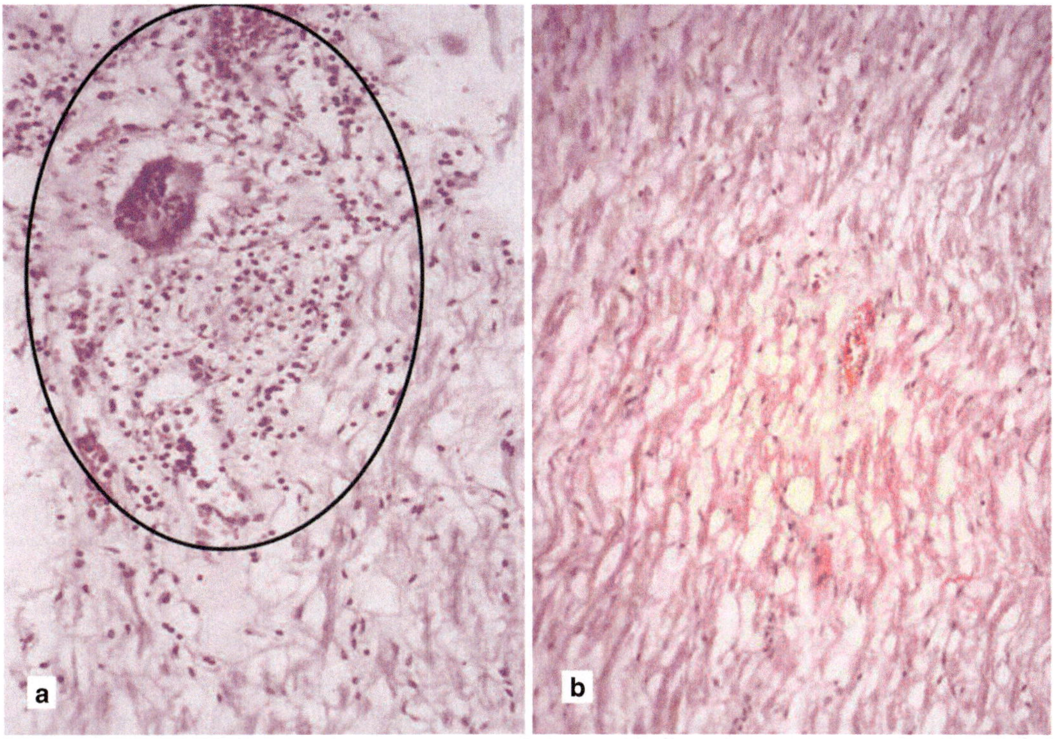

Fig. 13.28 Tuberculous lesions of the spinal cord. The root of the spinal nerve in the ponytail of the spinal cord. (**a**) Granuloma (circled by a round frame); (**b**) Pronounced edema. H-E × 200

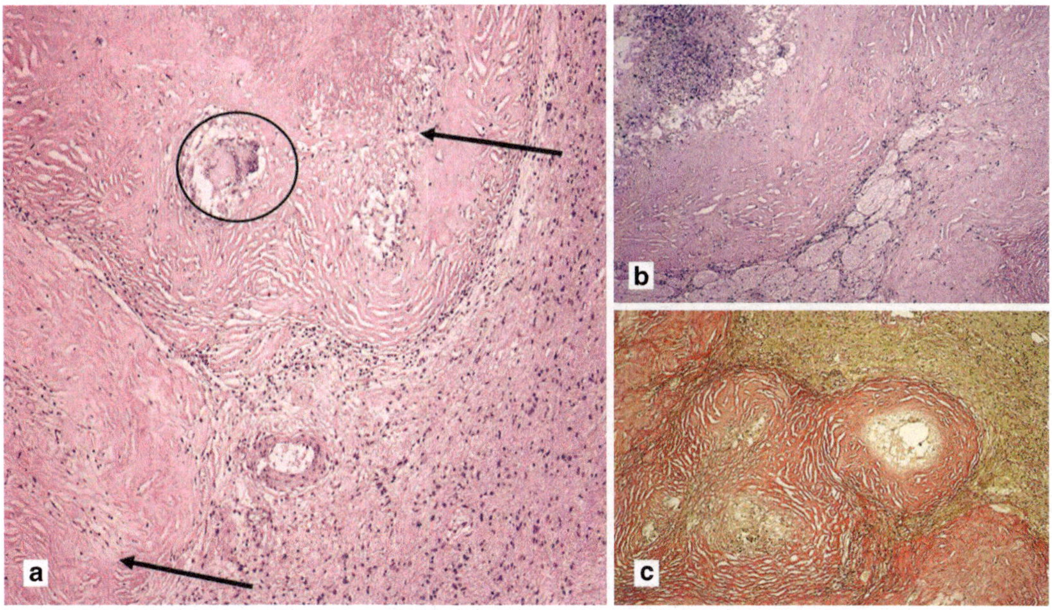

Fig. 13.29 Organized tuberculoma of the brain (indicated by arrows). (**a**) Granuloma with organized necrotic masses (the granuloma is surrounded by a round frame); (**b**) In organized necrotic masses, pulverized calcification (point basophilic inclusions); (**c**) Organized foci of caseous necrosis with hyalinosis (colored red). **a**, **b** – H-E. ×200; **b**-color by van Gieson. ×100

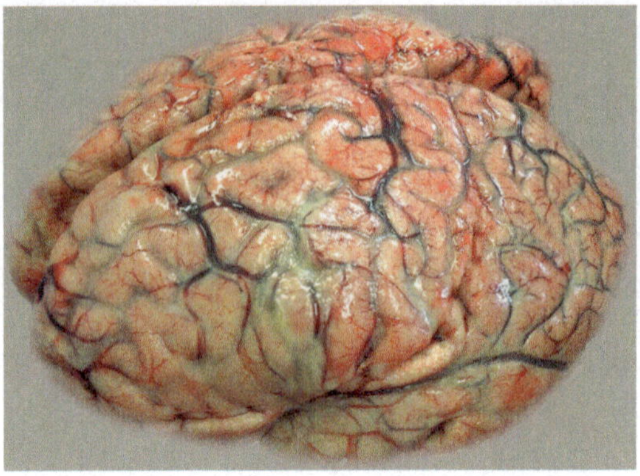

Fig. 13.30 Bacterial purulent leptomeningitis. Purulent impregnation of the soft medulla of the convexital surface of the brain. Unfixed macropreparation

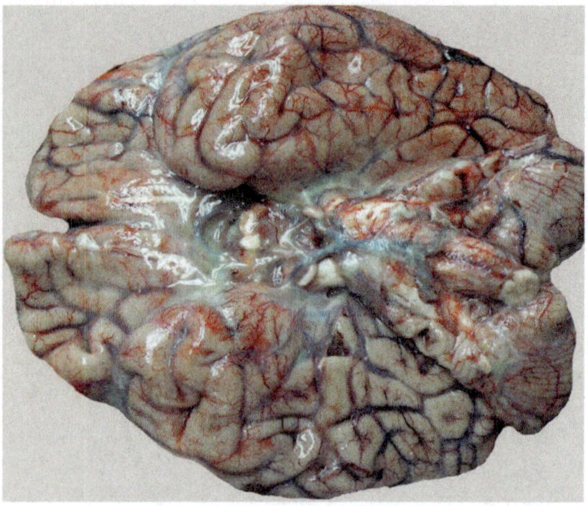

Fig. 13.31 Bacterial purulent leptomeningitis. Purulent penetration of the soft medulla of the base of the brain (along the vessels of the base of the brain, in the area of the chiasm of the optic nerve and with spread to the frontal and temporal lobes). Unfixed macropreparation

diagnosis of tuberculous meningitis is carried out with such diseases as acute serous lymphocytic meningitis (usually a viral lesion), purulent meningitis, meningism.

Serous meningitis of nontuberculosis origin (acute serous lymphocytic meningitis) is characterized by an acute onset with the severity of meningeal and course, rapid recovery with rapid regression of focal symptoms (paresis of the cranial nerves), without exacerbations and relapses. In the cerebrospinal fluid, lymphocytic cytosis is detected at normal glucose and chloride levels, and there is practically no film loss.

Purulent meningitis is usually caused by a purulent or mixed microflora, characterized by an acute and even lightning-fast onset, in the absence of damage to the cranial nerves (see also Chap. 10). The process involves the soft meninges of the predominantly convexital surfaces of the brain, although the basal parts are also affected. The shells have a yellowish-greenish tint due to purulent impregnation (with a total lesion of the soft medulla, the macroscopic picture is called a "purulent cap") (Figs. 13.30 and 13.31). Cerebrospinal fluid with high neutrophil pleocytosis ("purulent" CSF), elevated protein levels, and normal glucose levels. Microscopically, diffuse pronounced leukocyte infiltration were detected in the soft medulla (Fig. 13.32). In the absence of a lifetime study of the cerebrospinal fluid due to the impossibility of performing a lumbar puncture for any reason or the shortness of the patient's stay in the hospital, it is advisable to postmortem bacteriological examination of the cerebrospinal fluid, in which the causative agent of the disease is usually detected.

Meningism is observed in various acute diseases, it is manifested by edema of the membranes of the brain without the occurrence of the phenomena of their inflammation. Clinically, meningism is manifested by headache, vomiting, meningeal symptoms (rigidity of the occipital muscles, Kernig's symptoms). With a lumbar puncture, the flow of the cerebrospinal fluid under pressure is characteristic, but its composition remains normal. With successful treatment of the underlying disease, the phenomena of meningism disappear.

Tuberculous abscess of the brain often has to be differentiated from an abscess of a "nonspecific" nature caused by a purulent microflora (see also Chap. 11). The macroscopic picture of these diseases can be completely identical. If possible, the contents of the abscess should be taken at autopsy for bacteriological examination to determine the infectious agent. Moreover, the contents of the abscess may be more informative in bacteriological examination in comparison with the cerebrospinal fluid, since in the case of encysted and focal processes, the cerebrospinal fluid may

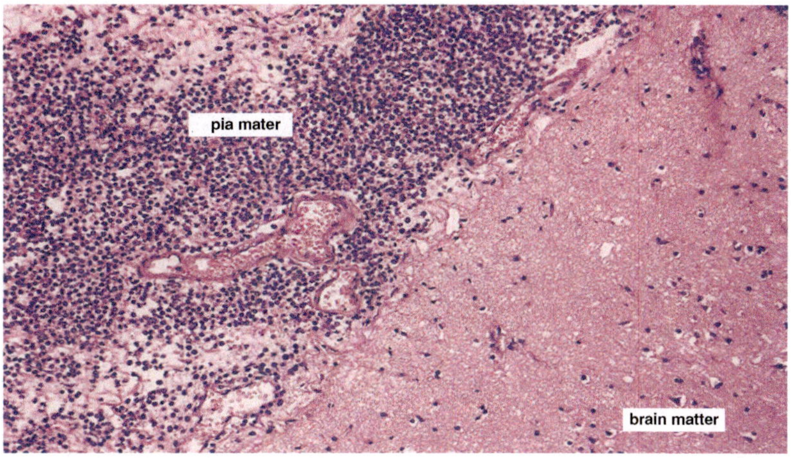

Fig. 13.32 Bacterial purulent leptomeningitis. In the soft medulla, there is a pronounced diffuse infiltration by neutrophilic leukocytes. H-E × 100

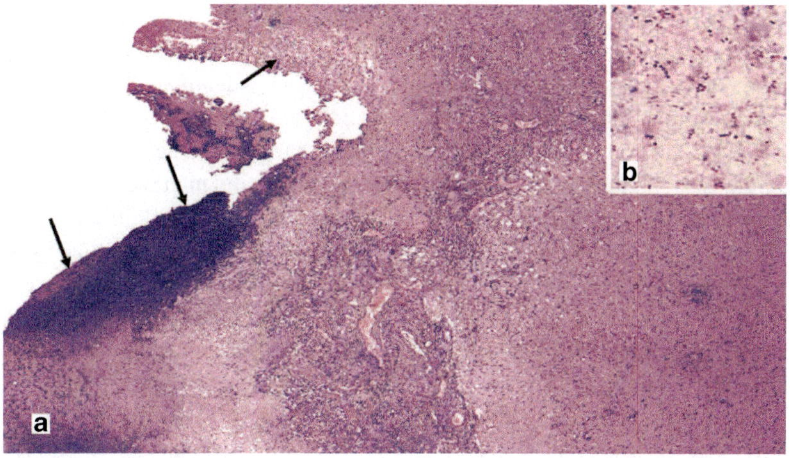

Fig. 13.33 Brain abscess. (**a**) The wall of the brain abscess (indicated by arrows) with uneven leukocyte infiltration of necrotic masses; (**b**) In the smearprint of the inner surface of the abscess wall, coccoid microflora. a-histological preparation; H-E × 100; b-cytological preparation; color according to Romanovsky-Giemsa. ×1000

be intact and sterile. Histological examination of the abscess wall showed purulent necrotic changes with an abundance of neutrophilic leukocytes in the absence of signs of granulomatous inflammation (Fig. 13.33a). For differential morphological diagnosis of brain abscess and tuberculous abscess, especially in cases of acute progressive tuberculosis or in immunosuppressive conditions with erased, minimal or absent granulomatous reaction, it is advisable to perform Z-N staining. In a "nonspecific" brain abscess, acid-resistant bacteria will not be detected, while in tuberculosis they can be detected. In the diagnostic search, it may be useful to conduct a histobacterioscopic examination for gram-positive and gram-negative flora, which is usually determined in a brain abscess of nontuberculosis origin (Gram, Gram-Weigert, Brown-Hopps, azur-eosine etc.). Cytological examination of the smear print of the abscess contents according to Romanovsky-Giemsa, methylene blue reveals different microbial flora, coccal, bacillary or mixed, depending on the pathogen that caused the purulent process in the brain (Fig. 13.33b). In the case of a tuberculous abscess, the cytological preparation color according to Z-N is determined by acid-resistant bacteria (see Fig. 13.8b).

During the differential diagnosis of tuberculous and mycotic abscesses, histobacterioscopic examination of the lesions of the brain with histological staining according to Z-N for acid-resistant bacteria and staining to identify the structures of the fungus (for example, according

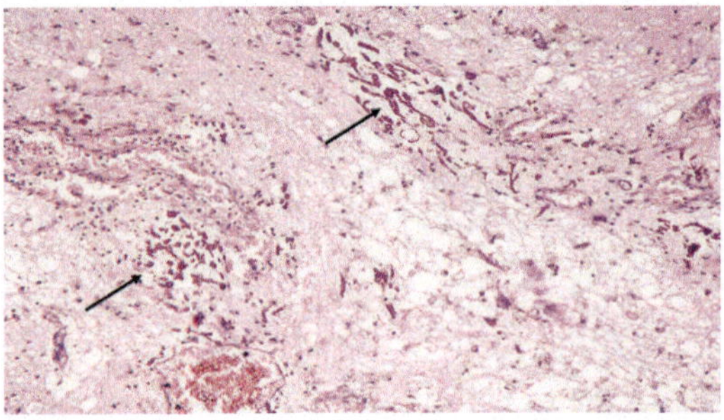

Fig. 13.34 Mycotic encephalitis. The structures of the mycelium of the fungus are colored crimson-red (indicated by arrows). PAS-reaction. ×200

to Grokott, PAS-reaction, etc.) is performed (Fig. 13.34). The Z-N staining in mycotic lesions will not reveal acid-resistant bacteria, but the cut may reveal fungal structures that will turn dark blue. Moreover, post-mortem examination of the cerebrospinal fluid, including using PCR, can confirm the mycotic etiology of the abscess, but in the case of calcified lesions, the cerebrospinal fluid may be intact and the culture will not reveal the growth of microflora (see also Sect. 14.1).

In the literature, there are indications of the need for a differential diagnosis of tuberculous meningitis with other diseases—viral encephalomyelitis, meningeal influenza, polio, brain tumors, and damage to the meninges in typhoid fever (see Chaps. 6 and 7, Sect. 12.5).

In rare cases, it is necessary to differentiate a tuberculous lesion from sarcoidosis of the brain. The most frequent (up to half of all cases) manifestation of neurosarcoidosis is neuropathy of the facial nerve, less often there is a lesion of other cranial nerves (visual, vestibular-cochlear and lingual pharyngeal), as well as the substance of the brain. It is possible that sarcoidosis involves the pituitary gland, soft meninges, spinal cord, peripheral nerves in mononeuropathy, polyneuropathy, or Guillain-Barre syndrome. The degree of brain damage in sarcoidosis and clinical manifestations depend on the localization of granulomatous inflammation in various parts of the brain and its membranes, their number (single or multiple) and size. In addition, changes of an ischemic nature may develop due to cerebral angiitis. The course of the disease is chronic, the rate of development of neurosarcoidosis can be either slow, with the gradual development of neurological symptoms and long-term remission, or fast with a steady progression of symptoms.

In our practice, there was a case of isolated neurosarcoidosis. A 54-year-old man was operated on for a brain neoplasm, pterionic craniotomy was performed on the right subtotal removal of the tumor from the chiasmal-sellar region.

In the surgical material of the brain, signs of granulomatous inflammation were revealed, and the granulomas were completely different. There were small forming macrophage epithelioid granulomas, some of which were with a structureless necrobiotic microfocus in the center (Fig. 13.35a). Larger epithelioid cell granulomas with necrosis in the center and a small number of destroyed white blood cells in the center were also identified. There is a moderate lymphoid reaction around the granulomas (Fig. 13.35b). The changes in the described areas were more consistent with the microscopic picture of tuberculous inflammation. In addition, in some fragments of the surgical material, organized granulomas with micronecrosis in the center were found (Fig. 13.36), as well as closely located, but not merging clearly defined organized granulomas of the "stamped type" typical for sarcoidosis (Fig. 13.37). In the substance of the brain, edema diffuse weakly or moderately pronounced lymphoid reaction, perivascular cuff-like lymphoid infiltration. Histobacterioscopy by Z-N did not reveal acid-resistant bacteria. PCR from the paraffin block was carried out, in which the DNA of Mycobacterium tuberculosis was not found.

However, despite the negative result of histobacterioscopy and PCR studies, according to the morphological study, there was a suspicion of a tuberculous etiology of the process—tuberculoma of the chiasmal-sellar region of the brain. A complete clinical phthisiological study, including a lumbar puncture with a study of the cerebrospinal fluid, could not be performed due to the severity of the patient's condition in the postoperative period. No changes were found in the lung and intra-thoracic lymph nodes during computed tomography; no acid-resistant bacteria were found in the pharyngeal swabs, as well as in the

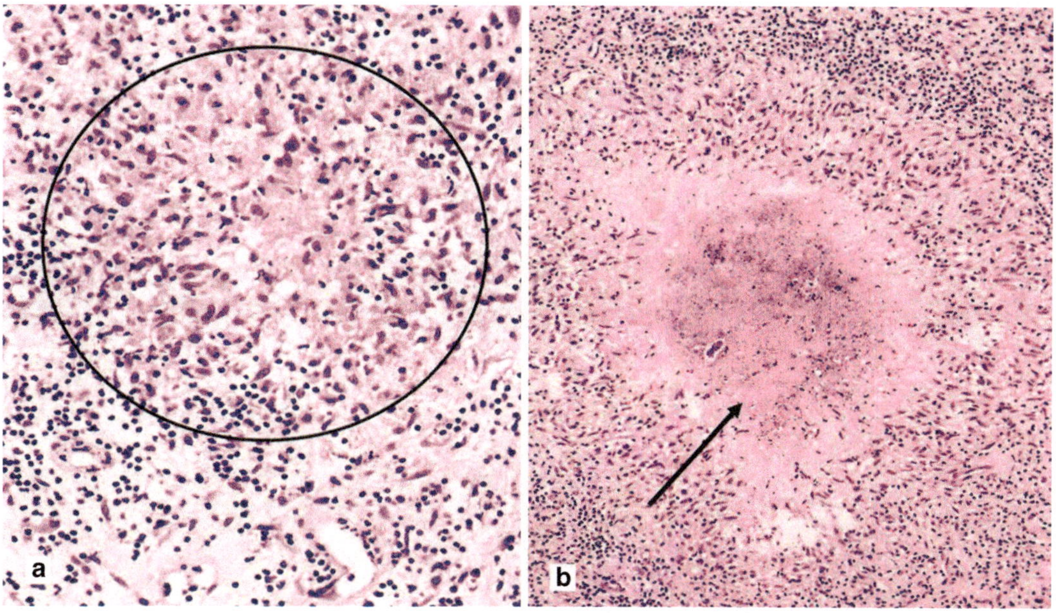

Fig. 13.35 Sarcoidosis of the brain. (**a**) Forming granuloma in the substance of the brain (circled by a round frame); (**b**) Granuloma with necrosis in the center (indicated by an arrow). H-E; **a** – ×200; **b** – ×100

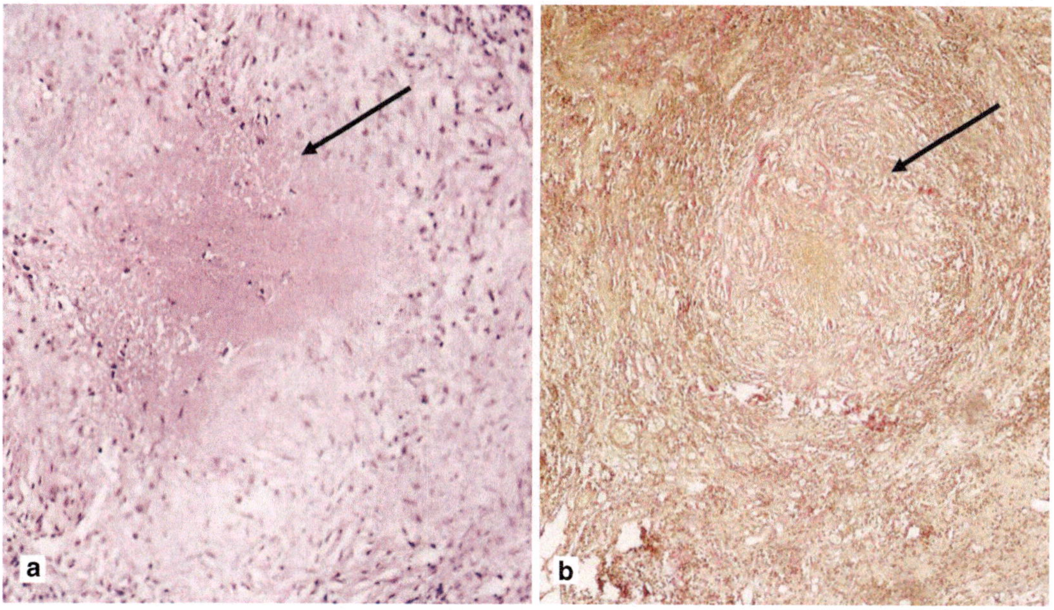

Fig. 13.36 Sarcoidosis of the brain. Organizing granulomas with micronecrosis in the center (indicated by arrows). **a** – H-E × 200; **b** – stained by van Gieson. ×100

urine and feces; skin tests (Mantoux reaction and Diaskin test were negative). A week after the surgery, an ischemic brain infarction developed, and the patient died.

At autopsy no signs of tuberculosis and sarcoidosis were found in any organ, including the brain. The material from various organs was examined microscopically, and by PCR with

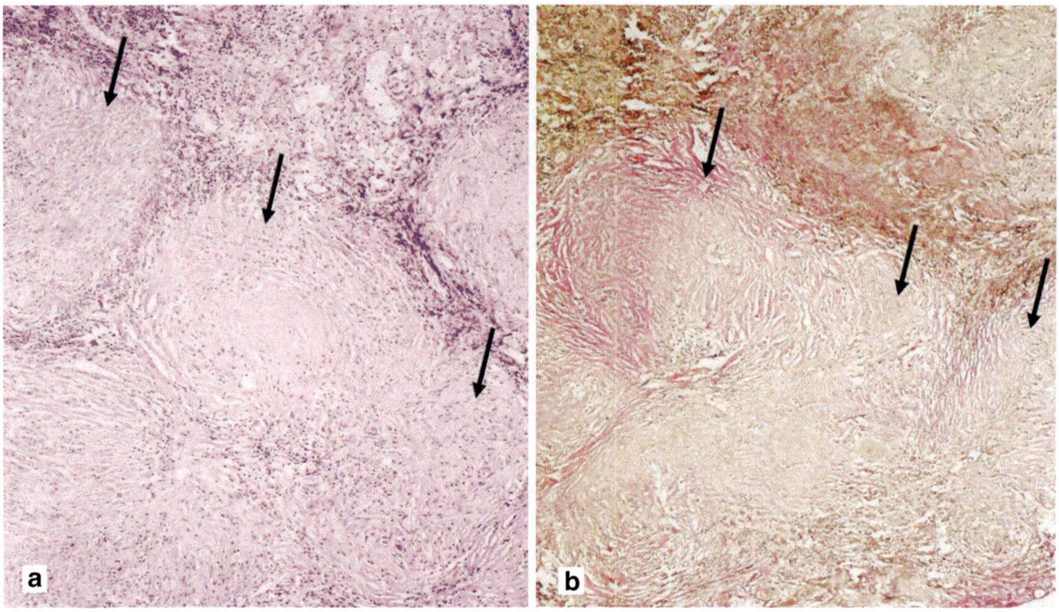

Fig. 13.37 Sarcoidosis of the brain. Organized granulomas (indicated by arrows). **a** H-E; ×100; **b** – stained by van Gieson. ×100

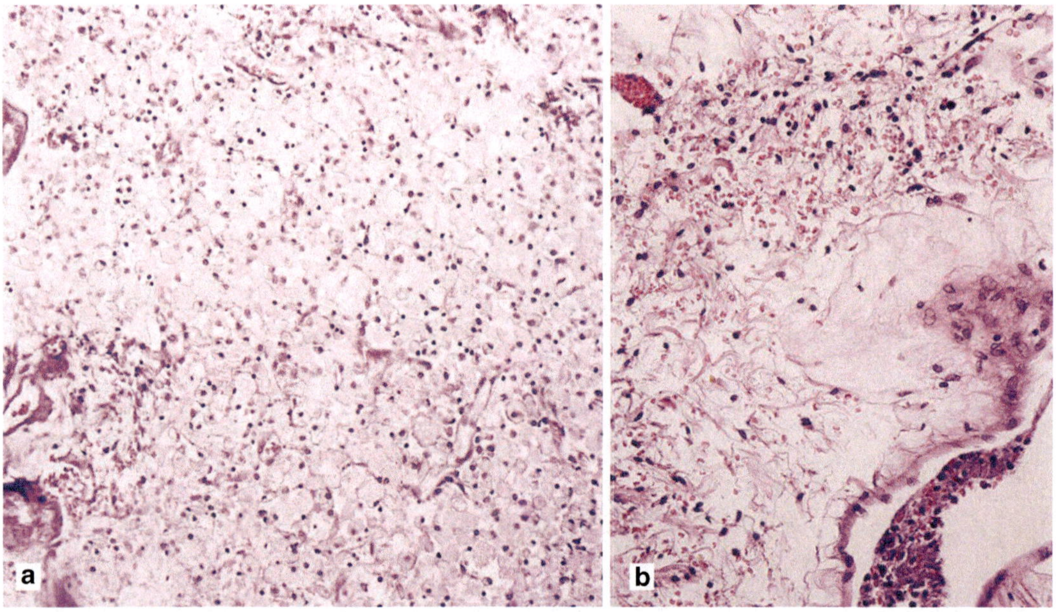

Fig. 13.38 (**a**) Ischemic infarction of the brain (cells of "granular balls"); (**b**) Serous meningitis. Stained with hematoxylin and eosin. ×100

negative result as well. Probably, the pathological focus was completely removed surgically. The study of the brain confirmed the presence of an ischemic infarction, and clusters of "granular ball" cells were also detected in the infarcted areas, which indicated a relapsing process (Fig. 13.38a). In addition to brain infarction, recurrent basal subarachnoid hemorrhage, productive epiduritis with a predominant lesion of the dura mater of the right hemisphere of the brain, and secondary serous meningitis were found (Fig.13.38b). The case was regarded as an isolated neurosarcoidosis with a lesion of the chiasmal-sellar region of the brain, a pseudotumor form.

13.1.3 Pathomorphology of Tuberculosis of the Central Nervous System in Children

There are significant difficulties both in the clinical and pathologic diagnosis of tuberculous lesions of the central nervous system in children. As an example, we give one of our observations from children's practice.

Roman N., 2 years and 7 months old, a visitor from Azerbaijan, was admitted to the Clinical Hospital on 3.01.1996 with a diagnosis of celiac disease? Exudative enteropathy? The newborn period without peculiarities, up to 6 months. he was breastfed, developed normally. There is no information about vaccination. According to the words, BCG vaccination in the maternity hospital. In 6 months, the disease with a rise in temperature, loose stools, convulsions, was treated in a hospital for 1.5 months, later lagging in psychomotor development. Since July 1995 constant diarrhea, copious loose stools, a sharp increase in the size of the abdomen, and progressive loss of appetite. Since November, cough with purulent sputum. Upon admission, the condition is severe, the child is extremely sluggish, the skin is dark, dry, sharp exhaustion, a sharply enlarged and dense abdomen, signs of sluggish current pneumonia, pronounced muscle hypotension and persistent fever. In connection with the diagnosis of celiac disease, he received an appropriate diet with antibiotics penicillin, gentamicin, kefzol. Despite the therapy, the child's condition progressively worsened, including an increase in protein, cytosis and sugar in the CSF. 31/01 according to the severity of the condition, he was transferred to the intensive care unit, the diagnosis remained unclear: "septic condition," "volume formation of the abdominal cavity," "generalized candidiasis against the background of hereditary enteropathy" were discussed. On radiographs of the lungs, infiltrative changes on the right in the cardiodiaphragmal corner and in the basal zone with positive dynamics. The Mantoux reaction was negative, the phthisiologist did not find any data for tuberculosis. The child did not come out of the coma, hypoxia, hypercapnia, and metabolic acidosis increased. 22/02 the child died.

The final clinical diagnosis: Celiac disease, the severe form. Complications of the underlying disease are secondary immunodeficiency, fungal-bacterial sepsis (meningoencephalitis, bilateral focal bronchopneumonia, enteritis, myocarditis? mesoadenitis); cachexia; severe psychomotor retardation. Concomitant disease— abdominal tumor? Intrauterine infection? Influenza A2?

As a result of detailed postmortem morphological and laboratory studies, the pathological diagnosis was formulated as follows:

Main disease: Primary progressive pulmonary tuberculosis with intracanalicular, lymphogenic and hematogenic generalization: exudative necrotic pleuropneumonia with encapsulation and sclerosis of the pleura, multiple bronchogenic and hematogenic foci of exudative-necrotic inflammation in both lungs; tuberculous lymphadenitis with bronchopulmonary and mesenteric lymph nodes in many necrotic miliary tubercles; miliary tubercles in the liver and spleen, ulcerative enteritis with multiple miliary tubercles in the submucosa and serosa, exudative-necrotic meningoencephalitis.

In connection with the topic of this book, we present the results of morphological studies of the brain. Macroscopically, the soft meninges were full-blooded, thickened at the base, cloudy, and greenish in color. The furrows are flattened, the brain tissue is flabby, spreading, bluish-gray. The lateral ventricles are dilated, their ependyma is swollen, dull with multiple small hemorrhages. Microscopic examination revealed exudative necrotic meningoencephalitis with extensive areas of caseous necrosis and mainly lymph-macrophage-leukocyte infiltration, vasculitis, perivasculitis, hemorrhage foci.

A retrospective analysis of this observation shows that it is extremely difficult in a number of cases to diagnose tuberculosis in children in time,

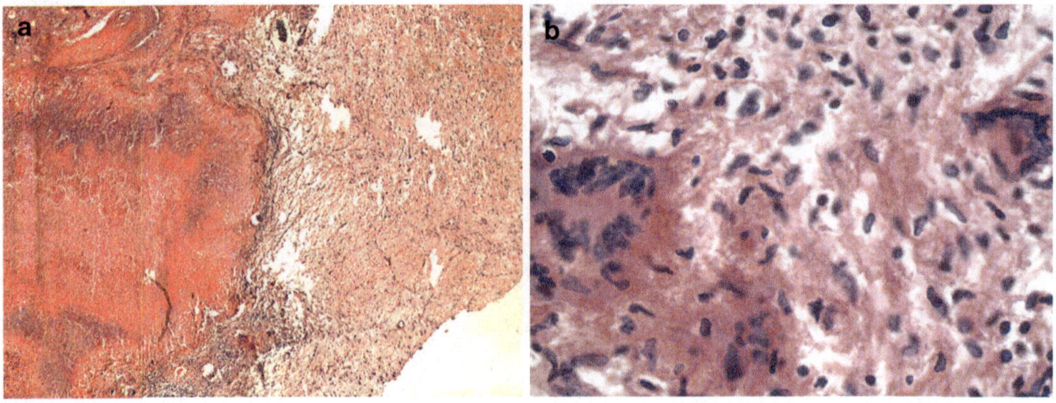

Fig. 13.39 Typical tuberculous granuloma in a child. H-E. (**a**) General view. ×100. (**b**) Detail. Giant Langhans cell. ×600

even if a fairly complete examination is carried out. Epidemiologically valuable information about the disease of the father was found out only by the pathologist.

Another example of post-mortem diagnosis of tuberculosis is our observation on the advisory material from Kaliningrad.

The girl Lyubov I. was born from the second pregnancy, the second birth from an HIV-infected mother, in connection with which BCG was not performed. There were no data for infection with the immunodeficiency virus. At 9 months, she suffered from bronchitis. The Mantoux reaction from 14.04.03–5 mm. She was hospitalized at the age of 1 year and 10 months in a moderate condition with suspected acute gastroenterocolitis. There were signs of bilateral lower lobe pneumonia and meningoencephalitis. There was a deterioration in the condition with the development of a brain coma. The issue of the connection of the detected pathology with HIV infection was discussed. Among the most diverse diagnostic assumptions, tuberculosis did not appear. On the 25th day of the hospital stay, the child died.

On autopsy—a picture of severe basal meningitis with abundant pus-like masses. Acute hyperplasia of the bronchial lymph nodes. Microscopic examination of the brain and its membranes shows widespread tuberculous lesions with pronounced caseous changes, sometimes with the formation of typical granulomas (Fig. 13.39). In bifurcation and peribronchial lymph nodes, tuberculous granulomatous lymphadenitis.

This observation demonstrates the objective difficulties of clinical and laboratory diagnosis of tuberculosis in children at present, especially those born to HIV-infected mothers.

13.1.4 Central Nervous System Damage in HIV-Associated Tuberculosis

Tuberculosis should now be considered the leading opportunistic disease in HIV infection: its various forms are detected in about half of the deceased (See also Sect. 8.2, Chap. 18). Tuberculosis can either precede or develop again on the background of HIV infection. The predominant lesion of the lymph nodes of different groups - mediastinum, abdominal cavity, neck, and other peripheral. They are in the form of large packets consisting of many nodes. At the same time, there are signs of generalization of tuberculosis with the involvement of the kidneys, spleen, liver, and other organs [2]. It is noteworthy that liver damage is not diagnosed in vivo. Quite often (up to half of the cases) there is a lesion of the intestine in the form of ulcerative ileocolitis. The meninges and brain matter are affected in almost a third of cases. In most cases, there are mainly alternative changes with minimal cellular response and significant accumulation of acid-resistant bacteria.

Clinical diagnosis of tuberculosis, even in the conditions of observation of patients by highly

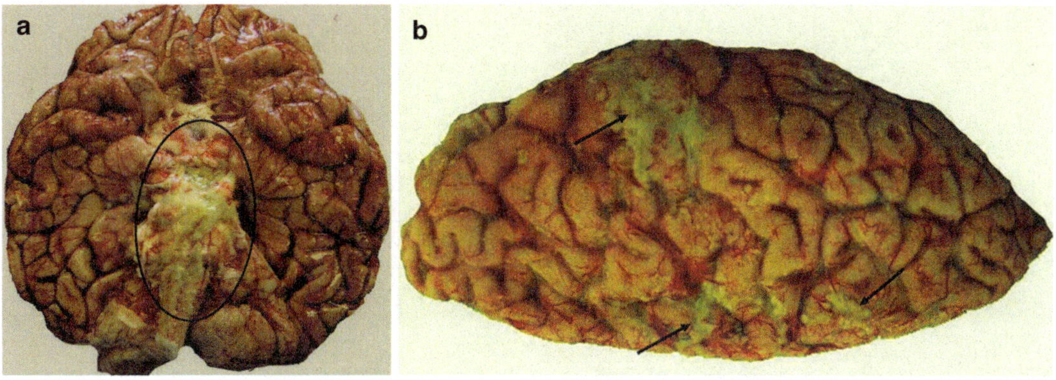

Fig. 13.40 HIV-associated tuberculous leptomeningitis, purulent infiltration of the soft meninges. (**a**) Damage to the basal parts of the brain; (**b**) Damage to the convexital surfaces of the hemispheres of the brain. Unfixed macropreparations

qualified phthisiologists, is objectively difficult and is largely based on assumptions. In half of the observations of HIV-infected people with neurotuberculosis, no changes in the brain substance are detected. The radiation semiotics of these nosological forms does not differ from the usual ones. Basal meningitis is typical, leading to deformation of the basal cisterns. Their diagnosis requires intravenous reinforcement. Tuberculomas, represented by focal lesions, the number of which varies from one to several\ many, deserve consideration. The localization is diverse: cortical-subcortical divisions, periventricular substance, subarachnoid, sub/epidural spaces. The foci are usually surrounded by perifocal edema, the severity of which varies from minimal to fairly pronounced, but always less than in the case of a bacterial abscess. The radiation pattern depends on the maturity of the tuberculoma. In CT, non-caseous tuberculoma is usually manifested by a low-density focus, isodense variants are possible; in MRI, hypo - on T1-VI and a hyperintensive signal on T2-VI. Post-contrast images are characterized by homogeneous gain. A liquid-centered caseous turbuloma is visualized as a hypodensal formation with a ring-shaped postcontrast enhancement. MRI shows a standard change in the signal, and after intravenous contrast, a ring - shaped gain. Caseous tuberculoma with a dense center is characterized by a heterogeneous central or ring-shaped enhancement after intravenous contrast, and by T2 – VI - iso/hypointensive signal. In 1/3 of cases, there is a centrally located petrification. The outcome of tuberculosis is atrophy.

Tuberculosis meningoencephalitis in the terminal stages of HIV infection is observed in a generalized progressive tuberculosis process and is characterized by a number of features. In HIV-associated tuberculosis meningitis, in addition to the typical tuberculosis lesion of the basal membranes of the brain, there was a more extensive spread of the process involving the membranes of the convexital surface. More often, there was purulent impregnation of the membranes, and they acquired a yellowish or yellowish-greenish color (like a "purulent cap"), which gave the impression of an inflammatory process caused by a purulent bacterial flora (Fig. 13.40b). Miliary lesions were observed quite rarely.

When dissecting the brain, foci of tuberculous inflammation were localized in all parts of the gray and white matter. There were both solitary and multiple foci of destruction. Macroscopically, they were yellowish, structureless, mush-like foci of various sizes, usually irregularly rounded in shape, and had the appearance of acute abscesses.

The lateral ventricles of the brain can be dilated, the cerebrospinal fluid from cloudy with a whitish tinge to pus-like. In the cerebrospinal

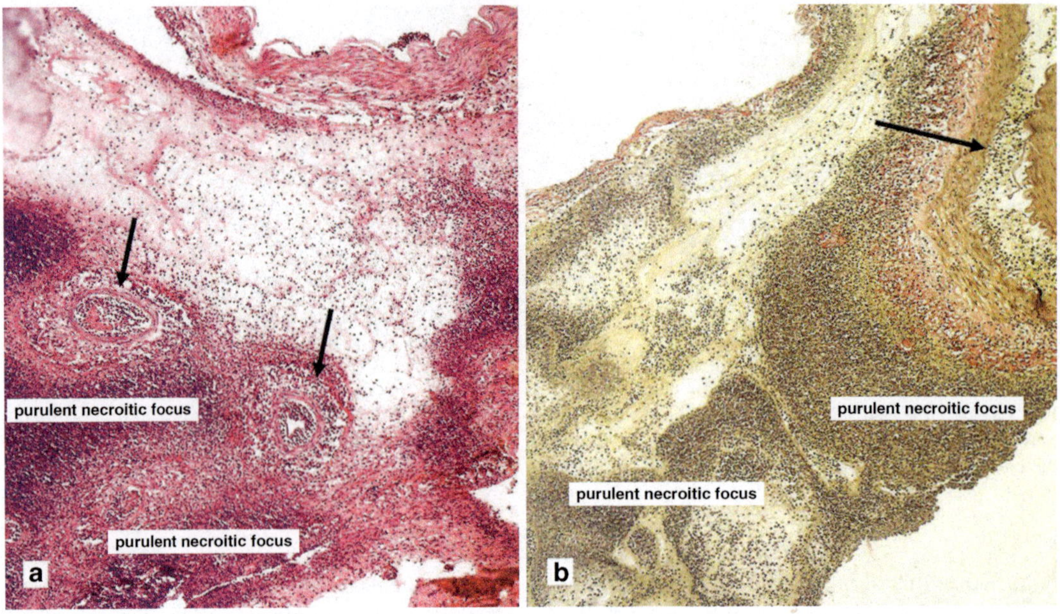

Fig. 13.41 HIV-associated tuberculosis leptomeningitis. Purulent-necrotic foci in the soft medulla without signs of granulomatous inflammation, without signs of organization; purulent panvasculitis (vessels are indicated by arrows). **a** – H-E. ×100; **b** – stained by van Gieson. ×200

fluid, high cytosis, neutrophilic type of smear is detected (for tuberculous meningitis without HIV infection, lymphocytic cerebrospinal fluid is more characteristic).

Quite often, with a pronounced morphological picture of encephalitis with extensive destructive changes, the lifetime neurological symptoms are very poor, for example, one of the following signs is determined - a small nystagmus, slight facial asymmetry, weakly pronounced tongue deviation, mild meningism, slight strabismus, transient headaches.

The microscopic picture of changes in HIV-associated tuberculosis has a number of features. It is characterized by the loss of the features of "specificity" of the morphological picture of tuberculous inflammation with the absence of a typical granulomatous inflammation. There are no signs of the undulating course of the process characteristic of tuberculosis in the form of foci of specific inflammation of various ages, which is noted in cases of tuberculosis without HIV infection. In HIV infection, the foci of tuberculous inflammation of the monomorphic structure which have the form of purulent necrotic foci, often located perivascularly. Alternative-exudative changes prevail in the absence or minimal manifestations of the productive component of inflammation. These changes indicate a violation of the processes of delineation and organization of foci of tuberculosis inflammation.

In the soft meninges of HIV-associated tuberculous meningitis, pronounced diffuse leukocyte infiltration is microscopically determined, that is, the histological picture is identical to the changes in purulent leptomeningitis caused by purulent microflora (Fig. 13.41). In some cases, single epithelioid cells or very small indistinct, almost indistinguishable epithelioid cell granulomas can be detected in individual fields of vision in the leukocyte infiltrate. When staining according to Z-N, a large number of acid-resistant bacteria are usually found. Purulent-necrotic vasculitis, panvasculitis (Fig. 13.42), and thrombovasculitis develop both reactive and tuberculous, with the detection of acid-resistant bacteria in the vascular wall and in the thrombotic masses (Fig. 13.43).

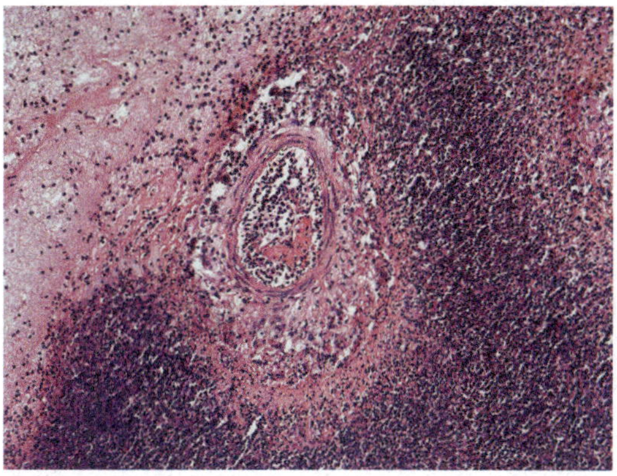

Fig. 13.42 HIV-associated tuberculosis leptomeningitis. Purulent panvasculitis in the soft medulla. Perivascularly purulent necrotic tuberculous focus, without signs of "specific" inflammation. H-E. ×200

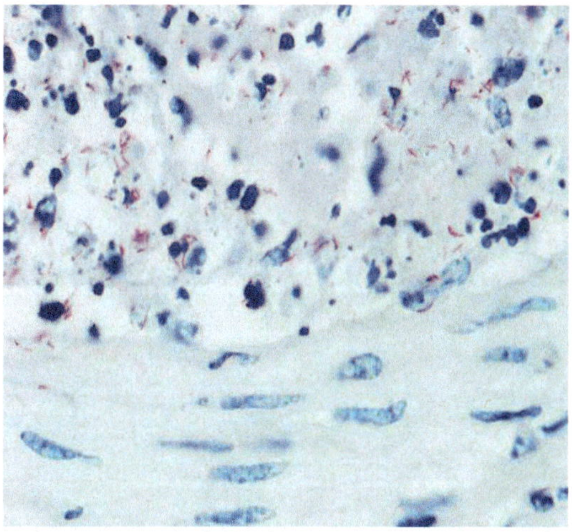

Fig. 13.43 Tuberculous thrombovasculitis. Acid-resistant bacteria in large numbers in the thrombotic masses and isolated in the vessel wall. Acid-resistant bacteria are colored red. Stained by Z-N. ×1000

In the study of autopsy material with tuberculosis encephalitis, the difficulty of morphological verification of the tuberculosis process may be due to the extremely small size of the foci of inflammation (submiliary dissemination), which are not detected by macroscopic examination. Moreover, as mentioned above, the microscopic picture of HIV-associated tuberculosis often has no signs of granulomatous inflammation and foci of tuberculosis inflammation are represented by necrotic masses with abundant infiltration by neutrophilic leukocytes, with purulent melting of necrotic masses (Fig. 13.44a). The walls of tuberculous abscesses are also represented by purulent-necrotic masses, without the formation of granulomatous inflammation. Purulent-necrotic foci of tuberculous inflammation and acute tuberculous abscesses in the late stages of HIV infection (purulent-necrotic foci) are practically indistinguishable from foci of purulent inflammation caused by purulent microbial flora. Signs of granulomatous inflammation are completely absent or there is a very poor reaction in the form of single epithelioid or multinucleated giant cells, small fuzzy granulomatous structures (Fig. 13.44b). The perifocal lymphoid response is sharply suppressed. Localization of foci of tuberculous inflammation is mainly perivascular, which is one of the signs of hematogenic generalization of the process characteristic of tuberculosis in the late stages of HIV infection.

It is also recommended to use cytological examination of smears prints of the soft meninges and lesions in the brain substance with the color of the preparations according to Zil-Nielsen (Fig. 13.45).

In the cerebrospinal fluid obtained at autopsy, during PCR examination, it is possible to detect the DNA of Mycobacterium tuberculosis, it is also possible to conduct a cytobacterioscopic examination or a luminescent microscopy of a cytological preparation from the sediment obtained by centrifugation of the cerebrospinal fluid.

In HIV-associated tuberculosis brain damage, the macro-and microscopic picture of the lesion is similar to other pathological processes (purulent meningoencephalitis caused by pyogenic flora, cryptococcosis (Fig. 13.46), candidiasis, and others) (see also Sects. 8.2 and 14.1, Chap. 18). For morphological differential diagnosis, it is necessary to use bacteriological, molecular-genetic examination of the cerebrospinal fluid obtained during autopsy, as well as histobacterioscopic staining of micropreparations, cytological preparations of smears prints (for example, Gram, Gram-Weigert, Brown-Hopps, Grokott, PAS-reaction), to identify the etiological factor of inflammation.

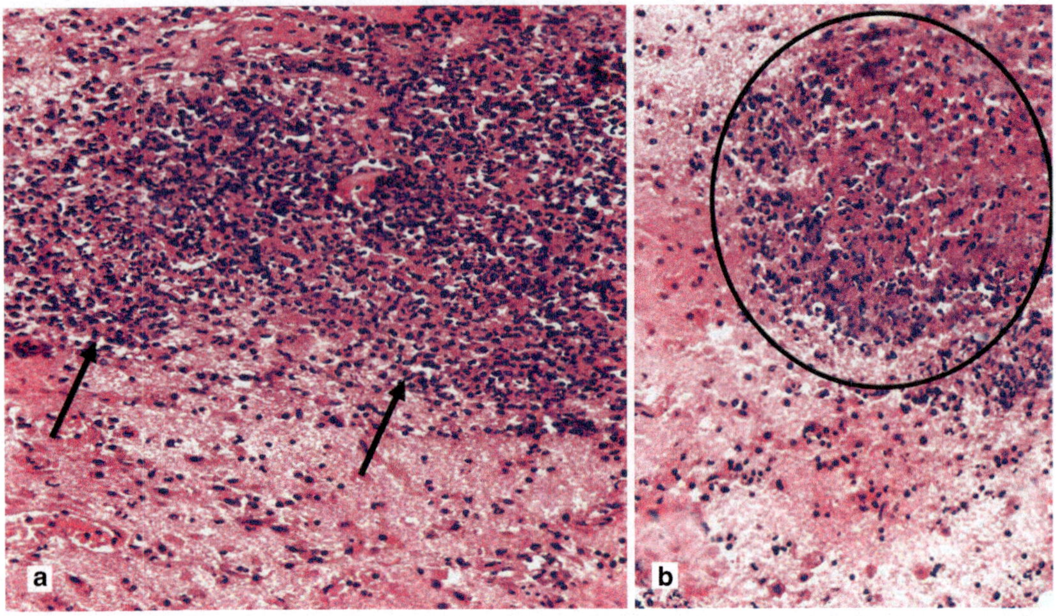

Fig. 13.44 HIV-associated tuberculosis encephalitis. (**a**) In the substance of the brain, a purulent-necrotic tuberculous focus, without signs of "specific" granulomatous inflammation; (**b**) In the substance of the brain, a fuzzy granulomatous structure of white blood cells and single epithelioid cells and lymphocytes. H-E. **a** – ×200; **b** – ×400

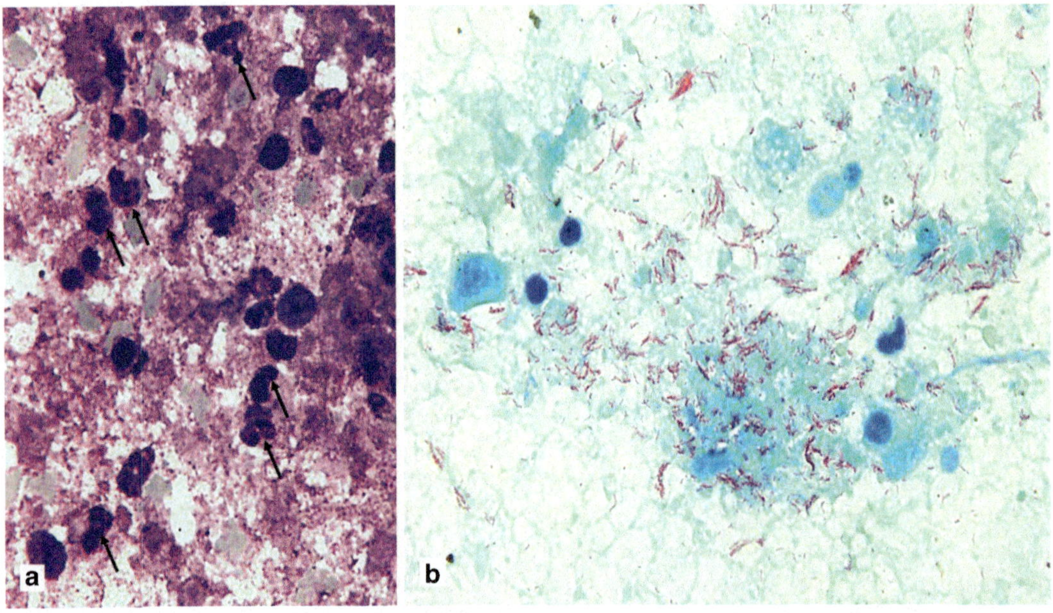

Fig. 13.45 HIV-associated tuberculous meningoencephalitis. (**a**) In the smearprint from the site of a tuberculous lesion of the brain, the purulent nature of the inflammation (some of the white blood cells are indicated by arrows); (**b**) A large number of acid-resistant bacteria in the smear print from the site of a tuberculous lesion of the brain. Cytological preparations. (**a**) stained according to Romanovsky-Giemsa; (**b**) stained according to Z-N. ×1000

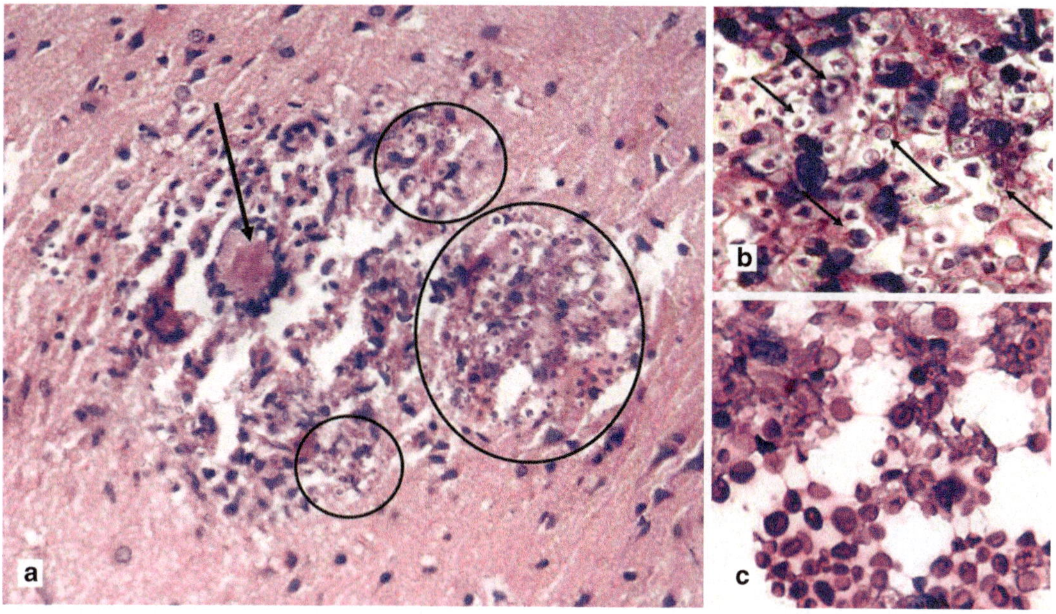

Fig. 13.46 HIV-associated cryptococcal meningoencephalitis. (**a**) Mycotic granuloma in the substance of the brain (mycotic structures in the granuloma are circled by round frames), the giant Langhans cell is indicated by an arrow; (**b**) Cryptococci (some of them are indicated by arrows); (**c**) Cryptococci (colored crimson-red). **a**, **b** – H-E; **c** – PAS-reaction. **a** – ×200; **b**, **c** – ×1000

13.2 Lesions of the Nervous System in Syphilis

Syphilis—(syphilis, lues, French disease, Italian disease, German disease, love plague)—chronic infectious disease, severe anthroponosis, caused by pale treponema (Treponema pallidum), transmitted mainly sexually, characterized by primary affect with damage to the mucous membranes and skin at the entrance gate of infection, with subsequent multi-organ lesions (involvement of internal organs, musculoskeletal system, nervous system), with a progressive stage recurrent progredient course (periods of manifestation, active manifestations alternate with periods of latency, latent states). There is a gradual change in the clinical and pathological picture towards more unfavorable manifestations. The variety of clinical manifestations and the chronic recurrent course of the disease is due to the combination of the virulent properties of the pathogen and the characteristics of the response of the immune system of the host to its introduction.

In Europe, the first epidemic of syphilis was registered in 1495 near Naples among the troops of the French King Charles VIII, besieging the city. Later, it spread to Switzerland, Germany and covered all European countries. For the first time, the possibility of syphilitic lesions of the nervous system drew the attention of the French doctor Johann Jean Astrou. In 1740 he reported on changes in the blood vessels of the brain in syphilis, noting that headache, dizziness, convulsive seizures, and paralysis in patients with syphilis can be caused by brain injuries and syphilitic lesions of the skull. Almost 130 years later, in 1834, these studies were continued in the works of Lallemann, who showed that syphilis causes damage to the membranes and substances of the brain. In the 40–50s of the nineteenth century, the doctrine of tabes dorsalis began to be created. Johann Jacobi was the first to establish the presence of a pathological process in the posterior cord in spinal cord dryness. Russian neurologists A. Ya. Kozhevnikov and P. I. Uspensky gave a detailed clinical and morphological description of tabes dorsalis. P. M. Petrov was one of the first to point out the possibility of syphilis of the sympathetic nervous system. In 1881, the French syphilidologist Jean Fournier published a monograph "Syphilis of the brain." At the end of the nineteenth century, the manifestations of neurosyphilis in children were described.

13.2.1 Etiology and Epidemiology

The causative agent of syphilis (Treponema pallidum, syn. Spirochaeta pallidum) belongs to the genus Treponema, the family Spirochaetaceae, the order Spirochaetales, the class Spirochaetia, the type Spirochaetes (Greek speira-spiral, chaite-hair). Treponemes (Greek. trepo-rotate, nema – thread) are thin spiral-shaped long microorganisms that have 8–12 whorls. The length of the cells is 8–20 microns, the diameter is 0.25–0.35 microns. In addition to the spirillary (spiral) form, the causative agent of syphilis has the form of cysts, L-forms, and polymembrane phagosomes. The cyst is a form of survival of pale treponema in unfavorable environmental conditions, the resting stage of T. pallidum which has antigenic activity. L-form is considered a way of survival of pale treponema, L-forms have weak antigenic activity. Polymembrane phagosomes are the result of incomplete phagocytosis of T. pallidum. The causes of long-term asymptomatic persistence of T. pallidum include incystation, L-transformation, and incomplete phagocytosis. The reversion of treponemas from the survival form to the pathogenic spiral form is the cause of relapse of syphilis [9–12]. In the modern literature there are no detailed descriptions of morphological changes.

There are several ways of infection with syphilis:

1. Contact—direct and indirect:
   direct (direct) contact with a sick person:
   - sexual way in which the infection occurs through damaged skin or mucous membranes, is the most common and typical route of infection,
   - household transmission, mainly in children through everyday contact with their parents, having syphilitic rashes on the skin and/or mucous membranes, rarely,
   - the professional path of transmission of infection of laboratory personnel working with experimental animals infected with syphilis, infection of medical workers (surgeons, obstetricians gynecologists, dentists, pathologists, and forensic medical experts) during the performance of professional duties.

   indirect (indirect) contact - through infected objects:
2. transplacental, characterized by the transmission of infection from the sick mother to the fetus through the placenta, which leads to the development of congenital syphilis,
3. transfusion with infection by blood transfusion from a donor with syphilis at any stage.

It is also considered possible to infect infants with syphilis through the milk of nursing women with syphilis. A woman who has syphilis and has specific rashes in the area of the nipple and areola can infect a baby while breastfeeding, but the infectivity of breast milk has not been proven. Infectious biological fluids include saliva and semen of patients with syphilis, which have clinical manifestations in the corresponding localizations. No cases of infection through sweat and urine were observed.

13.2.2 Clinical Manifestations

Infection with syphilis occurs through micro trauma of the skin or mucous membranes of the genital tract, mouth, and rectum. At the site of inoculation, intensive reproduction of T. pallidum begins, the features of the local tissue reaction to treponema determine the clinical characteristics of syphilis. Once inside the body, treponema interacts with fibronectin, which is a substrate for cell adhesion, and with other cellular receptors. Within a few minutes,

T. pallidum can enter the bloodstream and then attach to host cells, including epithelial, fibroblastic, and endothelial cells. After adhesion, helically rotating treponemes come into contact with the vascular endothelium, which can cause thrombosis, endoperiarteritis, necrosis, destructive changes in perivascular connective tissue, ulceration. There is a primary effect in the form of a compacted papule, the surface of which is necrotized with the formation of erosion or ulcers with clear boundaries. In this case, the pathogen persists in the interepithelial space, in the invaginations of endothelial cells, in lymphatic vessels and lymph nodes. Subsequently, there is a rapid lymphogenic and hematogenic spread of the process, penetration through the blood-brain and placental barriers, which determines the ability of T. pallidum to disseminate and spread infection to various human tissues and organs, which is accompanied by manifestations of syphilis that are distant from the primary affect.

Developing immune responses of the host prevent the further spread of the pathogen, but does not provide its complete elimination. In syphilis, infectious (non-sterile) immunity develops due to the presence of T. pallidum in the body, and disappears soon after its elimination as a result of treatment, that is, after the microbiological cure of syphilis reinfection is possible.

According to the WHO recommendations (2016), the classification of syphilis includes early (up to 2 years from the moment of infection) and late forms (more than 2 years from the moment of infection).

According to the classification of European Disease Prevention and Control, Centers for Disease Control and Prevention (USA):

- early (contagious) syphilis (acquired syphilis with a duration of less than 1 year or 1 year),
- late syphilis (acquired syphilis with a duration of more than 1 year),
- congenital syphilis.
  - early (the first 2 years of the child's life),
  - late.

In the classification according to the principles of stage of the disease and the nature of brain damage, the following forms are distinguished:

1. Early (mesenchymal) forms.
   - latent meningitis,
   - manifest meningitis,
   - vascular syphilis.
2. Transition forms.
   - pupillary monosyndrome,
   - late pupillary radicular symptoms.
3. Late (parenchymal) forms.
   - spinal cord tabes,
   - progressive paralysis,
   - amyotrophic spinal syphilis,
   - Erb's spastic spinal paralysis.

Neurosyphilis-symptom complexes that occur when the nervous system is affected by pale treponema, which, as the disease progresses, transform into one another or coexist in the form of a dynamic state; these lesions differ in the pathological picture, pathogenesis, clinic, course, prognosis and are related only by the unity of etiology.

Pale treponemas enter the nervous system hematogenically, lymphogenically, and over blood-brain barrier at an early stage of the disease. Already in the first days after infection, spirochetes are found in the nerve membranes and perineural lymphatic spaces, the pathogen can enter the central nervous system, migrating along the nerve fibers. It is believed that the invasion of the pathogen into the central nervous system occurs in 100% of cases of syphilis, with multiplication in the soft meninges and blood vessels, and the development of inflammation in the membranes of the brain and the substance of the brain. Infectious and allergic lesions of the cerebral arteries are accompanied by swelling of the intima and media with narrowing of the lumen of the vessel. Due to good vascularization, the hypothalamic region is primarily affected, which is accompanied by a violation of vegetative regulation, including changes in the vascular tone of the cerebral arteries with the development of local hypoxia with ischemia and metabolic acidosis. This leads to the death of cortical neurons with the proliferation of neuroglia.

Syphilitic damage to the nervous system can occur at any stage of the disease with various clinical manifestations. There are early and late neurological manifestations of syphilis.

Syphilis of the nervous system early (neurosyphilis, praecox), mesenchymal is diagnosed in patients with a confirmed diagnosis of syphilis in the presence of neurological/psychiatric symptoms corresponding to exudative inflammatory and proliferative processes in the meninges and vessels, and pathological changes in the cerebrospinal fluid or in the presence of only pathology of the cerebrospinal fluid (asymptomatic early neurosyphilis) and the duration of the disease up to 5 years. During this period, lymphoid plasmocytes infiltration is formed in the meninges, vessels (mesodermal structures) of the brain and spinal cord.

Syphilis of the nervous system late (neurosyphilis tarda) is diagnosed in patients with a confirmed diagnosis of syphilis in the presence of neurological/psychiatric symptoms corresponding to degenerative dystrophic processes in the parenchyma of the brain and/or spinal cord, and pathological changes in the cerebrospinal fluid or in the presence of only pathology of the cerebrospinal fluid (asymptomatic late neurosyphilis) and the duration of the disease is more than 5 years. In late forms of syphilis, a "specific" granuloma develops with secondary autoimmune damage to the vessels, the late neurosyphilis in most cases develops after five or more years from the moment of infection, although sometimes it is detected at an earlier time. Changes in the cerebrospinal fluid may not be accompanied by clinical symptoms (late latent specific meningitis) or there are non-pathognomonic symptoms of damage to the nervous system and visual organs. Degenerative-dystrophic processes in the brain and/or spinal cord tissue predominate in the form of demyelination followed by fibrosis (progressive paralysis, spinal tabes, taboparalysis, primary atrophy of the optic nerves). In parallel, inflammatory processes occur in the soft meninges (with the development of vasculitis and perivasculitis) and blood vessels—late meningovascular, vascular neurosyphilis, and gum of the central nervous system.

13.2.3 Early Neurosyphilis

Latent (asymptomatic) meningitis or "liquorosyphilis"—characterized by changes in the cerebrospinal fluid and positive serological reactions in the absence of meningeal symptoms. It is believed that syphilis is almost the only infection in which changes in the cerebrospinal fluid can be detected in the absence of meningeal symptoms. CSF flows out under pressure, characterized by lymphocytic pleocytosis, hyperalbuminosis, and positive serological reactions in the CSF. In some cases, there are mild general cerebral symptoms (mild headache, dizziness, general hyperesthesia) and so-called neurological microsymptoms (decreased bone conduction with auditory nerve damage, lengthening of the latent period in the reaction of the pupils to light, myosis, root-type hypoalgesia, etc.). Meningeal symptoms (symptoms of Kernig, Brudzinski) are usually absent. Microscopic examination of the soft meninges can reveal a weakly expressed focal or diffuse infiltration of lymphoid and plasma cells; the ependyma is intact. Hydrocephalus does not develop.

Acute (febrile) syphilitic meningitis manifests itself in the first 1–2 years after infection. Clinically, there are three forms of acute syphilitic meningitis: with a predominant lesion of the membranes at the base of the brain and a violation of the function of the cranial nerves; with a predominant lesion of the membranes of the convexital surface of the brain, accompanied by headache, vomiting, convulsive seizures, speech disorders, paralysis and mental disorders (signs of meningoencephalitis); acute syphilitic hydrocephalus with the development of stagnant changes in the fundus.

The process can develop as an acute infection, or gradually, with a prodromal period. Expressed meningeal syndrome, a variety of pathological reflexes, in 10% of cases, there is a spot-papular rash. Paresis or paralysis of the extremities, hydrocephalus with intracranial cerebrospinal fluid hypertension may occur. In the cerebrospinal fluid, lymphocytic pleocytosis is detected (150–1500 cells/μl), an increased protein content (0.6–1.2%), the pressure of the cerebrospinal fluid is usually increased to 500–800 mm of water. The Wasserman reaction in the blood and spinal fluid is usually positive.

Syphilitic lesions of the peripheral nervous system usually occur in the form of meningoradiculopathy and polyneuropathy. Characteristic is the lesion of the cervical thoracic and lumbosacral roots, the predominant disorders of sensitivity (without motor disorders). In the cerebrospinal fluid, there are changes of an inflammatory nature and positive serological reactions. Quite often, a lesion of the optic nerve is detected, the process is usually bilateral and leads to a decrease in visual acuity up to complete blindness. In clinical examination, the pathognomonic symptom of neurosyphilis is gray atrophy of the optic nerve.

Late pupillary radicular syndrome combines pupillary monosyndrome with loss of Achilles and knee reflexes, a violation of the surface sensitivity of the radicular type in the Gitzig zone (areas of innervation of the III–IV thoracic segments), C8-D1, L5-S1. This syndrome is regarded as progredient pretabes.

Clinically, there are three stages of tabes dorsalis:

1. neuralgic-predominant damage to nerve fibers and ganglia, there are shooting root pain (tabetic crisis), sensitivity disorders, decreased tendon reflexes, paresis and paralysis of the cranial nerves, primary atrophy of the optic nerves and pupillary disorders,
2. atactic static and dynamic ataxia, muscle hypotension, violation of the function of the pelvic organs (in the affected posterior columns of the spinal cord, the Gaulle and Burdach bundles pass, which are responsible for deep sensitivity),
3. paralytic areflexia of the tendons of the lower extremities, complete loss of deep muscle joint sensitivity, paresis and paralysis of the extremities are noted (moreover, there are no true paresis and paralysis, but due to severe ataxia, patients lose the ability to stand, walk, sit), trophic disorders (arthropathy of the lower extremities, Charcot joint, osteoporosis with painless fractures, ulcers on the soles, painless loss of teeth and nails), cachexia. In the cerebrospinal fluid, hyperalbuminosis and minor lymphocytic pleocytosis are detected, the serological reactions in the cerebrospinal fluid are 80% positive, in the blood, positive results are determined only in 30–50%.

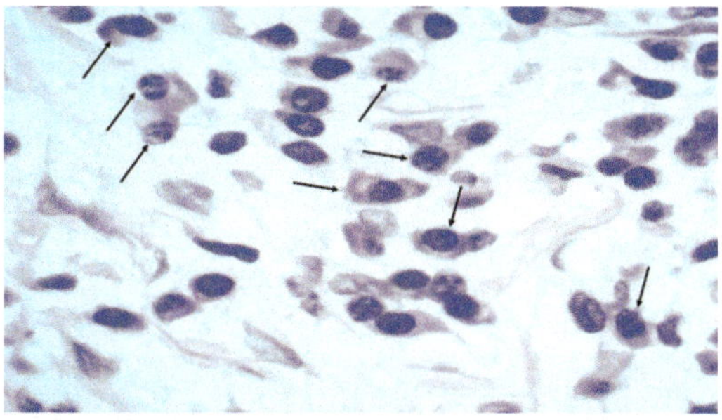

Fig. 13.47 Inflammatory infiltrate in syphilis with a predominance of Marshalko-Unna lymphoid and plasma cells (some plasma cells are indicated by arrows). H-E. ×1000

In recent years, tabes dorsalis has been benign. In congenital syphilis, tabes dorsalis is observed in childhood and adolescence.

Progressive paralysis, syphilitic encephalopathy, syphilitic dementia develops 10–20 years after infection, manifests itself in steadily progressive chronic meningoencephalitis and endarteritis, with a fatal outcome within a few months or years. It is believed that the changes are caused by the penetration of treponemes from the perivascular spaces into the brain cells. The patient slowly loses cognitive function up to dementia, various changes of a neurological nature, mental disorders (for example, agitation, manic and depressive states, delusions, hallucinations). In rare cases, a combination of progressive paralysis and spinal tabes (taboparalysis) is possible. In the liquor, there is an increase in the protein content to 0.45–0.6 g/l, positive Wasserman reaction.

13.2.4 Pathology of Neurosyphilis

In neurosyphilis, the following types of tissue reactions are distinguished:

1. diffuse (nonspecific)—inflammatory reactions with a predominance of plasma and lymphatic cells (Fig. 13.47),
2. granulomatous type with diffuse lesion of the meninges (gum meningitis) (Fig. 13.48),

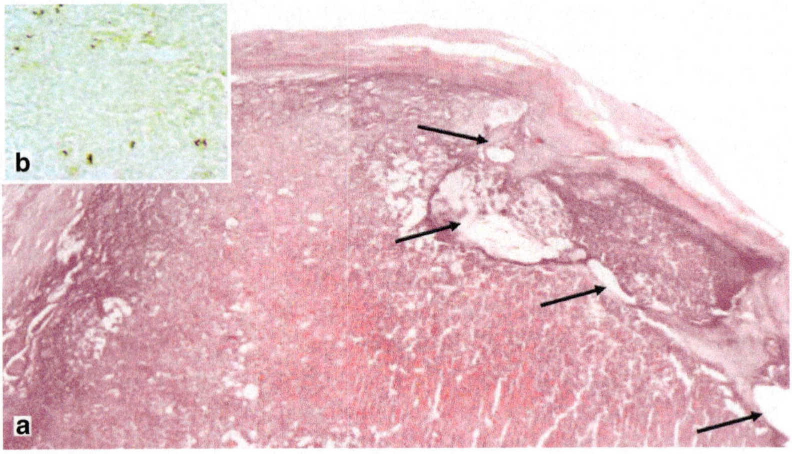

Fig. 13.48 (**a**) Syphilitic gumma is represented by a focus of necrosis surrounded by a fibrous capsule, multiple vessels in the capsule, and subcapsular (indicated by arrows); (**b**) Spirochetes with necrotic masses (colored black). H-E. ×100; **b**-stained by Warthin-Starry. ×1000

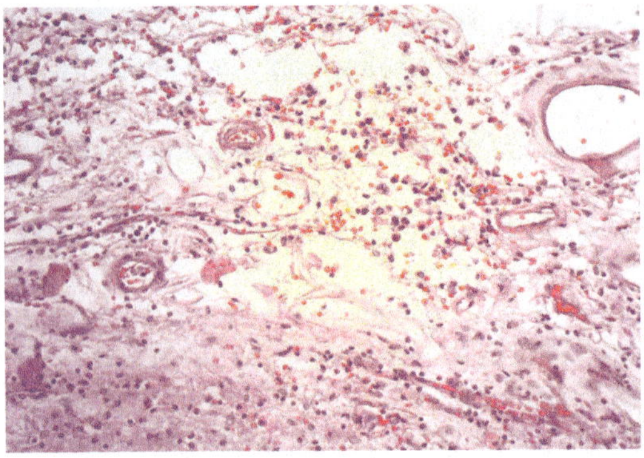

Fig. 13.49 Productive meningitis in syphilis. H-E. ×200

3. vascular type—arteritis, phlebitis with vascular obliteration, thrombosis (obliterating endarteritis),
4. changes in nerve cells, glia, and nerve fibers,
5. chronic meningitis in the late stages of the disease (Fig. 13.49).

Syphilitic granuloma (gumma) macroscopically represents a necrotic focus, necrotic mass of whitish-grayish color, viscous, resembling glue. "Gumma" comes from the Latin word gummi (Latin gummi-gum and Arabicus-Arabian, Arabian gum: a solid transparent resin consisting of the dried juice of some plants, an adhesive substance). The pathological focus got its name because of the similarity of the secretions from it with gum Arabic. Gumma is represented by an extensive focus of coagulation necrosis ("gum rods"), surrounded by a cellular infiltrate of lymphocytes, plasma, and epithelioid cells; giant Langhans cells are rare (Fig. 13.50). The plasma cells characteristic of syphilitic inflammation are called Marshalko-Unna cells (see Fig. 13.47). Plasma cells in the infiltrate can be detected by Brachet histochemical staining (Fig. 13.50), as well as by IHC examination with antibodies to plasma cells. In necrotic masses, it is possible to identify the outlines of small vessels with narrowed lumen due to the proliferation of endotheliocytes. For gum, a fairly rapid formation of connective tissue (capsule) with multiple vessels (see Fig. 13.48a) with proliferating endothelium (endovasculitis) is typical around the focus of necrosis, and obliterative changes in the vessels are characteristic. Perifocally, small granulomas identical to those in tuberculosis or granulomas of the sarcoidic type can be detected. In gummous infiltrates, a typical pattern is observed with the formation of perivascular inflammatory coupling, with the presence of Marshalko-Unna cells in the infiltrate.

In gums, histobacterioscopic examination (for example, with Warthin-Starry staining) can reveal treponema (see Figs. 13.48b and 13.50b). Methods of PCR and immunohistochemistry for the detection of pale treponema are very limited.

Classification of gum: by number—single (solitary) and multiple; by size—from microscopic, miliary (miliary gum) to large, with a diameter of several centimeters (3–6 cm). The outcome of gumma is sclerosis, scarring.

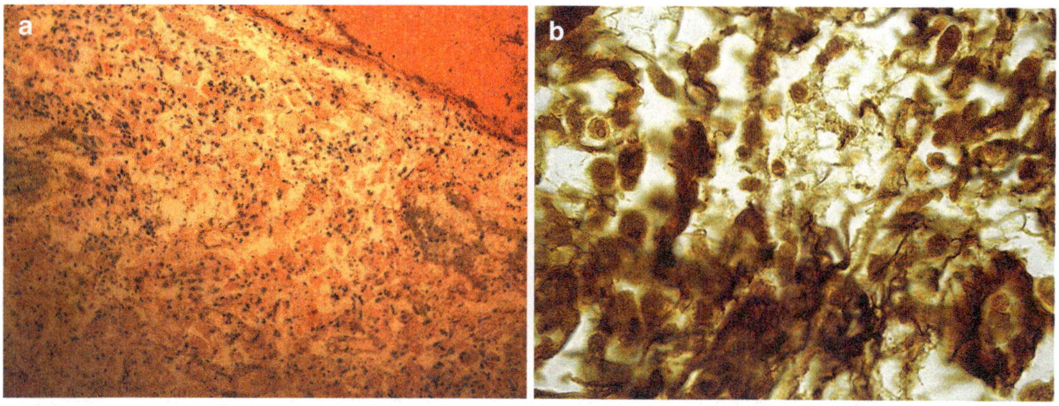

Fig. 13.50 Brain gumma. (**a**) General view H-E × 200; (**b**) Several pathogens. Silver impregnation. ×600

Syphilitic lesion of the central nervous system is also characterized by degenerative dystrophic, atrophic, demyelinating changes in the substance of the brain and spinal cord, roots. During histological examination, demyelination sites are identified using various histochemical stains on myelin.

Macroscopically in acute meningitis, the soft medulla is hyperemic and slightly edematous. The lesion is diffuse in nature, the inflammatory process often extends to the membranes covering the roots of the cranial nerves, as well as to the vascular plexuses of the ventricles (Figs. 13.51 and 13.52). Microscopically, dilatation and fullness of blood vessels, diffuse lymphoid-plasmocytic infiltration are detected. The final phase of ependymitis may be a pathological growth of subependymal neuroglia, the so-called "granular" ependymitis. Often involved in the pathological process of cranial nerves (visual, oculomotor, facial, auditory).

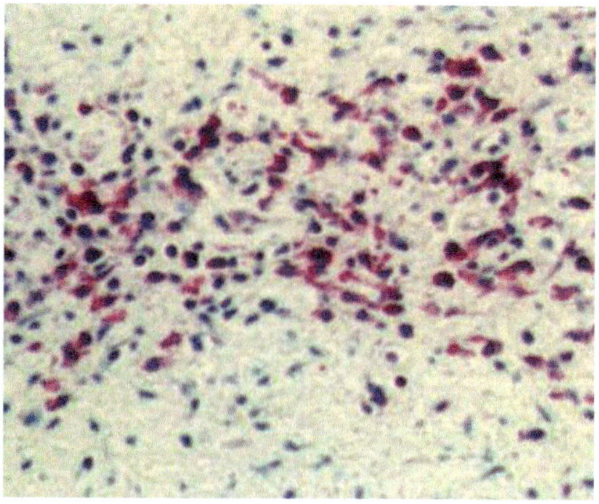

Fig. 13.51 Inflammatory infiltrate in syphilis, with a large number of Marshalko-Unna plasma cells (colored red). Stained by Brachet. ×200

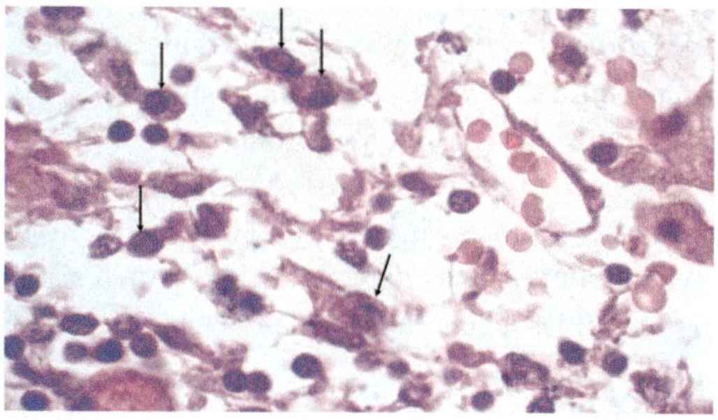

Fig. 13.52 Syphilitic ependymitis, lymphoid plasmocytic infiltrate (plasma cells are indicated by arrows). H-E. ×1000

Vascular neurosyphilis usually develops in the first 3 years after infection and is characterized by damage to the vessels of the brain and spinal cord. In cerebral vessels of all calibers, syphilitic endoarteritis develops, which leads to a concentric narrowing of the lumen of the arteries of the arteries. Syphilitic arteritis (Heubner obliterating arteritis) is characterized by lymphocytic infiltration of the adventitia and the muscular lining of the cerebral arteries, mainly of medium caliber (Fig. 13.53). Areas of stenosis and obliteration of blood vessels are formed with the development of foci of brain ischemia (when larger arteries are affected, a picture of ischemic, less often hemorrhagic brain infarction may occur), which is manifested by clinical polymorphism depending on the localization and degree of damage to the vessel (Figs. 13.54 and 13.55). More often, the

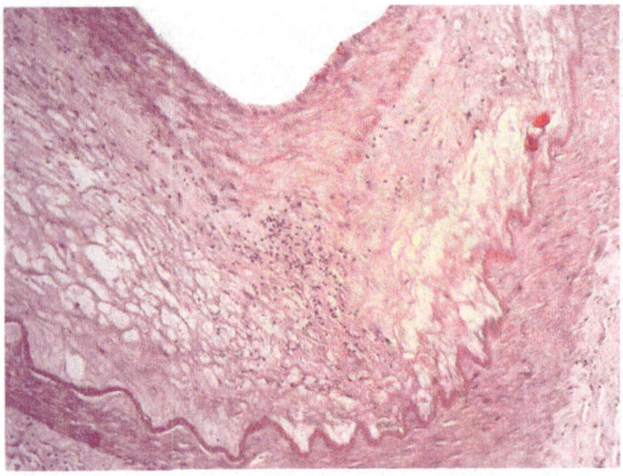

Fig. 13.53 Syphilitic obliterating endarteritis of the brain vessels. H-E. ×100

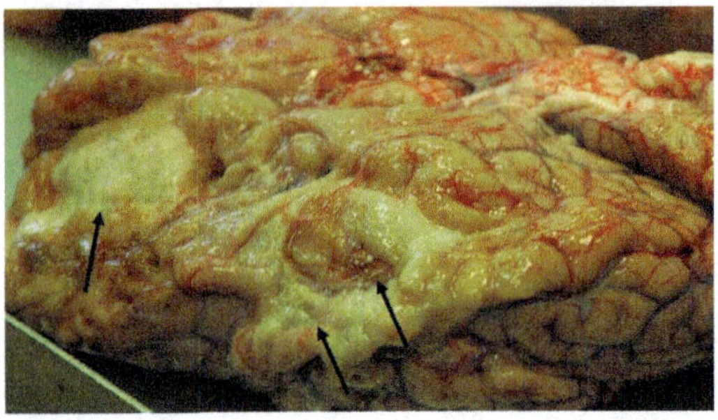

Fig. 13.54 Vascular neurosyphilis with the development of extensive ischemic infarction of the brain (the destruction site is indicated by arrows). Unfixed macropreparation

middle cerebral artery is involved in the process. The progression of the disease can lead to deep dementia. Since syphilitic endarteritis proceeds according to the type of meningovasculitis, both focal and meningeal symptoms are clinically established. In the cerebrospinal fluid, lymphocytic pleocytosis in the cerebrospinal fluid, hyperalbuminosis is detected. Membranes of the brain, with degenerative changes in the brain substance.

Spinal vascular neurosyphilis is characterized by damage to the membranes and vessels of the spinal cord (syphilitic endarteritis), which is manifested by meningoradiculopathy, spinal stroke, and chronic myelopathy. Spinal circulatory disorders can be acute or subacute, and the clinical and morphological picture is determined depending on the level of damage to the spinal cord, both in length and in diameter. In the case of localization of changes in the posterior spinal arteries, the picture may resemble spinal tabes in late neurosyphilis. In myelopathy, both the membranes of the spinal cord and the roots are usually involved in the process, with the development of meningomyeloradiculopathy. Involvement of the spinal vessels in the syphilitic process is usually secondary to meningeal inflammation.

Syphilitic meningomyelitis is characterized by slowly progressing lower spastic paraparesis, and in some cases, the changes develop acutely and asymmetrically, with the formation of Brown-Secar syndrome (a symptom complex observed in the lesion of half the diameter of the spinal cord: on the side of the lesion, central paralysis (or paresis) is noted with loss of muscle-joint and vibration sensitivity, on the opposite side—loss of pain and temperature sensitivity), which is more characteristic of thrombosis of the sulcate arteries—branches of the anterior spinal artery.

Cervical hypertrophic pachymeningitis refers to spinal meningeal syphilis, which was described by Charcot (extremely rare). In this form, fibrosis of the dura mater of the spinal cord develops and it merge with the surrounding tissues to form scars in the membranes of the spinal cord at the cervical level. The process develops slowly, over 1–2 years. Syphilis is more characterized by chronic hyperplastic pachymeningitis. Macroscopically, dura mater of the spinal cord is thickened due to impregnation with gelatinous exudates, yellowish-gray, and there may be adhesions with adjacent tissues. Histologically, granulomas (gummas) are detected.

Chronic syphilitic meningitis is clinically similar to early meningitis, but has a gradual development and a recurrent chronic course (Fig. 13.56). Neurologically, weakly expressed general cerebral and meningeal symptoms are determined. In this form of meningitis, the membranes at the base of the brain (basal leptomeningitis) are usually affected, with damage to the cranial nerves. More often, the oculomotor nerve, facial, trigeminal, and auditory nerves are involved in the process. CSF is characterized by hyperalbuminosis, lymphocytic pleocytosis, and positive serological reactions. Severe productive syphilitic leptomeningitis can lead to communi-

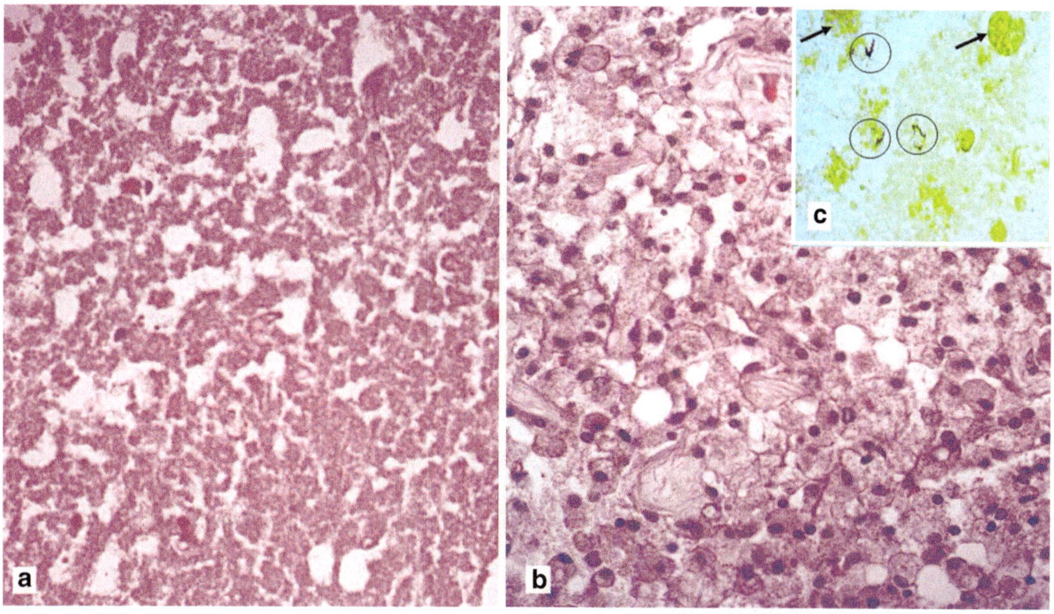

Fig. 13.55 Ischemic infarction in neurosyphilis. (**a**) The site of necrosis of the brain substance; (**b**) The cells of "granular balls" in the infarcted area of the brain; c) Spirochetes in the area of ischemic infarction of the brain in neurosyphilis (spirochetes are colored black (circled by round frames), the arrows indicate the cells of "granular balls." **a**, **b**-staining with H-E. ×400; **b** – stained by Warthin-Starry. ×1,000

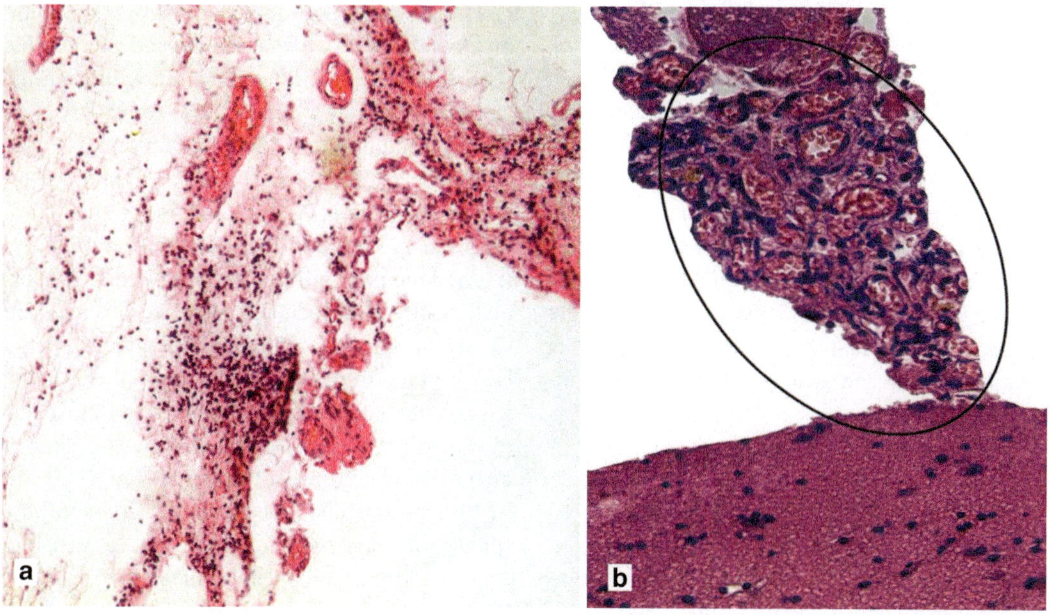

Fig. 13.56 Chronic productive syphilitic meningitis. H-E; **a** – ×40; **b** – ×100

cating or obstructive hydrocephalus as a result of obliteration of the subarachnoid space in the posterior cranial fossa or as a result of obstruction of the lumen opening. Late pupillary monosyndrome refers to the modern form of transitional neurosyphilis, currently usually found in isolation. Clinically determined anisocoria, bilateral pupil deformity, Argyle Robertson symptoms.

Gumma of the brain and spinal cord is extremely rare. It is most often localized in the

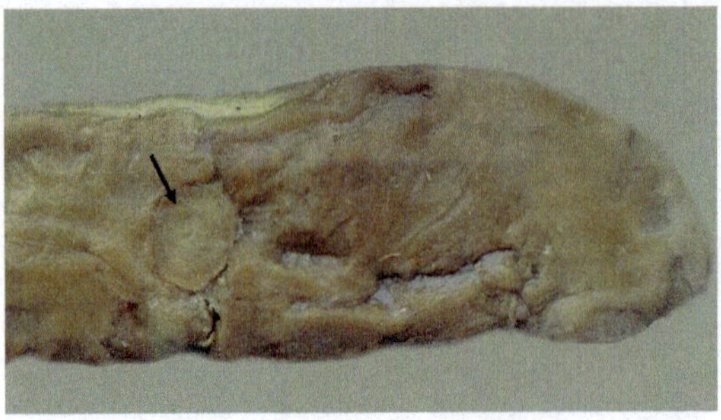

Fig. 13.57 Gumma of the brain (indicated by an arrow). Fixed macropreparation

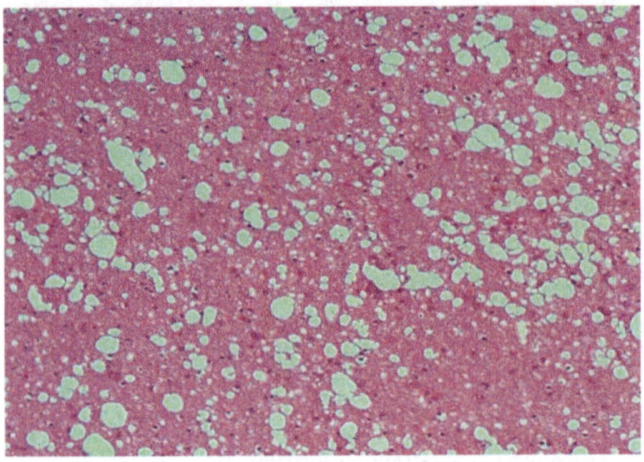

Fig. 13.58 Late neurosyphilis. Spongiose transformation of the brain substance. H-E; ×40

region of the base of the brain, less often - in the medulla (Fig. 13.57). The location of the gumma in the area of the basal liquid cisterns can lead to compression of the cranial nerves at the base of the brain, which clinically often simulates brain tumors. The gummas of the spinal meninges compress the spinal cord, causing partial or complete motor and sensory changes below the level of damage.

13.2.5 Late Neurosyphilis

Changes in the nervous tissue in late neurosyphilis are characterized by proliferative changes in astrocytic glia in the brain and spinal cord atrophic processes in the brain substance such as "laminar" or "pseudolaminar" loss of neurons, which leads to sponginess of the brain substance (status spongiosis) (Fig. 13.58) against the background of intense lymphocytic and plasmocytic infiltration (that is, there are pathological changes of an inflammatory and dystrophic nature). A diffuse vascular reaction develops in the form of syphilitic arteritis with necrotic changes in the intima (endovasculitis), fibrosis, and obliteration of the vessel lumen. Ischemic changes in the brain substance (foci of softening), mononuclear adventitial infiltrates are formed. Gummous nodules are formed, initially forming in the meninges, followed by spreading to the substance of the brain membranes and acquiring a multiple character.

The process involves nerve cells that conduct pathways, glia of the spinal cord and brain, and therefore late neurosyphilis is called "parenchymal," while early neurosyphilis is called "mesenchymal."

Clinical diagnosis of late neurosyphilis can be difficult, since serological reactions in the cerebrospinal fluid are not an absolute diagnostic, false-negative serological reactions in the cerebrospinal fluid occur in late neurosyphilis in 43.8% of patients.

Dorsal dryness tabes dorsalis syphilitic myelopathy refers to the late period of syphilis, occurs 10–15 years after infection with syphilis, and is currently extremely rare. In this form of syphilis, meningomyelitis develops with a predominant lesion of the posterior column, posterior horns, posterior roots of the spinal cord, cranial nerves (II and VIII), and the cerebral cortex, and the possibility of involvement of subcortical nodes is noted. Degenerative changes are slowly progressive. The pathological process begins in the spinal nerves and then spreads to the ganglia and subsequently passes to the substance of the spinal cord with a predominant lesion of the posterior column of the spinal cord.

Macroscopically, the posterior cords of the spinal cord and the posterior root are atrophic. The posterior columns are reduced in size, wrinkled, and the posterior surface of the spinal cord may be concave rather than convex. The spinal cord in the area of the posterior columns on the cross section is gray in color, translucent in appearance, different from the intact lateral and anterior columns. Changes in the posterior columns are found on transverse serial sections in

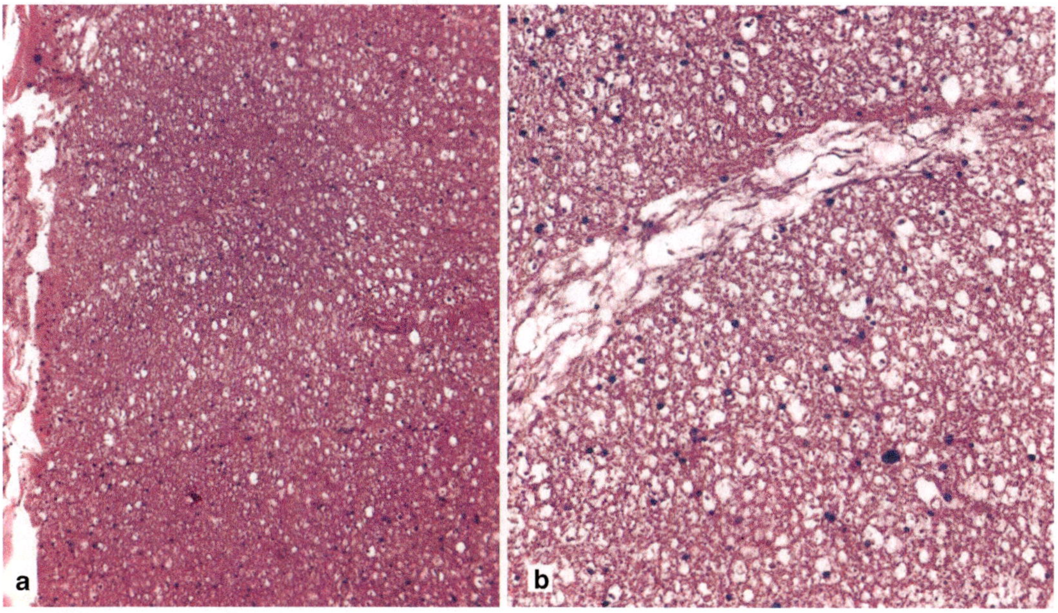

Fig. 13.59 Late neurosyphilis. Syphilitic myelopathy (spinal dryness). Spongiose transformation of the spinal cord substance. H-E; **a** – ×40; **b** – ×100

the thoracic and cervical segments, and remain limited by the Gaulle column up to the upper segments of the spinal cord. The soft medulla is thickened, reduced transparency, and cloudy, especially in the area of the posterior columns. The dura mater is thickened, there may be scarring, fusion of the dura mater with the roots. With a long-running process, the posterior roots of the ponytail are thinner and grayish in color, in contrast to the front roots. With the development of syphilitic atrophy of the optic nerve the optic nerves are thinned, atrophic, and gray in color, which is uncharacteristic for them. In the area of the optic nerves and chiasm sometimes develop adhesions. Other affected cranial nerves are also atrophic.

Microscopically, degenerative dystrophic, atrophic changes are detected in the posterior roots in the zone of their entry into the spinal cord, in the posterior horns of the spinal cord, in the posterior rope, in the Gaulle-Burdach pathways (chronic myeloradiculitis) (Figs. 13.59 and 13.60). When stained for myelin, normally myelin fibers are colored black or dark blue, and the affected areas with demyelination will be "discolored," pale gray-brown. In addition, a similar pattern is determined in some cranial nerves, prevertebral vegetative ganglia, and spinal nodes. In the soft medulla of the spinal cord, mainly on its posterior surface, changes of an inflammatory nature develop.

Morphological changes in progressive paralysis are characterized by atrophy of the cerebral cortex, thinning of the convolutions with laminar or pseudolaminar loss of neurons with the formation of "sponginess" of the brain parenchyma (status spongiosus), focal (focal) or diffuse demyelination, edema and necrosis/necrobiosis of neurons. In atrophied areas of the brain substance, inflammatory infiltration is weakly and moderately pronounced or completely absent. When impregnated with silver, spirochetes can be detected in small numbers, but in most cases they are not detected. Disorders of the cerebral circulation are the result of specific vasculitis, with a predominant lesion of small vessels, there are stenose and occlusion of vessels, proliferative changes in the intima of the capillaries of the cerebral cortex (Figs. 13.61, 13.62, 13.63). Mainly in the parietal region, clouding of the membranes of the brain, as well as their significant thickening due to fibrosis (Fig. 13.64).

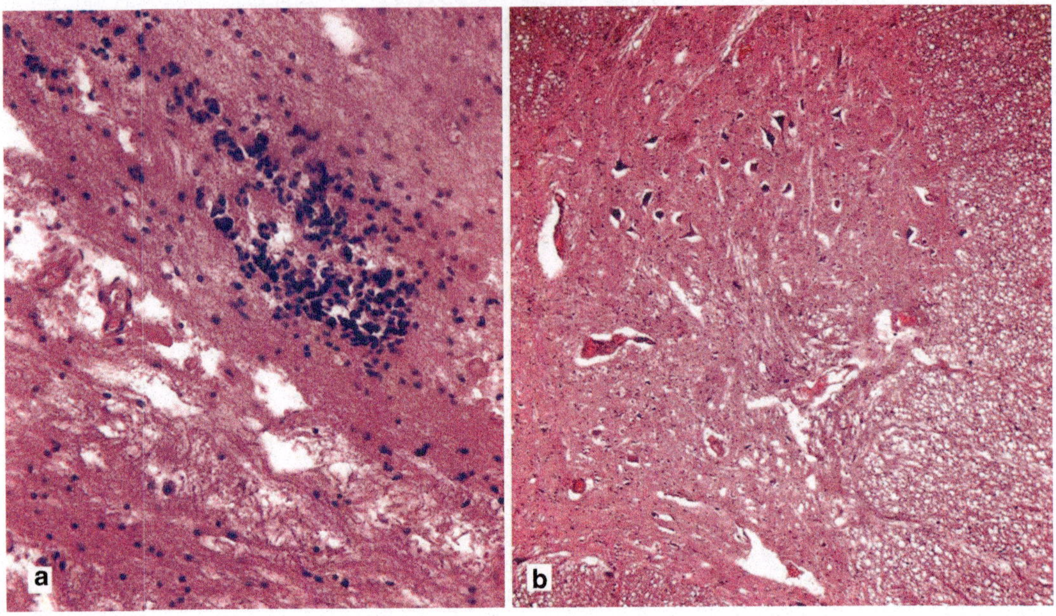

Fig. 13.60 Late neurosyphilis. Syphilitic myelopathy (spinal dryness). (**a**) Edema of the spinal cord; (**b**) Edema, spongy transformation of the spinal cord substance, atrophy of neurons. H-E; **a** – ×100; **b** – ×40

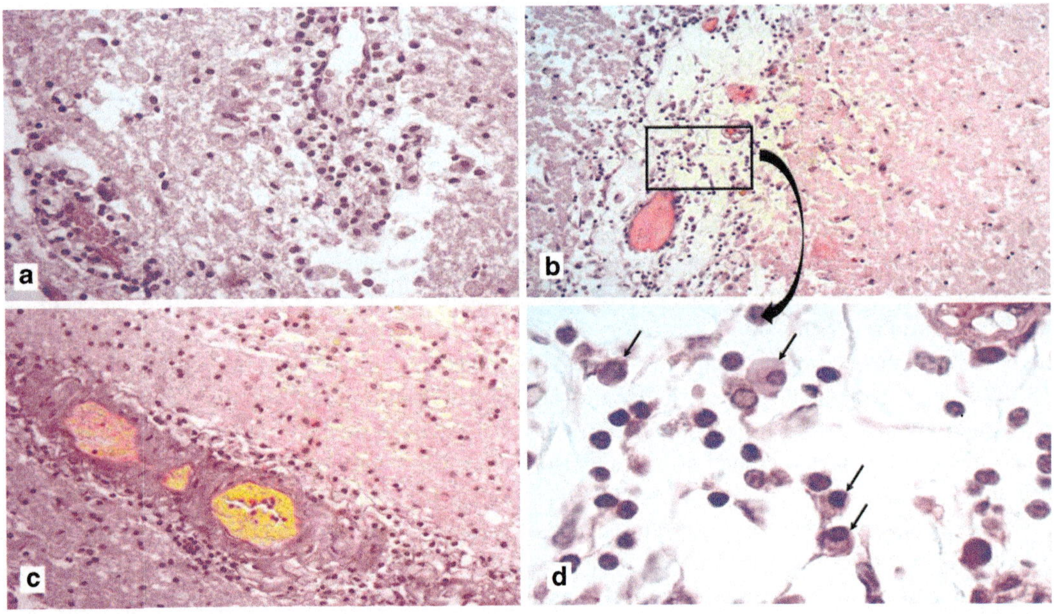

Fig. 13.61 Late neurosyphilis. Progressive paralysis, syphilitic encephalopathy. (**a**, **b**, **c**) Productive vasculitis in the substance of the brain in Fig. a-perivascular area of the brain with ischemic disorders; (**d**) Lymphoid plasmocytic infiltration in the vessel wall and perivascular, plasma cells are indicated by arrows (fragment of Fig. "**c**," the plot in the frame). H-E; **a**, **b**, **c** – ×100; **d** – ×400

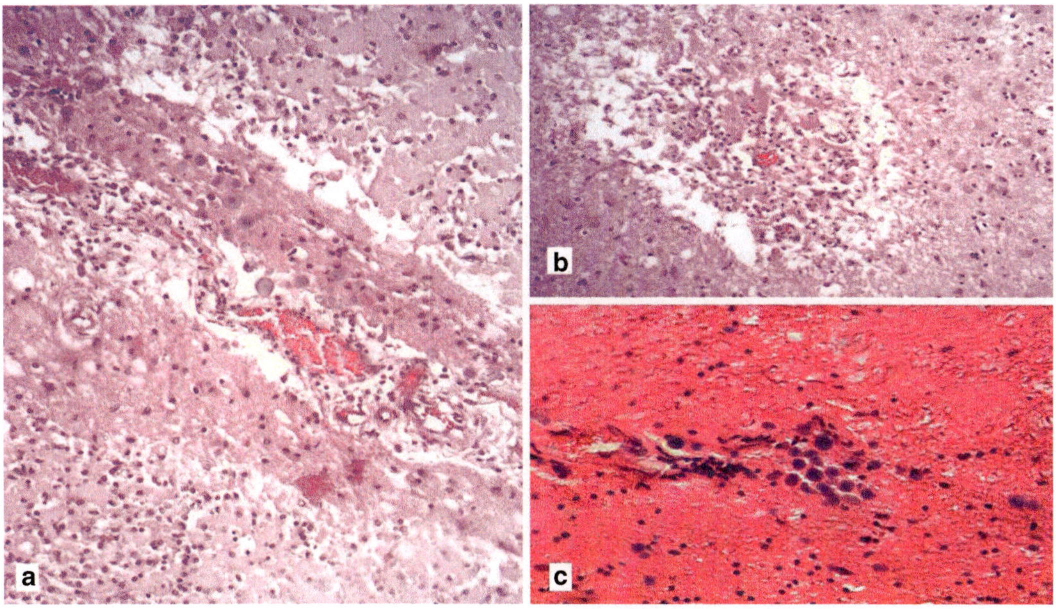

Fig. 13.62 Late neurosyphilis. Progressive paralysis, syphilitic encephalopathy. (**a**) Productive encephalitis, vasculitis; (**b**) Perivascular area of ischemia of the brain substance; (**c**) Dystrophic changes in the brain substance (perivascular basophilic globular structures). H-E; **a**, **b** – ×200; **b** – ×100

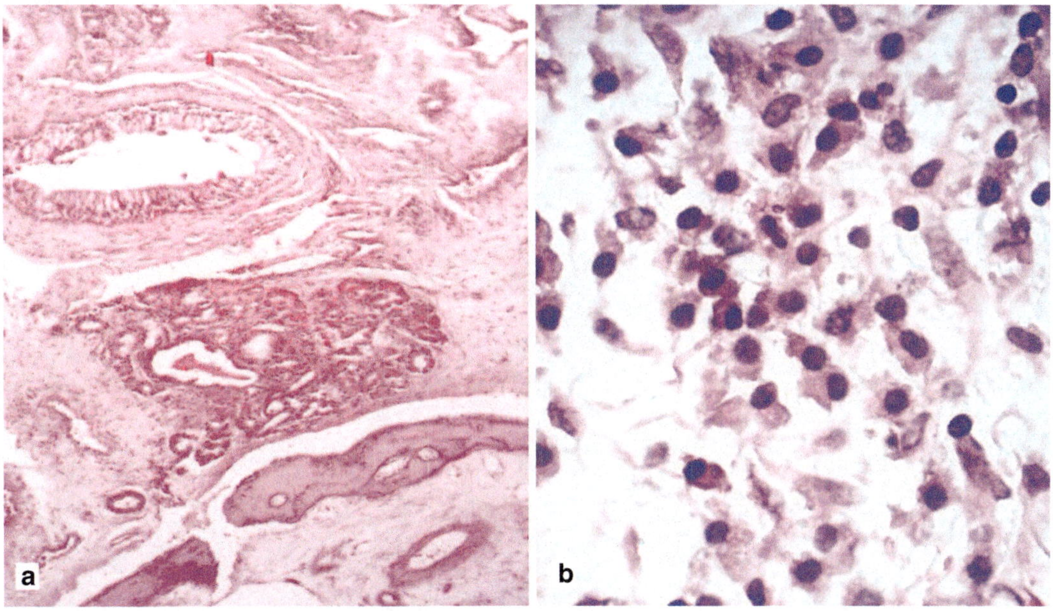

Fig. 13.63 Productive inflammation of the cranial sinus mucosa in late neurosyphilis. (**a**) Fibrosis, angiomatosis, and cellular infiltration; (**b**) The cellular composition of the inflammatory infiltrate with a significant predominance of plasma cells. H-E; **a** – ×40; **b** – ×400

Autopsies of the deceased with late neurosyphilis may also identify signs of late visceral syphilis, for example, cardiovascular syphilis (syphilitic mesaortitis, etc.) (Figs. 13.65 and 13.66).

In juvenile (congenital) syphilitic encephalopathy, the changes are identical to those in adult syphilitic encephalopathy, but more changes are detected in the cerebellum and brain stem.

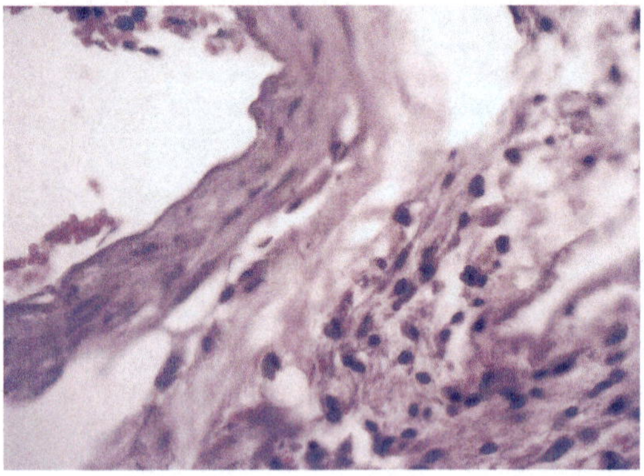

Fig. 13.64 Late neurosyphilis. Progressive paralysis, syphilitic encephalopathy. Fibrosis and mononuclear infiltration of the soft matter of the brain. H-E; ×200

Amyotrophic spinal syphilis is characterized by a slowly progressive degenerative inflammatory process in the anterior roots, motor neurons, and membranes of the spinal cord with a slow development of atrophy of the muscles of the hands, shoulder girdle and trunk, fasciculations. In the cerebrospinal fluid, positive serological reactions, there may be hyperalbuminosis and lymphocytic pleocytosis.

Erb's spastic paralysis develops 10–15 years after infection. The morphological substrate is chronic meningomyelitis with vasa endarteritis of the spinal cord, with the greatest lesion in the area of the pyramidal pathways of the lateral columns of the spinal cord.

Nissl—Alzheimer's neurosyphilis, Nissl Alzheimer's endarteritis is a form of brain syphilis in which a specific obliterating arteritis of small-caliber intracranial vessels develops with a predominant lesion of the cerebral cortex.

In the literature, there are other classifications of neurosyphilis that differ from the forms of neurosyphilis according to ICD-10, based on the clinical and morphological principles, including modern forms of syphilis of the ner-

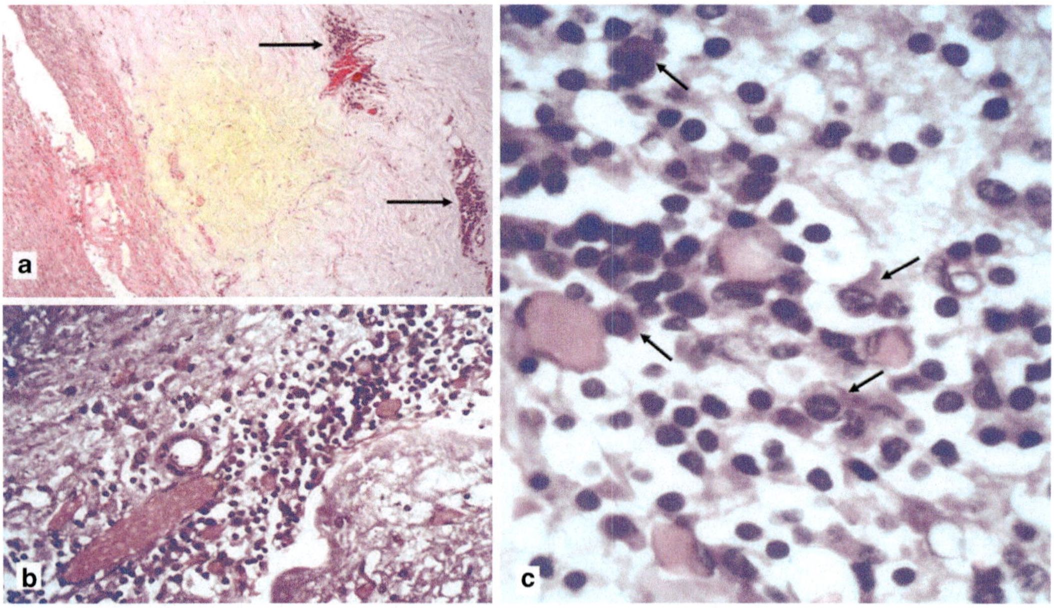

Fig. 13.65 Syphilitic mesaortitis. (**a**) Inflammation around vasa vasorum (indicated by arrows); (**b**) Perivascular infiltrate around vasa vasorum; (**c**) Cell composition of inflammatory infiltrate in syphilitic mesaortitis (lymphoid and plasma cells), some plasma cells are indicated by arrows H-E; (**a**) – X40; (**b**) – X100; (**c**) – ×400

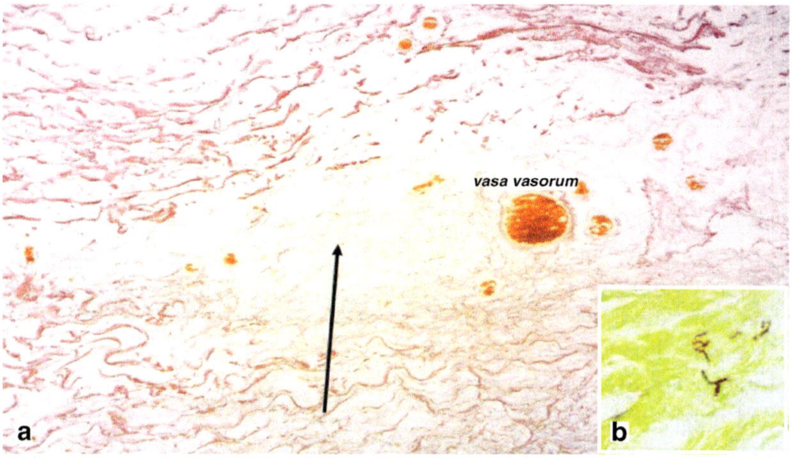

Fig. 13.66 Syphilitic mesaortitis. (**a**) Destruction of the elastic framework of the aorta in the areas of inflammation around the vasa vasorum (the area of destruction of elastic fibers is indicated by an arrow, the preserved elastic fibers are colored red-brown); (**b**) Spirochetes in the aortic wall around the vasa vasorum, spirochetes are colored black. a coloring with orsein on the elastic. X200; b-painting by Warthin-Starry. ×1000

vous system, which are the most common, excluding rare forms (syphilitic polyneuritis, syphilitic chronic polio, syphilitic paralysis of Erb, etc.), the specificity of which, according to the authors, in the light of modern ideas is questionable.

In congenital syphilitic lesions of the nervous system, clinical symptoms appear in the first year of life and in adolescence, characterized by symptoms of meningitis, hydrocephalus, deafness, epileptic seizures, atrophy of the optic nerves (see Sect. 16.2). Morphological manifestations are represented by the formation of microgyria, lobar sclerosis, inflammatory changes in the membranes of the brain, and cerebral endarteritis. Positive serological reactions are detected in the cerebrospinal fluid. In addition, in congenital syphilis, the Getchinson triad can be observed (interstitial keratitis, deformity of teeth with a semilunar defect, deafness). In adolescence, spinal cord tabes or taboparalysis may develop. Extremely rare, casually there are gummas of the brain and spinal cord, syphilitic cervical pachymeningitis.

Syphilis in HIV infection - an increase in the prevalence of neurosyphilis is probably associated with an increase in the aggressive course of syphilis in HIV infection, and a fairly rapid development of syphilitic lesions of the nervous system (see Sect. 8.2). In patients with HIV infection with syphilis, the probability of specific lesions of the nervous system, organs of vision, and hearing is 3–6 times higher than in HIV-negative patients. Although syphilis is typical in most patients with HIV infection, however, against the background of moderate and especially pronounced immunodeficiency (in the late stages of HIV infection, in the absence of highly active antiretroviral therapy), syphilis progresses rapidly. Such a special, atypical clinical picture of the development of the disease is called "malignant syphilis." Neurosyphilis, which develops against the background of severe HIV-induced immunosuppression, may differ in clinical polymorphisms, atypical clinical manifestations, and rapid progression of the process.

Differential diagnosis of neurosyphilis clinically or morphologically should be carried out with a variety of diseases: mental conditions, neurological pathology, meningitis of any etiology, sensorineural hearing loss of various origins, hypertensive crisis, myelitis of other etiologies, tumors of the brain (especially the frontal lobes) and spinal cord, vascular thrombosis of the spinal cord and brain, spinal form of multiple sclerosis, manic-depressive psychosis, schizophrenia, atherosclerosis, senile psychosis).

In case of spinal tabes, the differential diagnostic series should include brain and spinal cord injury, acute infectious diseases with damage to the nervous system (typhoid fever, influenza), long-term chronic intoxication (alcohol, chemicals for example, arsenic), polyneuropathies of various etiologies, Eidy syndrome.

Primary tabetic atrophy of the optic nerve is differentiated from atrophy of the optic nerve of another etiology, most often tuberculosis.

Gummous lesions of the central nervous system can simulate neoplasms of the brain and spinal cord, and brain tuberculosis.

Erb's spastic paralysis is differentiated from Strumpel's spastic paraplegia, amyotrophic lateral sclerosis, and spinal cord tumor.

To differentiate progressive paralysis from psychiatric conditions (manic–depressive psychosis), neoplasms of the frontal lobe, it is necessary to conduct studies of the cerebrospinal fluid.

In cases of differentiation of ischemic brain changes caused by syphilis with a stroke of different etiology, it is necessary to consider anamnestic data (for example, infertility and frequent miscarriages in women, the presence of other symptoms of neurosyphilis, positive serological reactions, changes in the cerebrospinal fluid—lymphocytic pleocytosis, hyperalbuminosis). Syphilis in anamnesis, positive serological reactions in the blood and liquor with a high degree of probability indicates a specific process in the blood vessels of the brain.

The features of the clinical course are a fairly rapid regression of the symptoms of a heart attack in syphilis and the recurrent nature of the process, this may be due to the young age of the patients and high compensatory functional ability.

References

1. Furin J, Cox H, Pai M. Tuberculosis. Lancet. 2019;393(10181):1642–56. https://doi.org/10.1016/S0140-6736(19)30308-3.
2. «The top 10 causes of death» https://www.who.int/news-room/fact-sheets/detail/the-top-10-causes-of-death
3. Zinserling VA (2021) Infectious pathology of the respiratory tract Springer International Publishing https://doi.org/10.1007/978-3-030-66325-4. ISBN 978-3—030-66324-7.
4. Kh KZ, Khokhlov IK, Savin AA, Batyrov FA. Clinical aspects, diagnosis and treatment of neurological complications of tuberculosis. Probl Tuberk. 2001;3:29–32.
5. Shaller MA, Wicke F, Foerch C, Weidauer S. Central nervous system tuberculosis: etiology, clinical manifestations and neuroradiologic features. Clin Neuroradiol. 2019;29(1):3–18. https://doi.org/10.1007/s0062-018-0726-9.
6. Davis AG, Rohlwink UK, Proust A, Figai AA, Wilkinson RJ. The pathogenesis of tuberculous meningitis. J Leucoc Biol. 2019;105(2):267–80. https://doi.org/10.1002/JLB.MR0318-102R.
7. Wilkinson RJ, Rohlwink U, Misra UK, et al. Tuberculous meningitis. Nat Rev Neurol. 2017;13(10):581–98.
8. Zinserling VA, Chukhlovina ML. Infectious lesions of nervous system. Issues of etiology, pathogenesis and diagnostics. Saint-Petersburg: ElbiSPb; 2011. p. 583. (in Russian)
9. Tampa M, Sarbu I, Matei C, Benea V, Georgescu SR. Brief history of syphilis. J Med Life. 2014;7(1):4–10.
10. Tsang SH, Sharma T. Syphilis. Adv Exp Med Biol. 2018;1085:219–21. https://doi.org/10.1007/978-3-319-95046-4_46.
11. Hook EW 3rd. Syphilis. Lancet. 2017;389(10078):1550–7. https://doi.org/10.1016/S0140-6736(16)32411-4.
12. Peeling RW, Mabey D, Kamb ML, et al. Syphilis. Nat Rev Dis Primers. 2017;3:17073. https://doi.org/10.1038/nrdp.2017.73.

Lesions Due to Fungi, Protozoa, and Helminthes (in Collaboration with Y.R. Zyuzya)

14

14.1 Damage to the Nervous System Caused by Certain Fungi

Brain lesions are described in a number of generalized mycoses that occur with immunodeficiency of various nature. In our material, such observations are extremely rare, except for brain cryptococcosis in HIV infection (see also Chap. 8).

14.1.1 Aspergillosis

Aspergillus, primarily Aspergillus fumigatus and A. flavus, reaches the brain by hematogenic route, usually from the lungs, less often from the gastrointestinal tract, paranasal sinuses, ears, skin, uterus appendages, or as a result of traumatic brain injury [1, 2]. In some cases, contact lesions are also possible. These pathogens are characterized by invasion of the arteries and veins with a picture of necrotic angiitis. Cerebral aspergillosis is a serious complication after organ transplantation and in hematological patients and is characterized by a high level of mortality. The immunosuppressive therapy carried out by such patients is also important for its development. The manifestation of cerebral aspergillosis may be focal neurological symptoms associated with the lesion of the basins of the anterior and middle cerebral arteries. In some cases, clinical symptoms may indicate a volumetric process. Among the symptoms usually indicate headache, hemiparesis, convulsions. Fever, paralysis of the cranial nerves, and abnormal plantar reflexes are also possible. In the part of the observations, signs of increased intracranial pressure and/or meningeal signs are determined. Neurological symptoms are usually regarded as nonspecific. In vivo diagnosis is extremely difficult. Pleocytosis in the CSF is usually less than 600 cl/mm^3, the protein level is only moderately elevated, the sugar content is normal, the pathogen in the CSF is usually not determined.

In postmortem morphological examination, macroscopically, foci of hemorrhagic necrosis or yellowish foci with a hemorrhagic component from 0.1 to 5 cm in diameter, resembling infarcts, are most often determined (Fig. 14.1). A thick fibrous capsule is determined only occasionally. Much less often, abscesses and granulomas form in the substance of the brain. The topography of the lesions may be different, including the hemispheres of the cerebellum. When microscopically examined, the most characteristic feature is vascular invasion and thrombosis (Fig. 14.2). At the same time, even when stained with hematoxylin-eosin, characteristic septic hyphae of the mycelium with a thickness of 4–12 microns, branching at an acute angle, are detected. According to our observations, the hyphae of mycelium in the brain tissue are less numerous and more subtle compared to the lungs (Fig. 14.3). Inflammatory infiltration in the early stages involves neutro-

V. Zinserling, *Infectious Lesions of the Central Nervous System*,
https://doi.org/10.1007/978-3-030-96260-9_14

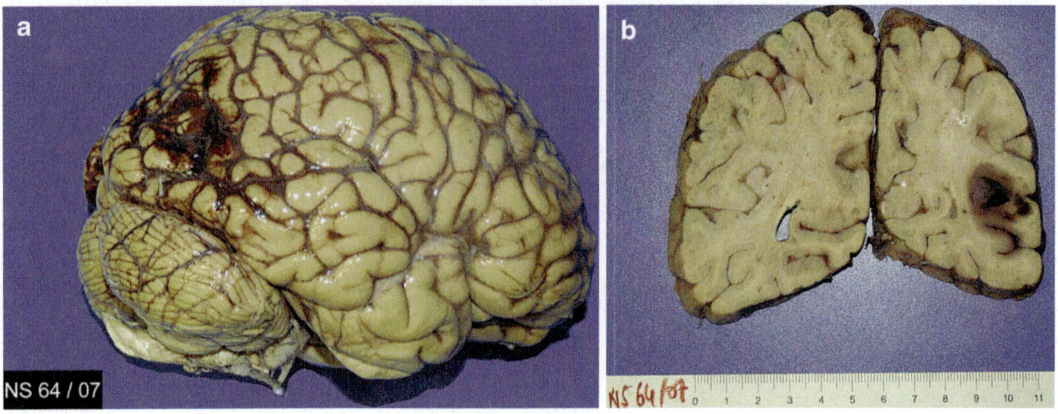

Fig. 14.1 Brain lesions in secondary aspergillosis in an oncohematological patient. Fixed macropreparation. Courtesy: Institute of Neuropathology, University of Münster, Germany. (**a**) General view; (**b**) Focus on a slice

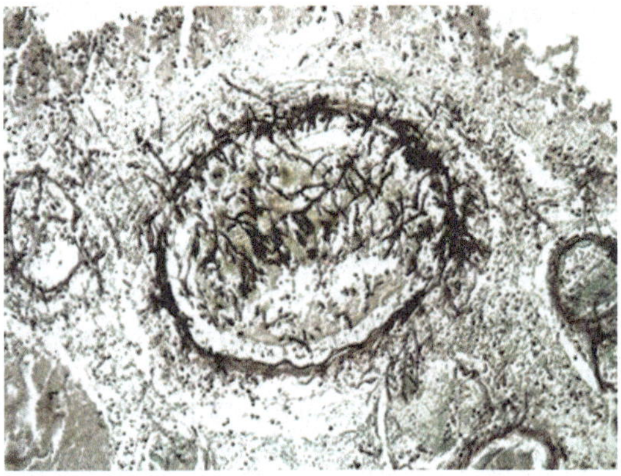

Fig. 14.2 Hyphae of Aspergillus in lumen and wall of brain vessel in a patient with HIV in AIDS stage. Impregnation by Grocott-Gomori. ×600

phils. In abscesses, free pus is located in the center, surrounded by neutrophil infiltration with an admixture of giant (Langhans type) and epithelioid cells. Granulomas are aggregates of lymphocytes, plasma, and epithelioid cells, as well as necrosis zones and collagen fibers.

14.1.2 Zygomycosis

Zygomycosis, most often caused by pathogens from the genera Rhizopus and Mucor, is often accompanied by brain lesions in usually immunecompromised individuals due to generalization from primary foci in the skin of the face, nasal mucosa, nasopharynx with damage to nearby parts, primarily the orbit, internal carotid artery, paranasal sinuses with very characteristic thrombosis [1, 3]. Hematogenous dissemination from the lungs and gastrointestinal tract is also possible. In the rhinocerebral form, the orbit is rapidly involved, which leads to unilateral ophthalmoplegia, proptosis, edema of the eyelids and cornea, and occasionally blindness. Headache, neck stiffness, and cramps may result from the involvement of the soft meninges. Severe vascular lesions lead to aphasia, hemiplegia, lethargy, disorientation, and coma. The disease can take a catastrophic course, leading to death within a few days. For diagnostics, the detection of wide, unsepted mycelial filaments from 6 to 15 microns in diameter with the possible appearance of sporangiospores and sporangia in the biopsy material is of leading importance (Fig. 14.4). The most frequent localization of lesions is the basal surface of the frontal lobes or the nodes of the base, more often in the form of hemorrhagic necrosis. Fungi are angiotropic and are detected around and in the walls of the blood vessels of the meninges and brain matter, leading to their obstruction and thrombosis. The inflammatory reaction is mixed, mainly neutrophilic, but it can be expressed minimally and practically absent. Occasionally, giant multinucleated cells can be detected, but the formation of granulomas is not characteristic.

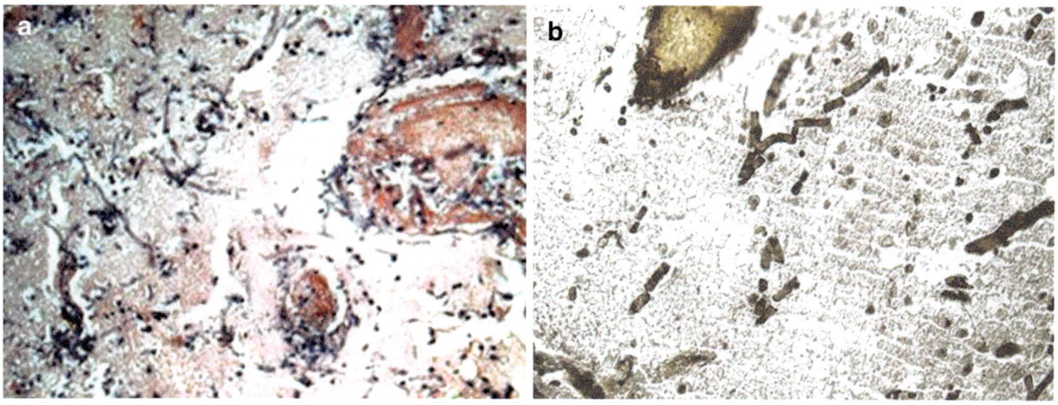

Fig. 14.3 Hyphae of Aspergillus in brain matter ×200. (**a**) H-E; (**b**) Impregnation by Grocott-Gomori

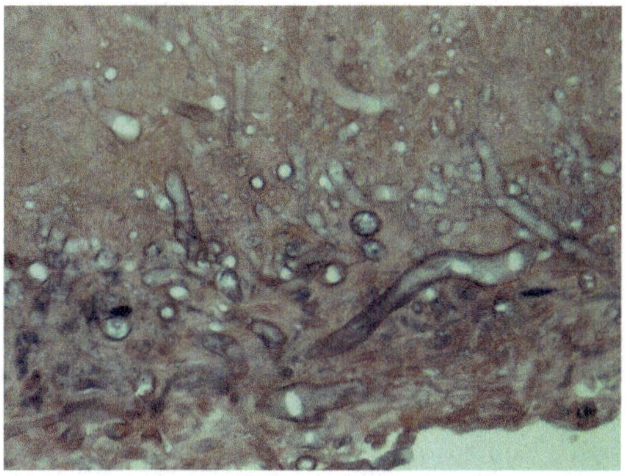

Fig. 14.4 Skin lesion by Zygomycetes of genus *Absidia*. H-E × 320

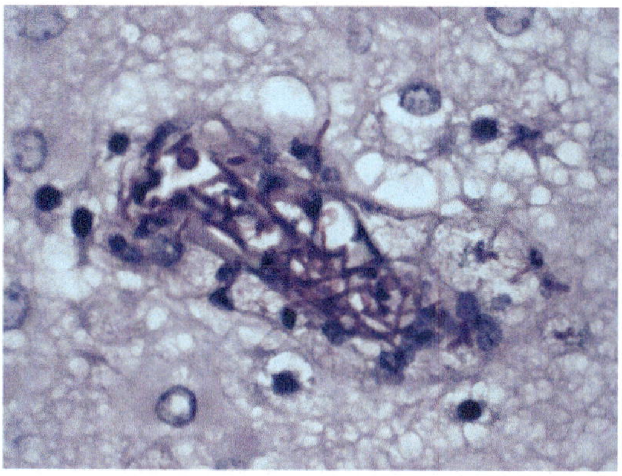

Fig. 14.5 Brain vessel lesion due to *Candida*. Note yeast-like forms and pseudomycelia, PAS reaction ×600

14.1.3 Candidiasis

Fungi of the genus Candida, primarily C. albicans, are the most common pathogens of mycosis in our condition. They are characterized in our condition at present primarily by the defeat of the mucous membranes of the esophagus, pharynx, and other parts of the digestive, as well as the urinary and reproductive systems. Much less often, it is possible to damage other organs, including the brain [1]. Such lesions are usually associated with sepsis or endocarditis, other variants of the onset of the disease are observed as casuistically rare. Nevertheless, there are descriptions of isolated cases with isolated brain lesions of fungi of the genus Candida. Clinically defined meningitis with a small predominantly lymphocytic pleocytosis. The basis for the diagnosis is the identification of the microorganism. The most characteristic variant of the lesion is microabscesses with the possible formation of microgranules. In the early stages, they can have the form of hemorrhagic heart attacks. In the future, such lesions take the form of abscesses and granulomas without central areas of necrosis. Perivascular lymphocytic couplings are characteristic. Yeast-like and pseudomycelial forms of the fungus are better detected by PAS reaction (Fig. 14.5) or silver impregnation. The cellular response may be represented by lymphocytes, single neutrophils, and giant cells, but may also be absent. Quite often, candidiasis of the central nervous system is a consequence of neurosurgical intervention. Candida spp. they are sown in children with hydrocephalus and operated with the imposition of a ventriculo-peritoneal shunt. Candidiasis of the central nervous system in children in the first year of life can be one of the manifestations of secondary nosocomial infection, which can be preceded by a variety of intrauterine, perinatal and iatrogenic lesions.

14.1.4 Cryptococcosis

Among the most important mycoses of the central nervous system is cryptococcosis. The causative agents are basidiomycete encapsulated yeast of the genus Cryptococcus of two species: Cryptococcus neoformans and C. gattii (synonyms: Cryptococcus hominis, Torula histolytica) [1, 4, 5]. C. neoformans includes three serotypes: C. neoformans var. grubii (serotype A), C. neoformans var. neoformans (serotype D) and hybrid (serotype AD). C. gattii includes serotypes B, B/C; also distinguish hybrids BD and AB). Capsule serotypes were determined by cross-reacting rabbit polyclonal antiserum. Rarely there are capsule-free isolates or capsules that cannot be serotyped. Cryptococcus is a common saprophyte of the skin and mucous membranes of some animals; cryptococcosis affects horses, cows, pigs, dogs, and cats.

In children, cryptococcal infection is much less common than in adults; however, serological studies indicate that by the age of two, most people are infected with cryptococcus; the frequency of subclinically occurring disease is unknown, as well as the localization of the pathogen in subclinically occurring infection. Some differences between variants of cryptococci are reflected in the literature. Thus, C. neoformans var. neoformans usually causes disease in immunodeficient patients, and var. gattii, on the contrary, causes infection in mainly immunocompetent individuals. C. neoformans var. neoformans is found everywhere in soil infected with birds (especially pigeons), and C. neoformans var. gattii is usually found in tropical and subtropical regions, often on eucalyptus trees.

The morphology of pseudohypha can vary from a chain of connected elongated yeast-like cells to hyphae-like structures bounded by partitions. These forms are rarely found in the host body and their biological significance is poorly understood. However, the so-called switching of the phenotype between yeast forms and pseudohyphs, which has been shown for some strains of C. neoformans, at the same time colonies other than smooth ones with yeast forms arise.

Cryptococcus is not a human commensal and its transmission from person to person is extremely rare, therefore it is believed that infection in humans is the final fatal event in the life cycle of the fungus.

Infectious particles are yeast forms (often acapsular) (≤4–5 microns in diameter), which strongly predominate among clinical and natural isolates; therefore, basidiospores are less likely as a source of infection. Yeast-like fungi not eliminated by the bronchial epithelium penetrate into the lumen of the alveoli, after which the onset of the disease is possible. Whether the disease and the dissemination of the pathogen into extrapulmonary foci will occur immediately or after the latent period depends both on the viability of the host's cellular defense and on the number and virulence of fungi. Primary lung infection is often asymptomatic; eradication of the pathogen or granuloma formation is possible.

From the lungs, C. neoformans can enter the bloodstream, where, as shown in in vitro experiments, polymorphonuclear leukocytes, monocytes and macrophages of monocytic origin kill yeast cells by intra- and extracellular mechanisms. In 10–20% of patients, hematogenic dissemination with lesions of the skin, prostate gland, organs of vision, bones, kidneys and other organs and systems is noted.

The spread of cryptococcus occurs, apparently, in a hematogenic way. Most often, the central nervous system is affected, then the lungs and other internal organs.

So far, the mechanism of overcoming the blood-brain barrier by T. C. neoformans has not been fully studied. Three BBB crossing paths for pathogenic microorganisms are described in the literature: 1 – transcellular; 2 – paracellular; 3 – Trojan Horse mechanism with the help of infected immune cells, such as macrophages (see Sect. 2.1).

It has also been shown that human fetal astrocytes activated by IL1ß and INFu in vitro inhibit the growth of cryptococci.

The probability of developing cryptococcosis is determined by the severity of immunodeficiency. The risk of developing cryptococcosis, as well as other opportunistic infections, increases significantly with CD4+ lymphocyte levels below 50–100 cells/ml of blood.

Laboratory diagnosis of cryptococcal infection does not present any particular difficulties in clinic today. In addition to indirect methods (lumbar puncture with general clinical and biochemical analysis of CSF, as well as determination of its pressure), the simplest, fastest and cheapest method is cytological examination of CSF, aspirates, secretions and other material.

The study of CSF reveals increased cytosis with a predominance of lymphocytes in HIV-negative patients. With HIV-associated meningitis, cytosis is lower, maybe even within the normal range. Protein is increased, glucose level is reduced.

For direct microscopy, smears are filled with 1–2 drops of carcass, against which encapsulated yeast cells are detected. The capsule does not miss the carcass particles and forms characteristic rims. The sensitivity of CSF microscopy with ink staining is 40–70%.

Cryptococcus neoformans is most often manifested by meningitis with a typical radiation pattern, complications in the form of hydrocephalus may develop. The formation of pseudocysts, manifested by the local expansion of Virchow-Robin spaces with a diameter of 3 mm or more, should be considered quite typical. Often the changes are two-sided. Usually the basal nuclei, the midbrain are affected, less often the rest of the brain is involved in the process. Mass effect and perifocal edema are absent. On CT images, the changes are isodensive, on MRI, they are isointensive to the cerebrospinal fluid. Pseudocysts do not respond to intravenous contrast.

With MRI, the picture varies depending on the structure of the focus (hypo- hyper-isointensive). Large cystic formations may have partitions. Typically nodular contrast enhancement. Mass effect, perifocal edema are possible, but not pronounced, significantly inferior in these parameters to the changes observed in toxoplasmosis. According to the MRC data on hydrogen, tuberculoma and cryptococcus have a similar MR spectrum of metabolites to toxoplasmosis, but the lactate peak is less pronounced.

The cells are usually spherical in shape, from 5 to 7 microns in diameter. The thickness of the capsule varies from a few micrometers to sizes equal to or greater than the size of cells, 50–60 microns. Cells of unusual sizes, from 2 to 15 microns, ellipsoid or capsule-free, can rarely be observed. A significant increase in the size of fungi was shown during infection. In tissue sections, when stained with hematoxylin–eosin, the causative agent of cryptococcosis is not clearly identified, it can deform during fixation. Encapsulated mushrooms are surrounded by a large empty space due to poor staining of capsule polysaccharides and deformation during the manufacture of slices. Detectable large-sized cryptococci (up to 14 microns) of bell-shaped, sickle-shaped and biconcave shape, without a capsule, are considered degenerating and dying.

We (together with A.M. Konstantinova) infection analyzed 20 observations of secondary cryptococcosis infection in HIV infection. Among the dead were 12 men (60%) and eight females (40%), average age was 36.3 years (20–51). Ten patient did not receive any antifungal or antiviral therapy; seven received antifungals (diflucan, amphotericin b, fungilab in one case); three received antiviral therapy, and antifungal drugs.

Among opportunistic infections, candidiasis of the mucous membranes was most common – 19 cases (95%), 11 cases (55%) were somewhat less common, cytomegalovirus infection and lesions caused by the herpes simplex virus – in 11 deceased (55%); tuberculosis was observed only in four cases (20%). In three of the deceased (15%), lesions caused by the Ebstein-Barr virus and brain lymphoma were detected, in two (10%), pneumocystosis and toxoplasmosis. In addition, nine of the deceased suffered from chronic viral hepatitis C; six – chronic viral hepatitis B; and in three cases, viral hepatitis was not deciphered.

At the time of diagnosis of cryptococcosis, the average level of CD 4+ lymphocytes was 51 cells per ml (from 4 to 138), and in 90% of the deceased their level was less than 100, in 10%—from 100 to 150.

The majority of patients had the following clinical manifestations: fever (85% of cases), positive meningeal signs (65%), coma (65%), severe headache (35%), focal neurological disorders (35%) and mental status disorders (35%),

The macroscopic picture in neurocriptococcosis is not very specific. The soft meninges involved in the process are edematous, thickened, dull, cloudy (Fig. 14.6). Focal changes in the brain were noted in isolated cases and looked like foci of a mushy yellowish consistency with loss of tissue structure, their sizes reached 1.5 cm.

The number of cryptococci in the meninges was different: abundant accumulations of pathogens were found in more than half of the cases; much less often pathogens were in moderate or minimal amounts. Massive accumulations of pathogens were found somewhat more often in the deceased who did not receive antifungal or antiviral therapy during their lifetime, and were accompanied by a minimal inflammatory reaction (Fig. 14.7), represented mainly by lymphocytes, less often by plasmocytes, histiocytes, often with an admixture of neutrophil leukocytes. Granulomatous type of inflammation was found with a much lower frequency (Fig. 14.8); pathogens were in moderate or small amounts. Multinucleated giant cells of the Langhans type or "foreign bodies" with phagocytic pathogens were noted in five cases: in four deceased who did not receive etiotropic therapy; and in one who only received antimycotics.

In the study of brain matter, focal encephalitis with microglial nodules and demyelination of white matter attracted attention; we associate these changes with HIV infection. In addition, contact necrotic cryptococcal encephalitis was often noted in the projection of the affected area of the meninges (Figs. 14.9, 14.10, 14.11). In the deeper parts of the brain substance, in almost all cases, pathogens were located mainly perivascularly, with the formation of peculiar "cryptococcal cysts" (Figs. 14.12 and 14.13), micromycetes in these zones in most cases were deformed, took different shapes: lemon-shaped, flattened, angular, etc., less often rounded. In four cases (20%), small "microcysts" were noted—zones of lysis of brain matter; deformed and rounded forms of cryptococci were found in them with the same frequency.

Certain information useful for analyzing the state of cryptocci and their structures can also semithin sections and electron microscopic examination (Fig. 14.14).

We conducted an experimental study with intravenous infection of mice with strains of cryptococcus of different virulence. The first, on the sixth day of the experiment, all mice infected with the highly virulent strain No. 1175 died. Mice infected with the other two strains did not die during the experiment and were sacrificed on day 7.

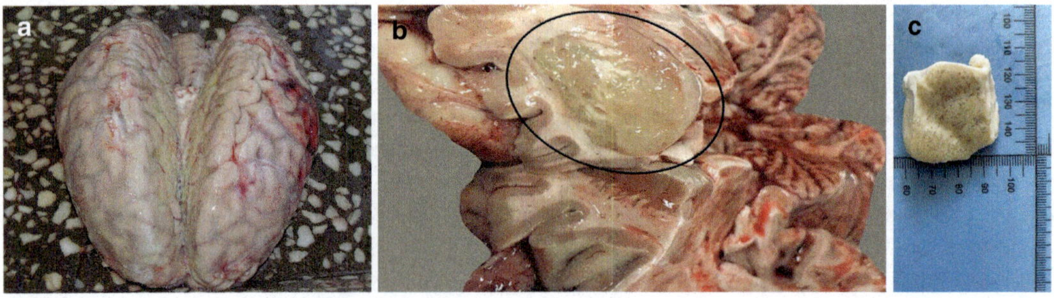

Fig. 14.6 Macroscopic changes in cryptococcal meningitis. Unfixed macropreparations. (**a**) General view; (**b**) The focus of cryptococcal brain damage (circled by a round frame); (**c**) Focal lesion with formation of small cyst-like lesions. (Courtesy of AN Isakov)

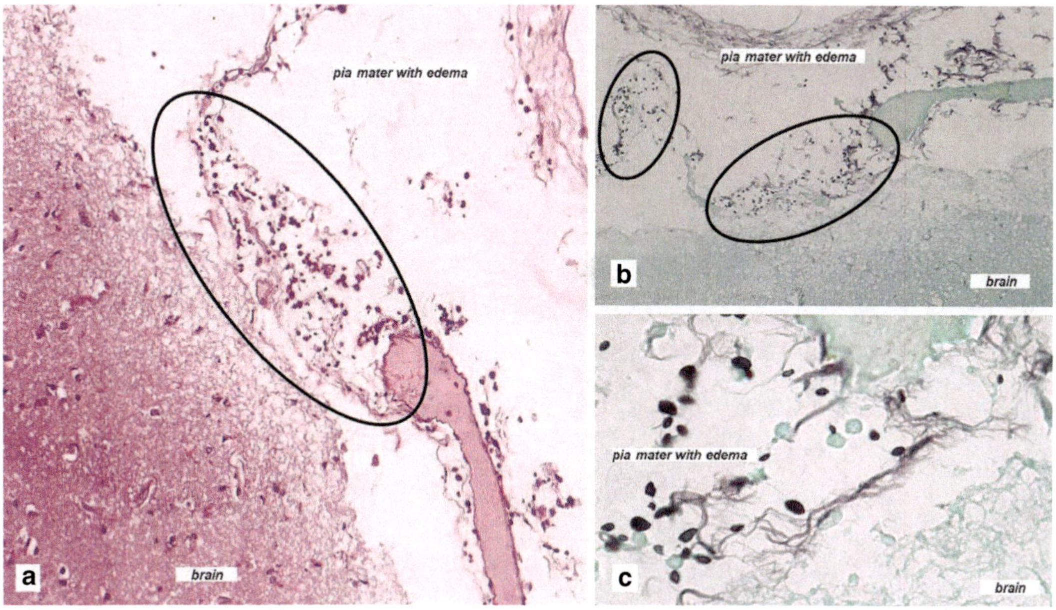

Fig. 14.7 Cryptococcal leptomeningitis (clusters of cryptococci are surrounded by oval frames). **a** – PAS-reaction. ×100; **b**, **c** – Grocott-Gomori impregnation. **b** – ×40; **c** – ×400

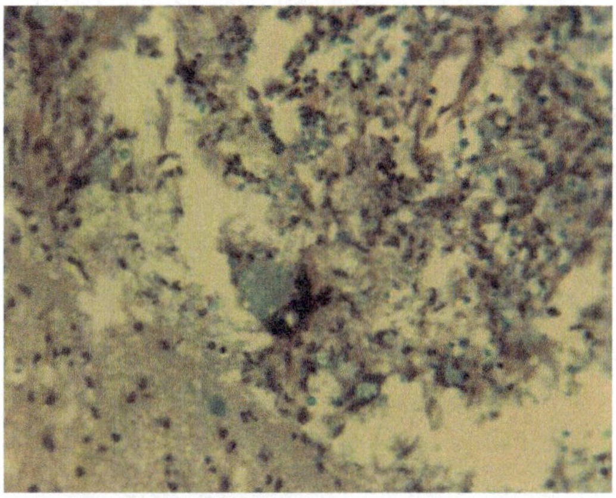

Fig. 14.8 Moderate inflammatory reaction in brain cryptococcosis. Note multinucleated cell. Stained by alcian blue+ PAS × 600

During histological examination of the internal organs of mice infected with strain No. 1175, on the third day after the start of the experiment, all five organs (lung, kidney, liver, spleen, brain) subjected to microscopy were affected. In mice infected with two other strains, only brain damage was noted during this period.

On the sixth day of the experiment, in mice infected with strain 1175, lesions caused by cryptococci were also found in all the organs studied.

Alterative changes in the form of the formation of peculiar foci of lysis were predominant in the histological picture in the brain, liver, kidneys and spleen of mice infected with various strains of C. neoformans (Fig. 14.15). In the zone of the greatest lysis, approximately equal proportions of cryptococci were rounded, encapsulated and deformed, devoid of capsules (lemon-shaped, flattened, etc.). In the zone of the least lysis, almost all micromycetes were deformed.

14.1.5 Generalized Mycoses with Brain Damage Caused by Other Fungi

Chromomycoses (chromoblastoses) are caused by various pigment fungi belonging to the genera *Cladosporidium*, *Hormodendrum*, and *Phialophora*. The skin is most often affected, especially the lower extremities, as well as the

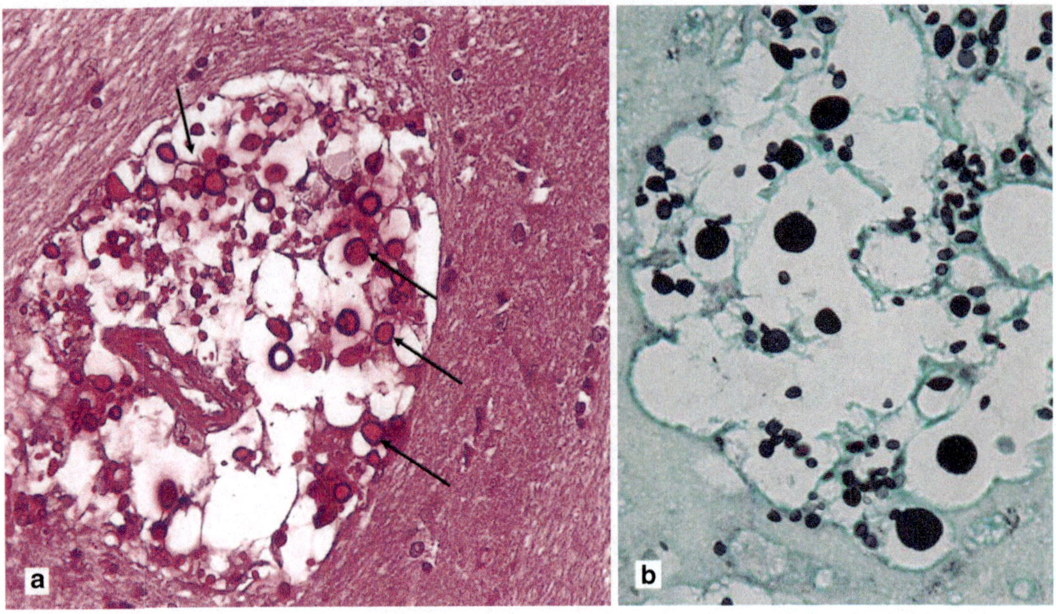

Fig. 14.9 Cryptococci in the substance of the brain. **a** – PAS-reaction. ×200; **b** – Grocott-Gomori impregnation. ×400

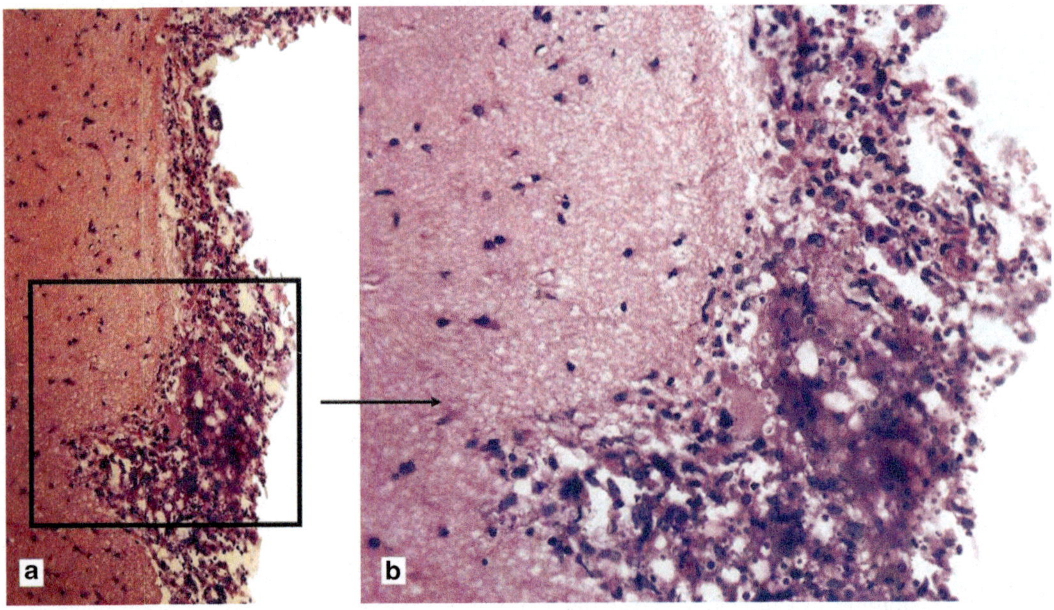

Fig. 14.10 Cryptococcal leptomeningitis. There is an abundance of cryptococci in the soft meninges. H-E. **a** – ×40; **b** – ×200

nasopharynx, lymph nodes, organs of the respiratory and digestive systems, and the brain. Most often, multiple small abscesses are formed in the substance of the brain with a minimal granulomatous reaction. Pigmented spores and hyphae are detected in the lesions [1].

Among the extremely rare variants of the lesion, mention should be made of allescheriosis

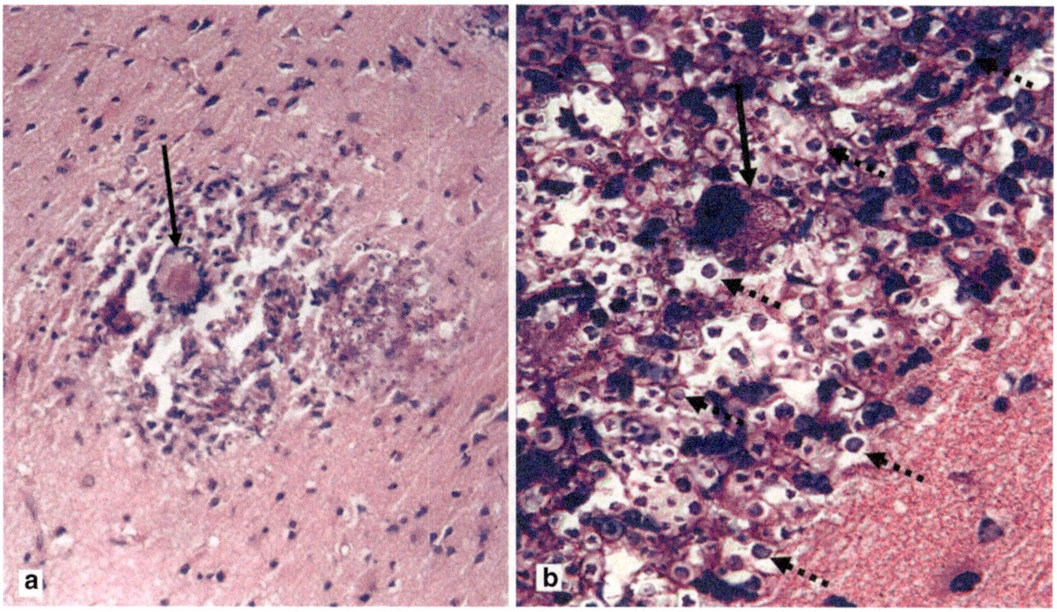

Fig. 14.11 Cryptococcal brain lesion. H-E; (**a**) A giant multinucleated cell of the Langhans type in the focus of a cryptococcal lesion (indicated by an arrow); (**b**) A giant multinucleated cell in the focus of a cryptococcal lesion (a giant cell is indicated by a solid arrow; individual cryptococci are indicated by dotted arrows). **a** – ×100; **b** – ×400

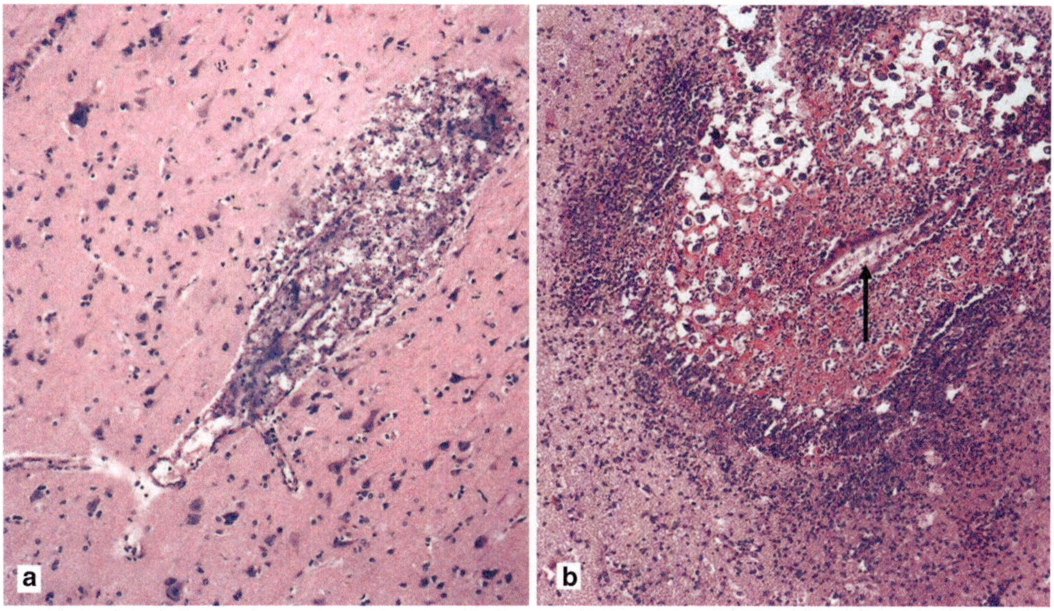

Fig. 14.12 (**a**) Cryptococcal vasculitis. The wall of the blood vessel is thickened, there is an abundance of cryptococci in the wall; (**b**) A perivascular focus of cryptococcosis (the vessel is indicated by an arrow). H-E. **a** – ×100; **b** – ×200

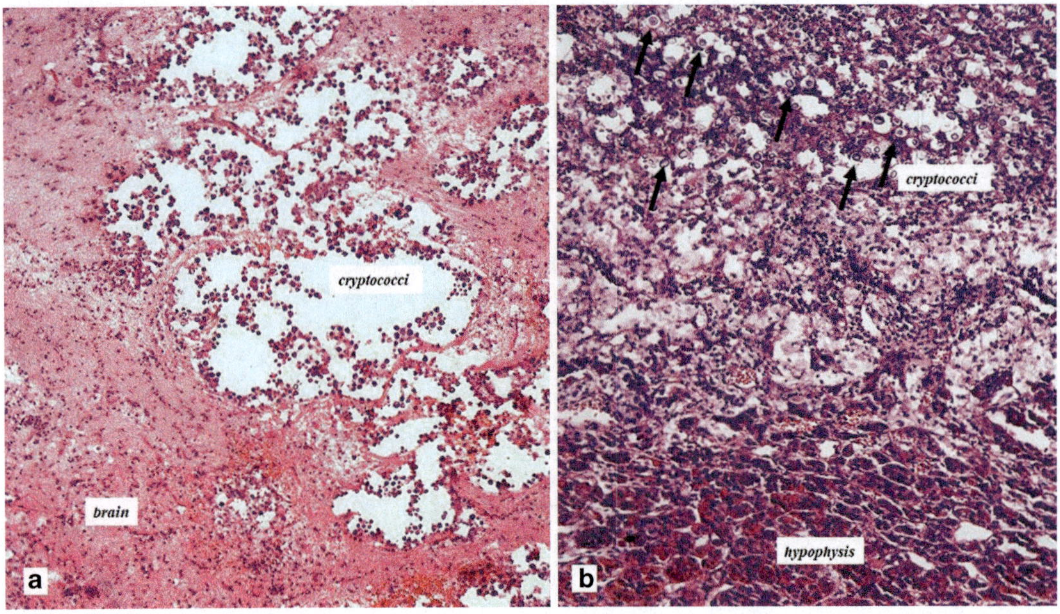

Fig. 14.13 (**a**) Brain cryptococcosis. Pituitary cryptococcal lesion (some of the cryptococci are indicated by arrows). H-E. **a** – ×100; **b** – ×200

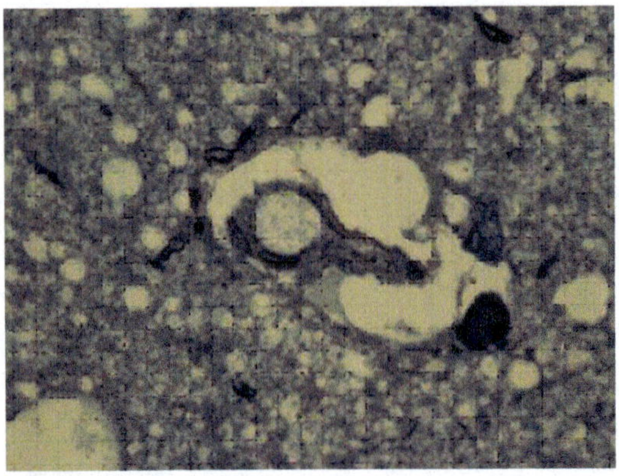

Fig. 14.14 Budding of cryptococcus in brain tissue. EM × 200

caused by *Allescheria boydii*. The pathogen belongs to the class Ascomycetes and is widespread everywhere as a soil saprophyte. The fungus penetrates the body through the skin and can cause damage to the respiratory system and central nervous system. In the brain, hemorrhagic infarcts are described, which can transform into abscesses that require surgical intervention. The pathogen is determined in the form of septic hyphae and chlamydospores. There are descriptions of rare brain lesions in individuals suffering from immunodeficiency fungi from the genus *Trichophyton*, usually causing onychomycosis. In extremely rare cases, the formation of granulomas in the brain substance is also described in some endemic mycoses of group 2 pathogenicity—coccidiomycosis, histoplasmosis, and North American blastomycosis. In the conditions of Russia, these diseases are currently not found.

14.2 Brain Lesions Caused by Protozoa

CNS infections caused by protozoa have become a serious problem in Europe and the North America. This is due to the processes of globalization, the development of business, mass tourism, in countries with a tropical climate. The influx of large numbers of migrants from countries where protozoal infections are widespread may also be a source of these diseases. The use of immunosuppressants is also important, which leads to the formation of immunodeficiency states and an increase in the possibility of developing an infectious disease in such patients.

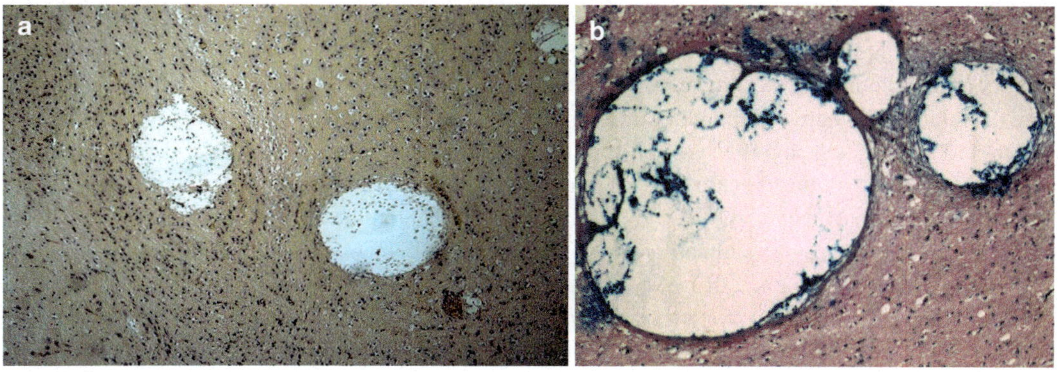

Fig. 14.15 Brain lesions in experimental cryptococcal infection in mice. Note numerous fungi in cysts. **a** – H-E × 100; **b** – Alcian blue ×200

14.2.1 Malaria

Malaria continues to be the most important parasitic infection in many regions of the world, mainly in hot climates, while it can be observed sporadically almost everywhere. In most cases, three-day malaria is reported. As the causative agents of malaria, four types of Plasmodium are described, but the most severe forms of human diseases are caused by Plasmodium falciparum. Among the most severe and life-threatening manifestations (complications) of malaria are certain brain lesions, often referred to as "cerebral malaria." There is evidence that up to 0.5 million children die from it every year in Africa alone. This form is also quite common in some countries of Asia and South America. The most up-to-date and complete data on cerebral malaria are given in the review by G. Turner [6].

Clinical manifestations are represented by diffuse, potentially reversible encephalopathy, associated with disorders of consciousness of various degrees. The patient can very quickly fall into unconsciousness and stop responding to pain, visual and verbal stimuli. Hemiplegia and lesions of the cranial nerves develop rarely. There are descriptions of isolated observations with cerebellar symptoms. The presence of symptoms such as opisthotonus and muscle rigidity is associated with an unfavorable prognosis. A characteristic clinical feature is the possibility of rapid reversibility of clinical symptoms. A child can wake up from a deep coma within an hour. Seizures in cerebral malaria are frequent and are associated with a poor prognosis. Cerebral malaria usually has a poor outcome, the mortality rate, even with active treatment and good care, reaches 30–50% [7].

The literature presents different opinions about the frequency of neurological complications in catamnesis. Initially, it was thought that they were extremely rare, but later careful observation of patients allowed to establish that at least 10% of convalescents have various complications, ranging from weakness and hearing impairment to tetraplegia, epilepsy and cortical blindness. In addition, children with convalescents of cerebral malaria may have difficulties in school education. Pathologic changes in cerebral malaria are highly variable, which probably depends on differences in the duration of the disease, treatment, and concomitant pathology of patients who died from malaria. It is impossible to exclude differences in the properties of Plasmodium in different geographical zones. The most characteristic feature of cerebral malaria is sequestration. Red blood cells infected with late maturing stages of plasmodium development (trophozoites/ring stage and schizonts) leave the free circulation. Red blood cells containing parasites are mainly located in the microcirculation vessels of vital organs (brain, lungs, gastrointestinal tract, heart), which in modern foreign literature is usually referred to as sequestration. Previously, it was believed that sequestration is determined only at the level of capillaries, but now it is shown that it can be observed in the venules of the brain. Quantitative clinical and morphological comparisons allowed us to confirm the relationship between the sequestration of infected red blood cells and the severity of clinical manifestations of the disease. At the same time, red blood cell sequestration can also be observed in the absence of a clinical picture of a brain coma. There is evidence that sequestration is more pronounced in the white matter compared to the gray matter and in the cerebellum compared to the hemispheres. Very characteristic of malaria are also hemorrhages, which can be of two types: point and ring-shaped. Pinpoint or petechial hemorrhages represented by ordinary red blood cells surrounding vessels with damaged walls are typical of cerebral malaria and are considered as an important diagnostic feature in macroscopic examination. Most often, such hemorrhages are detected in the white matter and topographically coincide with the most pronounced sequestration. Similar changes can be detected in many internal organs. It should be noted, however, that such hemorrhages are not strictly specific for malaria and can also be observed in severe asphyxia of various origins, barotrauma, or carbon monoxide poisoning. Ring-shaped hemorrhages are pathognomonic for malaria. Such lesions consist of a series of concentric rings surrounding a necrotic vessel located in the center. The outer ring is represented by a mixture of infected red blood cells and monocytes, some containing pigment. In the inner layer—uninfected red blood cells and gliocytes surrounding the vessel. It can be assumed that the mechanism of formation of such a hemorrhage is associated with "reperfusion" followed by rupture of the vessel, which was initially thrombosed with infected red blood cells. Such lesions are described in all parts of the brain, but not in other organs. Occasionally, they are described in the absence of a clinical picture of a brain coma. Another characteristic feature of brain damage in malaria is the so-called Durk's granulomas, first described in 1914. Marguelis, but the most fully characterized is Dürck. He described multiple rounded clusters of glial cells associated with damaged vessels and necrotic areas in the areas of hemorrhage, which were considered as a protective inflammatory process. At present, the exact mechanism of the formation of such granulomas is not established, a number of speculative assumptions have been made, among which the most likely is the point of view that Durk's granulomas are a consequence of annular hemorrhage. It is obvious that endothelial cells play a key role in the interactions between plasmodium and brain matter. Very characteristic of cerebral malaria are their changes in the form of degeneration, hyperplasia, and necrosis, most often in those areas where hemorrhage and granulomas are observed. The reasons for such changes can be very diverse and are not precisely studied. Modern IHC and EMR, included in model experiments on monkeys, confirm the activation of endothelial cells in cerebral malaria. In addition to these changes in cerebral malaria, areas of ischemic necrosis of nerve cells and perivascular edema are also described. Given the reversibility of coma, there is no reason to attach significant importance to these ischemic changes in the pathogenesis of brain damage in the cerebral form of malaria. Brain edema used to be considered as the leading cause of death in the cerebral form of malaria, but now the results of in vivo instrumental studies force us to assign it a much more modest role. For those who died from a malarial coma and survived it, deposits of malarial pigment (hemomelanin) are characteristic, which can be phagocytized by circulating monocytes and neutrophils, endothelial cells and naturally determined in the soft meninges and choroidal plexuses. It can be assumed that the amount of pigment correlates with the previous parasitic load. There is evidence that phagocytic pigments can have both toxic and stimulating effects on monocytes. It should be noted that the earliest and most complete pathological information about malaria was described in our country by M. V. Voino-Yasenetsky [8].

For many decades, experimental models of cerebral malaria have been developed in the world [9]. Most often, rats and mice, as well as monkeys, are used as experimental animals. In these studies, it was possible to confirm the importance of sequestration, cytokine release and the state of the host immune system in the pathogenesis of malaria. The model on monkeys is closer to the human disease but does not allow us to assess the effect of "switching off" certain genes on the course of the disease. There is abundant evidence that host molecules support the adhesion of infected red blood cells in organs affected by malaria.

A large number of studies have also been devoted to the study of hereditary factors determining human sensitivity to malarial plasmodia. Information about the increased resistance of erythrocytes in sickle cell anemia and thalassemia has been known for a long time. In recent years, the importance of the TNFa gene promoter region for sensitivity to cerebral malaria has been shown.

Currently, there are two alternative theories of the pathogenesis of cerebral malaria, according to the first, the main importance is attached to the local sequestration of plasmodium, and the second focuses on the "toxic phenomenon" caused by the mass release of parasites or the release of cytokines and mediators of the host, primarily TNFa and nitric oxide. It is possible that there is a combination of both mechanisms. A detailed study of these issues remains a matter of the future. Currently, there are indications of some mechanisms of adhesion of infected erythrocytes to endothelial cells. Thus, the role of thrombospondin (a glycoprotein of the trimeric extracellular matrix secreted by endothelial cells and involved in cell-matrix and matrix-matrix interactions), CD36 (glycoprotein expressed on the surface of platelets, monocytes and endothelial cells), ICAM-1 (an adhesive molecule from the Ig superfamily), E-selectin, VCAM-1, Chondroitin sulfate A. The study of ligands on the surface of plasmodium has also begun. The significance of pfEMP-1 molecules associated with the var. gene family determined on the surface of Plasmodium falciparum ligand-receptor interaction has been proved.

We studied several observations; studied macro- and microscopic changes were typical and corresponded to the above descriptions (Figs. 14.16, 14.17, 14.18, 14.19, 14.20, 14.21).

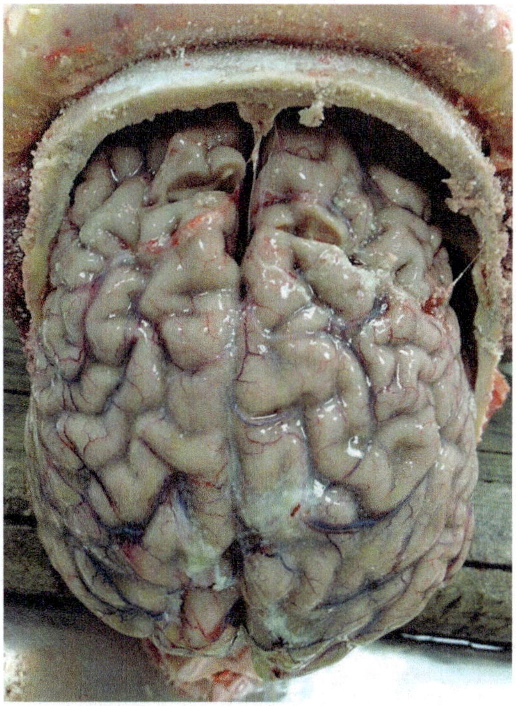

Fig. 14.16 Brain lesion in malaria. Unfixed macropreparation. (Courtesy of AN Isakov)

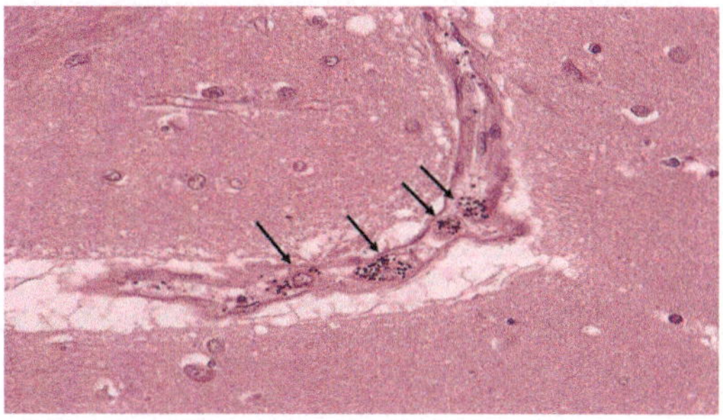

Fig. 14.17 Brain in malaria. There are multiple schizonts in the lumen of the blood vessel of the brain. H-E × 400

Cerebral coma was mainly associated with progressive hepatic insufficiency and, to a lesser extent, damage to the cerebral vessels by plasmodia, since their number in them was insignificant. Myocarditis and hepatic steatosis, probably associated with chronic alcoholism, had a certain significance in the genesis of death.

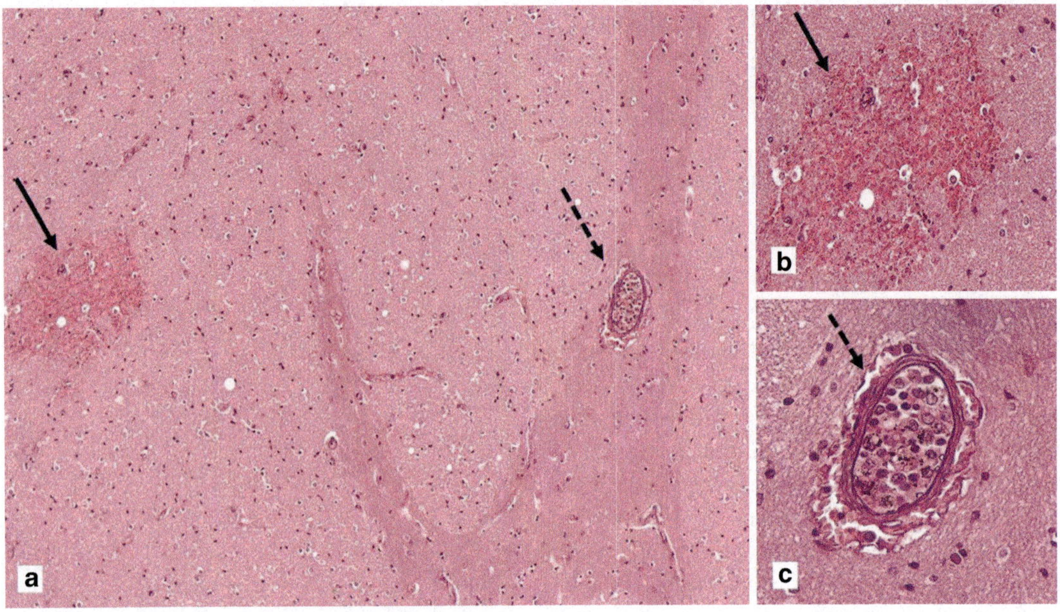

Fig. 14.18 Brain lesion in malaria. (**a**) Micro-hemorrhage in the brain substance (indicated by a solid arrow), schizonts in the lumen of the blood vessel (the vessel is indicated by an intermittent arrow), diapedesis of erythrocytes; (**b**, **c**) Fragments of Fig. "**a**." H-E. **a** – ×40; **b**, **c** – ×200

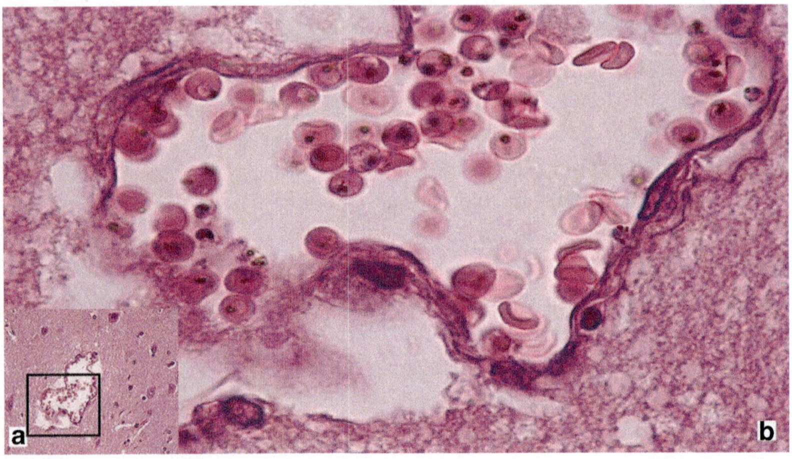

Fig. 14.19 Brain lesion in malaria. A blood vessel in the substance of the brain, red blood cells with schizonts in the lumen of the vessel. In Fig. "**b**" is a fragment of the Fig. "**a**" indicated by the frame. H-E. **a** – ×40; **b** – ×1000

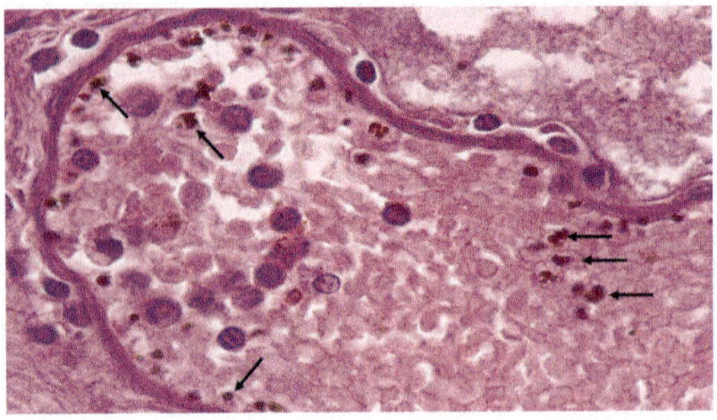

Fig. 14.20 Brain lesion in malaria. There are schizonts and pigment in the lumen of the vessel (indicated by arrows). H-E. ×1000

14.2.2 Brain Damage Caused by Toxoplasma

Toxoplasmosis is a zoonotic disease caused by intracellularly parasitizing protozoan Toxoplasma gondii and characterized mainly by an asymptomatic course, taking manifest forms in persons with reduced immunity [10]. Toxoplasma is an obligate intracellular parasite of humans and a wide range of animals. The final host of toxoplasmas is a domestic cat and other animals of this family, man

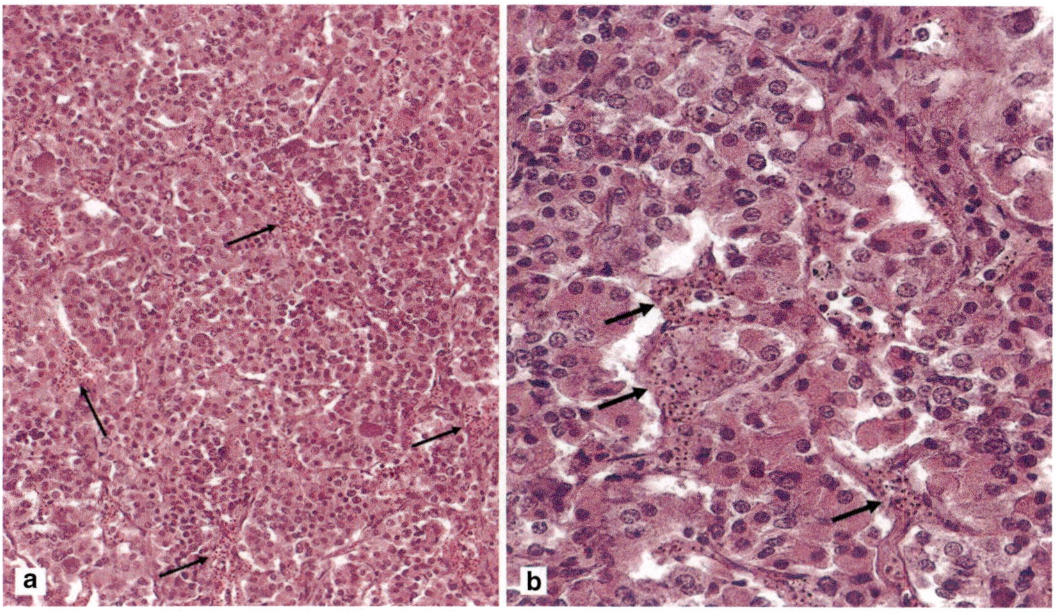

Fig. 14.21 Brain lesion in malaria. Parasitic stasis in the pituitary gland (indicated by arrows). Stained with hematoxylin and eosin. **a** – ×100; **b** – ×400

is an intermediate host, along with some mammals and birds. Toxoplasmas parasitizing in the intestinal cells of a cat are released with feces into the external environment, then invasive pathogen cysts mature, which can persist for several years in the external environment. Oocysts are formed as a result of sexual reproduction of the parasite in the cells of the intestinal mucosa, then after maturation in the environment and penetration into the human intestine, sporozoites are released. The latter are introduced into the intestinal tissues, and then into the mesenteric lymph nodes, where the pathogen multiplies with the development of mesadenitis. As a result of hematogenic dissemination, parasites are fixed in the internal organs and form cysts that persist for decades.

With the preserved immune status, the formation of specific antibodies occurs, which causes an asymptomatic course of the infectious process, prevents new infection. With the development of immunosuppression, there is a gradual release of toxoplasmas from cysts and their hematogenic spread. Thus, with HIV infection, toxoplasmosis develops with predominant damage to the brain, although generalized forms with damage to the liver, lungs, kidneys, and muscles are also found.

Human infection occurs in two main ways: (1) when swallowing oocysts present in the feces of cats; (2) when eating insufficiently heat-treated meat, eggs, milk of animals that are intermediate hosts for toxoplasmosis (more often beef). These products contain endozoites (trophozoites, the so-called tachyzoites) in pseudocysts and cysts of cystozoites (bradyzoites) of the parasite. With a chronic or latent course of the disease, the pathogen exists in the body of an intermediate host (human) in the form of cysts in which the pathogen persists in the form of bradyzoites. Infection of a person can take place in a transplacental way, and an asymptomatic course of the disease in the mother is possible. Brain lesions in intrauterine toxoplasma encephalitis are presented in Chap. 16.

On autopsy, in many parts of the brain, asymmetrically located areas of necrosis of various shapes are found, varying in number and size, resembling ischemic infarcts (foci of a porridge-like brownish-grayish color), in some cases with a reaction of hyperemia or hemorrhages along the periphery (Figs. 14.22 and 14.23).

Histological examination of the brain substance reveals necrotic foci with a macrophage reaction along the periphery (macrophages phagocytize parasites and necrotized brain

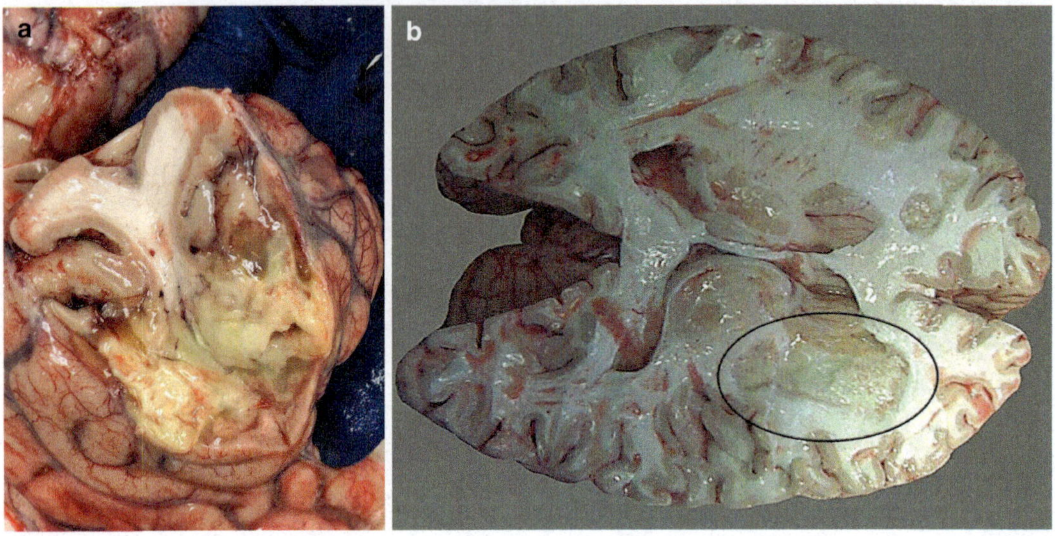

Fig. 14.22 Toxoplasmosis of the brain. Unfixed macropreparations. (**a**) General view (courtesy of AN Isakov); (**b**) An area of necrosis in the brain resembling an ischemic infarction (circled by an oval frame)

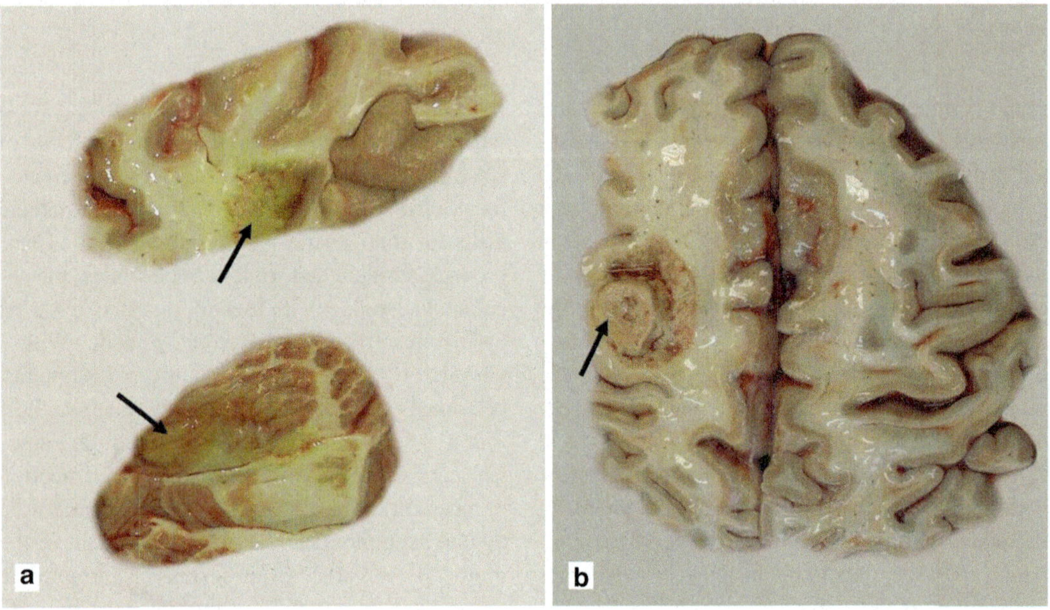

Fig. 14.23 Toxoplasmosis of the brain. (**a**) Areas of necrosis in various parts of the brain; (**b**) A site of necrosis in the brain resembling an ischemic infarction. Areas of necrosis are indicated by arrows. Not fixed macropreparations

tissue) (Fig. 14.24). Moderate exudative phenomena with leukocyte infiltration, erythrocyte stasis in the vessels with subsequent thrombosis and the development of secondary aseptic colliquation necrosis are noted perifocally. On the periphery of the foci of necrosis around the vessels, a lymphoid-histiocytic coupling reaction is noted. Reproduction of the parasite in the human body is best detected in nerve cells, which can accumulate up to 10–20 toxoplasmas and are called pseudocysts (Fig. 14.25). Rounded formations covered with a shell, which is formed by

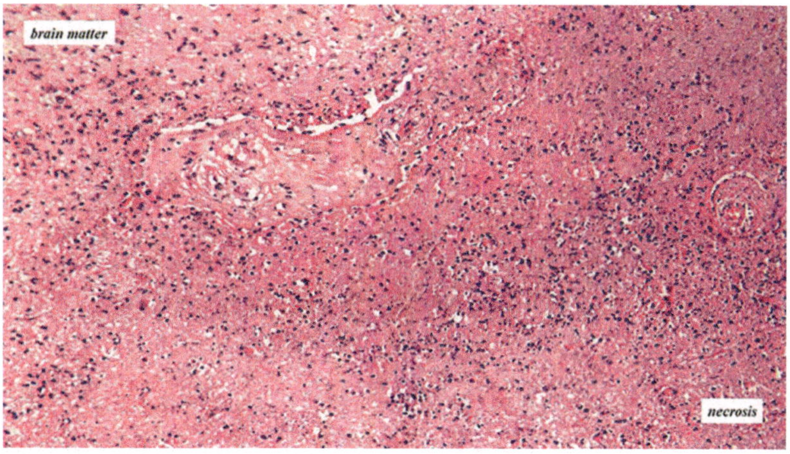

Fig. 14.24 Toxoplasmosis of the brain. The focus of necrosis, perifocally in the substance of the brain edema. H-E × 100

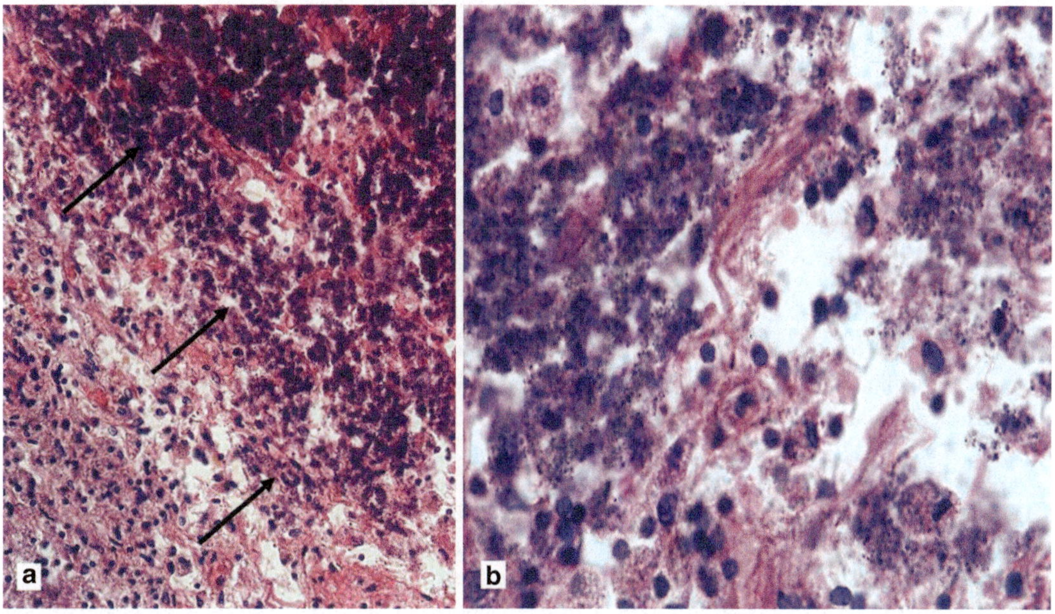

Fig. 14.25 Toxoplasmosis of the brain. (**a**) Toxoplasmic pseudocysts along the edge of necrosis (indicated by arrows); (**b**) Toxoplasmic pseudocysts (fragment of Fig. "**a**") loaded with toxoplasmas (small rounded basophilic inclusions. H-E. **a** – ×100; **b** – ×400

the pathogen itself, and containing several hundred parasites are true cysts (Fig. 14.26a). Toxoplasmas can also be freely located in the substance of the brain.

It is recommended to carry out microscopic diagnostics of smears of biological fluids (blood, cerebrospinal fluid), smears-prints of brain foci with the staining of cytological preparations according to Romanovsky. Toxoplasmas (trophozoites) have the shape of a crescent or an orange slice 4–7 × 1,5-2 microns.

In paraffin tissue sections, pathogens are usually rounded or oval, stained red with PAS staining (Fig. 14.26b). Toxoplasmas can be detected in tissues using immunofluorescence microscopy, when treated with luminescent serum, a specific glow of the toxoplasma antigen is visualized in a slice. Immunohistochemical examination of

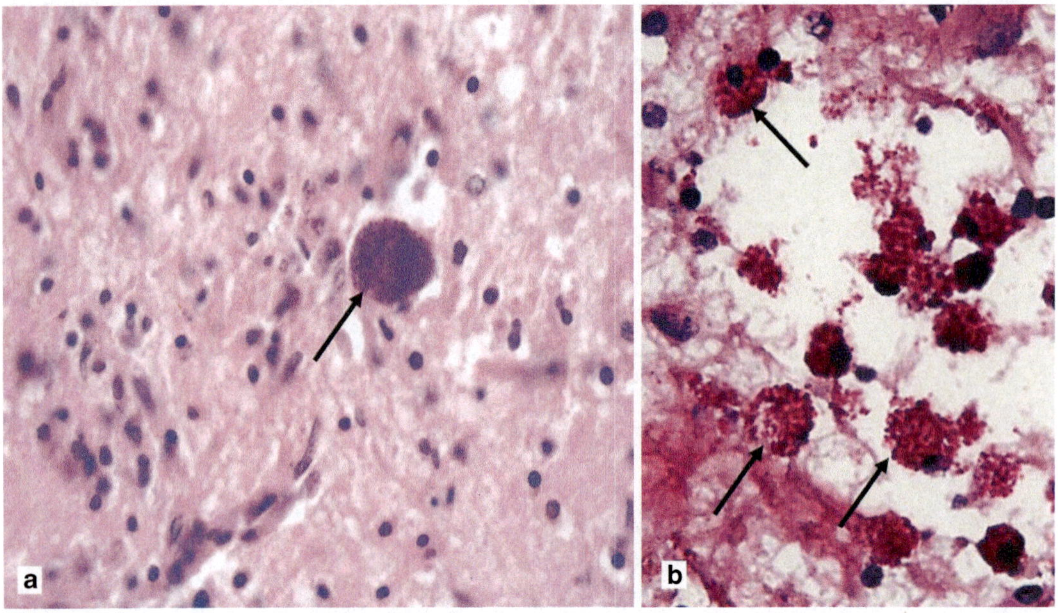

Fig. 14.26 Toxoplasmosis of the brain. Toxoplasma cysts (indicated by arrows). (**a**) H-E (toxoplasmas are colored purple); (**b**) PAS-reaction (toxoplasmas are colored crimson-red). ×1000

paraffin sections of an organ with polyclonal antibodies of Toxoplasma gondii also makes it possible to identify an infectious agent (Fig. 14.27). PCR-examination of native fragments of the brain, cerebrospinal fluid at the molecular level confirms the presence of the pathogen.

14.2.3 Brain Damage Caused by Amoeba

The most well-known and widespread form of amoebiasis in countries with hot climates is amoebic dysentery caused by Entamoeba histolytica. Against the background of severe ulcerative lesions of the large intestine, hematogenic dissemination of trophozoites-erythrophages with the development of foci in the liver, lungs, brain and other organs is possible [11]. Macroscopically, they resemble abscesses, microscopically represent foci of necrosis in the area of accumulation of the pathogen, surrounded by mixed cellular filtration with a significant number of eosinophils. "Abscesses" of the brain are relatively rare and they are usually secondary to lung damage.

Relatively rarely, mainly in immunocompromised individuals, lesions are observed caused by so-called free-living amoebas that have a trophicity to the central nervous system. Among them, Naegleria fowleri causes primary diffuse meningoencephalitis, and Acanthamoeba and Balamuthia mandrillaris cause granulomatous amoebic encephalitis. Isolated cases of this disease have been described in almost all countries of the world. Pathogens will enter the human body through the skin and mucous membranes when bathing in open reservoirs or in contact with the soil. Hematogenic entry of the pathogen into the brain is assumed. The most characteristic is the formation of granulomas with necrosis, mainly lympho-macrophage infiltration involving giant cells. Trophozoites and amoeba cysts are determined mainly perivascularly.

14.3 Brain Damage Caused by Helminths

Brain lesions, including tumor-like ones, can also be caused by some helminths [11]. Although the lesions caused by these pathogens are rare in

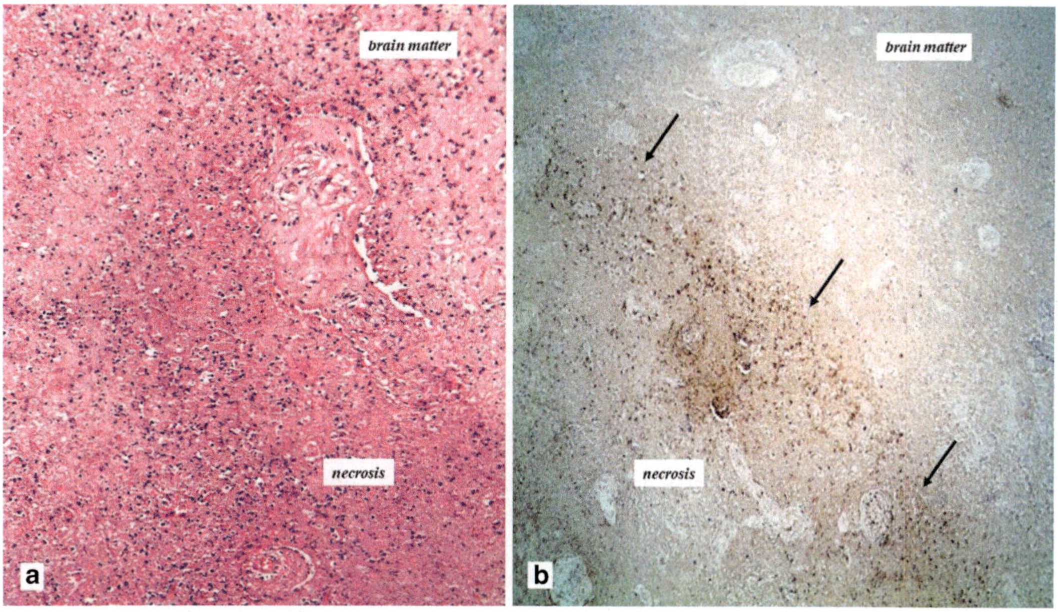

Fig. 14.27 Toxoplasmosis of the brain. The edge of the necrotic focus. Immunohistochemical examination revealed pseudocysts and macrophages with toxoplasmas, colored brown (indicated by arrows). (**a**) Staining with hematoxylin and eosin; (**b**) Immunohistochemical reaction with polyclonal antibodies of Toxoplasma Gondii. ×100

our country, but the population migration that has sharply increased in recent years makes it quite likely that tropical diseases that were not previously observed in our conditions will appear. We present data on the most fully studied helminthiasis, which is characterized by focal lesions of the brain.

Angiostrongylus cantonensis is a pathogen related to roundworms (Nematoda). The most common causes of diseases in Southeast Asia and Oceania, in particular in countries such as China (including Taiwan), India, Japan, Thailand, Vietnam, Sri Lanka, Reunion, Comoros, Fiji, the Philippines, Indonesia, Papua New Guinea, Samoa, as well as Egypt, Ivory Coast, Cuba. The final hosts are many species of rats, the intermediate hosts are gastropods, especially slugs and snails. Animals such as shrimps, crabs, planarians, cichlids, toads, and frogs may be intermediate hosts. Humans, primates, mice, and other mammals are random dead-end hosts. Human infection usually occurs when eating raw or insufficiently heat-treated snails, shrimps, crabs, frogs, and some endemic fish. In addition, infection can occur through unwashed vegetables, contaminated shellfish, and larval-infected drinking water. The incubation period for humans usually lasts from 12 to 28 days. Prodromal symptoms are usually reduced to vomiting with possible subsequent dehydration. Children are the most susceptible. When entering the blood-brain barrier, the development of eosinophilic meningitis or myelomeningoencephalitis is most characteristic. In the human brain, helminths can stay for a long time, causing severe damage and then dying. It is possible to damage other organs, in particular the eyes and lungs. Macroscopically, such lesions are characterized by thickening of the soft meninges on the basal surface and in the region of the cerebellum, subdural or subarachnoid hemorrhages involving adjacent areas of the cortex. On the sections of the brain, you can see focal necrosis and hemorrhage, corresponding to the movement of the helminth. Microscopically, living or dead helminths are found in the soft meninges, and sometimes in the blood vessels and perivascular spaces. Cellular responses to live worms are usually minimal but are expressed around the degenerating ones. Possible granulomatous, including giant cell reaction. Characteristic micro-cavities are "traces" of the movement of the helminth with cellular detritus. Eosinophilic infiltration is characteristic.

Among the long-known helminthiasis with brain damage is **cysticercosis**. It is caused by the plerocercoid of the widespread tapeworm Taenia solium cysticercus. Adults of this species live in the small intestine and have a length of 2–7 m. The ingress of eggs of this helminth into the intestine leads to the release of oncospheres, which penetrate through the mucous membrane, and then lymph - and hematogenically enter various organs, including the brain, where they form cysticerci. Cysticerci are milky-white, spherical or oval cysts that, when fully developed, reach 1 cm in diameter. Each cyst contains fluid and an invaginated protoscolex (Fig. 14.28). The protoscolex has four large spherical suckers and a proboscis with a double row of 22–36 large and small hooks. These structures can be detected in preparations stained with hematoxylin-eosin and are birefringent. The wall of the bladder consists of the shell, muscle cells, shell cells, and parenchyma. Most often, such lesions are detected in the brain, eyes, subcutaneously, as well as the heart, lungs, liver, kidneys, mammary gland, soft tissues, tongue, and skeletal muscles. Cerebral cysticercosis usually gives clinical symptoms and can be fatal. The nature and severity of the symptoms depends on the size, number, and location of the parasites. According to the localization, it is customary to distinguish between meningeal, ventricular, parenchymal (almost always with the involvement of gray matter) and mixed forms. Viable cysticerci practically do not cause an inflammatory reaction. Pronounced lympho-monocytic infiltration is formed with the dead pathogens. The substance of the brain also usually forms a thin fibrous capsule and a glial shaft.

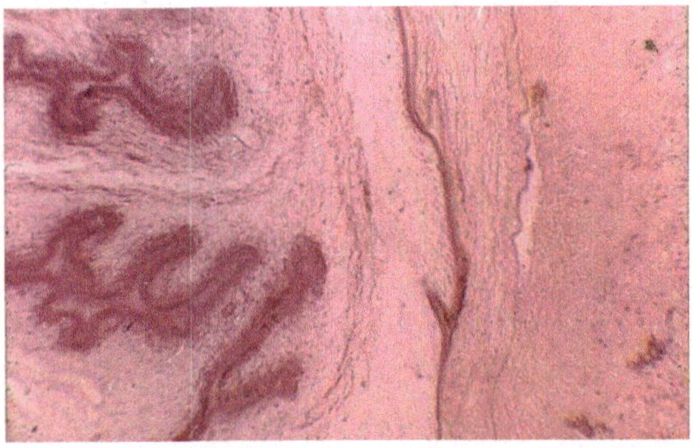

Fig. 14.28 Brain lesion in cysticercosis. H-E × 50

Cenurosis is a disease caused by a cenur cysticercus formed by Taenia multiceps or T. serial. The disease is more common in children in Africa, although isolated cases have been reported in sheep breeding areas in Europe, South America, the United States, and Canada. The final hosts of these helminths are carnivores from the canine family. The intermediate hosts are most often herbivores, primarily sheep and rabbits, but they can also be antelopes, chamois, cows, goats, horses, wild rodents, and yaks. Humans, especially young children, can become accidental intermediate hosts when eggs are ingested from the feces of the final host. In the intestine, eggs ripen release oncospheres, which actively penetrate the intestinal wall, and then into the bloodstream. Oncospheres are transformed into cenures in the brain, eyes, skeletal muscles, and subcutaneous tissue, which takes about 3 months. Brain damage is usually associated with T. multiceps. In the brain, cenures are usually localized in the subarachnoid space, causing basal arachnoiditis or ependymitis. The response to the parasite in the brain is often minimal and limited to a thin rim of fibrous tissue. The censors will easily get rid of the brain tissue when cutting a piece of tissue. Patients with a chronic form of the disease develop fibrosis of the soft meninges with a giant cell reaction around the cyst wall. After the death of the cenura, a pronounced inflammatory reaction develops with the infiltration of the larva mainly by eosinophils. On the background of degenerative changes in the cenura, the development of necrosis and a chronic inflammatory reaction, represented by lymphocytes, macrophages, and giant cells, is characteristic. Often there is perivascular inflammation and occasionally tissue eosinophilia. In the outcome, fibrosis and calcification are possible.

References

1. Góralska K, Blaszkowwska J, Dziekowiec M. Neuroinfections caused by fungi. Infection. 2018;46(4):443–59. https://doi.org/10.1007/s15010-018-1152-2.
2. Latgé JP, Chamilos G. Aspergillus fumigatus and Aspergillosis in 2019. Clin Microbiol Rev. 2019;33(1):e 00140-18. https://doi.org/10.1128/CMR.00140-18.
3. Bhandari J, Thada PK, Nagalli S. Rhinocerebral mucormycosis. In: StatPearls [internet]. TreasureIsland, FL: StatPeasrls Publishing; 2021.
4. Klock C, Cerski M, Goldani LZ. Histopathological aspects of neurocryptococcosis in HIV–infected patients: autopsy report of 45 patients int. J Surg Pathol. 2009;17(6):444–8.
5. Zinserling VA Konstantinova AM, Vassiljeva NV. Cryptococcal infection in springer encyclopedia of pathology, infectious disease and parasites/ Ed. P. Hoffman: 2016 82–86.
6. Turner G. Cerebral malaria. Brain Pathol. 1997;7(1):569–82. https://doi.org/10.1111/j1750-3639.1997.tb01075.x.
7. Varo R, Chaccour C, Bassat Q. Update on malaria Med. Clin (Barc). 2020;155(9):395–402. https://doi.org/10.1016/j.medcli.2020.05.010.
8. Voino-Yasenetski MV. Pathological anatomy of malaria. Arkh Patol. 1987;49(9):3–9. (in Russian)
9. Pasini EM, Zeeman AM, Voorberg-van der Wel A, Kocken CHM. Plasmodium knowlesi: a relevant, versatile experimental malaria model. Parasitology. 2018;145(1):56–70. https://doi.org/10.1017/S0031182016002286.
10. Lourido S. Toxoplasma gondii. Trends Parasitol. 2019;35(11):944–5. https://doi.org/10.1016/j.pt.2019.07.001.
11. Schmutzhard E. Parasitic diseases of the central nervous system. Nervenarzt. 2010;81(2):162–71.

15 Prion Neuroinfections

A separate essential problem is prion neuroinfections. Prions are proteins (PrP) encoded by the host and play a certain role for the secretory pathway. Prion protein gene is located on human chromosome 20 and encodes a protein of 253 amino acids; its possible polymorphism has been demonstrated. Recently, the concept of protein aggregation diseases, primarily neurodegenerative has appeared [1]. Prion is a non-nucleic, low-molecular-weight PrP^{C} cell protein that, upon conformation, becomes a pathogenic PrP^{Sc}. In principle, both exo- and endogenous formation of pathogenic prions is possible. The accumulation of pathogenic prions precedes the development of structural changes. PrP^{Sc} polymerizes into amyloid fibrils, which can lead to the formation of amyloid prion-containing plaques. After the accumulation of pathogenic prions, polymerization and formation of amyloid, it is deposited in the nervous tissue, causing activation of neuronal apoptosis; spongiose degeneration and damage to neurons are noted, mainly in the basal ganglia, cerebellum. Prion diseases are distinguished from other neurodegenerative diseases because they possess proven infectivity, have equivalents in animals, and they show a wide variety of phenotypes in humans and animals. We have to take into account that they may be also sporadic and have genetic origin. This group usually includes primarily transmissible spongiose encephalopathies caused by prions: kuru, Creutzfeldt-Jakob disease, Gerstmann-Sträussler-Scheinker disease affecting humans; scrapie, affecting sheep and transmissible encephalopathy of minks, "chronic debilitating disease" (deer and elk), spongiform encephalopathy of cattle, spongiform encephalopathy of cats, spongiform encephalopathy of exotic ungulates (African eland, oryx, kudu). In spite their modest practical role, they have been intensively studied; for modern reviews see [2, 3]. The main pathogenic feature seems to be transformation of cellular PrP^{C} into PrP^{Sc} playing leading role in development of scrapie – the best studied disease. Although the mechanisms underlying prion propagation and infectivity are now well established, many issues related to their toxicity and pathogenesis of diseases remain at least partly unclear. It was proved that in development and propagation of the diseases nearby deposition of abnormally folded protease-resistant PrP^{Sc} astrogliosis, microgliosis, and neurodegeneration are essential. Microglia are beneficial during prion diseases and critical to host defense against them. Reduction of microglia population accelerates disease and increases PrP^{Sc} burden in the CNS. Neurons and astrocytes are involved in prion replication and spread. Certain astrocytes, such as A1 reactive, might influence the progression of prion-associated neurodegeneration.

Similar clinicopathological changes can be due to slow neuroinfections caused by typical or atypical viruses: subacute sclerosing panenceph-

V. Zinserling, *Infectious Lesions of the Central Nervous System*,
https://doi.org/10.1007/978-3-030-96260-9_15

alitis and subacute post-measles leukoencephalitis – associated with the measles virus (see Sect. 7.4); progressive congenital rubella and progressive rubella panencephalitis (see Sects. 16.2 and 7.7); subacute and chronic herpetic encephalitis (see Chap. 5); subacute adenovirus encephalitis (see Sect. 7.2); progressive multifocal leukoencephalopathy associated with papova viruses JC, OB40; subacute brain lesions in CMV infection; epilepsy in tick-borne encephalitis (see Sect. 6.3); lymphocytic choriomeningitis caused by a virus from the arenavirus group; rabies (Sect. 6.5); brain damage in HIV infection (see Sect. 8.1). It is notable that HIV encephalopathy is characterized by spongioform transformation of white matter comparable in prion diseases. In animals, generally recognized slow viral neuroinfections include: visna, infectious anemia of horses, Born's disease, Aleutian mink disease, lymphocytic choriomeningitis of mice, rabies of dogs, African swine fever, slow-moving influenza infection in mice.

For the first time, diseases of this group caused by prions were isolated by the Icelandic researcher B. Sigurdson in 1954. The authors formulated their main characteristic features: a long incubation period (from several months to several years), a steady increase in clinical symptoms leading to death or severe disability, damage to one organ, and the presence of one host. Subsequently, thousands of studies were devoted to the diseases of this group in all countries of the world, detailing their etiology, clinic, and pathogenesis. It became obvious that humanity was faced with a fundamentally new class of infectious diseases caused by new pathogens prions. Transmission of the pathogen from one person to another has not been established. The fundamental work of S. B. Prusiner was awarded the Nobel Prize in 1997.

The morphological picture of slow neuroinfections is characterized by a significant variety. In viral cases, dystrophic changes in neurons with their subsequent loss, a widespread glial proliferative reaction, demyelination of fibers, and sometimes inflammatory changes are detected. Slow NI caused by prions is characterized by spongiform encephalopathy (pronounced vacuolization of dendrites, axons, and neuronal bodies), hypertrophy, and proliferation of astroglia, dystrophy, and loss of neurons. Signs of an exudative reaction are completely absent. In scrapie, kuru, and Creutzfeldt-Jakob disease, amyloid plaques are observed, although in different percentages of cases. Structural changes can vary significantly depending on the dose and nature of the pathogen, the state of the host, etc. Often, it is impossible to make an accurate etiological diagnosis based on morphological data. In some cases, the exact criteria for the diagnosis of "encephalitis" can be difficult to establish. From our point of view, the absence of perivascular inflammatory infiltration should not exclude the presence of a chronic infectious lesion of the central nervous system. From the point of view of diagnostics, in each case, it is necessary to use laboratory methods of research (molecular biological, serological, immunofluorescence, etc.).

Kuru refers to the exotic diseases of the central nervous system, first described by D. C. Gajdusek, V. Zigas in one of the aboriginal tribes of New Guinea with traditional cannibalism. D. C. Gajdusek received the Nobel Prize in 1976 for his outstanding achievements in the study of this disease. The clinical picture of kuru is characterized by cerebellar ataxia, tremor, turning into complete immobility. The earliest morphological sign of CNS lesions is hypertrophy and proliferation of astrocytes. The leading feature is the vacuolation of neurons and their processes, leading to a spongy transformation. The most up-to-date data on the pathological anatomy and pathogenesis of Kuru disease, based on the revision of archival materials, are given in the article by J. A. Hainfellner et al. [4], coauthors of which are also D. C. Gajdusek and one of the largest modern neurologists, H. Budka. The localization of prion protein (PrP) in the brain tissue of a deceased adolescent was studied using IHC. PrP was found in various parts of the brain, comparable to lesions in Creutzfeldt-Jakob disease, although its deposits were much more pronounced and fundamentally corresponded to spongiform changes and/or astrogliosis.

Scrapie, a lethal infection of sheep, known in the eighteenth century, occurs with a variety of symptoms, indicating the defeat of the central nervous system. In 1898, neuronal vacuolization was discovered in the brain of sheep suffering from scrapie. In recent decades, it has been established that the causative agent of scrapie is also prions. Sheep suffering from scrapie and mastitis secrete prions in milk and infect about 90% of suckling lambs [5]. The link between scrapie and bovine spongiform encephalopathy ("mad cow disease") has been traced, which has led to great difficulties in agriculture in a number of European countries in recent years. The nature of the structural changes detected in these diseases is generally close to those briefly described in kuru. The fact of fundamental similarity of structural changes in all prion diseases is generally recognized in the literature. Vacuolization followed by neuronal death and reactive astrocytosis in the absence of inflammatory changes are described. In the study of various morphological materials (autopsy observations of Creutzfeldt-Jakob disease, spontaneous scrapie in sheep and goats, experimental kurus, Creutzfeldt-Jakob disease, mink and scrapie encephalopathy) was shown that the vacuolation of neurons begins and develops intensively in the distal parts of the dendrites, the death of neurons can occur both by the type of cytolysis and pyknosis. According to their data, there is a reactive proliferation of all types of glia, including ependymar glia. In addition, there was an accumulation of microgliocytes, blood macrophages, pericytes, and lymphocytes both with diffuse infiltration of brain tissue and around degeneratively altered neurons. At the same time, the absence of an inflammatory reaction is noted.

In humans, the most common transmissible spongiose encephalopathy is Creutzfeldt-Jakob disease (CJD), described in 1920–1921. It is believed that it is characterized by features of anamnesis (dura mater transplantation, brain cell transplantation, eating prion-infected beef), a long incubation period that can last even decades, the development of extrapyramidal, pyramidal disorders in combination with severe cognitive disorders up to severe dementia, steady progression in most cases with a fatal outcome. There is evidence that more than 150 individuals in the UK have died from CJD acquired by eating meat infected with cow prions [6]. Currently, the nature of this disease, which is the most common representative of human diseases caused by unusual agent—prions, has been established. Currently, the classification of Creutzfeldt-Jakob disease is extremely complicated. It is customary to distinguish four forms: sporadic, iatrogenic (infectious), hereditary (with 15 genotypes) and "new," associated with bovine spongiform encephalopathy. The sporadic form is more common, but it is also a rare disease. The family form is inherited autosomally dominant, and mutations in the gene that encode the prion protein have been identified. The iatrogenic form is regarded as one of the greatest catastrophes in the history of medicine, as several hundred cases of CJD were associated with tissue transplantation (cornea, dura mater) or the appointment of pituitary hormones taken from individuals suffering from unrecognized spongiose encephalopathies. In recent times, the frequency of CJD decreased dramatically due to unclear causes.

References

1. Kretzschmar H, Tatzeit J. Prion disease: a tale of folds and strains. Brain Pathol. 2013;23:321–32. https://doi.org/10.1111/bpa.12045.
2. Carrol JA, Chesebro B. Neuroinflammation, microglia, and cell-association during prion diseases. Viruses. 2019;11:65.
3. Le NTT, Wu B, Harris DA. Prion neurotoxicity. Brain Pathol. 2019;29:263–77. https://doi.org/10.1111/bpa.12694.
4. Hainfellner JA, Liberski PP, Guiroy DC, Cervénaková L, Brown P, Gajdusek DC, Budka H. Pathology and immunocytochemistry of a kuru brain. Brain Pathol. 1997;7(1):547–53. https://doi.org/10.1111/j.1750-3639.1997.tb01072.x.
5. Ligios C, Cancedda MG, Carta A, et al. Sheep with scrapie and mastitis transmit infectious prions through the milk. J Virol. 2011;85(2):1136–9.
6. Goldberg AL. On prions, proteasomes, and mad cows disease. N Engl J Med. 2007;357(11):1150–2.

Brain Lesions in Perinatal Infections

16

The importance of special consideration of perinatal infectious brain lesions is related both to their high frequency (they are natural for all severe intrauterine infections) and their significance not only in the development of life-threatening conditions in the neonatal period, but also at a much older age. In addition, in many respects, the insufficiently studied specificity of the structural and functional features of the immature brain leads to significant differences in the clinical manifestations of infectious lesions compared to older children and adults, which significantly complicates their diagnosis [1, 2]. The morphological features of such lesions are not well known, the systematization of data on this issue was carried out seldom. This served as a basis for summarizing and analyzing the results of our long-term (1976–2021) research on this issue in comparison with the data of modern literature.

16.1 Morphological and Functional Features of the Brain of the Embryo and Fetus at Different Stages of Gestation

It is obvious that the features of the course of various pathological processes in the central nervous system, including infectious ones, in the embryo, fetus, and newborn, are largely determined by both structural and functional characteristics of the brain and spinal cord at certain stages of ontogenesis. Unfortunately, if the stages of morphological maturation of the brain are studied in some detail, then the data on the formation of its protective mechanisms are almost completely absent in the literature. In this regard, we give a brief summary of modern ideas about the stages of brain maturation. The most complete information in this regard is provided by J. C. Larroche et al. [3]. In the development of the central nervous system, it is customary to distinguish four periods: neurulation (3–4 weeks), the formation of brain bladders (4–7 weeks), corticogenesis (8–16 weeks), and maturation (starting from 16 weeks). Neurulation begins on the 18th day of intrauterine development (Carnegie stage 8) and is characterized by the transformation of the neuroectodermal plate into the neural tube. This rather complex multistage and insufficiently studied process was uploaded on day 26 (stage 12 according to Carnegie).

In the second period, during the 13–19 stages, the neural tube forms three brain bladders in its cranial part: prosencephalon, mesencephalon, and rhombencephalon. Soon the first of them is divided into the telencephalon (in turn, forming two lateral bladders the precursors of the cerebral hemispheres) and the diencephalon.

In the third period, the already formed structures increase in volume, and the corpus callosum appears. The most important events are the

V. Zinserling, *Infectious Lesions of the Central Nervous System*,
https://doi.org/10.1007/978-3-030-96260-9_16

appearance of the cortical plate, the formation of synapses, the biochemical maturation, and differentiation of glial cells.

In the fourth period, there are regular changes in the size, mass, configuration of the surface, stratification of the cortex, increased vascularization, and proliferation of glia. Myelination begins, which goes in the caudocephalic direction.

A number of guidelines provide standards for brain mass in different periods of gestation. It should be noted that there is a fairly significant spread of data (even in "healthy" fetuses) starting from the 32nd week of pregnancy. With formalin fixation, the brain mass increases by an average of 15–20%. There are no sexual differences.

The maximum growth rate is reached at the age of 35 weeks, then it slows down. The external configuration of the brain does not change significantly until 20 weeks. The hemispheres remain smooth without a pronounced pattern. The first furrow begins to appear at 14 weeks – the Sylvian. The first convolutions (Roland's and temporal) are formed at the age of 20 weeks. The corpus callosum begins to form from 12 weeks and from 18 weeks. Its anterior parts begin to be visualized by sonography. The hippocampal gyrus appears at 12–13 weeks, and since that time, it has acquired its characteristic form. Lateral ventricles up to 24 weeks. They are in a state of physiological hydrocephalus, while the occipital horn remains dilated up to 32–34 weeks. Vascular plexuses appear from 6 weeks in the roof of the rhomboid brain by duplicating the vascularized soft meninges and neuroepithelium. Primary vascular plexuses in the area of the lateral and third ventricles appear at 7 and 8 weeks, accordingly. They grow rapidly, differentiate, and almost completely fill the lateral ventricles by 11 weeks. In the first stage, their neuroepithelium is pseudo-multi-layer, then becomes cylindrical or cubic, surrounded by a richly vascularized loose mesenchyme. During this period, the stroma is quite often detected by ultrasound cysts, which disappear by the 24th day. The cerebral water supply and, to a lesser extent, the central canal of the spinal cord are also relatively dilated during this period (up to 24 weeks). The most complex differentiation processes occur in the cerebral cortex. In the period of 7–8 weeks the formation of layers of nerve cells begins. Approximately at this time, the differentiation of glial cells begins. Thus, astrocytes acquire the S100-protein antigen by week 8 and begin to contain GFAP (marking mature cells) from week 14, including in the immediate vicinity of the cerebral ventricles. Oligodendroglial cells begin to differentiate in the brain stem area from 17 weeks. During this period, the number of capillaries in the brain tissue is relatively small, and it is assumed that the supply of growing neurons with energy is mainly due to the glycogen-rich processes of glial cells.

After the beginning of the formation of the cortex in the brain, five layers can be identified. (1) The outer edge mesh layer (in future, the molecular or 1 layer), in which numerous terminals of growing axons and numerous synapses will be defined. (2) The cortical plate, consisting of immature bipolar neurons forming radial rays running parallel to the glial fibrils, undergoes gradual structural differentiation with the formation of dendrites and axons. (3) The subcortical layer, with respect to which there is the maximum number of unresolved issues, is represented by a loose mesh tissue with few neurons. Numerous synapses are also detected here, gamma aminobutyric acid and cholecystokinin are detected in excess, and fibronectin-like extracellular matrix molecules are richly represented. This layer is functionally evaluated as a transient "waiting" layer, but its true role remains unclear. The thickness of the subcortical layer grows faster than the cortex, but later in the fetal period, most of its neurons die. However, even at birth, individual neurons can be detected in the subcortical white matter. (4) The intermediate zone in the future, the white substance. (5) The periventricular zone or matrix contains a large number of cells with high mitotic activity. The arrangement of the cells in the form of columns is preserved. In the future, there is a thickening of the cortex, accompanied by an increase in the surface area of the hemispheres, which is associated with both an increase in the bodies of neurons and the formation of their dendrites and an increase in the number of spines and synapses of the latter, the development of axons, the growth of afferent fibers, the multiplication of glial cells and capillaries.

Starting from 16–18 weeks, a characteristic horizontal stratification of the cortex begins to be traced, which already allows us to obtain a cytoarchitectonic map. The most characteristic areas in the fetus of the second half of gestation are the motor and visual cortex. During the first weeks of pregnancy, most neurons leave the periventricular region to take their place in the cortex. Similarly, astrocytes migrate to the deep layers of the cortex and white matter. In this regard, normally the periventricular matrix layer loses its columnar structure and decreases quite quickly. Blast immature and glial cells can persist up to 32–33 weeks in three zones: the head of the caudate nucleus, in the area of the thalamostriatic fossa (groove), in the roof of the temporal horn, and in the outer wall of the occipital horn. These areas are usually referred to as the germinal matrix, in the area where hemorrhages are most often described in premature infants. Very little is also known about synaptogenesis in humans. The first axon-dendritic synapses were detected at 7 weeks by 10 weeks. Their number is already quite significant, especially in the area of the oldest cortex the hippocampus. Vascularization of the central nervous system begins in the medulla oblongata and spreads towards the terminal brain. Data on this issue is also quite scarce. Vascularization of the brain substance occurs by the formation of filopodia by capillaries of the soft meninges, which grow through the basement membrane and then form new capillaries in situ. Within a few weeks, the final formation of vascular and perivascular structures occurs. A primitive capillary consists of two to three endothelial cells and a pericyte that does not completely surround the capillary, temporarily lacking glial decoration. In the periventricular zone, endothelial cells are rich in endoplasmic reticulum, mitochondria, Golgi apparatus, vesicles, and various inclusions. Tight contacts are clearly identified. Occasionally, mitoses are detected. For about 12 weeks, the basal membrane becomes electron-dense and the glial processes surround the entire surface of the capillaries. From 8 to 16 weeks, there is a penetration of individual radial vessels into the terminal brain, the maximum number of them is determined in the periventricular zone. After 16 weeks, there is a significant increase in the vessels in the cortical zone compared to the matrix, which probably reflects the comparative changes in their metabolism.

Myelination begins in the second half of pregnancy after a period of proliferation and migration of neurons and continues until adolescence. The first signs of myelination are detected in the spinal cord in the fasciculus cuneatus at 24 weeks, fasciculus gracilis at 26 weeks. Myelination progresses quite quickly in the head direction and reaches the thalamus by 34 weeks. The fibers responsible for pain, temperature, and light sensitivity are myelinated later. Myelination of the ventral roots occurs earlier (22 weeks) than the dorsal root. In the brain stem, myelination of the statoacoustic system begins at 24 weeks, and it is progressing fast. Myelination of the corticospinal tracts of the bridge were determined from 36 weeks. In the cortex of the large hemispheres, the fibers of the extrapyramidal system are primarily myelinated (for 30 weeks). From 36 weeks myelination of the thalamocortical fibers occurs in the direction of the somatosensory gyrus. The optical system begins to be myelinated from 30 weeks. In the area of the optic chiasm, this process ends shortly after 36 weeks. Myelination of the fibers of the auditory analyzer and the corpus callosum occurs after birth.

The development of the cerebellum originates from the pterygoid plate of the posterior cerebral bladder and is also quite complex. Histologically, four stages of the formation of the cerebellum are determined. Stage of two layers (3–7 weeks): the outer molecular layer and the periventricular matrix are presented, between which the intermediate zone is located. Its outer part becomes more cellular and forms an inner granular layer. Stage of three layers (from 8 to 10 weeks): Cells migrating from the periventricular zone form a transient outer granular layer, where they divide. For 28 weeks, it consists of six to nine cells with neuronal differentiation and is thicker than the molecular layer. As a result of further migration, the cells of the outer layer together with the neurons migrating from the matrix zone form the inner granular layer. During the same period, the dentate nucleus and Purkinje cells are formed. Stage 5 layers (from 20 to 30–32 weeks). Beneath the molecular layer are cells separated from the inner granular layer by a distinct lamina dissecans structure consisting of dense plexuses of cellular processes. During this period, Purkinje cells become more visible on the surface of the inner granular layer. Stage 4 layers (from 32 to 40 weeks): lamina dissecans disappears, which is an important reference point for determining the gestational age. Thus, the cortex consists of an outer granular layer, a molecular layer, Purkinje cells, and an inner granular layer. There is a gradual thickening of the molecular layer and thinning of the outer granular layer. In a child aged 10–12 months, the histological structure of the cerebellum acquires an adult type: a wide molecular layer, Purkinje cells, and a granular layer. Unfortunately, it must be stated that the vast majority of researchers of embryonic and fetal brain development are not familiar with intrauterine infections, except for syphilis, toxoplasmosis, and rubella, and do not explain the criteria for selecting a "normal brain" in the material of abortion, artificial and spontaneous miscarriages.

16.2 Brain Damage in the Most Common Intrauterine Infections

A significant frequency of various intrauterine infections with a wide range of clinical and morphological changes is now generally recognized, summarized also by the author [4]. Lesions of the nervous system are naturally noted in any etiology of the process and all variants of infection. This is primarily due to the intensive metabolic processes in the brain and its priority blood supply in the embryo and fetus, as well as its immaturity, including the structure of the BBB and protective mechanisms. Due to a number of objective and subjective reasons, the etiology of intrauterine encephalitis often remains unknown. At the same time, focal perivascular, productive and productive necrotic inflammation is usually described, including the formation of granulomas and frequent involvement of the soft meninges in the process. A significant decrease in the vascular density of the paraventricular zone is considered characteristic. The problem of intrauterine brain lesions has another important aspect. In premature infants, intraventricular hemorrhages (IVH) are often noted. Most often, their causes are called anatomical and morphological features of the vascular bed of the periventricular region of the brain, as well as violations of the autoregulation of cerebral blood flow with changes in vascular pressure. In the pathogenesis of the development of IVH, the most significant are the effects of hypoxia and ischemia of the periventricular zone of various origins. We believe that in many studies insufficient importance is attached to infectious factors, taking into account that, when targeted, infectious complications and factors that contribute to infection during pregnancy and childbirth are observed in the vast majority of premature newborns who die from IVH. In addition, there are serious reasons to believe that part of the IVH may be associated with defects in the resuscitation aid.

In this book, we consider only those diseases that are most common in our practice, and described in sufficient detail.

16.2.1 Rubella

The causative agent of this disease is a virus of the genus *Rubivirus* from the family *Togaviridae*. The rubella virus has a diameter of about 70 nm, contains RNA, lipids in the shell, is sensitive to the action of chemical agents, persists for a long time at low temperatures, and is pathogenic for monkeys and small laboratory animals. The important role of rubella as an intrauterine infection is indicated in all numerous guidelines on perinatal infections [5]. For congenital rubella, Gregg's "classic triad"—cataracts, heart defects, and deafness was previously considered characteristic. Later on, it was found that other developmental abnormalities, including CNS lesions, are

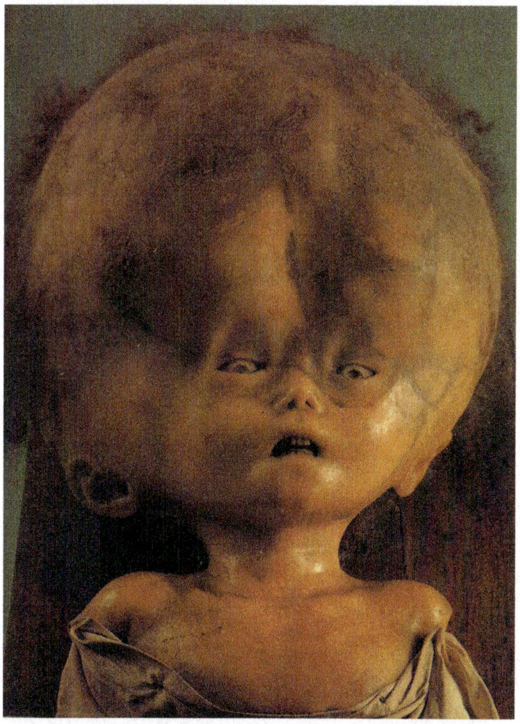

Fig. 16.1 Hydrocephaly. Wax macropreparation. Courtesy of G Nesi

often observed. In the first months of a child's life, lesions of the nervous system are manifested by changes in behavior—children are extremely sleepy or, on the contrary, sharply restless; then hyperkinesis, paralysis or paresis, and a pronounced decrease in intelligence to varying degrees are added. Very often observed in congenital rubella, deafness can be combined with vestibular dysfunction. Possible development of micro- and hydrocephalus is shown in Fig. 16.1. The pathogenesis of congenital rubella has not been definitively established. When a pregnant woman is infected from day 2, she develops viremia, which lasts 10–11 days. Then the virus enters the placenta, affects the endothelium of its capillaries, and spreads through the body to the blood of the embryo or fetus, causing the development of a chronic infection. The most dangerous infection of a pregnant woman is in the early stages of embryogenesis. Lesions of the nervous system in congenital rubella may be caused by the development of chronic meningoencephalitis. Neurological disorders may also be based on

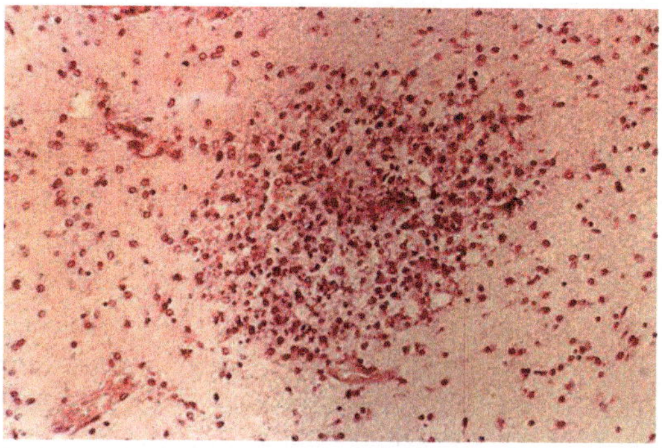

Fig. 16.2 Focal encephalitis in inborn rubella. H-E; ×100 Courtesy of TF Kogoi

chronic brain ischemia, which occurs as a result of vascular disorders. It is shown that long-term persistence of the virus is possible in rubella encephalitis. The possible role of rubella virus in the development of panencephalitis is discussed.

In intrauterine rubella productive necrotic encephalitis (Fig. 16.2), productive leptomeningitis, necrosis with the formation of cysts and calcifications, productive vasculitis, and small foci of glial proliferation mainly in the white matter was observed. Along with this, there was productive necrotic endoophthalmitis with retinal detachment, foci of necrosis, productive uveitis, homogenization of the lens fibers with the formation of cysts in it, desquamation and proliferation of the epithelium. Productive dermatitis with perivascular lymphohistiocytic infiltrates, hyperkeratosis, and hemorrhage in the dermis were detected in the skin. Interstitial productive pneumonia with giant cell metamorphosis of alveolocytes was present in the lungs. In some organs, focal lymphohistiocytic infiltrates were also detected, as well as focal hematopoiesis. We did not observe intrauterine rubella in the autopsy material of St. Petersburg in recent years.

16.2.2 Toxoplasmosis

Toxoplasma (*Toxoplasma gondii*) is an obligate intracellular parasite belonging to the tissue cyst-forming coccidia, a class of spores (see Sect. 14.2). The frequency of intrauterine toxoplasmosis, according to various authors, ranges from 1 to 6 cases per 1000 newborns. In the smears of their fluids, the toxoplasmas have a semilunar shape. Intracellularly, especially in paraffin sections of tissues, they are often rounded or oval, the size of a large coccus, and are best PAS-stained. The longitudinal intracellular division of toxoplasmas is best detected in nerve cells. The manifestations of toxoplasmosis in the early stages of development are generalized. At this time, small areas of necrosis occur in all affected organs in the location of toxoplasmas. Here, in the interstitial tissue, more common infiltrates are visible, consisting of lymphocytes, histiocytes, as well as plasmocytes, neutrophils, and eosinophilic leukocytes. The most often described is liver damage. It is an interstitial hepatitis with small areas of necrosis and pronounced periportal infiltration, followed later by fibrosis. Along with this, extra-medullary hematopoiesis was detected. The spleen is hyperplastic, and its moderate infiltration by eosinophilic leukocytes is possible. In the myocardium, respiratory organs, adrenal glands, and, less often, in other internal organs, small areas of necrosis and infiltration of the intervertebral tissue are noted. Typical exanthema has the character of a roseolous or macular papular rash. Similar focal changes occur in the brain and eyes. At this time, toxoplasmas are detected in the substance of the brain, both in nerve cells and extracellularly (Fig. 16.3). In the brain, dystrophic and then necrotic changes occur. The leukocyte exudative reaction is very weak. Macrophages phagocytize pathogens and decay products of necrotic brain tissue. In the blood vessels, there is stasis, swelling of the endothelium, proliferation of adventitia cells, and often thrombosis. As a result of vascular damage, secondary focal aseptic colliquation necrosis of the brain tissue occurs. The foci of necrosis are located in the brain asymmetrically, mainly in the cortex of the large hemispheres and in the subependymal zone of the lateral ventricles, both in gray and white matter. They can vary in size and number. With the greatest severity of the process, these foci merge into solid yellowish stripes running along the convolutions of the cerebral cortex. On the walls of the ventricles, ependymal defects may be detected. The vascular plexuses and cerebral ventricles are often thickened, whitish or yellowish in color. In the later stages of intrauterine toxoplasmosis, a few months or years after birth brain damage is sharply predominant.

The necrotic tissue resolves with the formation of cysts (Fig. 16.4). Especially, often they are located on the border between the gray and white matter of the large hemispheres. In the cavities there is a cerebrospinal fluid, and on their walls macrophages are found, containing in the cytoplasm the products of the breakdown of brain tissue. The areas of necrosis are delimited by glial growth, as a result of which the brain substance surrounding the cysts is devoid of the usual structure and sharply compacted. Sclerosis also

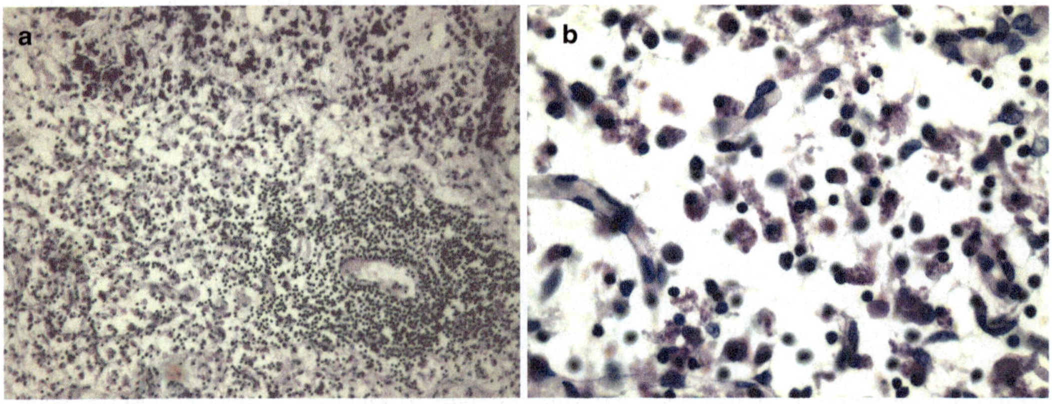

Fig. 16.3 Brain lesion in inborn toxoplasmosis. PAS (**a**) Massive inflammation and numerous necrosis ×600; (**b**) Numerous predominantly intracellular PAS-positive inclusions—toxoplasms. ×1000

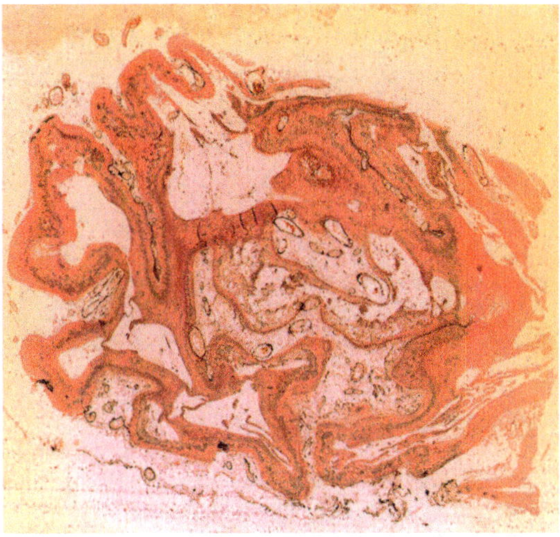

Fig. 16.4 Cysts as outcomes of chronic inborn toxoplasmosis. H-E 25

affects the vascular plexuses and soft meninges. In connection with the violation of the outflow of the cerebrospinal fluid, internal hydrops of the brain develops. In parallel with this, calcification occurs with pulverized or granular, and sometimes massive lime deposition. Calcification is not specific to toxoplasmosis, so it cannot be diagnosed on the basis of a single focal calcification. At the same stage of toxoplasmosis, changes in the eyes can also be detected—chorioretinitis, which manifests itself in focal infiltration of the membranes of the eyes and the development of small areas of necrosis. This leads to a thickening of the reticular and vascular membranes. Less often, other areas of the eye are affected. Later, granulation tissue develops here and synechiae are formed.

Sometimes, skin lesions are possible. On the trunk, surface and deep perivascular infiltrates are detected, consisting mainly of lymphocytes and histiocytes, as well as macrophages, plasmocytes, and eosinophils. In addition, there are hemorrhages and sometimes allergic vasculitis. Calcification, sometimes diffuse, of the surface layers of the skin is also possible. Macroscopically, the foci have the character of papulo-hemorrhagic, papulo-nodular, and infiltrative necrotic elements. Intrauterine toxoplasmosis is often accompanied by a violation of the development of the brain, expressed to varying degrees. There may be an underdevelopment of one lobe and even the large hemispheres of the brain as a whole. There are descriptions of the association with toxoplasmosis with other malformations. Currently, such lesions are extremely rare.

16.2.3 Cytomegaly

Cytomegalovirus (cytomegalovirus, herpes virus 4) is one of the most important pathogens of human diseases, the study of which is devoted to many thousands of publications in recent decades (see Chap. 5 and Sect. 8.2). Intrauterine cytomegalovirus infection is among the most frequent and well-studied. In the United States, every year 3000–4000 children are born with a clinically pronounced disease; a large number of children suffer from its late manifestations, including hearing loss, blindness, and delayed psychomotor development. Many important features of intrauterine cytomegaly were recently summarized by [2]. It occurs in 0.25–2.4% of seropositive mothers; as a rule, these are individuals with recent seroconversion. It was found that the presence of antibodies in the mother, especially the IgG class, does not significantly affect the embryo. An infected mother most often gives birth to a healthy child. In pregnant women acute cytomegalic infection is diagnosed by IgM class antibodies. They noted the threat of termination of pregnancy and repeated blood tests in the third trimester of pregnancy revealed seroconversion in 1.4%. In three of them, the pathogen was found in the placenta. Two of them were diagnosed with intrauterine pathology: microcephaly and hearing loss.

The penetration of CMV to the fetus in acute cytomegalic infection is incomparably higher and is 45%, including 2–4% of children developing severe generalized cytomegaly. Intrauterine cytomegaly is characterized by a lesion of the central nervous system, and therefore the most serious complication of this disease is mental retardation. It was shown that intrauterine cytomegaly can lead to both the formation of intrauterine malformations and various inflammatory changes similar to those described in intrauterine herpes. Many authors note that in children with CMV infection, cellular immunity is suppressed. This can be considered as a state of tolerance in response to early antigen penetration, when immunity has not yet been established. In any pathway of infection, the virus multiplies in cells of epithelial origin. In childhood, cytomegalovirus can also cause encephalitis. In adults, this pathogen usually causes neuropathy, polyradiculoneuropathies. More often, cytomegalovirus lesions of the nervous system occur as a result of intrauterine infection and are manifested by hydrocephalus, microcephaly, microgyria, porencephaly. Damage to the nervous system is detected in the first days of a child's life or occurs acutely a few months after birth. The clinical picture is dominated by hypertension hydrocephalus and convulsive syndromes. In the cerebrospinal fluid, moderate pleocytosis is detected, mainly of a lymphocytic nature. Differential diagnosis of cytomegalovirus encephalitis presents significant difficulties. With intrauterine infection at 3–5 months of pregnancy in a newborn, X-ray examination of the skull can reveal calcifications located periventricularly, in contrast to toxoplasma encephalitis, in which they are more often located in the cortex of the large hemispheres. Cytomegalovirus cells can be found in saliva, urine, CSF. They emphasize the importance of repeated examination of saliva and urine: they examine two to three samples daily for 3–4 days. Currently, along with the use of virological and serological methods in the diagnosis of cytomegalovirus infection, enzyme immunoassay techniques and PCR are used.

Pathologically, pathognomonic for cytomegalovirus infection is the formation of giant cells with nuclear and cytoplasmic inclusions. Most often, such cytomegals are formed in epithelial tissue, less often in muscle and nervous tissue (Fig. 16.5). The development of productive necrotic meningoencephalitis is characteristic (Fig. 16.6). Following variants of lesions are distinguished as well: damage to the vessel wall, ischemia, leukomalacia, deposition of calcium salts until the formation of mineralizing vasculopathy, defeat of the germinal matrix, violation of neuronal migration with the development of lissencephalopathy, polymicrogyria, ependymitis, water pipe stenosis with hydrocephalus, subependicular cysts. Often the damage is caused by indirect exposure to toxins-necrosis, cysts, calcium deposition, atrophy, leukoencephalopathy. If infection occurs in the first to second trimester, then the formation of malformations of development, the deposition of calcium salts is typical. During infection in the first trimester, the formation of destructive changes, calcification, and ventricular dilatation were observed.

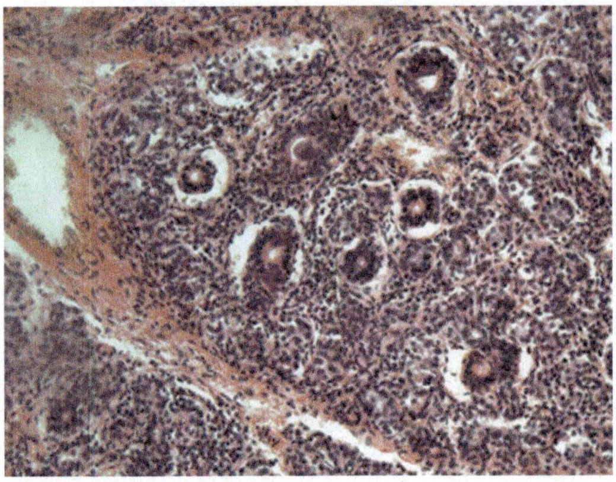

Fig. 16.5 Typical "owl eye" like intranuclear inclusion in salivary gland in inborn cytomegaly H-E × 600

16.2.4 Herpes

Herpes certainly belongs to the most common intrauterine infections caused by herpes simplex virus 2, and probably 1 type (see Chap. 5). Many important features of intrauterine herpes were recently summarized [2]. Its diagnosis should be based not only on the identification of characteristic skin rashes at the time of birth (which are determined very rarely), but, above all, on the results of qualified virological and morphological studies. Pregnant women are highly sensitive to herpetic infection. During pregnancy, 55.6% of women have herpetic rashes on the skin and mucous membranes. Herpetic infection can be transmitted transplacentally to the fetus, infection of the newborn is possible during the passage of the birth canal of the mother suffering from

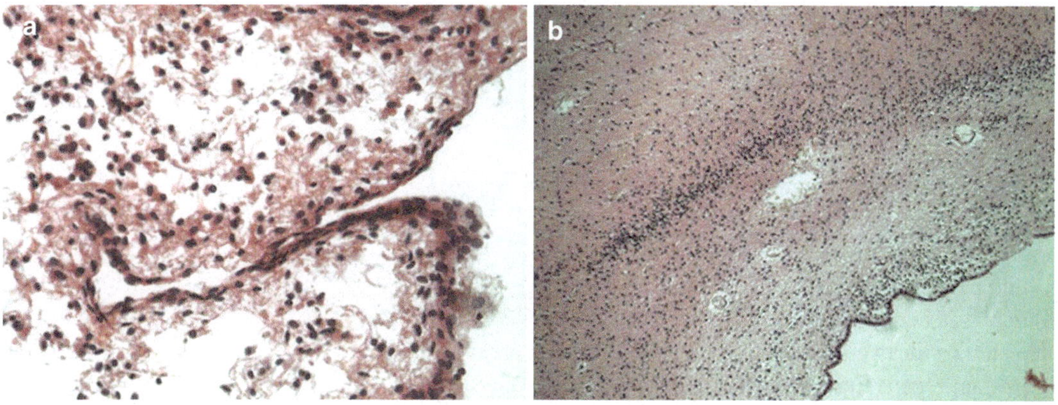

Fig. 16.6 Brain lesion in inborn cytomegaly H-E. (**a**) Diffuse infiltration and proliferation of arachnoendothelial cells in meninges ×600; (**b**) subependymal gliosis ×100

genital herpes. The development of the latter in 20–40% of cases is associated with HSV-1, in 50–70% of cases with HSV-2.

Genital herpes, the most common infection among sexually transmitted infections, in most cases, proceeds without clinical manifestations. It is established that 60–80% of newborns with neonatal herpes are born from mothers with an asymptomatic carrier of this infection. It is believed that the outcome of a herpetic infection that has developed in a pregnant woman with the fetus depends on the timing of the primary infection or relapse of the disease in the mother: if it occurs in the first trimester, a miscarriage is possible; in the second semester—malformations, in case of their incompatibility with life—stillbirth; in the third semester, the development of a congenital herpetic infection.

An important role in the formation of herpetic lesions of the nervous system in the fetus is played by immune mechanisms. The herpes virus contains antigenic determinants similar to one of the fragments of the nerve growth factor; as a result, when a herpetic infection is activated, antibodies to this neurotrophic factor appear in a pregnant woman. With an increase in the level of antibodies to the nerve growth factor above 0.74–1.43 units, the mother has a high probability of a stillborn fetus. It is appropriate to note that the detection of characteristic intracranial inclusions in smears or paraffin sections (Cawdry type 1 bodies) is considered an internationally recognized absolute proof of the herpetic etiology of the process of any localization, sufficient for the appointment of specific antiviral therapy.

In recent years, the importance of confirming the diagnosis using molecular biological methods has been emphasized. Depending on the fullness of the compensatory processes in the afterbirth, different variants of the further course of the disease in the fetus (child) are possible – from severe antenatal herpes to the birth of a healthy child. Infection can also occur intranatally, especially in the presence of genital herpes in the mother. There is an increase in spontaneous abortions and premature births against the background of herpes in the mother. The most likely route of infection in the development of severe forms of the disease with damage to the skin conjunctiva of the eye, as well as the mucous membranes of the genitals, is contact when the child passes through the infected birth canal of the mother. At the same time, it should be noted that 70% of mothers whose children were born with disseminated intrauterine herpes did not show signs of genital lesions during childbirth, and 52% did not even have a history of it. Along with this, postnatal infection of the newborn is also possible.

The frequency of neonatal herpes remains unclear, and the figures vary significantly even in countries where laboratory tests are conducted to search for this disease (from 1 in 1500 births in the United States, to 1 in 33,000 births in the United Kingdom. The frequency of neonatal herpes varies in the range of 1: 5000 to 1:7500 births. Very high mortality rates of children in this age period: without treatment from 18% (local form with skin and mucosal lesions) to 90% (disseminated form); when treated with acyclovir, the mortality rate in the disseminated form decreases to 57%. It should be noted that under seemingly equal conditions, the lesions of the organs of the newborn can differ dramatically. Clinical variants of herpetic lesions may include panencephalitis with an outcome of multicystic encephalomalacia; periventricular encephalitis with the formation of cystic forms of periventricular leukomalacia; as well as intraventricular and periventricular hemorrhages. It should be noted that there was a good correlation between the results of intravital and postmortem studies in the fatal cases. Vegetative state, severe forms of cerebral palsy, oligophrenia, atrophy of the optic nerves, sensorineural hearing loss, mental development disorders, and hydrocephalus are described as neurological consequences of such lesions. At the same time, it is noted that focal cortical subcortical encephalitis, meningitis, ventriculitis, and choroiditis of herpetic etiology, diagnosed and treated in the neonatal period, are currently controlled pathology with relatively favorable neurological outcomes. In congenital herpetic encephalitis, changes are usually localized in the medial part of the temporal lobes, the parietal-occipital region, and the lower frontal gyri. MRI is a more sensitive method than CT. The radiation semiotics of herpetic encephalitis does not differ from the changes observed in other cases. When a contrast agent is administered, the signal intensity changes throughout the entire volume or only in the gray matter of the affected area. In 80% of cases, the changes are two-sided and symmetrical. In 75% of patients, a pronounced mass effect is observed, in 15% of cases, a hemorrhagic component is traced, due to pronounced necrosis of the brain substance. However, in the early stages, there are difficulties in differentiating minor edema from unmyelinated white matter. Within a few weeks, the substance is destroyed, encephalomalacia zones are formed. Residual changes are usually represented by the expansion of the ventricles and furrows, periventricular calcifications are possible.

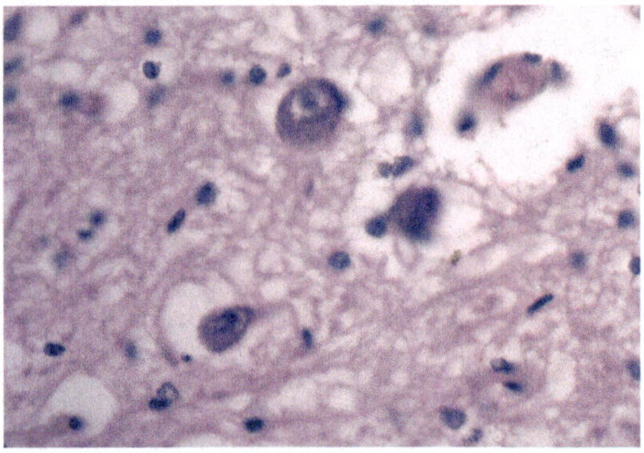

Fig. 16.7 Brain lesion in inborn herpes. Note large intranuclear basophilic inclusions. H-E; ×600

Morphological examination in the early stages of brain damage against the background of generalized herpes reveals swelling of individual neurons and glial cells in the nuclei of which large basophilic inclusions are detected (Fig. 16.7). Hyperchromatosis of the nuclei with fragmentation and the marginal location of the nuclear substance is often visible. In addition, there are signs of subependimar gliosis of various degrees of severity. Macroscopically, such a brain is moderately flabby. With a longer duration of the process, with its progression, necrotic meningoencephalitis occurs with widespread foci of necrosis mainly in the subperpendicular zones and in the frontal lobes. There are cell changes around that are identical to those described above. There are also foci of gliosis, located mainly subependimar, more often in the area of the visual tubercles. They are represented by diffuse or perivascular clusters of poorly differentiated glial cells. The walls of small blood vessels in the substance of the brain are often thickened due to the proliferation of the endothelium, some of the cells of which undergo giant cell transformation. Similar changes in blood vessels are detected in other organs. Were described also a reactive necrosis, necrosis with perifocal lymphoplasmocytic infiltration, foci of gliosis, more often periventricular, swelling of the cytoplasm of neurons, degenerative changes in them with eosinophilic intracranial inclusions. It is proved that the epidemic source can be not only the mother, but also the father. Herpes simplex infection in children was divided into three groups, depending on the age and the most likely time of the disease: (1) intrauterine herpes – newborns aged 2–24 days; (2) presumably intrauterine children were ill from birth and died in 1–7 months of life; (3) children who became ill in the postnatal period and died in 4–8 months [4]. It was found that herpetic infection with a fatal outcome is diagnosed in children in the first year of life quite often—in 4.7% of cases. The disease was caused in most cases by HSV-2, which is associated with mainly intrauterine infection in this age group. In postnatal herpes, lung damage prevailed, which is probably explained by the aerogenic infection of such children. In children of the first year of life, herpes was characterized by a generalized character with lesions nearby with the brain and spinal cord of the liver, lungs. Clinical manifestations were characterized by a predominance of general cerebral symptoms, only by 3–4 months of life symptoms of focal damage to the nervous system were detected. The latter can be explained by the immaturity of the brain structures, the presence of mixed infection (association of herpes with cytomegalovirus, mycoplasma, chlamydia), which prevents the development of characteristic clinical manifestations.

Lesions in chronic probably intrauterine herpes encephalitis have been described in Sect. 5.5.

16.2.5 Mycoplasmosis

Among the numerous pathogens of the *Mycoplasmataceae* family, the role of *M. incognitus, M. hominis, M. genitalium, M. fermentans, M. penetrans, M. pirum, Ureaplasma urealitycum, U. parvum*, and *Acholeplasma laidbawii* is discussed in connection with urogenital and intrauterine infections. In practice, given the objective and subjective difficulties of laboratory diagnostics, the role of *Mycoplasma hominis, Ureaplasma urealitycum*, and, much less frequently, *M. genitalium* is usually discussed. The ability of mycoplasmas to cause intrauterine infection was shown by foreign researchers in the descriptions of single observations in the late 1960s, early 1970s of the twentieth century. The most complete information about intrauterine mycoplasmosis was obtained in Russia in the 1970s by various teams in Leningrad, Moscow, Kishinev as a result of studying a variety of autopsy and experimental materials. Unfortunately, in the future, due to a number of objective and subjective reasons, less attention to this pathology was paid. A small number of similar publications abroad have prompted to express doubts about the practical significance of this problem. At the same time, our data allow us, despite the sharply deteriorated laboratory capabilities in the diagnosis of genital mycoplasmosis, to talk about the preservation of this infection with an important role in the etiology of intrauterine infections at present. The question of the location of mycoplasmas is currently being discussed. Many authors, focusing on American publications, especially those of previous years, consider mycoplasmas as an extracellular pathogen located on the surface of cell membranes. In numerous domestic studies, including those performed with the help of EM, the ability of mycoplasmas to both intracellular (in the most severe course of the disease) and extracellular location (in mild forms) has been repeatedly proven. According to our data, the most characteristic feature of intrauterine mycoplasmosis is the multiplication of mycoplasmas in epithelial cells [4]. In the respiratory organs, changes in alveolocytes are particularly typical; along with this, protein masses, red blood cells and sometimes a small number of granular white blood cells are found in the lumen of the alveoli and small bronchi. There are also circulatory disorders in the form of increased blood filling of vessels of all calibers, hemorrhage in the alveoli, and sometimes thrombosis of blood vessels. Moderate lymphohistiocytic infiltration is often detected, as well as fibrosis of the peribronchial and, to a lesser extent, perivascular and interalveolar interstitial tissue. Macroscopic changes are moderate and nonspecific. In the brain, the histological study shows the fullness of the soft meninges, an increase in the number of macrophage cells in them. The vacuolated cytoplasm of many of them contains mycoplasmas. There is no clear stratification in the cortex of the large hemispheres, and poorly differentiated elements predominate among their cells. Many neurons of the cortex, as well as the nodes of the base, are colored pale and undergo the metamorphosis characteristic of mycoplasmosis. Nerve cells with "ischemic" changes are also identified. However, there is no pronounced glial reaction. Ependymocytes are often incorrectly oriented in the cytoplasm, some of them there are mycoplasmas. Similar changes are naturally determined in the cells of the choroidal plexus lining. There may be clusters of poorly differentiated glial elements around the ventricular system. Macroscopically, puffiness and fullness of the soft meninges, flabbiness of the brain substance are detected, and small hemorrhages can also be noted, mainly in the disease caused by M. pneumoniae. As an example of intrauterine mycoplasmosis with severe lesions of the nervous system in the perinatal period, we present our following observation. Example: the twin sisters of M., who died after 15 hours and 4 days in the clinic of the Pediatric Institute. They were born at 32 weeks. Pregnancy one with a weight of 1350 and a height of 38 cm and the other with a weight of 1190 and a height of 34 cm. The pregnancy of a young primiparous mother was accompanied by a severe form of nephropathy. The fetal bladder opened prematurely. The girls were born with severe asphyxia. Independent breathing in both appeared only after intubation. Despite intensive treatment, it was not possible to achieve respiratory stabilization. The girl, who was born with a large weight, died in 15 hours, and her sister in 4 days after birth. The clinical diagnosis of both sisters was intrauterine asphyxia, complicated by aspiration pneumonia with hyaline membranes on the background of prematurity. On macroscopic examination, the morphological changes in both girls were similar and were reduced to densification of the posterior part of the lungs and small-point hemorrhages of different localization. On the part of the brain, only puffiness and fullness of the MMO, flabby consistency of the brain, and lack of clear differentiation into gray and white matter were noted. Cytological examination of lung scrapings in both cases revealed a large number of alveolocytes with cytoplasm with focal clearance containing mycoplasmas. During a bacteriological study in the bacteriological laboratory of the Pediatric Institute using conventional nutrient media, pathogenic microflora could not be detected. During a special microbiological study at the Influenza Research Institute using media for growing mycoplasmas in both cases, it was possible to isolate *Mycoplasma hominis* from the brain, lungs, liver, and in one of the observations also from the kidney. In an IF study of lung scrapings and liver sections, serum for *M. hominis* was detected; studies with sera for respiratory viruses of lung smears were negative. Histological examination of both children in many areas of the lungs shows uneven fullness and airiness of the lung tissue due to the alternation of dystelectases with small areas of acute emphysema. The lumen of the alveoli contains a small amount of loose protein masses, quite numerous red blood cells, quite numerous red blood cells, single white blood cells, and macrophages. There are also quite a lot of desquamated, partly nuclear-free large alveolocytes with a light foamy cytoplasm. Sharply enlarged alveolocytes with a light foamy cytoplasm containing mycoplasmas are often seen on the walls of the alveoli. In both cases, hyaline membranes were also detected, which were more pronounced in the deceased 15 h after birth. In the liver, in addition to congestive fullness, there are hemorrhages in the connective tissue layers. Kupffer cells are mostly hyperplastic, and the circular sinusoid spaces are expanded. Discoplexation of the hepatic beams, pronounced vacuolization and protein dystrophy, and even necrotic changes in hepatocytes were detected. In many hepatocytes, intracellular PAS- and azur-positive inclusions are detected, some of which glow when treated with luminescent serum to *M. hominis*. Naturally, there is an expansion of the bile capillaries, especially in areas with the most pronounced alternative changes in hepatocytes. In the kidneys, there are dystrophic changes, vacuolization, and an increase in the size of nephrothelial cells, mainly convoluted tubules. Their cytoplasm, and sometimes in the lumen of the tubules, contains small basophilic PAS-positive bodies containing the *M. hominis* antigen. Damaged nephrothelial cells are partially exfoliated. In those areas where they are absent, regenerating cells of a flattened shape are visible. The lumen of part of the tubules is significantly increased.

Blood vessels are dilated, and their endothelium is often swollen. The histological picture of the brain of both girls was also similar. The soft medulla was full-blooded, containing a slightly increased number of macrophage cells, some of which contained azuro- and PAS-positive inclusions in the vacuolated cytoplasm. In the cortex of the large hemispheres, there were no pronounced layers among the cells; small, poorly differentiated ones prevailed. Among the larger nerve cells of the cortex, as well as the nodes of the base, many were very pale colored with thionine by Nissl and contained in their cytoplasm a significant number of the above-described inclusions, often surrounded by clearances. The outlines of such cells were mostly indistinct. A pronounced glial reaction to these changes could not be detected. In addition, there were also "ischemic" changes in nerve cells. Clusters of poorly differentiated glial elements were observed around the ventricular system. Ependymocytes in many places looked dark, lay in several layers, were incorrectly oriented in their cytoplasm, in some cases it was possible to detect the above-described inclusions. The pathological diagnosis was formulated as a generalized mycoplasma infection with damage to the liver, lungs, brain, and kidneys, complicated by multiple hemorrhages in the internal organs and hyaline membranes in combination with intrauterine asphyxia.

In recent years, intrauterine mycoplasmosis with lesions of many organs, including the brain, continues to be systematically diagnosed on the basis of clinical and morphological data, as well as the results of an IF study. Thus in recent years, according to St. Petersburg, mycoplasmosis (caused by M. *hominis* and *M. urealyticum*) accounts for about 10% of intrauterine infections, which are determined in total in 10–17% of fetuses and newborns. Despite the presence in the literature of indications about the ability of mycoplasmas to survive for a long time in humans and experimental animals, there are practically no descriptions of reliably proven intrauterine mycoplasmosis caused by *M. hominis* in children who have come out of the perinatal period. We present our observation [6]. The girl M. was born from two births, five pregnancies with an Apgar score of 7/9, with a body weight of 3350 g, height of 51 cm. The neonatal period was uneventful. The extremely unfavorable obstetric history of the mother drew attention to itself: the first pregnancy ended in stillbirth at 34–35 weeks, while the child's weight deficit was more than 40%, the second, third, and fourth ended in miscarriages at 7–8 weeks. The last pregnancy occurred with the threat of termination at the terms of 7–8, 23, and 37 weeks. In this connection, the woman was on inpatient treatment for 16 weeks. During pregnancy, from the mother was isolated *M. hominis*, for which she received treatment.

After discharge on the eighth day of life from the maternity hospital, the girl was breastfed, the psychomotor development of the child corresponded to the age. Attention was drawn to the excess weight (in 3 months, 6900) by 15% with an age-appropriate height. At the age of 3 months, the girl was hospitalized for a mild form of acute respiratory infection, on the 18th day of the disease, she had convulsive twitching in the handles. At the age of 4 months, the child became ill again, with anxiety, excessive salivation, nasal mucus discharge, pharyngeal hyperemia, and hard breathing, and the girl was hospitalized again. During the examination, attention was drawn to the presence of a number of dysmorphs in the child (a square-shaped skull with a high forehead, deformity of the auricles, Gothic palate, facial asymmetry, short neck), which, in comparison with the anamnesis data, allowed us to think about the presence of an intrauterine infection in the girl. The condition was assessed as moderate. After 2.5 h after admission, the child had reversible seizures with a turn of the head to the left, fixing the gaze to the left, and excessive salivation. A large fontanelle with a size of 1 × 1 cm, its voltage is normal. Then there were convulsive twitches in the left arm, and later in the left leg. With the introduction of antiepileptic drugs, convulsive seizures stopped and did not recur later. Upon subsequent examination by a neurologist, the absence of rigidity of the occipital muscles was noted. During lumbar puncture, CSF flowed out in rapid drops, cytosis was 289×10^9 cl/l, including 89% lymphocytes, 12.5% neutrophils, 2.5% monocytes, 0.33 g/l protein,

2.16 mmol/l sugar. Blood test: Hb 140 g/l, er. 4, 12×10^{12}/l, ESR 4 mm/h. A biochemical study of the blood revealed a decrease in the content of γ - globulins to 8.6% (at the norm of 12–18%) and, accordingly, an increase in the A/G index to 2.0 (at the norm of 1.0-1.2). In the urine analysis, there are traces of protein, 6–10 white blood cells in the field of vision. The child was transferred to the infectious hospital with suspected serous meningitis. Upon admission, the child's condition was assessed as serious. The fontanelle did not bulge, the heart, tones were rhythmic, but muted, and the lower border of the liver protruded 2 cm from under the edge of the costal arch. The next day after admission, the child resumed convulsive twitching, which was repeated 4 times, over the next day, the phenomenon of respiratory failure increased, and therefore, in an extremely serious condition, the girl was transferred to the intensive care unit. At lumbar puncture, cytosis was in the range of 184×10^{12}–314×10^{12} cl/mcl with a predominance of neutrophils protein 0.99–3.0 g/l. In the blood, leukocytosis was observed up to 13×10^9/L with a sharp shift to the left; ESR 10 mm/h. The EEG revealed gross violation of bioelectric activity of the epileptiform type, and the EchoEG showed signs of intracranial hypertension. All results of the bacteriological study were negative. The child underwent complex antibacterial therapy, prednisone (5 mg/kg), blood transfusions, anti-influenza globulin, dehydration, antiepileptic and symptomatic therapy. Despite the treatment, the girl's condition continued to deteriorate, the neurological symptoms worsened, the phenomena of respiratory and cardiovascular insufficiency increased, in connection with which the child was transferred to artificial ventilation, and in the last day the phenomenon of acute renal failure joined. On the seventh day of her stay in the hospital, the girl died. Clinically, the disease was regarded as meningoencephalitis of unclear etiology, complicated by bilateral bronchopneumonia, cardiovascular and acute renal failure, DIC. Possible intrauterine infection, perinatal encephalopathy, acute respiratory viral infection, and bilateral otitis media were considered as concomitant diseases. During the pathological examination, along with the above-described dysmorphic changes, a number of other dysplastic changes were revealed: unevenly located and often double pyramids in both kidneys, hypoplasia of the white matter of the occipital lobes of the brain, deep longitudinal and transverse furrows in the spleen. The lungs, especially in the basal parts, were of a doughy consistency with individual punctate subpleural hemorrhages, and on the incision – with grayish-reddish foci. On the liver section, yellowish-grayish areas in the area of the center of the liver lobes attracted attention. In other organs, dystrophic changes were noted. The soft meninges were thickened due to edema. The thymus gland was 9 g in weight, of a very flabby consistency. Cytological examination revealed a significant number of cells with enlarged vacuolated cytoplasm containing small inclusions in smears from various parts of the lung, soft meninges, and middle ear. IF examination revealed a distinct positive glow with serum for *M. hominis*, as well as parainfluenza, in smears from the lungs and soft meninges. During the bacteriological study, the pathogenic flora was not isolated. Serological examination of the blood antibodies to parainfluenza virus type 2–1: 20. Antibodies to *M. hominis* were not detected due to the absence of the necessary antigen in the laboratory.

Histological examination revealed a typical morphological picture of intrauterine mycoplasmosis with the development of changes typical for this disease in the liver, lungs, kidneys, heart, spleen, thymus gland, lymph nodes, salivary glands, and intestines in the form of the appearance of cells in an enlarged foamy, containing PAS- and azur-positive inclusions of the cytoplasm, corresponding to the descriptions available in the literature [5]. Of particular interest were changes in the brain, where, along with the typical changes described above in meningocytes, ependymocytes of the choroidal plexus and lateral ventricles, as well as nerve cells, a moderate focal proliferation of glia was also revealed. Thus, these data served as the basis for the diagnosis of a generalized intrauterine mycoplasma infection in the deceased girl, which was associated with both direct lesions of a number of internal organs, including the immune system, which caused some signs of secondary immunodeficiency in the clinic, and pronounced dysplastic changes that allow us to consider these changes as early fetopathy. It can be assumed that since the mother received treatment during pregnancy, the massiveness of infection of the fetus was relatively moderate, and therefore the disease in the first months of life was little manifest. Subsequently, due to the superinfection of parainfluenza and, possibly, bacterial infection, a significant exacerbation of the course of mycoplasmosis occurred.

16.2.6 Syphilis

In recent years, the problem of congenital syphilis remains actual. The morphological manifestations of congenital syphilis are similar to those described in adult syphilis [4]. Since the infection of the fetus occurs hematogenically, congenital syphilis has similarities with secondary syphilis (see Chap. 13). In the central nervous system, chronic productive leptomeningitis, meningoencephalitis, and ependymatitis are detected. It is possible to develop gum and progressive hydrocephalus. Eye lesions in the form of chorioretinitis ("salt and pepper" on the periphery of the fundus), uveitis, glaucoma, and atrophy of the ocular nerve are quite characteristic.

The course of neurosyphilis has its own characteristics in children. It is believed that in children, congenital syphilis is more common, due to placental transmission of the pathogen during pregnancy. Infection of the fetus is possible from the moment of formation of the placenta: from 9–10 weeks of intrauterine development by introducing spirochetes through the umbilical vein, the lymphatic slits of the umbilical vessels, with maternal blood with increased placental permeability. In recent years, it has been proven that pregnant women with syphilis can give birth to a child with congenital syphilis even after a full course of therapy. This is possible if a pregnant woman has an early stage of syphilis, while maintaining a high titer of serological reactions during therapy and childbirth, in case of a short time interval between therapeutic measures and childbirth, with a gestational age of the newborn less than 36 weeks. It is proved that the most contagious for the fetus is secondary syphilis in the mother. The study of placental histopathology in congenital syphilis revealed necrotic changes, expansion, and acute inflammation of the chorionic villi; large infiltrates consisting of neutrophils, macrophages, and plasmocytes are located mainly around the foci of necrosis in the basal plate and extraplacental membranes [4]. In rare cases, children can become infected with domestic contact with a patient with syphilis, with a transfusion of infected blood. There are congenital syphilis of infancy, congenital syphilis of early childhood, and late congenital syphilis. It should be emphasized that due to the neurotropism of treponema, 60% of newborns with congenital syphilis have neurosyphilis. Pathological studies indicate that in congenital syphilis, spirochetes are present in the liver, intestines, membranes of the brain of newborns.

It should be emphasized that the diagnosis of congenital syphilis in newborns is difficult due to the non-specificity and erasure of clinical manifestations, the high frequency of negative serological reactions.

Often a severe manifestation of congenital syphilis is hydrocephalus. In its occurrence, increased production of CSF and occlusion of CSF spaces are important, which is associated with syphilitic lesions of the membranes and ependyma of the ventricles. Hydrocephalus in patients with congenital syphilis can develop acutely or gradually. Meningeal symptoms are not pronounced or absent, often affecting the visual, oculomotor, facial, auditory, and trigeminal nerves. Differential diagnosis is performed with congenital toxoplasmosis in the chronic phase of the disease, in which hydrocephalus is combined with chorioretinitis, foci of calcification on X-rays of the skull.

In addition, in children with congenital syphilis of infancy, along with damage to the nervous system, various lesions of the skin, mucous membranes, bones, and internal organs are noted. The most important for the diagnosis of congenital syphilis was previously considered the classical Hutchinson triad (parenchymal keratitis, labyrinth deafness, Hutchinson teeth—the upper middle incisors have an irregular shape with a semilunar notch, with convex lateral edges), which is currently detected infrequently. In addition, there may be radial scars around the lips, a saddle-shaped nose, enlarged frontal bumps, saber-shaped shins, and an increase in the size of the liver, and spleen.

Lesions of the nervous system in congenital syphilis at the age of 1–2 years usually appear in the form of a vascular form. Specific endarteritis leads to vascular obliteration with the development of ischemia of the nervous tissue. As a result, such children over the age of 5–6 months develop central spastic hemiplegia. Paralysis can be accompanied by partial or generalized seizures, mental retardation. In the vascular form, Argyle Robertson's symptoms, anisocoria, ptosis, strabismus, and optic nerve atrophy may also occur. At the same time, in children of 3–4 months of age, Peters described paresis and paralysis of the hands, developing immediately or within a short time. Paresis is peripheral, with low muscle tone, with a decrease or absence of deep reflexes. The affected limbs take a fin position, there is a pronation of the hands that are taken outwards. Specific treatment leads to a rapid reverse development of paralysis. In clinical practice, Peters' palsy must be differentiated from Parrot's pseudoparalysis, which occurs in the first weeks of life and is rare after 4 months. It was established that the basis of Parrot's pseudoparalysis is syphilitic osteochondritis, leading to resorption of epiphysis more often in the area of the elbow and wrist joints. At the same time, there is swelling of the joints, pain in passive movements, restriction of movements due to the presence of pain syndrome. Such children are sometimes misdiagnosed flaccid paresis of the upper or lower extremities. At the same time, spontaneous activity is sharply reduced; when the doctor tries to conduct passive movements, the child cries and screams. However, in Parrot's pseudoparalysis, physiological reflexes are triggered, sensitivity is preserved, atrophy and changes in the electrical excitability of the muscles do not develop. The correct diagnosis in these cases helps radiography of both forearms with the distal end of the humerus and both shins with the distal end of the femur: at the border between the epiphysis and the diaphysis, a dark, 2-4 mm wide rarefaction band is symmetrically visible, indicating osteochondrosis.

It should be noted that lesions of the nervous system in congenital syphilis can occur with remission and deterioration or progrediently. The course depends on the activity of the syphilitic process, on the presence of associations with syphilis of various intrauterine infections. Severity of damage to the child's nervous system and prognosis are determined by a combination of congenital syphilis with herpes, cytomegaly, and other intrauterine neuroinfections, which requires examination to exclude associated pathogenic agents.

Late (parenchymal) forms of neurosyphilis, with congenital disease, can manifest as Jackson's epilepsy, atrophy of the optic nerves, ataxia, and mental retardation. At the same time, spinal cord dryness in children with congenital syphilis is rare, mainly in patients older than 10 years. The early symptoms of spinal cord dryness in congenital syphilis include primary atrophy of the optic nerves, which develops slowly, gradually. In some patients, the symptom of Argyle Robertson is detected, anisocoria and irregular shape of the pupils are often found. Pelvic disorders are characteristic: at the beginning of the disease, imperative urges are expressed with incontinence at night, then daytime enuresis is also noted. Gradually, there is a decrease in knee and Achilles reflexes. It should be emphasized that coordination disorders, diabetic crises, and trophic disorders in children are rare, and their severity is much less than in adults. Progressive paralysis is not typical for young children. In patients with congenital syphilis, the juvenile form of progressive paralysis may occur after 12 years. In cases of acquired syphilis, a childhood form of progressive paralysis may develop. Progressive paralysis develops slowly in children. The clinical picture is dominated by mental and physical development delays. The child becomes inattentive, indifferent, irritable, tearful. There is impulsivity, malice, disinhibition of drive, behavior becomes antisocial. Patients commit theft, arson; hypersexuality is observed. In the future, progressive dementia is noted; in the final stage, speech is lost, and, in the absence of treatment, mental insanity occurs. In the symptom complex of mental disorders in children, unlike adults, delusions of greatness are less often observed. In the neurological picture, there may be a symptom of Argyle Robertson, areflexia; there may be convulsive seizures. The duration of the course of progressive paralysis in children in untreated cases is on average 5 years. The diagnosis of progressive paralysis in children is quite complex. The latter is due to the fact that this form of neurosyphilis begins most often on the background of congenital syphilis, which causes damage to the child's brain, changing the clinical manifestations.

In congenital syphilitic lesions of the nervous system, clinical symptoms appear in the first year of life and in adolescence, characterized by symptoms of meningitis, hydrocephalus, deafness, epileptic seizures, atrophy of the optic nerves. Morphological manifestations are represented by the formation of microgyria, lobar sclerosis, inflammatory changes in the membranes of the brain, and cerebral endarteritis. Positive serological reactions are detected in the cerebrospinal fluid. In addition, in congenital syphilis, the Hutchinson triad can be observed (interstitial keratitis, deformity of teeth with a semilunar defect, deafness). In adolescence, spinal cord dryness or taboparalysis may develop. Extremely rare, casually, there are gummas of the brain and spinal cord, syphilitic cervical pachymeningitis.

16.2.7 Brain Lesions in Intrauterine Chlamydiosis (IUC)

Chlamydiosis is a widespread infection that in humans is caused mainly by three pathogens *Chlamydia trachomatis, C. psittaci, C. pneumoniae*, capable of causing a variety of lesions, including generalized diseases, in various ways of infection. One of the most fully studied problems is urogenital chlamydia, which can lead to the development of intrauterine infection.

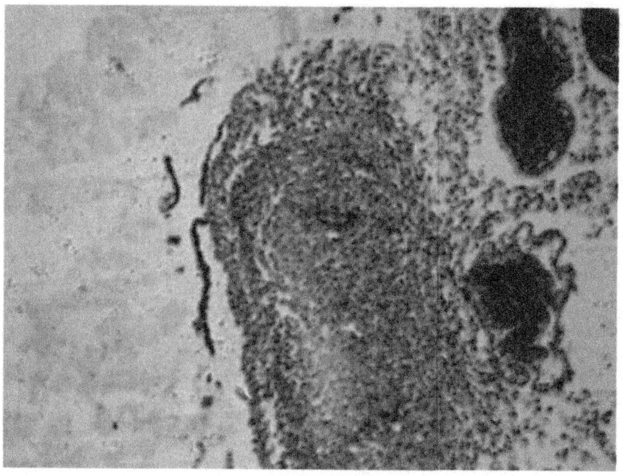

Fig. 16.8 Meningeal granuloma in inborn chlamydiosis. H-E × 100

From the first days of life, children infected with chlamydia have symptoms of central nervous system damage. They have a sleep disorder, tremor of the arms and legs, changes in muscle tone, increased reactivity, inhibition of tendon reflexes. In the following days, functional disorders of the central nervous system persist. Children are prone to rapid hypothermia, local cyanosis is pronounced, "marbling" of the skin. In some cases, neurological symptoms increase, the so-called chlamydial choriomeningitis develops, occurring with fever, vomiting, swelling of the cerebellum, meningeal phenomena, red dermographism. It is possible to develop meningoencephalitis with repeated attacks of clonic tonic seizures and apnea. CNS lesions in newborns are similar to those of hypoxic and/or traumatic genesis. It should also be noted the possibility of infection with chlamydia and the absence and minimal severity of neurological manifestations.

Currently, the attention of a number of Russian researchers from the Ural region in intrauterine chlamydia attracts brain damage, especially soft meninges (Fig. 16.8). The authors describe the appearance of peculiar granulomas in them, which are already determined macroscopically on the convexital surface of the brain in the form of "cotton-like" formations. Using EM, chlamydia was determined inside the cells of these granulomas. On our material, such pronounced changes in the meninges were not determined. It can be assumed that these differences in MMO

Fig. 16.9 Chlamydia antigen in nervous cells in inborn infection. Luminescent microscopy ×1000

lesions may be related to differences in the properties of strains circulating in different regions.

According to our data, with generalized intrauterine chlamydia in the brain and spinal cord, there is a characteristic transformation of the cells of the soft meninges, choroidal plexuses, endotheliocytes (Fig. 16.9). It is impossible to exclude the possibility of direct damage to nerve and glial cells.

Chlamydiosis is often not accompanied by expressed symptoms during the newborn period. In the first year of life, these infections are diagnosed with a delay in psychomotor development, respiratory and intestinal infections. In older children, infections are masked by other diseases of the central nervous system, aggravating or imitating their course, while in some the inflammatory process from birth has a sluggish character, in others clinical manifestations debut a few years after "recovery" from perinatal encephalopathy, probably under the influence of an intercurrent process or superinfection. Based on clinical-laboratory and MRI comparisons, it was suggested that sluggish perinatal encephalitis has features of an inflammatory-degenerative process, and immunopathological reactions associated with IUC can contribute to neurodegeneration.

In our common study with Y.I. Vainshenker [7] among children and adolescents (3–15 years old) who were diagnosed with perinatal encephalopathy in infancy and had various noninfectious neurological and psychoneurological diagnoses at the time of the examination, 93% (39/42) revealed (culturally and PCR) various low-manifest infectious pathogens in various combinations and in various biological materials, including *Chlamydia* spp. in 71% (30/42), *Mycoplasma* spp. in 31% (13/42)., *Ureaplasma* spp. (*U. urealyticum*) in 14% (6/42). A significant increase in the frequency of occurrence of *Chlamydia* spp. was revealed in the presence of HHV-6 and VEB. As a monoinfection of *Chlamydia* spp. (with various combinations of *C. trachomatis*, *C. rpeimopiae*, *C. psittaci*) was detected in 27% (8/30) of cases of infection.

The participation of the detected infections in the central nervous system damage was confirmed by the positive dynamics of neuropsychiatric and neurological symptoms during etiotropic antibacterial therapy. Retrospectively, the leading clinical manifestations of low-manifest infections with CNS damage were identified: asthenia and psychoneurological disorders, stem symptoms, extrapyramidal, as well as pyramidal and cerebellar syndromes. There could be an epileptic syndrome with polymorphic seizures, diencephalic syndrome, a headache of a shell-vascular nature. At the same time, the areas of the central nervous system that are mainly involved in the infectious and inflammatory process in the central nervous system were identified (topical neurological diagnosis): the frontal lobes, basal ganglia, diencephalic region and oral parts of the brain stem, as well as the temporal and parietal lobes and the brain membranes.

Low-manifest infections can presumably contribute to the violation of embryogenesis. But taking into account the low-symptom manifestations, their participation in the formation of undifferentiated connective tissue dysplasia is likely. A number of combined signs of connective tissue dysplasia (arachnoid cysts, cranio-vertebral dysplasia in combination with cerebral vascular dysplasia or internal organs) were accompanied in 100% of cases by infection with VUI pathogens (*Chlamydia* spp., *Mycoplasma* spp., *U. urealyticum*).

16.2.8 Respiratory Viral Infections

Among intrauterine infections, a certain place is occupied by the processes caused by influenza, parainfluenza, RS viruses, and adenoviruses [4]. Although these infections are among the most common, they are rarely associated with the death or disability of children. In intrauterine viral respiratory infections, we specifically studied brain lesions, which, as a rule, were localized in the periventricular areas of the anterior horns of the lateral ventricles of the brain and were characterized by circulatory disorders and cell proliferation of varying intensity. Circulatory disorders were detected in the form of hyperemia, stasis, and hemorrhage. In some cases, erythrocyte "sludge" and hyaline blood clots were observed in the lumen of the vessels. At the same time, circulatory disorders were more widespread in the white matter of the brain than cellular proliferating and occupied a larger area. They were accompanied by necrobiosis and necrosis of the walls of blood vessels and capillaries. There was pycnosis and lysis of the capillary endothelium, disintegration of the basal membranes. In addition, diffuse and perivascular edema was observed. Proliferates consisting of neuroglia cells and elements of vascular walls were quite characteristic. They were mainly perivascular in nature and were localized in the periventricular region in the zone of the subependimar matrix. In some children, such proliferations spread deep into the white matter towards the cerebral cortex. The changes described above generally did not extend beyond the white matter of the brain around the lateral ventricles. However, in some cases, with a mixed viral-bacterial infection, pathological changes spread to the cerebral cortex, where there was a loss of nerve cells with focal nodular proliferation of glia. In some cases, circulatory disorders and small focal proliferations spread to the cerebellum and spinal cord. In the vascular plexuses of the brain, hyperemia, hemorrhage, and edema were detected. On the part of the choroidal plexus epithelium, endotheliocytes, and ependymocytes, dystrophic and necrobiotic changes were observed with a violation of the integrity of the lining in certain areas. In addition, there was a proliferation of ependymal glia in the ventricles of the brain, as a result of which it became multilayered. In the soft meninges, meningitis was often diagnosed with edema, hyperemia, hemorrhage, and infiltration by lymphoid, monocyte, and macrophage cells, including cytoplasm transformed in a typical influenza manner. In some cases, the formation of leptomeningeal hematomas with damage to the underlying brain structures was noted. In the EM study of various parts of the brain (trunk, periventricular zone of the lateral ventricles, cortex of the hemispheres) [8], the accumulation of viruses in the periventricular zone is described. The virions of influenza A and B viruses had a characteristic structure and did not differ in their morphology from the virions of similar viruses in the lungs of children. They were located freely in the edematous intercellular spaces and on the cell membranes with signs of dystrophic changes. During the influenza epidemic caused by the influenza A H1N1 California virus (swine) in 2009, in many regions of Russia, a particularly severe course of the disease was noted in pregnant women with a very likely development of intrauterine influenza in fetuses.

Changes in the brain in intrauterine parainfluenza are usually localized. They form around the lateral ventricles of the brain in the form of focal cell proliferation and circulatory disorders. In isolated cases, there are indistinct papillary proliferations on the part of ependymocytes and the epithelium of the choroidal plexus.

Changes in the brain in intrauterine RS infection are usually localized. They are located around the lateral ventricles of the brain in the form of focal cell proliferation and circulatory disorders. In isolated cases, indistinct papillary proliferations were observed on the part of ependymocytes and the epithelium of the chorial plexus.

Changes in the brain in intrauterine adenovirus infection are also usually local. They form around the lateral ventricles of the brain in the form of focal cell proliferation and circulatory disorders. In single cells, intracranial basophilic inclusions are noted. In intrauterine adenovirus infection, along with the above-described hemo- and cerebrospinal fluid changes, the appearance of cells with characteristic intracranial inclusions can be noted, primarily in the meninges, as well as in the choroidal plexuses and in the brain substance. It is extremely difficult to judge the frequency of such lesions, since their clinical and laboratory diagnostics are practically not carried out anywhere in the world, and deaths in recent years are extremely rare.

References

1. Kurent JE, Sever JL. Pathogenesis of intrauterine infections of the brain. In: Biology of brain dysfunction, vol. 3. NewYork: Pleneim Publishing Corp; 1975. p. 307–41.
2. De Vries LS. Viral infections and the neonatal brain. Semin Pediatr Neurol. 2020;32:100769.
3. Larroche JC, Amiel-Tisson C, Dreyfus Brisae C. In: Aladujem S, Brown AK, Surcau S, editors. Fetal and neonatal brain: clinical perinatology. London: St-Louis-Toronto; 1980. p. 116–59.
4. Zinserling VA, Melnikova VF. Perinatal Infections: issues of pathogenesis, morphological diagnostic and clinic-pathological correlations. Manual for doctors. 2002. "Elbi-SPb", 351 p (In Russian).
5. Leung AKCV, Hon KL, Leong KF. Rubella (German measles) revisited. Hong Kong Med J. 2019;25(2):134–41. https://doi.org/10.12809/hkmj187785.
6. Tsinzerling VA, Gorelik ND, Naglenko BP. Intrauterine mycoplasmosis in child of 4 months. Vopr Okhr Mat Det. 1985;10:65–8.
7. Vaĭnshenker II, Kalinina OV, Nuralova IV, Ivchenko IM, Meliucheva LA, Tsinzerling VA. Low-manifest infections in children and adolescents with consequences of perinatal damage of nervous system. Zh Mikrobiol Epidfemiol Immunobiol. 2012;5:77–80.
8. Erman BA, Shabunina NR, Tulakina LG, Poluisakhtova MV, Golovko VD. Central nervous system lesions in fetuses and newborns in intrauterine infection caused by respiratory viruses. Arkh Patol. 1998;60(2):27–31.

17 Hidden Encephalitis in Prolonged Disorders of Consciousness (in Collaboration with Y.I. Vainshenker)

17.1 Problems of Prolonged Disorders of Consciousness from the Standpoint of Infectious Pathology

Prolonged disorders of consciousness, PDoC[1] is a severe consequence of traumatic brain injury or acute nontraumatic brain injury (hypoxia, stroke, etc.), in which, after coming out of a coma, the consciousness of patients remains "quantitatively" disturbed: in the presence of wakefulness, awareness is absent (vegetative state, VS) or minimal (minimally conscious state "minus"/ "plus", MCS (−)/(+)) [1].

Infectious pathology is one of the most frequent complications of traumatic brain injuries, as well as other severe acute brain lesions. The most well-known are severe intra- and extracranial purulent-septic complications. They usually develop in the acute period after brain damage and largely determine the high mortality of patients in a coma and in the first months after coming out of it. They manifest a vivid clinical picture of inflammation and endogenous intoxication [2].

Over time, chronic inflammatory processes come to the fore—infectious-associated "attributes" of bedridden, severely disabled patients with swallowing disorders and numerous stomas. Typical are chronically recurrent inflammatory diseases of the urinary tract, tracheobronchial tree, and other internal organs, as well as trophic disorders with the formation of bedsores [3]. The infectious component is often not studied. It is obvious that exogenous infection (including within the framework of a hospital infection), activation of its own local dormant infection, and translocation of the intestinal microbiota can be important. Taking into account the general chronically severe condition of patients, it is not surprising that 98% of patients have general immunity disorders [4].

In addition to the above, patients may have various syndromes [3, 5] that do not exclude infectious genesis. Indirectly, this is evidenced by the frequent resistance to symptomatic therapy, the failure of surgical treatment, and so on. Such conditions include hydrocephalus (often from impaired resorption or partially obstructing the ventricles), symptomatic epilepsy, sympathetic hyperactivity, violation of thermoregulation, and so on. In addition, patients have rapidly progressive brain atrophy [3], which can only partially be explained by reactive changes as a consequence of trauma.

Note that the pathogenesis of PDoC (as well as prognosis and treatment) as a whole remains

[1] Note. PDoC is set at a time > 28 days after brain damage, but VS and MCS can last indefinitely, up to decades. Chronic VS refers to cases of VS lasting >12 months from the moment of traumatic and > 3 months from nontraumatic brain injury (if chronic VS lasts 6 and 3 months, respectively, it is considered permanent) [1]

V. Zinserling, *Infectious Lesions of the Central Nervous System*,
https://doi.org/10.1007/978-3-030-96260-9_17

poorly understood. The main direction of fundamental research of PDoC is realized within the framework of the search for the structural and functional foundations of disturbed consciousness with an insignificant role of comorbid states (and their causes). This applies to both lifetime and postmortem studies [3, 5]. A possible infectious aspect is terra incognita, despite the fact that infectious pathology, in particular occult infections, is listed among other factors that negatively affect the effectiveness of rehabilitation [6].

A little more attention is paid to infection in the study of other neurodegenerative processes, in the final of which patients may also end up in VS [7]. In the pathogenesis of CNS diseases with "quantitative" or "qualitative" impairment of consciousness (Alzheimer's disease, Parkinson's disease, schizophrenia, autism, etc.), as well as autoimmune diseases, infection is considered as an initiating or provoking factor (See Chap. 20). The main attention is paid to chronic, often asymptomatic infections. Based on factors such as widespread prevalence, contagiousness, diverse transmission routes, biological properties, including the ability to persist and modulate apoptosis for a long time, experimental and morphological studies, bacteria with an intracellular development cycle (especially Chlamydia spp.) and herpes viruses are considered likely pathogens. Other pathogens are also being discussed – fungal hyphae and so on.

Taking into account the above features, we (Y.I. Vainshenker in collaboration with I.V. Nuralova, et al.) conducted a study of clinically low-symptomatic (otherwise hidden) infectious pathology in PDoC, in comparison with other noncommunicable diseases of the central nervous system. Below are the most important results of this unique pilot long-term study concerning PDoC [[4, 8], and unpublished data]. It is based on the analysis of a comprehensive step-by-step examination of 68 patients in PDoC (a solid sample), of which 50 are traumatic, 18 are nontraumatic. By the time the examination began, 1 month had passed in all patients since coming out of the coma. By the time the examination began, 1 month had passed in all patients since coming out of the coma up to 10 years, while they were in VS – 43 (of which in chronic VS – 15, according to the terms already corresponding to permanent), in MCS – 25. Cerebrospinal fluid (CSF), blood, nasopharyngeal mucosal scrapings, and conjunctiva, and, if necessary, other biomaterials were examined in vivo. Culturally and/or using PCR in all biomaterials – CSF, blood, scrapings from the mucous membranes of the nasopharynx and conjunctiva, as well as others, various representatives of bacterial, including those with intracellular development cycles, fungal and viral infections were determined. Markers of immunopathological conditions were detected in the CSF and blood serum. At the same time, the level of consciousness and the data of neurophysiological studies, including positron emission tomography, were recorded. All studies were carried out regardless of the presence/absence of typical manifestations of the inflammatory process (in vivo and during autopsy).

17.2 Identification of Infectious Agents and their Tropicity to the Central Nervous System

Cases of purulent-septic complications of the early period of trauma, which occurred according to the anamnesis in almost all patients, are not considered in this work.

Despite the absence of typical signs of a generalized infectious process in the vast majority of patients, only 5% of the examined patients had sterile CSF and blood, and all of them suffered a traumatic brain injury ($p < 0.001$). In the remaining 95% of patients, different pathogens in different combinations were detected in the CSF and/or blood during an in-depth study (Table 17.1). Taking into account the study of other biomaterials, the absence of various pathogens was found in 2% of patients, while the remaining 97% of patients were infected.

Nosocomial bacterial pathogens (*Staphylococcus hyicus*, *S. aureus*, MRSA, *Pseudomonas aeruginosa*), as well as *Candida* spp., were rare in the CSF/blood, in 6% of patients ($p < 0.001$). Clinically,

Table 17.1 Hidden pathogens at PDoC: infection cases (%) and tropism to different biomaterials

Hidden pathogens and number of examined, n	Pathogen revealed ≥1 biomaterial	
	Number of cases, %	Relation of detection – CSF: blood: mucous membranes (nasopharynx, conjunctiva)
I intestinal microbiota located extraintestinally Capsular forms of *Bacteroides fragilis*, n = 68	59%	1,2: 1: 1,2
II *chlamydia/mycoplasma/Ureaplasma* spp. (≥ *1*), *n* = 68	84%	–
Chlamydia spp.	56%	1,2: 1,2: 1
Mycoplasma spp.	38%	1: 1,2: 1,2
Ureaplasma spp.	28%	1,3: 1: 1,4
III. *Herpesviridae* 1–6 (≥ *1*), *n* = 62	76%	–
Herpes simplex virus 1,2	11%	0: 1: 7
Epstein Barr virus	42%	1: 13: 18
Human herpes virus type 6	56%	1: 2: 6
Cytomegalovirus	27%	1: 2: 6
Varicella zoster virus	3%	0: 1: 0
I/ II/III (or/and), *n* = 62	97%	–

all these cases were manifest, diagnosed within 3–6 months after traumatic brain injury. In flushes from the tracheobronchial tree, in urine, especially with exacerbation of the corresponding inflammatory processes, these and other commensal bacteria and fungi were detected in almost all of the examined cases (data are not provided).

Both in purulent-septic and in other cases, regardless of clinical manifestation, three conditional groups of pathogens were identified in biomaterials: (a) representatives of the intestinal microbiota—pathogenic (capsular) *Bacteroides fragilis*; (b) bacteria with an intracellular development cycle – *Chlamydia* spp. *Mycoplasma* spp., *Ureaplasma* spp., (c) viruses of the *Herpesviridae* family 1–6.

Only in 3% of cases, these pathogens themselves (*B. fragilis* and *C. psittaci*), without the participation of ordinary commensal bacteria and fungi, were associated with purulent focal meningoencephalitis. The pathology was revealed accidentally, with a planned magnetic resonance imaging (MRI) with contrast, 7 and 13 months after a traumatic brain injury. The clinical picture was not special for PDoC: sympathetic hyperactivity with a violation of thermoregulation, as well as spasticity-dystonia with retrolaterocollis and muscle spasms (after etiotropic treatment, sympathetic hyperactivity, muscle spasms, and retrocollis regressed). Taking into account the relatively (for PDoC) erased clinical picture described, all these pathogens as a whole were called hidden pathogens.

The spectrum of hidden pathogens in PDoC is presented in Table 17.1. The most common (taking into account the occurrence in the CSF and/or blood) were *Chlamydia* spp. and capsular (pathogenic) forms of *B. fragilis*. These pathogens were detected with equal frequency and were typically detected in the CSF/intrathecally. *Ureaplasma* spp. were also tropic to the central nervous system and to a lesser extent *Mycoplasma* spp. At the same time, *Herpesviridae* 1–6 were rarely detected in the CSF ($p < 0.001$).

Hidden pathogens ($n = 62$) typically occurred in the form of associations. As a rule (81% of cases, $p < 0.001$), different groups of pathogens were combined: *Chlamydia*/*Mycoplasma*/*Ureaplasma* spp. with *Herpesviridae* 1–6 and/or with B. fragilis (all three groups were found together in 24%). In addition, in 76% of cases there were different combinations of herpesviruses, and in 84% there were combinations of different genera (*Chlamydia* spp., *Mycoplasma* spp., *Ureaplasma* spp.) and/or bacterial species with an intracellular development cycle among themselves. For example, *Chlamydia* spp. in the CSF/intrathecally ($n = 18$), the ratio *C. trachomatis*: *C. pneumoniae*: *C. psittaci* was represented equal 10:9:4 (3:2:1).

To detect *Chlamydia* spp., *Mycoplasma* spp., *Ureaplasma* spp. repeated laboratory and even morphological studies were often required. Such difficult-to-diagnose "veiled forms" of pathogens in the central nervous system have been found in *Chlamydia* spp. – in 23%, in *Mycoplasma* spp. – 35%, in *Ureaplasma* spp. – 43% of cases. The presence of these forms correlated: with the presence in the CSF of ≥2 genera of bacteria with an intracellular development cycle ($p < 0.01$, RR = 35); with the cystic-adhesive process in the brain ($p < 0.05$); with a period of 2–4 months after nonspecific antibacterial therapy ($p < 0.05$). However, the presence of antibodies to *Chlamydia* spp. in the CSF strictly reflected the existence of the pathogen itself in the central nervous system (p < 0.01).

17.3 Immune Effector Reactions of Hidden Pathogens

Ninety-three percent of patients in PDoC had significantly elevated levels of the myelin basic protein in the CSF. The fact, although established by us for the first time, did not cause surprise: the myelin basic protein is an indicator of nonspecific demyelination and was expected in patients with brain damage and progression of its atrophy.

In addition to the myelin basic protein, 89% of patients had markers of autoimmune processes: inflammatory demyelination (in 68%) and/or systemic autoimmune disorder (in 71%). The presence of both intrathecal (inflammatory demyelination) and systemic autoimmune disorder was demonstrated in 47% of patients. Cases of increased content of the myelin basic protein did not correlate with autoimmune disorders ($p > 0.05$).

Autoimmune indicators of both the intrathecal and systemic response were polymorphic and occurred in various combinations. In absolute values, they, as a rule, only slightly exceeded the control values. Inflammatory demyelination (≥ 1 indicator) included: oligoclonal IgGs types 2,3,4 (32%), kappa free light chains (12%), lambda free light chains (60%). Systemic autoimmune disorder (≥1 indicator): antinuclear factor (antibodies) (16%), beta-2 glycoprotein 1 antibody (16%), anti-endothelial cell antibodies (26%), anticomplement 1q antibody (8%), cryoglobulins (23%), circulating immune complexes (35%). In addition, 51% had significantly increased levels of c-reactive protein.

A reliable association of hidden pathogens with laboratory markers of inflammatory demyelination (excluding the myelin basic protein) and systemic autoimmune disorder has been established. It is important to emphasize that hidden pathogens individually had not only direct but also inverse correlations with effector reactions ($p < 0.05$–$p < 0.01$), and a modulation of the relative risk (↓↑ RR = 2.9–10) of effector reactions could be observed in a pair, including "immunologically indifferent" pathogens. The same pathogen can have a number of effector reactions, manifested depending on the localization of the pathogen (CSF, blood).

Among the microorganisms directly correlating with inflammatory demyelination, the most significant were *Chlamydia*/*Mycoplasma*/*Ureaplasma* spp. when they are in the CSF/intrathecally, especially *Chlamydia* spp. (including "veiled forms"). The leading pathogen (pathogens) for the development of systemic autoimmune disorder has not been established.

17.4 Diagnostic Capabilities and Morphological Confirmation

As already noted, since PDoC almost completely revealed hidden pathogens and associated immune responses, it was not possible to identify their clinical features, perhaps, taking into account the features of the clinical picture of PDoC. Perhaps, taking into account the features of the clinical picture of PDoC.

Classical CSF and neuroimaging signs of CNS infection were not observed in the vast majority of cases ($p < 0.001$). Thus, moderate cytosis in the CSF ([Me =52] cells /3 μl, N = 0–15 cells/3 μl) associated with these pathogens was present only in 5% of cases. Moderate protein-cell dissociation was usually detected with/without a decrease/increase in glucose, as well as with a decrease in

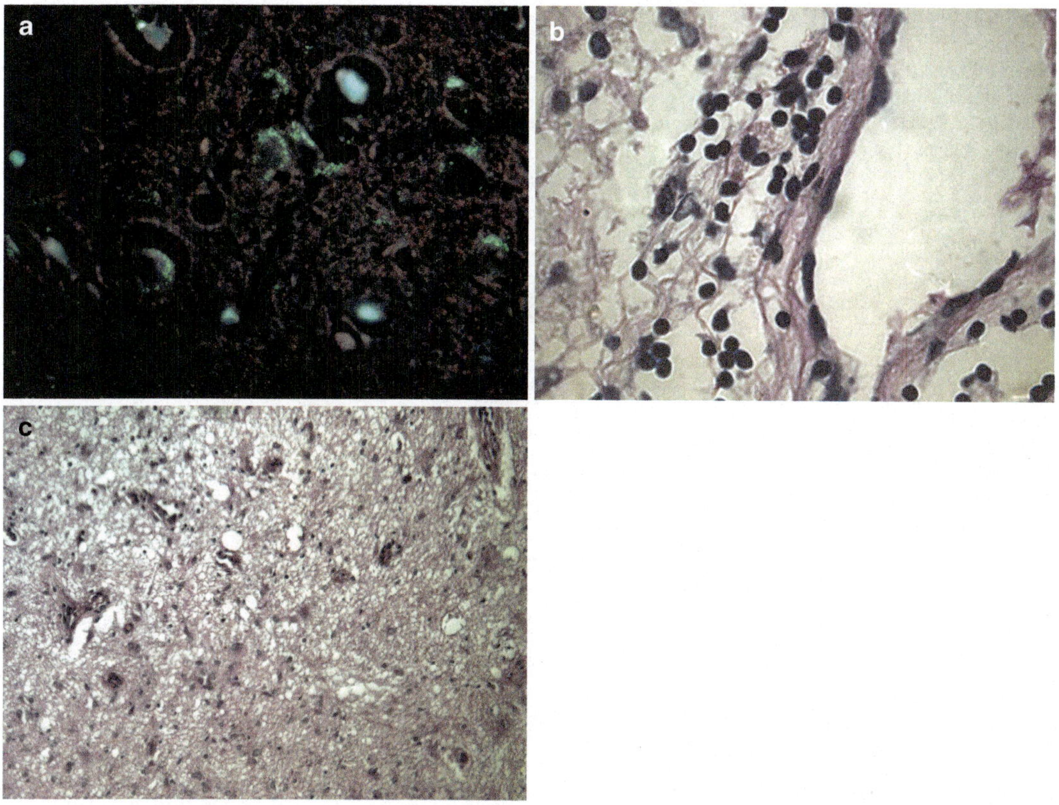

Fig. 17.1 Microscopic examination of the brain in PDoC patients who were not treated against hidden pathogens. (**a**) Lightening of Chlamydia antigen in nervous cells luminescent microscopy ×1000. (**b**) Brain vasculitis. Small PAS-positive inclusions in vacuolated cytoplasm of perivascular macrophages. PAS-staining. ×1000. (**c**) Focal demyelination. H-E. ×200

chlorides. Contrast-enhanced MRI revealed only cases of purulent focal meningoencephalitis (which was rare), as well as cases of acute transient demyelination. The latter was also extremely rare (in 5% of patients with laboratory-confirmed inflammatory demyelination).

The only but absolute proof of the presence of a hidden infectious-immunopathological process in the brain was an in-depth morphological study (conducted by V. Zinserling). We emphasize that in the presence of only hidden encephalitis, macroscopic signs of an inflammatory process in the brain were usually not observed.

In patients who did not receive targeted etiotropic therapy from hidden pathogens, the following pathogens were found in the brain: *Chlamydia* spp. and other pathogens, their "veiled forms," widespread vasculitis, and demyelination (confirmed by lifetime laboratory data). In addition to brain damage, there were also signs of the presence of the infection under discussion in other organs and tissues (Fig. 17.1). On the contrary, after effective treatment of hidden pathogens with regression of autoimmune laboratory parameters, no microbial agents or signs of immunopathology were detected at autopsy (death as a result of sudden cardiac arrest unrelated to treatment).

17.5 Infectious Pathology as a Participant in the Pathogenesis of Prolonged Disorders of Consciousness

The occurrence of hidden pathogens did not depend significantly on the etiology, nature of brain damage, and other factors associated with "surgical" infection. The exception was the fact

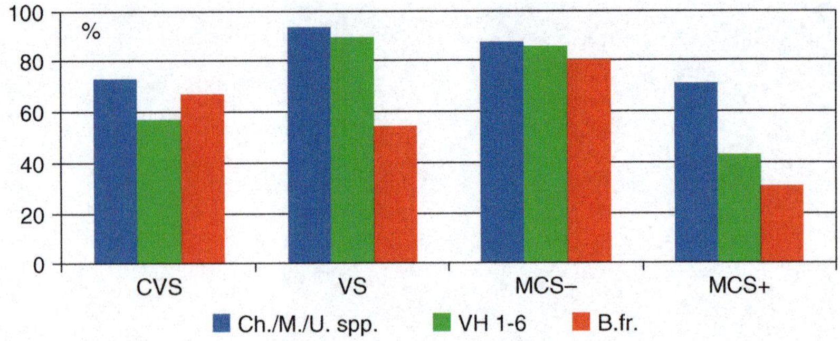

Fig. 17.2 Frequency of detection of different groups of hidden pathogens in patients in PDoC at different levels of consciousness with the release of chronic VS.

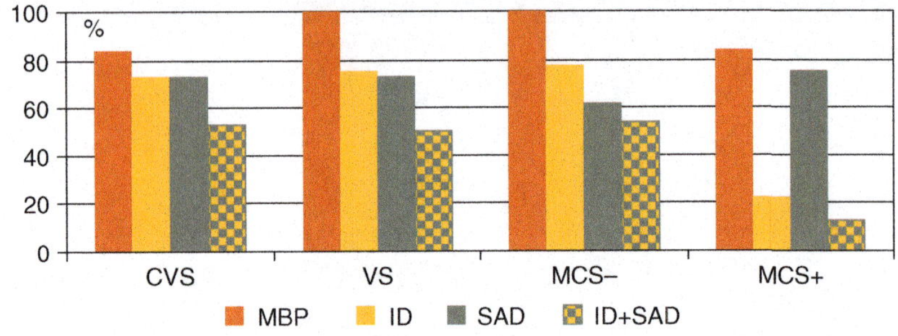

Fig. 17.3 Frequency of detection of laboratory markers of autoimmune disorders in PDoC patients at different levels of consciousness with the release of chronic VS)

that lymphotropic viruses in the CSF and blood prevailed in patients who had previously suffered sepsis and severe intracranial purulent-septic complications ($p < 0.05$).

Significant correlations were established between the detectability of hidden pathogens (according to the study of CSF, blood and mucous membranes) and the levels of disturbed consciousness, as well as the timing of VS (chronic, non-chronic) (Fig. 17.2).

The occurrence of *B. fragilis*, despite the jump of detection at the first stages of recovery from coma, decreased to a minimum with MCS(+) ($p < 0.01$). For intracellular bacteria and herpesviruses (with some differences in individual pathogens), the occurrence was maximal with non-chronic VS and MCS(−), decreasing ($p < 0.05$, $p < 0.01$, respectively) both with chronic VS and with the improvement of consciousness to MCS(+). As it was found, in addition to individual microorganisms, combinations of hidden pathogens associated with inflammatory demyelination had functional significance. Intracellular bacteria (especially *Chlamydia spp.* in CSF) always played a negative role, while the contribution of the others was not so unambiguous.

Like hidden pathogens, inflammatory demyelination (≥1 indicator collectively) also did not correlate with the etiology of brain damage. Its occurrence (and/or absolute values of indicators) usually decreased only starting from the second year of PDoC and became minimal with the improvement of consciousness – MCS(+) ($p < 0.05$). (Figure 17.3) Note that the degree of increase in myelin basic protein was greater in traumatic brain injury (compared with other etiology) ($p < 0.01$), which is natural for a nonspecific indicator. Nevertheless, its maximum absolute value was observed at non-chronic VS ($p < 0.05$), and isolated cases of norm corresponded to long-term PDoC ($p < 0.05$) – chronic VS and MCS(+).In contrast to demyelination, systemic autoimmune disorder (≥1 indicator cumulatively) was more common in non-traumatic PDoC ($p < 0.05$). In addition, the dependence on the duration of PDoC and the level of consciousness of patients was not established ($p > 0.05$), although some trends were outlined for individual indicators. The increase in c-reactive protein prevailed in terms up to 3 months PDoC ($p < 0.01$).

The combination of both inflammatory demyelination and systemic autoimmune disorder was more common in nontraumatic PDoC ($p < 0.01$) and during the first year of PDoC ($p < 0.05$); less common in patients with MCS(+) compared with VS and MCS(−) ($p < 0.05$). (Figure 17.3).

A comparison of the treatment results of two groups of patients (a) who received standard therapy—the ST group ($n = 26$) and (b) who received in addition to the standard treatment for all hidden pathogens—the HPT group ($n = 24$) confirmed the above results. Note that, if necessary, treatment for nosocomial infections was carried out as part of standard therapy.

During repeated sampling of biomaterial, it was found that as all hidden pathogens (HPT group) were treated, "veiled" forms of pathogens began to appear as a stage, immunopathological reactions gradually regressed (laboratory data). This was not observed in the ST group ($p < 0.05$).

However, the most significant result was a change in consciousness associated with treatment from hidden pathogens.

In the first 1–3 months from the start of therapy in the HPT group, the improvement of consciousness was more significant than in the ST group, in which both an increase and a decrease in the level of consciousness relative to the baseline level were noted ($p < 0.01$). The improvement in the HPT group in both patients in VS and patients in MCS was realized due to mobility, visual responsiveness, and auditory comprehension ($p < 0.01$). There was no significant difference between the groups in the improvement of respiration ($p = 0.055$) and verbal communication. Within the HPT group, the result was better ($p < 0.01$) if the patients were in MCS (compared to VS), which corresponds to well-known ideas about the prognosis of PDoC (Fig. 17.4). There is no significant difference within the ST group.

Along with clinical improvement, positive dynamics of electrophysiological parameters (electroencephalography (EEG); evoked brain potentials), as well as improvement of glucose metabolism (positron emission tomography, PET) in certain areas of its initial violation were noted in the same time frame. Sometimes, neurophysiological indicators preceded clinical improve-

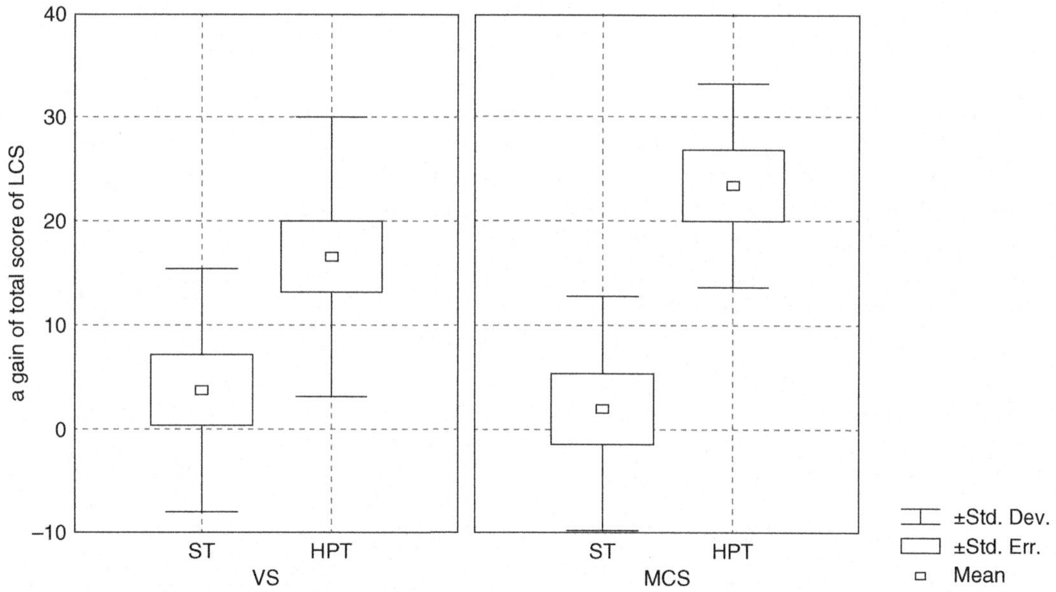

Fig. 17.4 Change of consciousness (a gain of total score of Loewenstein communication scale, LCS [9]) in patients in VS and MCS after 1–3 months of standard therapy (ST, $n = 26$) and with additional treatment of hidden pathogens (HPT, $n = 24$). Explanation in the text

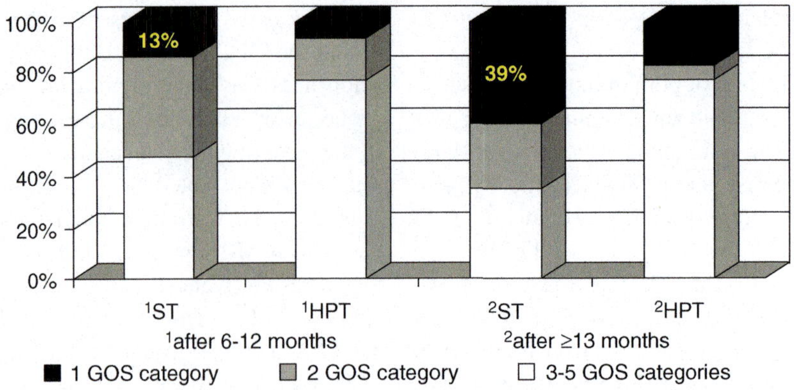

Fig. 17.5 PDoC outcomes after standard therapy (ST, $n = 23$) and with additional treatment of hidden pathogens (HPT, $n = 18$). Explanation in the text. *GOS* Glasgow Outcome scale. Categories of GOS: 1 – dead; 2 – vegetative state; 3,4,5 – severely, moderately disabled, and good recovery (combined here)

ment. Areas of improvement (EEG, PET) corresponded to neurological manifestations.

The further state of patients from the HPT group was also more optimistic than patients from the ST group (Fig. 17.5): there were more cases of improvement of consciousness to MCS and higher—both after 6–12 months ($p < 0.05$) and later ($p < 0.01$). Within the ST group, an increase ($p < 0.05$) in mortality was observed over time.

It should be noted that in addition to improving the functional state of the brain and consciousness (the HPT group), there were improvement in the general condition of patients, in some cases – clinical and EEG remission of epileptic syndrome, a decrease in the severity of sympathetic hyperactivity, muscle spasms, severity of pathological muscular hypertonicity (especially with a spastic posture "resembling" meningeal syndrome), violent crying, etc.

17.6 Conclusion

Of course, there are many questions, especially from the standpoint of infectious pathology. However, it is already obvious that hidden pathogenic microorganisms, as well as their effector reactions, cannot be considered separately (with at least PDoC). The pilot data obtained indicate that there is a single clinically erased infectious process (hidden infection) provided by different pathogens affiliated with each other.

The study of hidden infection that disrupts the functional state of the brain in PDoC is a new direction in the study of these conditions. The data we have provided indicate the prospects of such an approach. At the same time, the involvement of the translocated intestinal microbiota in the process of the consciousness changing confirms the idea of the relationship between the state of the body and the state of the brain, even at the microbiological level. It is obvious that the detection of hidden encephalitis (especially with the participation of bacteria with intracellular type of development and inflammatory demyelination), although formally aggravates the severity of the condition of patients, including potentiating neurodegeneration, in fact it is a favorable prognostic factor (taking into account further targeted etiotropic treatment). At the same time, the good news is that most patients have this opportunity, regardless of the length of stay in PDoC .

References

1. Royal College of Physicians. Prolonged disorders of consciousness following sudden onset brain injury: national clinical guidelines report of the 2020 working group. London: RCP; 2020. p. 200.
2. Scheld WM, Whitley RJ, Marra CM, editors. Infections of the central nervous system. 4th ed. Philadelphia: Walters Kluwer Health, LWW; 2014. p. 875.
3. Dolce G, Sazbon L, editors. The post-traumatic vegetative state. Stuttgart, New York: Thieme; 2002. p. 158.

4. Vainshenker YI, Ivchenko IM, Tsinzerling VA, Nuralova IV, et al. Low manifest infections with CNS damage in patients in prolonged unconscious state of non-inflammatory etiology. J Mikrobiol Epidemiol Immunobiol. 2011;6:85–9. [in Russian.]
5. Giacino JT, Fins JJ, Laureys S, Schiff ND. Disorders of consciousness after acquired brain injury: the state of science. Nat Rev Neurol. 2014;10(2):99–114.
6. Giacino JT, White J, Nakase-Richardson R, Katz DI, Arciniegas DB, et al. Minimum competency recommendations for programs that provide rehabilitation services for persons with disorders of consciousness: a position statement of the American Congress of Rehabilitation Medicine and the National Institute on disability, independent living and rehabilitation research traumatic brain injury model systems. Arch Phys Med Rehabil. 2020;101:1072–89.
7. Wainshenker Yu.I. [*Vainshenker Yu.I.*], Nuralova I.V., Onishchenko L.S. Chlamydial infection of the central nervous system. Laboratory diagnosis and clinic and morphological features. Arkh Patologii 2014; 76 (1): 57–62. [in Russian.]
8. Vaynshenker J. [*Vainshenker Yu.I.*], Ivchenko I.M., Tsinserling V.A., Korotkov A.D., Melucheva L.A. Infectious factors of brain damage in prolonged unconscious states. Ann Clin Exp Neurol. 2014; 8(3): 21–29.[in Russian.]
9. Borer-Alafi N, Gil M, Sazbon L, Korn C. Loewenstein communication scale for the minimally responsive patients. Brain Inj. 2002;16(7):593–609.

18 Problems of Neuroinfections of Mixed Etiology

Despite the considerable importance of viral-bacterial associations in pathology, especially in childhood [1], including respiratory infections [2], the study of this issue in neuroinfections has almost not been conducted. The possibility to detect simultaneously several pathogens behind BBB was also noted by WI Lipkin and M Hornig [3]. There are only a few publications devoted to the description of individual cases of a combination of meningococcal infection or purulent meningitis with influenza or herpes. There are also isolated descriptions of the combined influenza-herpetic etiology of acute encephalitis.

Some of the most intriguing concepts in viral pathogenesis involve complex mechanisms that include infections with other microbes (other viruses, bacteria, or parasites), immunogenic variations, or a timing component. The most straightforward instances are those where viral infection results in immunosuppression that enables opportunistic infections. The most dramatic example is HIV. When speaking about brain complications, we mention encephalitis due to *Toxoplasma gondii,* cytomegalovirus (Fig.18.1), *Cryptococcus neoformans* (see also Chaps. 7 and 13). We do not possess data concerning frequency and clinical relevance of such combinations. We can only assume that several pathogens meeting in one tissue can lead to different results as it was discussed in the example of respiratory infections [2].

18.1 Clinical Data

It was suggested that the frequency of viral-bacterial associations in purulent meningitis may be significant, and they may cause long-term subfebrility on the background of successful antibacterial therapy. In joint studies with M. A. Dadiomova [4], we analyzed the features of the clinical manifestations of Meningococcal infection (MI) in the case of viral-bacterial associations. The results of clinical and laboratory comparisons indicate a significantly more severe course of MI in the case of its combination with ARVI. It should be noted that the main criteria for the diagnosis of ARVI were the results of virological (serological and IF) studies. Among viral infections, influenza of various serological variants was the most naturally diagnosed. Clinical manifestations of the disease were variable and often moderately pronounced.

18.2 Morphological Data

To identify viral brain lesions, we [4] conducted a detailed comprehensive study of 94 children who died from hypertoxic forms of meningococcal infection and 57 children who died from purulent meningitis and meningoencephalitis of non-meningococcal etiology. The diagnosis of meningococcal infection in all cases was based

V. Zinserling, *Infectious Lesions of the Central Nervous System*,
https://doi.org/10.1007/978-3-030-96260-9_18

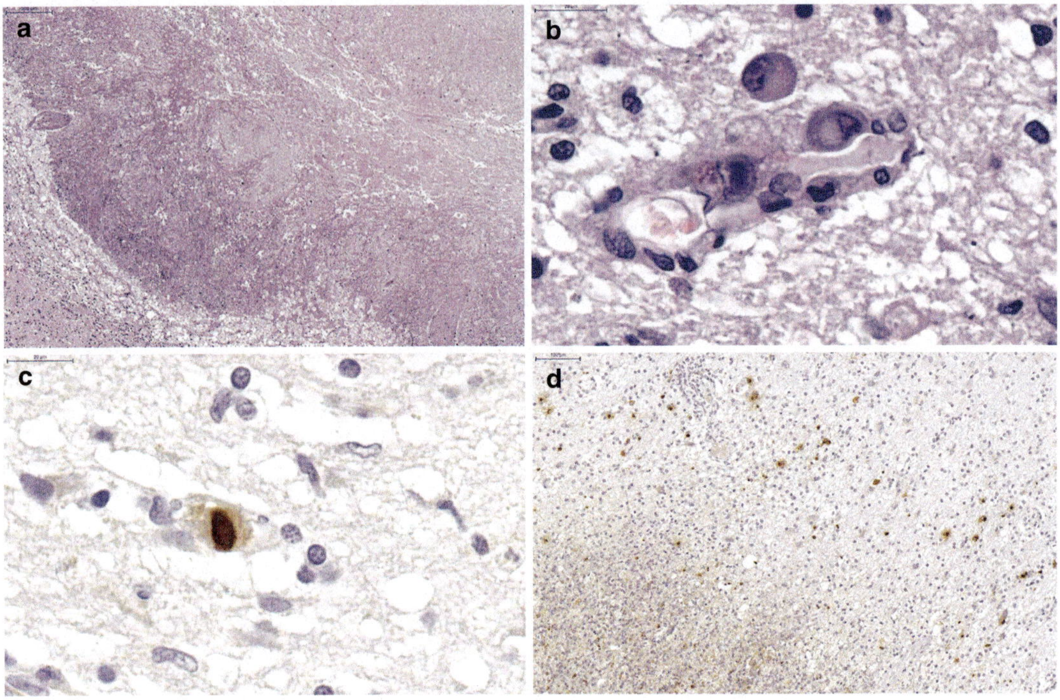

Fig. 18.1 Mixed infection CMV + toxoplasmosis in a patient with HIV infection. (**a**) general view. H-E × 40, (**b**) intracellelar toxoplams PAS-reaction × 400, (**c**) positive IHC reaction with CMV antigen × 400; (**d**) positive IHC reaction with toxoplasma antigen × 100. (Courtesy of J.R. Zyuzya)

on clinical, morphological, and bacterioscopic data, and in 19 cases on bacteriological seeding (in 7 cases—*Neisseria meningitidis* A and in 12 cases B). Among the dead children were 53 boys and 41 girls. From the age of 1 to 6 months, 13 people died; from 6 to 11 months – 23; from 1 to 3 years – 32; from 3 to 7 years – 26 and over 7 years – 7 people. The immediate cause of death in 62 children (66%) was bilateral hemorrhagic necrosis of the adrenal glands against the background of generalized thrombohemorrhagic syndrome. In 13 children, bilateral cortical necrosis in the kidneys was detected. Some of the children died from brain edema, respiratory and cardiovascular insufficiency, pneumonia, as well as other causes. Forty-five children were diagnosed with a mixed form of MI (meningococcemia +meningitis). Special attention was paid to the detection of acute viral respiratory infections, which were diagnosed in the vast majority of children who died from meningococcal infection – 88 (98%). Most often, it was influenza A (27 cases), less often influenza B (11 cases), Ad infection (4 times), parainfluenza, and MS infection (3 times each). Mixed RVIs were detected in 40 cases, including 22 cases involving influenza A. As a result of the analysis of laboratory and morphological data, the heterogeneity of the studied observations was revealed. In 51 cases, there were signs of fresh generalization of VRI with brain damage. In 13 cases, laboratory morphological comparisons made it possible to diagnose the presence of an isolated, long-existing brain lesion due to respiratory viruses. In 30 observations, there were no signs of RV brain damage. When comparing groups of children who died from MI with the presence and absence of RV brain damage, it was possible to identify a tendency to some differences. Thus, the average age of children who did not have CNS lesions with viruses was somewhat higher (almost 3 years), compared with the age of children who had such lesions (about 2 years). In the case of clinically pronounced RI before the onset of meningococcemia in children with viral brain lesions, the duration of respiratory manifestations was longer than in children of the compared group (6.4 days compared to 4.8). Most frequently, brain lesions occurred in combined RI. A subsequent analysis of 51 observations with signs of fresh generalization of VRI in the brain revealed heterogeneity of this group. If laboratory-morphological comparisons allowed us to speak about the generalization of preexisting viral infections against the background of meningococcemia in all cases, then anamnestic information about their manifestations was ambiguous. In the medical records of only 19 children, there were indications of respiratory infections of any severity that was tolerated before the development of meningococcemia. In 32 observations, such data were absent. Thus, the detailed analysis [3] allowed to conclude that viral-bacterial coinfections are present in majority of cases, clinical manifestations of viral respiratory infection are usually moderate or even absent. This phenomenon needs further study.

18.3 Results of Experimental Studies

To confirm the facts obtained on the sectional material and to study in depth the pathogenesis of influenza meningococcal infection, we [V. A. Zinserling] together with E. A. Murina, O. A. Aksenov, N. A. Korzhueva, and N. V. Berezina conducted experimental studies. In the first series of experiments, 150 white mongrel mice weighing 6–8 g were infected with influenza A0 virus and meningococcus A under light anesthesia at intervals of 1–72 h. The infecting dose for the influenza virus not adapted to mice was 100–200 LD50 and 1000 microbial cells of freshly isolated or lyophilized meningococcus. The effectiveness of the model was judged primarily on the basis of comparing animals infected with only one of the pathogens and when they were coadministered. Reproduction of the influenza virus in the lungs in the compared groups indicates a more severe course of infection in animals with combined infection, primarily due to greater reproduction of the influenza virus. The results of bacterioscopic and histobacterioscopic studies suggest a certain increase in the reproduction of meningococcus in this group.

Morphological studies were performed on 72 white mice, of which 12 animals were infected intranasally with the influenza A0 virus (1 control group); 24 mice were infected intranasally with meningococci of strains 208 and 44 (2 control group); 12 animals were once intranasally injected with saline solution (3 control group); 12 the same was done twice (4 control group). Three mice from the same batch were examined without any effects (5 control group). The main experiment was conducted on 24 animals that were administered intranasally with both influenza A0 virus and meningococci of both above strains. The animals were examined 2 h, 1, 2, and 5 days after infection (six mice for each term). Most of the animals were slaughtered with ether, only three mice were opened shortly after their fall on the fifth day after infection with influenza virus and meningococcus. The main experimental group – mice infected with both influenza virus, unadapted to the brain, and meningococci. Two hours after infection, a moderate amount of diplococci was detected in the lungs (small bronchi and alveolar passages). Here, the appearance of small but numerous accumulations of neutrophilic leukocytes was also noted. In addition, dystrophic changes in the bronchial epithelium, focal fullness, and distelectases were detected. Meninges were moderately full-blooded in all animals. On day 1, all animals had loose, mainly leukocyte infiltrates that occupied 15–20% of the lung area in the studied areas. In the area of these foci and outside of them, there were a significant number of small, mostly paired cocci. Dystrophic changes in bronchial epithelial cells were detected with an increase in individual cells in size. Moderate fullness of the lung tissue and significant fullness of both the brain substance and the MMO and vascular plexuses were also detected. On day 2, the changes remained the same, but became more common. The number of diplococci remained quite significant, with many of them continuing to be located freely. From the side of the lung vessels, there is an expansion, edema of the wall, and aggregation of part of the red blood cells in their lumen. Individual diplococci were detected on such red blood cells. Changes of a similar nature were observed on the part of the vessels of the soft meninges of the brain, as well as the vascular plexus. On the part of the substance of the brain itself, only fullness was detected. On the fifth day after infection, the changes were most pronounced. In the respiratory organs of all animals, a sharp fullness was determined, the accumulation of serous exudates in both the respiratory tract and alveoli, and the occurrence of large foci of pneumonia with mainly leukocyte exudates, which occupied an area of 10–70% of lung square. Diplococci, mostly free-lying, were detected in approximately the same amount as on day 2. In one mouse, their number was much larger and they were located in large clusters. Along with this, there were widespread and quite severe changes in the bronchial and alveolar epithelium. Most of its cells underwent dystrophic changes, significantly increased in size, and desquamated. Changes in the brain were similar to those detected on day 2 (Fig. 18.2). They consisted in pronounced changes on the part of the blood vessels, in which the aggregation of red blood cells continued to be detected, and diplococci were found on their surface. As before, there was no clear leukocyte reaction.

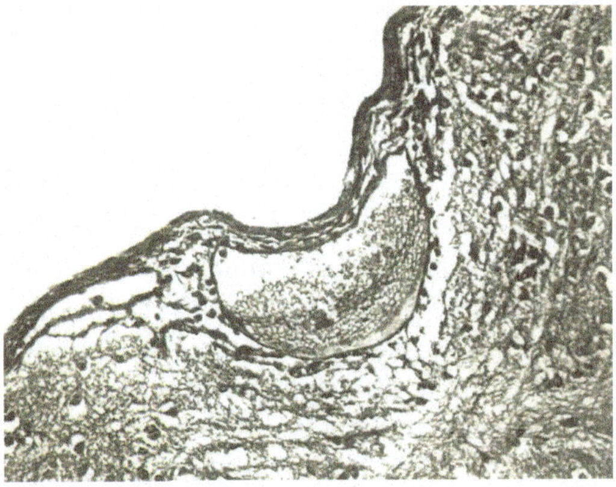

Fig. 18.2 Sharp fullnes and mixed infiltration in soft meninges in mouse on the 2 day after challenge with neurotropic strain of influenza virus and meningococcus. H-E × 600

In 1 control group, mice infected only with A influenza virus (see also Chap. 7). After 2 h, they had only focal uneven fullness of the lungs and MMO. After day 1, along with this, there were dystrophic changes in the cells of the bronchial epithelium with an increase in their size, mainly due to the cytoplasm. On day 2, the severity of changes in the respiratory tract became even greater, dystrophic changes in the epithelium grew, and quite common peribronchial lymphocytic infiltrates appeared. In the same areas, an increase in the size of individual alveolocytes was observed, mainly due to basophilic stained cytoplasm. Some of these cells were exfoliated into the lumen of the alveoli. Along with this, there was also a little serous exudate. Changes in the brain were not detected. On day 5, there was a moderate progression of the same changes in the lungs, which consisted in a significant increase in the number of affected alveolocytes, a greater accumulation of serous exudates in the lumen of the alveoli, and greater vascular fullness. In some of them, the aggregation of red blood cells occurred. The airiness of the lungs remained, and distelectases were noted in some places. On the part of the brain, only moderately pronounced circulatory disorders were noted.

In group 2, mice infected with meningococci alone. The changes detected when using both strains of Meningococcus turned out to be of the same type both qualitatively and quantitatively, which allows them to be described in summary. After 2 hours after infection, a rather sharp fullness was detected in the lungs in one mouse with widespread hemorrhage. In addition, there were small but widespread mainly perivascular accumulations of neutrophilic leukocytes and histiocytes. In the small bronchi, alveolar passages, and alveoli, in particular, in those areas where infiltration was noted, small groups of small and paired cocci were also found. In the brain of two out of six animals, there was a moderate fullness of meninges. Microbes were not detected here. After 1 day, only rare diplococci were detected in the lungs of all animals, and the severity of the leukocyte reaction was less than before. The area of airless foci was 5–10%. The brain changes remained the same. On day 2, only a small number of mainly phagocyted diplococci remained in the lungs. The volume of airless foci did not change, but macrophages began to significantly predominate in them, while the number of neutrophilic leukocytes significantly decreased. Along with this, edema of the walls of small blood vessels, the formation of small blood clots in their lumen, and minor hemorrhages were noted. In the brain, uneven fullness, moderate edema of the walls of blood vessels, occasionally very small lymphocytic infiltration of the soft meninges. On the fifth day, the area of airless foci in the lungs decreased to 2–5% in the studied areas. Loose macrophage exudates prevailed here. The germs were almost gone. The changes on the part of the lung vessels remained the same. In the brain of two out of six mice, focal fullness of meninges was noted; in the remaining animals, no structural changes were detected. Control groups 3 and 4 were mice with intranasal saline injection. Both with a single and double administration of it, only a slight focal fullness of the lungs was noted, and irregularly. There were no changes on the part of the brain. In 5 control group, intact mice. No significant morphological changes were detected.

Thus, in the case of combined influenza-meningococcal infection, a largely different course of the disease was observed compared to monoinfections. It is distinguished, first of all, by more severe manifestations of the infectious process, and in the first days mainly bacterial, and later mainly viral. There are also significantly more diplococci that persist longer in the lungs. Along with this, their dissemination also occurs in the brain, in the vessels of which, especially in the meninges and vascular plexuses, there is an aggregation of red blood cells with the presence of diplococci on them.

We also conducted a simulation of mixed influenza-meninococcal infection using a strain of influenza A0 virus adapted to the brain of mice. Information about the morphological manifestations of monoinfection is given in Sect. 7.1.3. Histological examination on day 1 in the lungs of animals showed pronounced dystrophic changes in the cells of the bronchial epithelium, distinct fullness, and serous edema. Diffuse

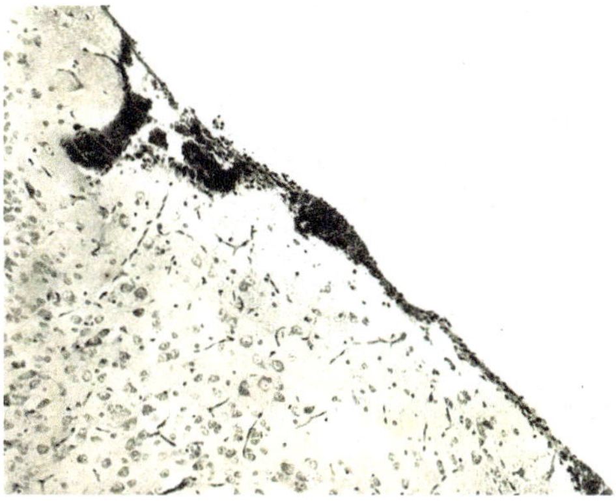

Fig. 18.3 Sharp fullness, perivascular hemorrhages and moderate lymphocytic infiltration in mouse on the fifth day after simultaneous challenge with influenza virus and meningococcus. H-E, × 200

leuco-lymphocytic infiltration captured up to one-third of the cut area. We also conducted modeling of mixed influenza-meninococcal infection using a strain of influenza A0 virus adapted to the brain of mice. In the brain, there is sometimes a significant fullness of meninges and its very moderate mainly lymphocytic infiltration. A sharp fullness of the choroidal plexus vessels and pronounced dystrophic changes in the ependymocytes of their lining. Significant dystrophic changes in nerve cells, up to the loss of some of them. On the second day after infection, there is an incipient peribronchial and perivascular lymphoplasmocytic infiltration in the lungs, covering up to half of the cut area. In the lumen of the alveoli, there is a moderate amount of "flu-like" alveolocytes. Histobacterioscopically, a few mainly phagocytic diplococci are visible. In the brain, there is a pronounced fullness meninges and their moderate, mainly lymphocytic infiltration (Fig. 18.3). Part of the arachnoendothelial cells has an enlarged dark-colored cytoplasm. In the lumen of individual vessels, and less often perivascularly, small diplococci are visible. Choroidal plexuses are full-blooded, ependymocytes of their lining, have undergone pronounced dystrophic changes, often having a loose, basophilic stained cytoplasm, and small diplococci lie on the surface of some of them. In one of the animals, a small cluster of glial cells were detected subperpendicularly near the choroidal plexus. In

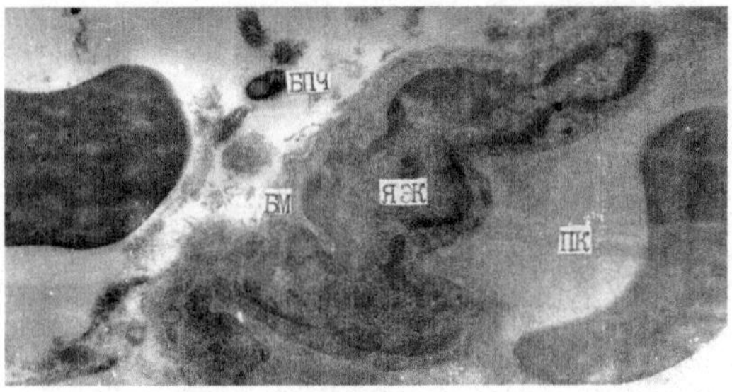

Fig. 18.4 Brain changes on the 3 day after combined challenge of mice with influenza virus and mernigococcus. Oval bodies probably are transformed menigococci. Electron microscopy × 54000 BM – basal membrane (БМ), NEC – nucleus of endothelial cell (ЯЭК), LC – lumen of capillary (ПК) BLB – bacterial-like bodies (БПЧ)

the IF study, the specific lightening was determined in single ependymocytes of the vascular plexus, lateral ventricles, as well as single cells in the substance of the brain. On the third day after infection, changes were found in the lungs, brain, thymus gland, and spleen that were fundamentally similar to those described on the second day. Only a slightly higher prevalence of pneumonic infiltration can be noted. In EM, quite pronounced changes were detected. The lumen of the capillaries was quite significantly expanded, and the endothelial lining was thinned. Endothelial cells were characterized by irregular nuclei with peripheral chromatin arrangement, absence of pinocyte vesicles, and shortening of specialized contacts. The basal membrane had scalloped borders and was formed mainly by electron-dense material with a few irregularly oriented light fibrils. The perivascular zone of the processes of astrocytic cells was mainly represented by a poorly structured electron-light material with single organoids. Virus-like structures are found in the area of the capillary basal membranes and the perivascular space. There is also the presence of oval bodies with a size of 0.1–0.2 microns, inside which there is a lighter rounded homogeneous structure, possibly representing transformed meningococci (Fig. 18.4). Individual red blood cells were also detected in the perivascular space. In the cytoplasm of the cells surrounding probable meningococci, the number of ribosomes was sharply reduced, and the mitochondria had an electron-dense matrix and swollen intracrystal gaps.

Thus, the conducted set of experimental studies confirmed a much more severe course of influenza combined with meningococcal infection. This is supported by both increased animal mortality and the results of virological, histological, IF, and EM studies. In conditions of combined infection, the pathogens most easily enter the brain, even with intranasal infection, with the development of distinct structural changes in it in many cases. The more severe course of combined infections could to some extent be associated with the well-known local and general immunosuppressive effect of the influenza virus. This facilitated the subsequent replication in the lungs of mice of meningococcus, which normally does not reproduce here. In addition, it was possible to show that the influenza virus, when combined with meningococcus in animals, changes its properties and becomes more neurotropic and acquires the ability to enter the brain during intranasal infection.

References

1. Zinserling AV, Zinserling VA. Modern infections: pathologic anatomy and issues of pathogenesis: A guide. SPb: Sotis. 2002. 346 p. (In Russ.)
2. Zinserling VA. Infectious pathology of the respiratory tract. Springer International Publishing; 2021. https://doi.org/10.1007/978-3-030-66325-4. ISBN 978-3—030-66324-7
3. Lipkin WI, Hornig M. Diagnostics and discovery in viral central nervous infections. Brain Pathol. 2015;25:600–4.
4. Zinserling VA, Chukhlovina ML. Infectious lesions of nervous system. Issues of etiology, pathogenesis and diagnostics. Saint-Petersburg: ElbiSPb; 2011. p. 583. (In Russian)

19 Differential Diagnostics in Clinical Pathology

Brain biopsies nowadays are investigated practically inclusively in order to confirm clinical and radiological diagnosis of the tumor, put the most exact morphological diagnosis corresponding the modern classification, and evaluate genetical characteristics in order to elaborate the optimal curative tactics. Similar tasks are to be solved by pathologists while studying material. Issues of neurooncopathology are the topics of special manuals and are not discussed in the present book. Clinical neurosurgery pathology was most fully summarized and illustrated by Russian D.E. Matsko [1]. Clinical pathology of neurosurgery specimen during treatment of certain form of epilepsy also allows sometimes suspect infectious and inflammatory processes [2, 3].

In several, relative rare cases, the preliminary clinical diagnosis of tumor is not confirmed by pathologists. We intend to remind what focal brain lesions can simulate tumors. Certain aspects of the problem have been discussed previously [4], but we tried to add certain issues basing upon our own experience.

As casuistic case can be regarded observation when instead of probable encephalitis at the autopsy was found brain metastasis of melanoma, primary locus of which remained unclear (Fig. 19.1).

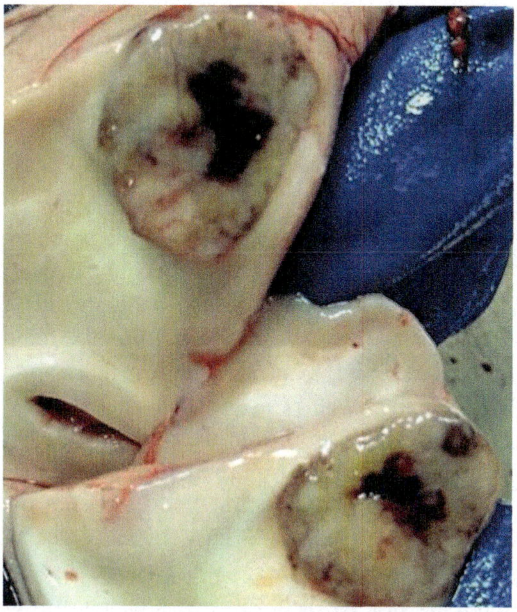

Fig. 19.1 Brain metastasis of melanoma from unknown primary node. Unexpected finding at the autopsy. Fresh macropreparation. Courtesy of AN Isakov

It should also be noted that in many cases we have to deal with a combined pathology – infectious lesions can coexist with tumors, ischemic injuries, injuries, malformations. Sometimes, such combinations can have pathogenetic significance. Below we present only those manifestations of infectious brain lesions that are of interest to neurosurgeons (focal and volumetric processes).

V. Zinserling, *Infectious Lesions of the Central Nervous System*,
https://doi.org/10.1007/978-3-030-96260-9_19

19.1 **Abscess** (See Also Chap. 11)

Among intracranial volume formations, brain abscesses account for 2–8%. In children, brain abscesses account for about 1.4% of all CNS diseases and 4.4% of neurosurgical pathology. According to the mechanism of occurrence, it is customary to distinguish between brain abscesses that have developed by contact (more often in otorhinolaryngological pathology), posttraumatic, metastatic, and post-encephalitic. In approximately 22–27% of cases, the mechanism of abscess development remains unknown. Metastatic brain abscesses of pulmonary origin are the most common in clinical practice. The localization of abscesses is predominantly supratentorial. In a third of the cases (33.3%), they are localized in the frontal lobe, slightly less often (24%) in the parietal, even less often in the temporal (13.6%) and occipital (7.6%) lobes. There are initial, manifest, and latent stages, during which the abscess is separated from the brain tissue and a capsule is formed. Usually, it takes from 4 to 6 weeks for its formation. It should be emphasized that often for a long time the brain abscess has no clinical manifestations, and the patient's well-being remains satisfactory. Diagnosis of an abscess in the initial and latent stages is quite difficult, and sometimes at the prehospital stage is almost impossible. Before the introduction of brain CT into clinical practice, the diagnosis of abscesses was usually late, the mortality rate reached 30–50%; after the use of modern neuroimaging methods, this indicator decreased to 24%. Characteristic CT and MRI signs of a formed brain abscess are: a rounded formation with a thin-walled capsule that intensively accumulates contrast material – the phenomenon of a "ring" with clear and smooth internal contours. However, with small abscess sizes, even an MRI of the brain may not be informative enough. The most common pathogens of the disease are *Staphylococcus aureus* and white staphylococcus, streptococcus, in the second place – strict anaerobes (usually bacteroids, fusobacteria, anaerobic streptococci), which can be isolated in 65% of cases. In almost half of the cases, it is possible to determine the otogenic origin of the abscess, in 15% of its development is preceded by various bronchopulmonary pathologies—abscesses, bronchiectasis, empyema, pneumonia, more often caused by fusobacteria. In 8% of cases, the development of abscesses is preceded by inflammatory processes in the sinuses of the frontal and main bones, most often caused by *B. fragilis*. Pathological examination reveals both calcified abscesses and formations that are in the encephalitic stage. In the cavity of the abscess, liquid and gas are usually detected. Histological examination reveals the focal proliferation of mainly astrocytic glia forming a capsule, as well as perivascular infiltration by neutrophilic leukocytes.

19.2 **Tuberculosis**

Tuberculosis remains important in clinical practice in many countries, among the various forms of which an important role is played by brain lesions (see Chap. 13). Along with the most frequent and relatively easy to diagnose basal meningitis/meningoencephalitis on the background of early or late hematogenous dissemination, there are also significantly more difficult cases in terms of diagnosis. Correct recognition of the nature of the process is facilitated by indications of a history of tuberculosis, prolonged contact with tuberculosis patients, the presence of tuberculosis lesions in other organs, combined with the picture of intracranial neoplasms, acute infectious diseases, respiratory diseases, and the appearance of the first symptoms of brain damage after these infections. The presence of the prodromal period of the disease, subfebrile temperature, children's and youth age of patients, subtentorial localization of the process, the presence of symptoms of multifocal brain damage, positive tuberculin reactions, increased protein in the cerebrospinal fluid and pleocytosis, mainly lymphocytic, are important. Prior to the introduction of modern methods of neuroimaging into clinical practice, in vivo recognition of brain tuberculosis occurred in 17.6% of cases. Currently, tuberculomas of the brain in adults occur in 0.87–8.8% in pulmonary tuberculosis and in 12.2% in tuberculous lesions of the central nervous system. Patients with tuberculomas of the brain are admitted to neurological or neurosurgical departments with directional diagnoses: intracranial hypertension, volume formation of the brain, acute circulatory disorders of the brain. According to the clinical course, brain tuberculomas can simulate any volume formation in the cranial cavity. During the 25 years of operation of the neurosurgical department of the Mariinsky Hospital of St. Petersburg, among 2000 patients operated on for tumors of the central nervous system, brain tuberculoma was detected in four cases [5]. Solitary tuberculomas are most often detected in the cerebellum, brain stem, and meninges, and are less often found in the large hemispheres. Histologically, the tuberculoma is a weakly vascularized granuloma with giant multinucleated cells, often with a curd-like degeneration in the center, prone to calcification.

19.3 Gumma

Neurosyphilis is one of the most well-known forms of this disease (see Sect. 13.2). At the same time, detailed descriptions of the structural changes caused by it are completely absent in the literature of the last decades. In a retrospective analysis of the materials of the Botkin Hospital's autopsy department for the post-war period, we also failed to identify any reliable observations. At the same time, given the significant increase in syphilis, we can predict a new appearance of neurosyphilis on autopsy material. We briefly present the characteristics of neurosyphilis, based on studies provided in the 20–30th of the XX century. Surely, it is impossible to fully agree with all concepts expressed in those years. According to these data, neurosyphilis was the cause of death for 42% of those who died from syphilis. In the structure of deaths from nervous and mental diseases, neurosyphilis accounted for up to 20%. It was proposed to distinguish six forms of neurosyphilis: syphilis of the cerebral vessels; syphilitic meningitis; gumma of the brain; progressive paralysis; spinal dryness; syphilitic myelitis. Syphilitic meningitis affects the base of the brain as much as possible and is considered in three variants: acute or subacute serous (with predominantly lymph-monocytic infiltration of soft meningitis); chronic (with fibrosis similar to tuberculosis); gummous (limited or diffuse with lymph-plasmocytic infiltration around sclerosed vessels and nerves). Syphilitic meningitis was considered to develop during the first year after infection. Brain gummas were more often combined with infiltrates in meninges and were tumor-like nodes of yellowish-gray or gray-pink color up to 1.5–2 cm in diameter, usually irregular in shape with indistinct borders. Spirochetes were identified in their peripheral zone. The main differential diagnosis was recommended to be carried out with solitary tuberculomas.

19.4 Focal Lesions of Viral Etiology

In this group of focal injuries of the nervous system, the first place belongs to herpesviridae family. This is due to both the widespread prevalence of herpetic viruses and the severity of the damage to the nervous tissue caused by them (see Chap. 5). At the same time, the herpesvirus has the ability to persist for many years in the sensitive ganglia, mainly in the ganglia of the trigeminal nerve, remaining in a latent form and causing exacerbations in the presence of various resolving factors. Acute focal necrotic encephalitis with intracranial inclusions in nerve and glial cells is considered as the most typical and frequent. Among other variants of herpes lesions – tumor-like encephalitis has to be mentioned. Typical inclusions are rounded, eosinophilic, homogeneous, or granular, and are more commonly referred to as Cowdry bodies of type A (a or 1). For a long time, they were considered the "gold standard" for the diagnosis of herpetic encephalitis in biopsies. Currently, PCR is considered as the most reliable method of clinical diagnosis. Due to the fact that herpetic rashes on the skin in such patients are rare, carrying out a differential diagnosis causes significant difficulties. Quite often, these patients with directional diagnoses: acute cerebrovascular accident, subarachnoid hemorrhage are hospitalized in neurological departments instead of infectious hospitals. As a result, modern laboratory diagnostics of herpes were not carried out at an early stage, which does not allow timely prescribing antiviral drugs. It should be remembered that with herpetic encephalitis, the cerebrospinal fluid may not differ from the norm. In cases of herpetic meningoencephalitis, pleocytosis with a predominance of lymphocytes (up to several hundred in 1 μl), hyperalbuminosis (up to 2–3 g/l) is detected. When studying the biopsy and surgical material, it is occasionally possible to establish the herpetic etiology of focal encephalitis. In these cases, patients were operated on due to an erroneous diagnosis of a brain tumor. The latter is due to the fact that herpetic necrotic encephalitis can occur under the guise of glial brain tumors. Only a brain biopsy allowed the diagnosis of acute necrotic encephalitis to be established also had to deal with observations of the tumor-like course of herpetic on our own material (Fig. 19.2).

Focal encephalitis can also be caused by other viruses. We have evidence that such lesions, especially in childhood, may be associated with cytomegalovirus. Unfortunately, there is no reliable data on their true frequency. In neuroinfections caused by tick-borne encephalitis, viruses, ECHO, Coxsackie, chlamydia, and mycoplasma, tumor-like lesions are considered uncharacteristic and have not been observed in our material, although this possibility cannot be completely excluded. At the same time, the possibility of detecting focal lesions in these diseases may make it necessary to conduct a differential diagnosis during histological examination. The fact that the etiological interpretation of encephalitis is difficult is well known.

19.5 Focal Lesions of Fungal Origin

Among pathogenic micromycetes, most pathogens are able to affect the brain, leading, in some cases, to the formation of focal changes. In our conditions, these are primarily fungi of the genus *Candida, Cryptococcus, Aspergillus*, as well as various and differentiable only in cultural mycological studies, pathogens of chromomycosis and zygomycosis. It should be noted, however, that such lesions almost always develop as manifestations of a severe generalized infection, often against the background of immunodeficiency, which facilitates clinical diagnosis. The diagnosis is made on the basis of the general principles accepted in clinical mycology, a combination of clinical, laboratory, and radiological data with the isolation of the pathogen. In the case of morphological examination of biopsy or autopsy material, significant importance is attached to the identification of fungi in the tissues. To do this, in

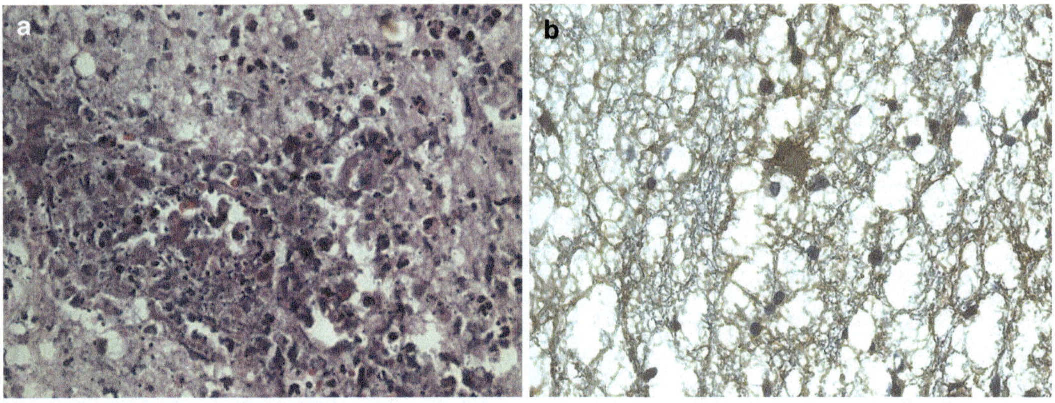

Fig. 19.2 Histological findings in a case of clinically suspected glial tumor, which appeared to be focal herpes encephalitis. (**a**) Hyperchromatosis and karyorexis of numerous cells typical for herpes infection. H-E, ×600; (**b**) Antigen of HSV1 in nervous cell. IHC ×600

most cases, in addition to staining with hematoxylin-eosin, it is enough to use a PAS reaction (it is especially important for detecting *Candida* and cryptococci). In some cases, impregnation by Gomori–Grokkot and staining with alcyan blue by Mowry may be useful. Aspergillus, primarily *Aspergillus fumigatus* and *A. flavus*, reach the brain by a hematogenic route, usually from the lungs, less often from the gastrointestinal tract, paranasal sinuses, ears, skin, uterus appendages, or as a result of traumatic brain injury. In some cases, contact lesions are also possible. These pathogens are very characterized by invasion of the arteries and veins with a picture of necrotic angiitis. The manifestation of cerebral aspergillosis may be focal neurological symptoms associated with the lesion of the basins of the anterior and middle cerebral arteries. In some cases, clinical symptoms may indicate a volumetric process. The symptoms are usually headache, hemiparesis, convulsions. Fever, paralysis of the cranial nerves, and abnormal plantar reflexes are also possible. In the part of the observations, signs of increased intracranial pressure and/or meningeal signs are determined. Neurological symptoms are usually regarded as nonspecific. In vivo diagnosis is extremely difficult. Pleocytosis in the CSF is usually less than 600 cl / mm3, the protein level is only moderately elevated, the sugar content is normal, the pathogen in the CSF is usually not determined. In postmortem morphological examination, macroscopically, foci of hemorrhagic necrosis or yellowish foci with a hemorrhagic component from 0.1 to 5 cm in diameter, resembling infarcts, are most often determined. A thick fibrous capsule is determined only occasionally. Much less often, abscesses and granulomas form in the substance of the brain. The topography of the lesions may be different, including the hemispheres of the cerebellum. When microscopically examined, the most characteristic feature is vascular invasion and thrombosis. At the same time, even when stained with hematoxylin-eosin, characteristic septic hyphae of the mycelium with a thickness of 4–12 microns, branching at an acute angle, are detected. According to our observations, the hyphae of mycelium in the brain tissue are less numerous and more subtle compared to the lungs. Inflammatory infiltration in the early stages involves neutrophils. In abscesses, free pus is located in the center, surrounded by neutrophil infiltration with an admixture of giant (Langhans type) and epithelioid cells. Granulomas are clusters of lymphocytes, plasma cells, and epithelioid cells, as well as areas of necrosis and collagen fibers. Zygomycosis, most often caused by pathogens from the genus *Rhizopus* and *Mucor*, is often accompanied by brain lesions in usually immunecompromised individuals due to generalization from primary foci in the skin of the face, nasal mucosa, nasopharynx with damage to nearby parts, primarily the orbit, internal carotid artery, paranasal sinuses with very characteristic thrombosis. Hematogenous dissemination from the lungs and gastrointestinal tract is also possible. In the rhinocerebral form, the orbit is rapidly involved, which leads to unilateral ophthalmoplegia, edema of the eyelids and cornea, and sometimes blindness. Headache, neck stiffness, and cramps may result from the involvement of the soft meninges. Severe vascular lesions lead to aphasia, hemiplegia, disorientation, coma, and lethargy. The disease can take an extremely severe course, leading to death within a few days. For diagnostics, the detection of wide, nonsegregated mycelial filaments from 6 to 15 microns in diameter with the possible appearance of sporangiospores and sporangia is of leading importance in the biopsy material. The most frequent localization of lesions is the basal surface of the frontal lobes or the nodes of the base, more often in the form of hemorrhagic necrosis. Fungi are angiotropic and are detected around and in the walls of the blood vessels of the meninges and brain matter, leading to their obstruction and thrombosis. The inflammatory reaction is mixed, mainly neutrophilic, but it can be expressed minimally or practically absent. Occasionally, giant multinucleated cells can be detected, but the formation of granulomas is not characteristic. Fungi of the genus *Candida*, primarily *C. albicans*, are the most common pathogens of mycosis in our conditions. They are characterized in our condition at present primarily by the defeat of the mucous membranes of the esophagus, pharynx, and other parts of the digestive, urinary, and reproductive systems.

Much less often, it is possible to damage other organs, including the brain. Such lesions are usually associated with sepsis or endocarditis, other variants of the onset of the disease are observed as casuistically rare. Meningitis with a small predominantly lymphocytic pleiocytosis in the cerebrospinal fluid is clinically determined. The basis for the diagnosis is the identification of the microorganism. The most characteristic variant of the lesion is microabscesses with the possible formation of microgranules. In the early stages, they can have the form of hemorrhagic focuses. Later on, such lesions take the form of abscesses and granulomas without central areas of necrosis. Perivascular lymphocytic couplings are characteristic. Yeast-like and pseudomycelial forms of the fungus are better detected by PAS reaction or silver impregnation. The cellular response may be represented by lymphocytes, single neutrophils, and giant cells, but may also be absent. Cryptococcosis-deep visceral mycosis with distinct neurotropy, usually caused by *Cryptococcus neoformans*, most often affects immunocompromised individuals, especially those suffering from HIV infection in the AIDS stage. Morphological manifestations can be of two types. More often, fungal accumulations are detected in the soft meninges, microcysts, and in the substance of the brain in the absence or minimal cellular response. In another rarer variant, focal lesions are determined—cryptococcomas. Such lesions are usually described in individuals without serious resistance defects, measuring 2–3 microns in diameter, usually close to blood vessels, and resembling tuberculomas, including on MRI. Histologically, such foci consist of lymphocytes, plasma cells, eosinophils, fibroblasts, and giant multinucleated cells. Numerous pathogens are also detected, weakly stained with hematoxylin-eosin and much better PAS reaction, mucicarmine, alcyan blue, and impregnated with silver salts. Chromomycoses (chromoblastoses) are caused by various pigment fungi belonging to the genera Cladosporium, Hormodendrum, and Phialophora. Most often, multiple small abscesses are formed in the substance of the brain with a minimal granulomatous reaction. Pigmented spores and hyphae are detected in the lesions. Among the extremely rare variants of the lesion, should be mentioned allescheriosis caused by *Allescheria boydii*. The pathogen belongs to the class Ascomycetes and is widespread everywhere as a soil saprophyte. The fungus penetrates the body through the skin and can cause damage to the respiratory system and central nervous system. In the brain, hemorrhagic infarcts are described, which can transform into abscesses that require surgical intervention. The pathogen is determined in the form of septic hyphae and chlamydospores. In extremely rare cases, the formation of granulomas in the brain substance is also described in some endemic mycoses of group 2 pathogenicity—coccidiomycosis, histoplasmosis, and North American blastomycosis.

19.6 Amoebiasis

The most well-known and common form of amoebiasis in countries with hot climates is amoebic dysentery caused by *Entamoeba hystolytica*. Against the background of severe ulcerative lesions of the large intestine, hematogenic dissemination of trophozoites erythrophages with the development of foci in the liver, lungs, brain, and other organs is possible. Macroscopically, they resemble abscesses, microscopically they are foci of necrosis in the area of accumulation of the pathogen, surrounded by mixed cell filtration with a significant number of eosinophils. "Abscesses" of the brain are relatively rare and they are usually secondary to lung damage.

Relatively rare, mainly in immunocompromised individuals, there are lesions caused by so-called free-living amoebas that have tropicity to the central nervous system. Among them, *Naegleria fowleri* causes primary diffuse meningoencephalitis, and *Acanthamoeba* and *Balamuthia mandrillaris* cause granulomatous amoebic encephalitis. Isolated cases of this disease are described in almost all countries of the world. Pathogens enter the human body through the skin and mucous membranes when bathing in open water or in contact with the soil. It is assumed that the pathogen enters the brain hematogenically. The most characteristic is the formation of granulomas with necrosis, mainly lymph-macrophage infiltration with the participation of giant cells. Trophozoites and cysts of amoebas are usually determined perivascularly.

19.7 Toxoplasmosis

Toxoplasmosis is caused by *Toxoplasma gondii*, which is an obligate intracellular parasite belonging to the tissue cyst-forming coccidia, a class of spores (see Sects. 14.2 and 16.2). The final host is the animals of the cat family, the intermediate one is man and a number of other mammals and birds. Based on the results of the serological study, an extremely high frequency of infection in the population is indicated (one fourth to one third of all people). Clinically important forms of the disease are observed mainly in newborns (born to mothers with acute infection) and in immunocompromised individuals, primarily patients with HIV infection in the AIDS stage. In the smears of patient's fluids, toxoplasmas have a semilunar shape, are located intracellularly (especially in paraffin sections of tissues), and are PAS-stained. The longitudinal intracellular division of toxoplasmas is best detected in nerve cells. In brain lesions, toxoplasmas are found both in the substance of the brain and in nerve cells, with the appearance of dystrophic and then necrotic changes. The leukocyte exudative reaction is very weak. Macrophages phagocytize pathogens and decay products of necrotic brain tissue. In the blood vessels, there is stasis, swelling of the endothelium, proliferation of adventitia cells, and often thrombosis. As a result of vascular damage, secondary focal aseptic colliquation necrosis of the brain substance occurs. The foci of necrosis are located in the brain asymmetrically, mainly in the cortex of the large hemispheres and in the subependimar zone of the lateral ventricles. They can vary in size and number. With the greatest severity of the process, these foci merge into solid yellowish stripes running along the convolutions of the cerebral cortex. On the walls of the ventricles, ependymal defects may be detected. The vascular plexuses and cerebral ventricles are often thickened, whitish, or yellowish in color. In the later stages of toxoplasmosis, the necrotic tissue resolves to form cysts. Especially often they are located on the border between the gray and white matter of the large hemispheres. In the cavities there is a cerebrospinal fluid, and on their walls macrophages are found, containing in the cytoplasm the products of the breakdown of brain tissue. The areas of necrosis are delimited by glial growth, as a result of which the brain substance surrounding the cysts is devoid of the usual structure and sharply compacted. Sclerosis also affects the vascular plexuses and the soft meninges. In connection with the violation of the outflow of the cerebrospinal fluid, internal drops of the brain develops. In parallel with this, calcification occurs with pulverized or granular, and sometimes massive lime deposition. Calcification is not specific to toxoplasmosis, so it cannot be diagnosed on the basis of a single focal calcification. Along with brain damage, it is possible to involve the liver, lymph nodes, and other internal organs in the pathological process.

19.8 Helminthiasis

Focal brain lesions, including tumor-like ones, can be caused by certain helminths (see Sect. 14.3) Although the lesions caused by these pathogens are rare in moderate climate, the population migration that has sharply increased in recent years makes it quite likely that tropical diseases that were not previously observed in our conditions will appear in our country. We present data on the most fully studied helminthiasis, which is characterized by focal lesions of the brain. *Angiostrongylus cantonensis* is a pathogen related to roundworms (*Nematoda*). The most common diseases due to helminthes are in Southeast Asia and Oceania, in particular in countries such as China (including Taiwan), India, Japan, Thailand, Vietnam, Sri Lanka, Reunion, Comoros, Fiji, the Philippines, Indonesia, Papua New Guinea, Samoa, as well as Egypt, Ivory Coast, Cuba. Animals such as shrimps, crabs, planarians, cichlids, toads, and frogs may be intermediate hosts. Humans, primates, mice, and other mammals are random dead-end hosts. Human infection usually occurs when eating raw or insufficiently heat-treated snails, shrimps, crabs, frogs, and some endemic fish. In addition, infection can occur through unwashed vegetables, contaminated shellfish, and larval-infected drinking water. The incubation period for humans usually lasts from 12 to 28 days. Prodromal symptoms are usually reduced to vomiting with possible subsequent dehydration. Children are the most susceptible. When crossing the blood-brain barrier, the development of eosinophilic meningitis or myelomeningoencephalitis is most characteristic. In the human brain, helminths can stay for a long time, causing severe damage and then leading to death. It is possible to damage other organs, in particular the eyes and lungs. Macroscopically, such lesions are characterized by: thickening of the soft meninges on the basal surface and in the region of the cerebellum; subdural or subarachnoid hemorrhages involving adjacent areas of the cortex. On the sections of the brain, one can see focal necrosis and hemorrhage, corresponding to the movement of the helminth. Microscopically, living or dead helminths are found in the soft meninges, and sometimes in the blood vessels and perivascular spaces. Cellular responses to live worms are usually minimal and are significantly pronounced around the dying ones. Possible granulomatous, including giant cell reaction, is typical. Characteristic micro-cavities are "traces" of the movement of the helminth with cellular detritus. Eosinophilic infiltration in pathological foci is typical. Among the long-known helminthiasis in our country with brain damage is cysticercosis. This is a disease in the spread of which social factors are of great importance. The most affected population group is rural residents. In cities, people who work in slaughterhouses and food processing centers, including the use of raw or insufficiently roasted pork meat, usually get sick.

Cystecyrcosis is caused by the plerocercoid of the widespread tapeworm *Taenia solium* cysticercus. Adults of this species live in the small intestine and have a length of 2–7 m. The ingress of eggs of this helminth into the intestine leads to the release of oncospheres, which penetrate through the mucous membrane, and then lymphogenically and hematogenically enter various organs, including the brain, where they form cysticerci. They are milky-white, spherical, or oval cysts that, when fully developed, reach 1 cm in diameter. Each cyst contains fluid and an invaginated protoscolex. The protoscolex has four large spherical suckers and a proboscis with a double row of 22–36 large and small hooks. These structures can be detected in preparations stained with hematoxylin-eosin and are birefringent. The wall of the bladder consists of the shell, muscle cells, shell cells, and parenchyma. The number of cysticerci developing in the brain depends on the number of oncospheres that have simultaneously entered the body. With multiple cysticercosis, there can be up to 1000 or more parasites in the brain. In rare cases, single cysticerci of the brain may occur. With combined lesions, simultaneous cysticercosis of the brain and eyes is most often observed. There are frequent combinations of cysticercosis of the central nervous system with cysticercosis of subcutaneous tissue, muscles, liver, and lungs. The pathogenesis of the disease is diverse. The local effect is due to the mechanical effect of cysticercus as a volume formation on the brain tissue and the pathways of cerebrospinal fluid circulation. The general effect of cysticerca on the central nervous system is associated with the entry into the blood and cerebrospinal fluid of toxic products of cysticerca metabolism, in particular succinic acid, which causes inflammatory reactions at a distance from the parasite. Anatomical and clinical classification includes the following variants: parenchymal; meningobasal; hydrocephalus; spinal. There are four main localization of cysticercosis: large hemispheres; ventricular system; brain base; mixed form. And, finally, single cysticerci (simple, cellular) and racemose (complex, cluster-shaped, multi-bubble) are distinguished. With surgical removal of cysticerci, the bladders of parasites may rupture and their contents may leak into the subarachnoid slits, which often leads to the development of aseptic meningitis in the postoperative period. Viable cysticerci practically do not cause an inflammatory reaction. Pronounced lymphocytic monocytic infiltration is formed with the dead pathogens. The substance of the brain also usually forms a thin fibrous capsule and a glial shaft.

Cenurosis is a disease caused by a cenur cysticercus formed by *Taenia multiceps* or *T. serialis*. The disease is more common in children in Africa, although isolated cases have been reported in sheep-breeding areas in Europe, South America, the United States, and Canada. The final hosts of these helminths are carnivores from the canine family. The intermediate hosts are most often herbivores, primarily sheep and rabbits, but they can also be antelopes, chamois, cows, goats, horses, wild rodents, and yaks. Humans, especially young children, can become accidental intermediate hosts when eggs are ingested from the feces of the final host. In the intestine, eggs ripen releasing oncospheres, which actively penetrate the intestinal wall, and then into the bloodstream. Oncospheres are transformed into cenures in the brain, eyes, skeletal muscles, and subcutaneous tissue, which takes about 3 months. Brain damage is usually associated with *T. multiceps*. In the brain, cenures are usually localized in the subarachnoid space, causing basal arachnoiditis or ependymitis. The response to the parasite in the brain is often minimal and limited to a thin rim of fibrous tissue. The censors will easily get rid of the brain tissue when cutting a piece of tissue. Patients with a chronic form of the disease develop fibrosis of the soft meninges with a giant cell reaction around the cyst wall. After the death of the cenura, a pronounced inflammatory reaction develops with the infiltration of the larva mainly by eosinophils. On the background of degenerative changes in the cenura, the development of necrosis and a chronic inflammatory reaction, represented by lymphocytes, macrophages, and giant cells, is characteristic. Often there is perivascular inflammation and occasionally tissue eosinophilia. In the outcome, fibrosis and calcification are possible. Echinococcosis of the central nervous system is a disease that occurs as a result of the development in the human body of the larval stage of a canine tapeworm (*Echinococcus granulosus*). There are echinococcoses of soft tissues, bones, visceral organs, and the central nervous system. Most people who are engaged in animal husbandry, as well as those who have direct contact with dogs, get sick. The cestode of *Echinococcus granulosus* consists of a scolex (head), a neck, and three to four segments (proglottids). In the sexually mature state, these helminths live in the small intestine of dogs, wolves, jackals, less often foxes. In size, the dimensions are 2–6 mm in length. At the anterior end of the helminth, there is a head (scolex), which is armed with four muscular suckers and a crown of two rows of hooks, on which it is embedded in the intestinal mucosa. An echinococcal cyst consists of an outer coarse chitinous layer and an inner thin, germinal one. Echinococcal cysts are single-chamber (hydatidous) and multichamber (alveolar). They are more often solitary and are mainly localized in the lateral ventricles and in the white matter of the frontal lobes. There are two main forms of Echinococcus—solitary and racemous. In the first case, there are single cysts, often reaching very large sizes (in diameter up to 5–6 cm or more). In racemous echinococcosis, clusters of blisters are located in the brain and spinal cord tissue, around which there are pronounced reactive changes. A connective tissue capsule is formed around the echinococcus, surrounded by a shaft of inflammatory-altered brain tissue, and foci of softening and hemorrhage are found. Inflammatory changes are present in the area of the echinococcal bladder, as well as in the membranes of the brain.

19.9 Differential Diagnostics of Hemorrhages

In the clinical autopsies, especially in cases with short time of clinical observation and limited data related to disease history occasionally are found different not expected changes, hemorrhagic first of all. Although macroscopic diagnosis can be relatively easy (Figs. 19.3 and 19.4), the reconstruction of the chain of events that caused them frequently appears very difficult. In certain cases, they may be result of brain trauma in other due to aneurisms of brain vessels or their malforma-

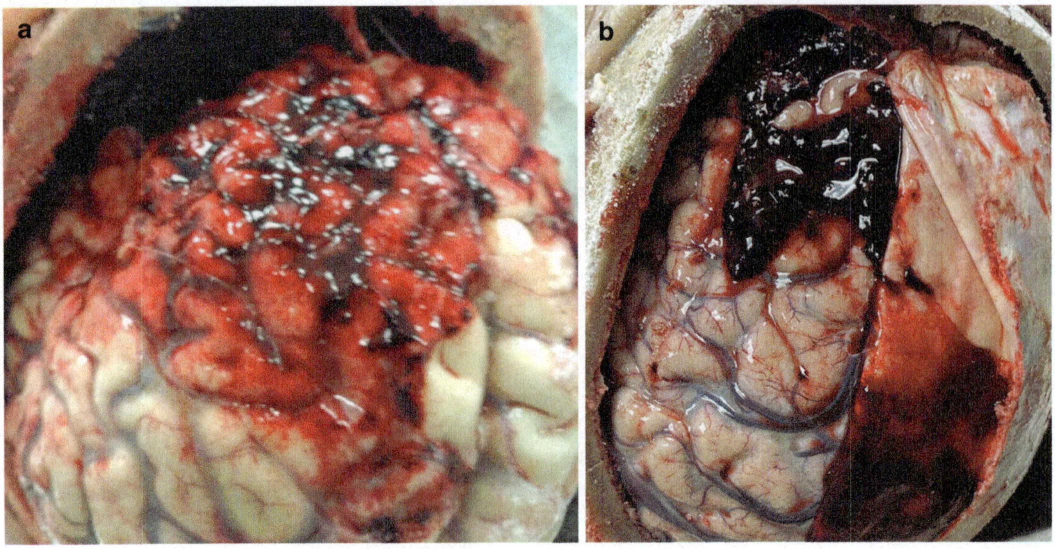

Fig. 19.3 (**a**, **b**) Different variants of subdural hematoma of unclear origin as unexpected finding at autopsy. Fresh macropreparations. Courtesy of N.A. Lugovskya and AM Isakov

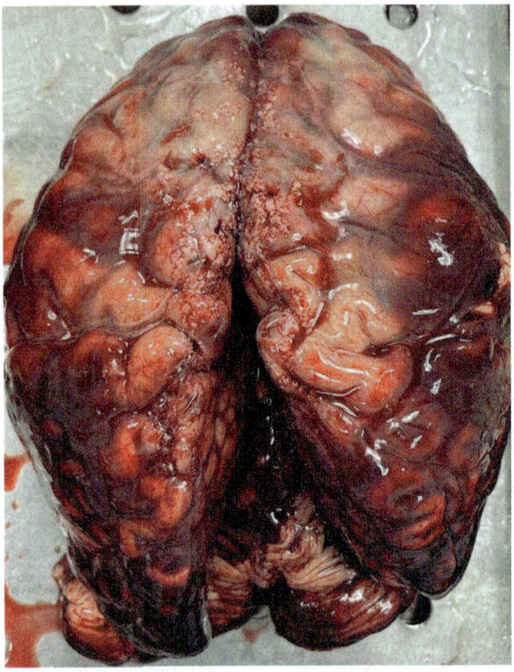

Fig. 19.4 Subarachnoidal hematoma of unclear origin as unexpected finding at autopsy. Fresh macropreparation. Courtesy of N.A. Lugovskya

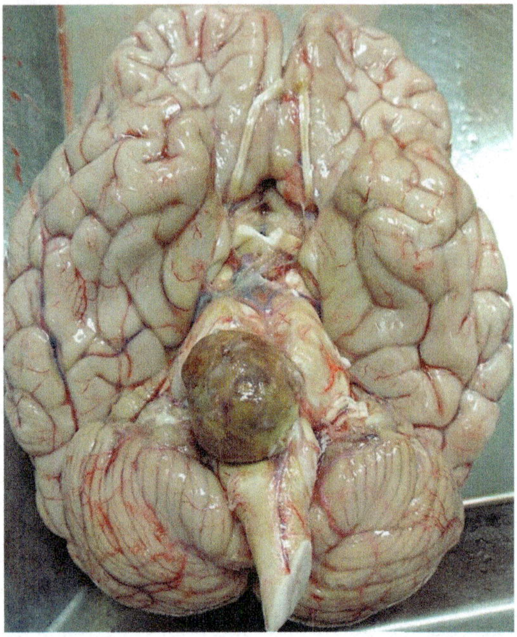

Fig. 19.5 Aneurism of brain basal artery as unexpected finding at autopsy. Fresh macropreparation. Courtesy of N.A. Lugovskasya

tions, disturbances of blood coagulation of different origin, brain infarctions. Hemorrhagic meningitis and meningoencephalitis are quite typical for the plague and anthrax. Brain aneurism if intact is evident during macroscopic investigation (Fig. 19.5), but when ruptured make for pathologist more difficult task. It should be mentioned that detecting series of "subarachnoid hemorrhages of unclear origin" allowed pathologists of Sverdlovsk (now Ekaterinburg) to suspect the outbreak of anthrax in 1979, later confirmed bacteriologically [6]. Hemorrhagic encephalitis has been also described as typical for influenza.

References

1. Matsko DE (2015) Neurosurgical pathology Manual. SPb AL Polenov Research neurosurgical Institute. (In Russian).
2. Vezzani A, Fujinami RS, White HS, et al. Infections, inflammation and epilepsy. Acta Neuropathol. 2016;131(2):211–34. https://doi.org/10.1007/s00401-015-1481-5.
3. Thomas DL, Pierson CR. Neuropathology of surgically managed epilepsy specimen. Neurosurgery. 2020;88(1):1–4. https://doi.org/10.1093/neuros/nyaa366.
4. Rapalino O, Mullins ME. Intracranial infections and inflammatory diseases presenting as neurosurgical pathologies. Neurosurgery. 2017;81(1):10–28. https://doi.org/10.1093/neuros/nyx201.
5. Zinserling VA, Chukhlovina ML. Infectious lesions of nervous system. Issues of etiology, pathogenesis and diagnostics. Saint-Petersburg: ElbiSPb; 2011. p. 583. (In Russian)
6. Abramova FA, Grinberg LM, Yampolskaya OV, Walker DH. Pathology of inhalational antrax in 42 cases from Sverdlovsk outbreak in 1979 proc. Natl Acad Sci USA. 1993;90(6):2291–4. https://doi.org/10.1073/pnas.90.6/2291.

20 Some Noncommunicable Diseases of the Central Nervous System with a Possible Infectious Etiology (in Collaboration with V.A. Orlova, I.I. Mikhailova, A.A. Garbuzov, D.A. Khavkina, P.V. Chukhliaev, T.A. Ruzhentsova I. L. Naidenova, A. B. Danilov, A.V. Simonova, E.G. Filatova, I.A. Pavlovsky, O.V. Bystrova, A.M. Zatevalov, S.L. Bezrodny, T.Sh. Sadekov)

Currently, it is obvious that biological pathogens can cause not only acute and chronic infections, but also play a role in the development of noncommunicable diseases, such as diabetes mellitus, coronary heart disease, rheumatic diseases, bronchial asthma, and many others. Their role for the occurrence of a number of neoplasms is also discussed. The pathogenesis mechanisms of the development of such diseases are poorly understood. It is obvious that under conditions of persistence of the pathogen, especially in persons with a genetic predisposition, mechanisms associated with cell reprogramming and various autoimmune mechanisms can contribute to pathogenesis. It is possible that the disease may persist and even progress after the elimination of the pathogen. This question has not only theoretical significance, but in many situations it has also practical importance, since it implies modification of the therapy being carried out.

In many diseases of the nervous system, the etiological and/or in pathogenetic role of various biological pathogens is also periodically discussed. It should be noted that relatively few neurologists, psychiatrists, neurosurgeons, and neuropathologists are interested in these issues. This chapter, prepared with the participation of many colleagues from Moscow, provides both literary and own data on a number of diseases. Unfortunately, we do not have sufficient experience and our own material to represent various forms of epilepsy, multiple sclerosis, Parkinson's disease, CNS tumors, in which some authors do not exclude the pathogenetic role of the infectious factor.

20.1 Schizophrenia and Schizoaffective Psychosis. Possible Etiopathogenetic Role of Infection[1]

Schizophrenia is very common (affecting up to 1% of the population), and in a significant proportion of cases a chronic progressive mental illness, the causes of which have not yet been precisely established. The disease is characterized by disharmony and loss of unity of mental functions (thinking, emotions, motor skills), continuous or paroxysmal course, and different severity of positive (the most important—delusions, hallucinations, mental automatisms) and negative disorders leading to personality changes in the form of autism, a decrease in energy potential, emotional

[1]With collaboration of V.A. Orlova and I.I. Mikhailova.

V. Zinserling, *Infectious Lesions of the Central Nervous System*,
https://doi.org/10.1007/978-3-030-96260-9_20

impoverishment, and increasing invertedness. Forms of schizophrenia are diverse. The course of the disease can be chronic or episodic with progression or stability of disorders, one or more episodes of the disease with complete or incomplete remission are possible. During the disease, mood disorders are observed—depressive, manic, but episodic disorders in which schizophrenic symptoms and mood disorders are equally expressed, observed simultaneously or sequentially during the same episode, according to the 10th International Classification of Diseases (ICD), are referred to as schizoaffective psychosis (SHAP). SHAP still remains one of the most controversial nosological categories in psychiatry; its definition in textbooks and manuals of many countries is uncertain and diagnosis is traditionally carried out within the framework of either affective or schizophrenic diseases [1]. In ICD-9, SHAP was considered as a schizoaffective type of recurrent schizophrenia. In ICD-10, adapted to the Russian classification, the SHAP is referred to as schizoaffective variants of paroxysmal schizophrenia [1]. In accordance with this, in this work, the SHAP is considered as a marginal favorable variant of recurrent schizophrenia, transitional to affective disorders.

The structural features of the brain in schizophrenia are established by both postmortem and lifetime morphological studies.

Macroscopically, the brain in schizophrenia does not have any characteristic features with the exception of a kind of swelling. The characteristic features of the microscopic picture are well known and described in the manuals on psychiatry [2, 3]. Microscopic cellular changes are polymorphic: along with a decrease in the number of neurons, their atrophy, wrinkling, loading with lipofuscin, swelling, the formation of shadow cells, in cells are also detected swelling with changes in organelles. A characteristic feature of this disease is the absence of astrogliosis, atrophic microglia, and regressive changes in oligodendroglia in the absence of classical manifestations of vasculitis. Subtle violations of cytoarchitectonics are described, manifested by a change in the location density of the cells, the orientation of neurons and their processes, the distortion of the branching of processes. Changes in interneuron connections at the synaptic level were revealed. Both the cortex and other parts of the brain (subcortical structures, brain stem, hypothalamus, cerebellum) are involved in the pathological process. An important feature of the pathological picture of the brain in schizophrenia is the small-scale tissue lesion, as well as a wide range of possible changes in brain tissue – from cases where even microscopically detected disorders of brain structures are minimal, to pronounced pictures of damage to cellular elements. A very common point of view is that described brain abnormalities in schizophrenia have to be regarded as encephalopathy, expressed by diffuse dystrophic changes of a toxic-hypoxic nature and caused by metabolic changes in the body or within the nervous system itself (in particular, as a result of a violation of the of mediators metabolism).

When conducting lifetime studies (computed tomography, magnetic resonance imaging – MRI) in patients with schizophrenia, the most common is the expansion of the lateral and III ventricles of the brain, reduction of the frontal and temporal cortex, changes in the basal ganglia, hippocampal-amygdala complex, a decrease in the volume of the cerebellum [4–8].

For a long time, dominated the opinion that morphological changes in the brain in schizophrenia are formed even before the onset of the disease and reflect the pathology of brain development [9–11]. This opinion was confirmed by their stability according to a number of catamnesis tomographic studies [12–15], as well as the absence of replacement gliosis in the foci of nerve cell loss [2, 3].

However, the data gradually accumulated indicate the current pathological process in the brain. It was reported about the aggravation of neuropathological changes in patients after repeated attacks of the disease [6, 16, 17]. In some ultramicroscopic studies was revealed a correlation between the degree of dystrophic changes in oligodendroglia and the severity of deficient psychopathological symptoms [18].

There was also a unitary point of view, combining the two considered approaches to assessing the genesis of neuropathological changes in schizophrenia [18–21]. It is based, on the one hand, on the establishment of relatives of patients with similar, although less pronounced changes in MRI characteristics of the brain, and on the other hand, the presence of correlations between MRI parameters of brain structures and the severity of clinical manifestations of the disease in patients, their relationship with the duration of the disease. The use of specific morphometric MRI indices aimed at differentiating primary hydrocephalus and the current atrophic process [22] confirms this point of view, revealing in patients with schizophrenia nearby primary hydrocephaly developing central atrophy of the hemispheres.

20.1.1 Schizophrenia as a Multifactorial Disease

Like most human diseases, schizophrenia belongs to the group of so-called multifactorial diseases, the genesis of which involves both environmental and genetic factors. The frequency of occurrence of manifest forms of schizophrenia in relatives of patients ranges from 4.4% to 16% [21–23], which significantly exceeds the noted population indicator. The familial liability to schizophrenia is neither extremely non-specific nor extremely specific [24]. Despite the high concordance in homozygous twin pairs, the incidence of the disease never reaches 100% [25] and usually not exceeding 28% [26]. Risk factors for schizophrenia are age—the first symptoms of the disease are most often observed at the age of about 20 years; sex—in men, the disease is diagnosed earlier and more severe than in women; the birth season—in persons born in the spring-winter period, schizophrenia develops more often [27, 28], nutritional insufficiency in the prenatal period [29]; burdened obstetric history (birth injuries, asphyxia) [30], infectious diseases of the mother during gestation [31–34], the presence of older sibs [35]; places of residence – mainly large cities [36]; climatic zones of residence (relatively low incidence in the tropics and high in countries with a cold climate) [37]. For example, in the north of Sweden, the incidence of schizophrenia reaches 17 cases per 1000 people of population [38]; low socioeconomic level [39], as well as unsatisfactory housing conditions (living of a large number of people in a limited area) [40].

Some viruses, acting on the expression of genes associated with genetic predisposition, increase the risk of developing psychosis. Epidemiological analysis showed that influenza [31], herpetic [32], and rubella [33] infections suffered by a woman during pregnancy increase the risk of developing schizophrenia in offspring by 3–7 times. A large study conducted in Sweden, covering 1.2 million people born from 1973 to 1985, showed that cytomegalovirus and mumps infections transferred in childhood (0—12 years) significantly increase the risk of developing psychosis [34].

Thus, the study of the causes and pathogenic features of the development of schizophrenia is aimed not only at the genetic aspects of predisposition to the disease, but also at environmental factors, including infectious ones. The role of the latter as the causes of mental illness was assumed in the nineteenth century [41, 42] in connection with observations of the seasonal nature of exacerbations of mental disorders, the relationship of their occurrence, and exacerbations with various infectious diseases. Since corpuscles similar to viral particles were described in the cerebrospinal fluid and nasal secretion of schizophrenic patients in 1954 [43], a targeted search for viruses in the brains of patients with schizophrenia has been conducted, but its results have been uncertain.

As we analyzed earlier [44], recent interest in the role of infectious agents in the pathogenesis of mental diseases, including schizophrenia and SHAP, has increased significantly. This was facilitated by research conducted within the framework of the international Human Microbiome Project (HMP), which aims to better understand the importance of the body's microflora for human health and related problems. The microbiome (microbiota) is a complex dynamic system that actively affects human health at both the local and systemic levels, up to the influence on its cognitive functions. The HMP outlines new ways to determine health and predisposition to diseases, specifies the parameters for creating, evaluating, and applying a strategy for conscious management of microflora in order to achieve a qualitatively new level of optimal physiological health [45]. Important components of HMP have been the study of the microbial community using metagenomic methods, as well as the determination of the total human genome. The work carried out in this direction has become a new epicenter of mental health research and is considered as a new, vital determinant of the processes of neuroimmunoregulation, brain development, emotional manifestations, cognition, and behavior [46]. HMP is associated with another global project, Global Virom Project, started by an international team of scientists in 2016, studying the effects of viruses on the occurrence of various human diseases [47]. To date, a number of works have substantiated the possible mechanisms by which viruses can participate in the etiopathogenesis of schizophrenia.

1. Predisposition to schizophrenia is determined by a number of genes whose protein products are involved in the functioning of the signaling systems responsible for glutamatergic neurotransmission, oligodendrocyte function, neuroplasticity, and oxidative stress processes. At the same time, they are associated with the life cycle of pathogens such as *herpes simplex viruses* (HSV), *cytomegalovirus* (CMV), *rubella, influenza, bornaviridae, polioviruses,* as well as *Toxoplasma* and *Chlamydia* [48]. For example, the signaling pathway of neuregulin 1 (NRG1), responsible for glutamatergic transmission and function of oligodendrocytes, is associated with the release of the EUR1 factor, which inhibits the replication of the *Influenza virus A*.
2. The mutagenic influence of viruses can be realized due to ability of a number of them, including herpetic ones, to integrate into human DNA [49–51]. Being integrated into the genetic apparatus, viral genetic material changes the metabolism of the cell, and also becomes an endogenous factor for the body and can be transmitted from generation to generation. This circumstance served as a justification for the virogenetic hypothesis of schizophrenia [52].
3. The interaction of the virus with the genetic apparatus provokes the expression of abnormal genetic structures. For example, "exogenous" viral infections can activate genes in the structure of which a particular virus is embedded (including one that has been introduced since ancient times and spreads by vertical transmission to offspring) [53].
4. Sensitization of microglia [54] under the influence of various stimuli, including those associated with neurodegeneration and inflammation [55]: like cells of the immune system, microglia have memory and retain their activated status for a long time, which leads to an enhanced immune response to subsequent weak stimuli. Small systemic inflammation or stress leads to proliferation of microglia and increased production of pro-inflammatory cytokines [56], which, in turn, can lead to an exacerbation of inflammatory pathology in the brain. Changes in neuroimmune processes and activation of microglia inherent in schizophrenia are possible under the influence of infections, including intrauterine [57, 58].
5. The effect of viral proteins (in particular, *influenza*, CMV) on glutamatergic signaling pathways is involved in the pathogenesis of schizophrenia [59].
6. The effect of viruses on serotonin metabolism. IF γ, IL1ß, and TNFα, whose levels rise in response to viral infection, stimulate the expression and activity of the tryptophan-cleaving enzyme indolamine-2,3-dioxygenase (IDO), and IL-4 and IL-10, in turn, inhibit the activity of IDO [60]. This changes the concentration of the precursor of serotonin – tryptophan and the product of its metabolism -N-formylkinurenin, a precursor of kynurenic acid, the level of which in schizophrenia increases, as well as picolinic acid—an endogenous antagonist of nicotinic, acetylcholine, and NMDA receptors [61].This effect can be caused by a cascade of inflammatory reactions in response to infection, which, in turn, contributes to neurotransmitter imbalance, which underlies the symptoms of many mental diseases [62].

7. Violation under the influence of viral infection of the process of methylation of the protein extracellular matrix of reelin [63], which is responsible for the processes of repair of nervous tissue.
8. The direct effect of viruses on the elements of nervous tissue (neurons, glial cells, myelin) and the vascular endothelium [64, 65], disrupting the processes of neurotransmission. Many viruses, in particular, *herpesviruses*, have a pronounced tropism to the cells of the endothelium of blood vessels and the nervous system, are able to persist for life in a latent state in the autonomic ganglia, reactivate and restore infectious properties, and also cause not only dangerous acute inflammatory reactions and neurodegenerative diseases, but also low-symptomatic neuroinfectious processes (see Chap. 5). Thus, *varicella zoster virus* (VZV) can be an etiological factor of two independent diseases—chickenpox and herpes zoster infection that occurs after endogenous reactivation of the virus [66, 67]. Prolonged persistence of VZV in the central nervous system contributes to the development of angiopathy and cascades of inflammatory processes in the brain, which can underlie many neurological and mental diseases. In an experimental model of schizophrenia obtained by prenatal infection of mice with *Influenza virus A,* the development of a number of morphological disorders in the brain similar to those in patients is shown – thinning of the cortex and hippocampus, impaired migration of neurons, atrophy of pyramidal neurons, decreased expression of reelin [68]. The discovery of chronic influenza infection [69] showed that with a slow course of the disease, primary degenerative changes in the brain are possible in the absence of inflammatory reactions (see Chap. 7). Here it is appropriate to recall the absence of classical signs of inflammatory reactions in the brain tissue in patients with schizophrenia. In addition, it is now believed that in the form of a slow infection, herpesvirus infection can also occur (see Chap. 15).
9. Damage to brain tissue during autoimmune reactions arising from the similarity of individual proteins or amino acid sequences of viruses with the structures of human tissues, that is, molecular mimicry [70–72].

20.1.2 Further Development of the Infectious Hypothesis of Schizophrenia

As we noted earlier [44], a significant part of the studies indicating that the symptoms of schizophrenia may reflect the current infectious process were performed using an immunological approach. In particular, the elevated levels of specific antiviral antibodies identified in most studies suggested that some viruses were an etiopathogenetic factor[2] of schizophrenia. The works focused on individual members of the family *Herpesviridae* predominate, which is not accidental. All herpesviruses are neuropathogenic, tropic to all tissues of the human body (panthropic), all immunosuppressive (see also Chap. 5). Systemic herpesvirus infections that can maintain chronic persistence in the body for life or occur in a latent form, when reactivated, cause a pronounced clinical manifestation, up to the development of severe meningoencephalitis or other diseases, and with moderate or mild course—chronic recurrent or asymptomatic chronic infection [73].

In most of the performed studies, was obtained immunological confirmation of the presence of herpesvirus infection in patients with schizophrenia. Contradictory data [74–76] are few and may be associated with a number of methodological disadvantages such as: examination of patients without taking into account the stage of the infectious process, insufficient number of observations (8 patients with the study

[2] According to modern ideas about multifactorial diseases, which include schizophrenia, the concept of risk factor (environmental, genetic) coincides with the concept of etiopathogenetic factor. However, at present, the question of removing a number of diseases of this group into the category of atypical slow infections has been raised.

[74]) and without differentiation in forms and activity of the process, insufficient consideration of the somatic state of mentally healthy persons of control groups. In a number of studies, when as control group are regarded the patients of primary medical care centers where herpes viruses are widespread and are involved in the pathogenesis of many somatic diseases, including their variants with latent and subclinical course, the results appear incorrect. Analytical emphasis only on seropositive cases, difficulties in assessing serological indicators (in particular, the lack of an increase in specific antibodies) may be associated with a weakening of immunity, which does not allow developing an adequate immune reaction, the effect on the results may cause associations of viruses with other microflora, the use of limited methods for diagnosing infections, the interpretation of data regardless of modern views about the significance of a particular serological indicator also allows us to consider the conclusions to be not evidence based. At the current level of science, the diagnosis of the infectious process faces a number of problems. Especially difficult is the diagnosis of latent, persistent, atypical infections in which the virus "escapes" from diagnostic techniques due to a defective form or integration into the cell genome. Modern studies changed the traditional interpretation of the serological studies: an increase in specific IgG is estimated now as an exacerbation of a chronic infectious process; absence of an increase in specific IgM does not exclude the transition to the acute phase of the persistent infectious process [77, 78].

It is shown that in the blood serum of patients with schizophrenia, high titers of antibodies to *herpes simplex virus* (HSV), *Epstein-Barr virus* (EBV) and *cytomegalovirus* (CMV) are determined, significantly exceeding the corresponding indicators in persons not suffering from this disease [79–84]. Similar differences were found in relation to IgG antibodies to CMV in the cerebrospinal fluid of patients and persons of control groups [79, 85]. In addition, correlative links were established between the occurrence of primary cytomegalovirus infection, diagnosed by the presence in the blood serum of low-avid IgG- and (or) IgM to CMV, in patients with the first episode of schizophrenia and the formation of their resistance to haloperidol and clozapine therapy [86]. Increase in schizophrenia of serum IgM, which is an indicator of the acute infectious process (to CMV, as well as to HSV-2), is reported by other researchers [82, 83]. Associative links between schizophrenia and HSV type 2 (HSV-2) infection have been established [87], as well as with human *herpes virus type 6* (HHV-6) [88]. A number of studies have demonstrated a relationship between the level of antibodies to HSV type 1 (HSV-1), *human herpesvirus-8* (HHV-8) and EBV and the severity of some psychopathological symptoms [80, 89, 90].

In a number of studies was found a reliable relationship between the seropositivity of patients with schizophrenia to HSV-1, and thinking disorders, as well as morphological changes in the gray matter of the cerebral cortex and hippocampus [91, 92]. In studies by DJ Schretlen et al. [92], KM Prasad et al., a progressive reduction of the brain's gray matter (singular gyrus, cerebellum) associated with HSV-1 persistence was demonstrated, detected in catamnesis studies.

Herpes viruses, as well as *influenza*, are able to activate HERV-W from the family of retroviruses that make up 9.3% of the human genome [93]. Activation of HERV-W stimulates proinflammatory and neurotoxic cascades. It was reported that antibodies to these viral agents in the serum of patients with schizophrenia are detected much more often than in mentally healthy individuals from control groups, and the level of reverse transcriptase (a marker of retroviruses) is increased in the cerebrospinal fluid, both in the early stages and in the long-term chronic course of schizophrenia [94]. Nucleotide sequences of the genome of retroviruses, proteins of their shell and capsid, as well as increased transcription (stage of the reproductive cycle) of elements of these viruses were detected in samples of cerebrospinal fluid, blood, and brain of persons diagnosed with schizophrenia [95]. As a component of the human genome, retroviruses can be a link between heredity, immunity, and adverse environmental factors [96, 97].

In combination with elevated levels of antibodies to herpesviruses, indirect signs of persistent viral infection in patients with schizophrenia can serve as increased levels of autoantibodies to neuroantigens [98], signs of nonspecific inflammation of the nervous tissue [99], as well as changes in immunity, including its lymphocytic link, and their relationship with a number of clinical parameters of schizophrenia [100, 101]. To this should be added the relatively recently identified MR-angiographic signs of brain abnormalities, reflecting the complex functional and anatomical pathology of cerebral circulation in the system of cerebral collectors, large vessels and capillary network, which may be related to inflammatory and destructive processes in the walls of cerebral vessels and brain tissue [102].

It seems important to conduct research that integrates the above-discussed issues. Thus, we undertook a multidisciplinary study aimed at establishing etiological and pathogenic factors and their causal interactions in patients with schizophrenic spectrum disorders (schizophrenia, SHAP), as well as the allocation of significant biological characteristics to determine the strategy of a personalized therapeutic approach. The research focused on the study of basic structural-functional and immune anomalies, as well as the detection and determination of the activity of pathogens with clarification of their clinical significance in patients of this contingent, and the features of their interaction. A group of herpetic viruses (HSV-1 and HSV-2, CMV and EBV) was chosen as a research object.

In total, 212 patients with schizophrenia and SHAP (94 men, 118 women) aged 17 to 50 years in the phase of exacerbation of the disease, in a state of acute psychosis, were examined, undergoing inpatient treatment in the clinic "Mental Health" (head – Prof. V.L. Minutko). Among the examined patients, there were 30 with episodic paranoid schizophrenia with a tendency to transition to a continuous course and increasing defect (F20.00-20.01), 88 – episodic paranoid schizophrenia with remissions of higher quality with the preservation of rudimentary subpsychotic symptoms and stable defect (F20.02), 32 – paranoid remittent schizophrenia (remissions without positive and negative symptoms) (F20.03), and 62 – SHAP (F25). The study of individual indicators and their relationships was carried out on groups of patients of smaller numbers included in the described sample. The analysis included the study of parameters differentially in different forms of schizophrenia, with patients with one form or another of the disease serving as a control group in relation to patients of another group. In some aspects of the study, control groups of mentally healthy individuals were used. Since immunological studies were conducted in highly qualified laboratories certified for medical laboratory services with the results interpretation in comparison with reference values these interpretations were also taken into account.

The exclusion criteria were: the presence in the history and (or) at the time of the study of periods of abuse of narcotic and medicinal substances, the presence of clinical signs of somatic and neurological diseases, as well as the presence at the time of examination of classical signs of the infectious process of any etiology and localization.

The study covers simultaneously psychopathological, morphological, electrophysiological, immunological, microbiological, and virological aspects. Within the framework of the integrative picture of the studied parameters, not only deviating but also normative were analyzed. This approach allows us to assess the diagnostic significance of a number of laboratory indicators in schizophrenia, taking into account the immunity anomalies characteristic of these patients.

Research methods included:

1. *Clinical and psychopathological.* Diagnosis was carried out according to ICD-10. When making a diagnosis, data from both psychiatric and psychological examinations were taken into account. Psychometry was performed using the BPRS scale.
2. *Serological.* Serum antibodies to HSV-1, HSV2, CMV, and EBV in peripheral blood were determined.
3. *Immunological.* The state of innate and acquired immunity was assessed (21 indicators of immune screening "assessment of immune status").
4. *Immunochemical.* To determine the serum content of 12 autoantibodies to microstructures of nervous tissue, ELI-Neurotest-12 was used.

5. *Electrophysiological.* The parameters of latency and amplitude of auditory cognitive evoked potentials (EP, SKVP, P300) and latency of long-latent auditory VP (DSVP) were studied.
6. *Morphological.* Structural MRI of the brain with contrast-free MR angiography was performed.

Statistical data processing included calculation of average values and standard deviations of indicators, determination of the frequency of occurrence of multilevel features in the studied sample. Determination of the reliability of differences in the frequency of occurrence of features in the selected groups (Fisher coefficient). Methods of nonparametric statistics (Statistika 10 program): (1) Calculation of the Spearman rank correlation coefficient to establish the relationship between various traits in the entire sample and within the groups of patients identified by cluster analysis. (2) Nonparametric method of intergroup comparison for two and more independent Mann-Whitney and Kraskel-Wallis groups.

Statistical analysis was carried out jointly with Prof. A.A. Romanyukha.

20.1.3 Results

Serological, immunological, and morphological indicators and their relationships with each other and with the symptoms of mental disorder were studied on the same sample in 80 patients with paranoid schizophrenia (35 men and 45 women), which included 52 patients with paranoid paroxysmal schizophrenia with a stable and increasing defect and preservation in remission of residual psychotic symptoms (F20.01-02) and 28 with paranoid episodic remitting schizophrenia with complete or actually complete remissions between psychotic episodes (F20.03), with the duration of the disease: 0–5 years – in 45 pts, 6–15 years – in 29 pts, more than 15 years – 6 pts.

Serological examination revealed in all patients an increase in IgG levels to HSV-1 and EBV (general). Their average levels exceeded the reference values by 1.5 and 3.8 times, respectively. In 20 patients (25%), IgG to CMV were increased, with an excess of the average value relative to the reference value by 1.5 times. IgM to all studied viruses were detected closer to its upper limit of the reference interval. It is important to note that in samples from 74 patients, in all respects comparable to the described, compared with the control group of 10 mentally healthy individuals, statistically significantly higher levels of IgM to EBV and HSV-2, which were predominantly normative in both groups [103], were revealed.

Immune screening showed the presence of deviant indicators of the lymphocytic populations in 69% of patients.

In particular, the cluster analysis in a group of 70 patients identified four clusters that significantly differ in the level of preservation of different components of the immune response to the infectious process. So, if patients of the first cluster (8 people) were distinguished by increased indicators of cellular immunity and maximum (within the normal range) values of the phagocytic indicator, then in patients of the third (22 people) and fourth (19 people) clusters revealed partial insufficiency of certain components of the immune status, and the second cluster (21 people) was characterized by a pronounced decrease in the immune response (indicators of the cellular immunity are lower than normative, phagocytic index is minimal within normal limits).

Along with the cluster analysis, the entire sample of 80 people was divided into groups on the basis characteristic of all patients from this group, and not found in others. Thus, the first group (28 people) was selected on the basis of relative lymphocytosis, the second (25 people)—by reduced values of T-helpers, and the third (27 people)—by the absence of indicators deviating from the norm [104].

The data of Table 20.1 show significant intergroup differences in laboratory parameters. So, if patients in the first and third groups can be conditionally designated as immunocompetent, then representatives of the second group clearly demonstrate immune compromise, especially pronounced in the lymphocytic populations.

Table 20.1 The average values of the parameters of cellular, humoral immunity, and BPRS scale in the studied groups of patients with schizophrenia, having a significant intergroup difference in Mann-Whitney *U*-test at $p < 0.05$

Parameters	The reference value	(M ± p)		
		1 group (N=28)	2 group (N=25)	3 group (N=27)
Leucocytes, 10`9/l	4,5-9,5	5,5 ± 1,6*	4,9 ± 1*	**6,5** ±1,6**
Lymphocytes %	18-38	**46,5** ± 5,6**	27,3 ± 4,3**	32,8 ± 4,8**
Lymphocytes (10^9/l)	0,8-3,6	**2,7** ± 1**	1,3 ± 0,2**	2,1 ± 0,5**
Neutrophiles, 10`9/l	1,9-6,5	3 ± 1**	3,6 ± 0,9**	**4,4** ± 1,4**
CD3+ (T-lymphocytes)%	55-80	64,3 ± 5,6*	61,6 ± 4,7**	64,8 ± 6,5*
CD3+ (T-lymphocytes) Cells/mkl	800-2200	**1680** ± 723**	796 ± 116**	1390 ± 329**
CD3+CD4+(T-helpers) Cells/mkl	600-1600	**1043** ± 453**	483 ± 62**	843 ± 173**
CD3+CD8+(cytotoxic cells) Cells/mkl	300-800	648 ± 302*	314 ± 64**	555 ± 154*
CD3-CD16+56+ (natural killers) Cells/mkl	100-500	**370** ± 148**	185 ± 68**	295 ± 100**
CD19+ (B-lymphocytes) Cells/mkl	100-500	343 ± 227*	148 ± 42**	293 ± 94*
IgA, g/l	0,5-3,5	1,7 ± 0,8*	2,0 ± 0,8*	1,8 ± 0,9
IgG CMV positivity coefficient	<6	4 ± 2,4*	**7** ± 4,5**	4 ± 3*
IgG EBV positivity coefficient	<1	3 ± 1,8*	**5** ± 3,2*	3,2 ± 2,2
Paranoid factor BPRS points	<10	17 ± 4,2*	**18,9** ± 2,8**	17,4 ± 4,2*

**asterisks of the same color indicate pairs of reliably different indicators.*

The calculation of the lymphocytic index (LI) in patients showed increased values in the first (0.85 ± 0.2) and third (0.51 ± 0.1) groups and mainly normative values in the second (0.41 ± 0.16), which indicates the presence of a viral infection. The normativity of values in the second group can be associated with its characteristic lymphopenia.

The combination of these indicators of LI and elevated IgG levels to CMV and EBV reflects the presence of a sample of herpes infection in patients. In its favor is the presence of correlations between the levels of antibodies to the studied herpesviruses and indicators of immune screening (Tables 20.2 and 20.3).

Differences in correlations in groups may reflect the presence of characteristic features of the inflammatory process for each group.

Despite the identified heterogeneity of the samples, correlations of antibody levels with immune screening indicators were revealed, reflecting the general patterns in the samples (Table 20.3).

The data of Table 20.3 correspond to the literature data on the immunosuppressive effects of herpesviruses, especially CMV.

The analyzed material indicates the presence of herpes infection in patients of the sampling group. The data obtained in the same group on the conjugation of serological and immunologi-

Table 20.2 Correlations of levels of antibodies to herpes viruses with cellular and nonspecific immunity parameters in groups of patients with schizophrenia

Levels of antibodies to herpes viruses	(M ± p)	Nonspecific immunity parameters	(M ± p)	*r*
1 group (*N* = 28)				
IgG HSV2	3.2 ± 2.6	CD3-CD 16 56 (natural killers) %	14.7 ± 4.5	−0.45
		Leucocytes, 10`9/l	5.5 ± 1.6	−0.47
		Neutrophiles, 10`9/l	3 ± 1	−0.42
IgM EBV	0.9 ± 0.4	CD19+(B-lymphocytes) %	12.7 ± 3.9	0.43
IgG HSV 1	15.6 ± 8.3	CIC with 4% PEG	0.07 ± 0.0	−0.43
IgM CMV	0.8 ± 0.1	IgG (joint)	12.4 ± 2.9	0.5
		Leucocytes. 10`9/l	5.5 ± 1.6	0.43
IgG EBV	3 ± 1.8	Lymphocytes %	46.5 ± 5.6	−0.51*
2 group (*N* = 25)				
IgG HSV 1	15.1 ± 10.9	CIC with 4% PEG	0.07 ± 0.0	−0.45
IgM HSV 1	0.8 ± 0.1	CD3+CD8+(cytotoxic cells) %	24 ± 2.8	0.46
IgG HSV 2	3.6 ± 3.7	IgM (joint)	1.6 ± 0.8	−0.41
IgM HSV 2	0.8 ± 0.1	CD19+(B-lymphocytes) %	11.6 ± 3.1	0.49
IgM EBV	0.8 ± 0.2	IgM (joint)	1.6 ± 0.8	0.48
3 group (*N* = 27)				
IgG HSV 1	16.2 ± 11	CD3+(T-lymphocytes) Cells/mkl	1390 ± 329	0.4
		CD3+CD4+ (T-helpers) Cells/mkl	843 ± 173	0.44
IgG HSV 2	3.0 ± 2.9	CD3+(T-lymphocytes) %	64.8 ± 6.5	0.52*
		CD3+CD4+ (T-helpers) %	39.2 ± 3.8	0.4
		Neutrophiles **10 * 9/l**	**4.4** ± 1.4	−0.43
IgM HSV 2	0.7 ± 0.2	IgM (joint)	1.1 ± 0.4	−0.44
IgG HSV 2	3.0 ± 2.9	Leucocytes, 109/l	**6.5** ± 1.6	−0.46

*$p < 0.005$

Table 20.3 Correlations of AT levels to herpesviruses with indicators of immune screening in a sample of studied patients with schizophrenia

AT levels to herpesviruses	M ± p	Indicators of immune screening	M ± p	*r*
IgG HSV 1	15.7 ± 10	CIC with 4% PEG	0.07 ± 0.00	−0.34**
IgG EBV	3.7 ± 2.5	Lymphocytes %	35.9 ± 9.3	−0.31*
IgG CMV	5 ± 3.7	Lymphocytes 10*9\л	2.1 ± 0.9	−0.37**
		CD3+(T-lymphocytes) cells/mkl	1306 ± 578	−0.35**
		CD3+CD4+ (T-helpers) cells/mkl	799 ± 356	−0.39**
		CD3+CD8+ (cytotoxic cells) cells/mkl	513 ± 238	−0.33*
		CD19 (B-lymphocytes) cells/mkl	261 ± 161	−0.33*
		CD3-CD 16 56 (natural killers) cells/mkl	288 ± 131	−0.3*

*$p < 0.01$;**$p < 0.005$

cal indicators with symptoms of a mental disorder at the time of the examination (Table 20.4) reflect, at least, the pathogenetic relationship between infectious and psychopathological processes, with the presence of its specifics in each group.

The correlations given in Table 20.4 in each group of patients have their own characteristics.

In patients of group 1 with symptoms of schizophrenia, mainly indicators of humoral, mainly specific immunity are associated. The cell changes are represented by indicators of the percentage of

Table 20.4 Correlations of serological and immunological parameters with BPRS parameters in the studied groups of patients with schizophrenia

BPRS parameters	Immunological parameters	*r*
1 group		
Depressive mood	IgG HSV 1	0.41
Hostility		−0.41
Motor retardation	IgM HSV 1	0.47
Conceptual disorganization	IgM HSV 2	0.4
Mannerism and posture	IgM CMV	−0.45
Anxiety	IgG EBV	0.5
Hallucination		0.43
Noncooperation		0.42
Points total		0.47
The paranoia factor	CIC with 3% PEG	0.38
Acute psychotic factor	Lymphocytes %	−0.38
2 group		
Somatic anxiety	CD3+CD8+(cytotoxic cells)%	0.4
	CD3+ (T-lymphocytes)%	0.5
	CIC with 3% PEG	0.4
Tension	IgG CMV	−0.59**
	CIC with 4% PEG	−0.41
Feeling of guilt	IgG CMV	−0.53*
	CIC with 3% PEG	−0.41
	IgG (joint)	0.44
	IgM (joint)	0.59**
Megalomania	IgM (joint)	0.4
	IgA (joint)	0.46
Depressive mood	IgG (joint)	0.42
Motor retardation	CD3-CD 16 56 (natural killers) cells/mkl	0.45
	CD3-CD 16 56 (natural killers)%	0.4
Mannerism and posture	IgG EBV	0.61**
	Neutrophiles, 10`9/l	0.045
	Phagocytic indicator	0.49
Hostility	CD3+ (T-lymphocytes) cells/mkl	−0.45
Excitement		−0.51*
	CD3+CD4+ (T-helpers) cells/mkl	−0.45
	CD3+CD8+(cytotoxic cells)%	−0.43
	CIC with 3% PEG	−0.43
	lymphocytes 10*9/л	−0.42
Conceptual disorganization	CIC with 3% PEG	−0.43
Suspicious	CD3+CD8+(cytotoxic cells)%	−0.47
Points total	IgM HSV 2	−0.45
The paranoid factor	IgM(joint)	0.53*
The paranoia factor	CD3+ (T-lymphocytes) cells/mkl	−0.42
	CD3+CD8+(cytotoxic cells)%	−0.41
	CD3+CD8+(cytotoxic cells) cells/mkl	−0.4
Anxiety-depressive factor	IgG CMV	−0.53*
Acute psychotic factor	CIC with 3% PEG	−0.5

(continued)

Table 20.4 (continued)

BPRS parameters	Immunological parameters	*r*
3 group		
Hostility	IgG HSV 1	0.4
Megalomania	IgG HSV 2	−0.42
Feeling of guilt	IgM CMV	0.6**
	IgM EBV	0.52
	CD3+ (T-lymphocytes) cells/mkl	−0.42
	CD3+CD4+ (T-helpers) cells/mkl	−0.44
	CD3+CD8+ (cytotoxic cells) cells/mkl	−0.4
Anxiety	CD3+ (T-lymphocytes) cells/mkl	−0.6**
	CD3+CD4+ (T-helpers) cells/mkl	−0.63**
	CD3+CD8+ (cytotoxic cells) cells/mkl	−0.46
	CD19+ (B-lymphocytes) cells/mkl	−0.48
	Lymphocytes 10*9/л	−0.5
Tension	Phagocytic index	0.44
Depressive mood	CD3-CD 16 56 (natural killers)%	0.42
	Lymphocytes %	−0.46
Noncooperation		−0.47
Points total	Phagocytic index	0.41
	Lymphocytes %	−0.4
Anxiety-depressive factor	Lymphocytes %	−0.4
	CD3+ (T-lymphocytes) cells/mkl	−0.42
	CD3+CD4+ (T-helpers) cells/mkl	−0.46
	CD3-CD 16 56 (natural killers)%	0.4
	Phagocytic index	0.47

$*p < 0.01$; $**p < 0.005$

lymphocytes, their average values are increased, the percentage of T-helpers and number of natural killers, the values of which correspond to the norm (see Table 20.1). Thus, in this group, the association of psychopathological symptoms with the tension of the immune system within the framework of herpetic infection with a predominance of HSV-1, CMV, and EBV was revealed.

In the second group, with the symptoms of schizophrenia, the indicators of all components of the immune response correlate, with the predominance of its cellular component. Participation in correlations of the total number of lymphocytes and their populations, as well as neutrophils, can indicate their increased consumption in conditions of high viral load and, accordingly, the depletion of the immune response. This assumption is confirmed by a decrease in the average values of the number of T-helpers in patients of this group relative to the norm, and the remaining indicators of the total number of T- and B lymphocytes compared with other groups (these indicators are close to the lower limit of the norm) (see Table 20.1). Correlations of symptoms of schizophrenia with the total number of neutrophils can indicate both the accession of bacterial and (or) fungal infection, and a significant amount of cells damaged by pathogens, as well as pronounced intoxication processes. Since the activation and secretory degranulation of neutrophilic leukocytes is associated with leukocyte elastase—a marker of chronic and acute inflammatory diseases, the positive nature of the correlation of the total number of neutrophils with the severity of symptoms of schizophrenia may reflect the relationship of the latter with the inflammatory process.

Thus, in the second group, the symptoms of schizophrenia appear to be associated with a more severe viral process with a predominant role of HSV-2 and EBV, possibly with the accession of a bacterial infection, with the depletion of the immune response.

In the third group, the indicators of all links of antiviral immunity correlate with BPRS parameters. Participation in these correlations of the total number of T- and B lymphocytes also indicates depletion of immunity. However, in this group it is compensated, as evidenced by the normative average levels of these indicators (Table 20.4). In this group, the symptoms of schizophrenia are associated with infection with a predominance of CMV and EBV in conditions of compensated depletion of immunity.

These data suggest that in the three groups studied, herpes infection in individuals comparable in age and duration of the disease has significant differences in the consistency of the antiviral immune response. In the first group, he is wealthy, in the second with signs of obvious exhaustion, and in the third hidden, compensated.

The connection of the infectious process with the symptoms of a mental disorder does not yet prove its cerebral localization. The presence of inflammatory-degenerative processes in the brain of the examined patients associated with herpes infection reflects data on the conjugation of immunological, serological, and clinical indicators with abnormal signs of structural MRI and MR angiography and electrophysiological indicators, as well as the relationship with these indicators of autoantibodies levels to the nervous tissue.

In the course of the study, any MR indicators reflecting anomalies of the brain and its vascular network were identified in almost all the patients examined. The frequency of occurrence of the most significant of them was as follows. The expansion of perivascular spaces was determined in 65.8% of cases, of which most often (48.7%)—in the basal nuclei. The expansion of subarachnoid convexital spaces, mainly in the frontoparietal region, was detected in 67.9% of cases. Expansion of the furrows of the cortex was noted in 20.5% of cases. The expansion of certain parts of the lateral ventricles was detected in 57.1% of patients. Disorders of blood circulation were noted in 49% of patients, of which the pathology of venous sinuses (mainly transverse and sigmoid) was detected in 28% of patients. The predominance of left-sided localization of anomalies of these sinuses (narrowing, signal attenuation) was established.

As illustrations to the above material, MRI images from the collection of tomograms that served are presented (Fig. 20.1).

Comparison of the parameters of the BPRS scale and immunological indicators in patients with specific MR anomalies and without them determined the relationship of structural changes in the brain and cerebral circulation with the characteristics of specific and nonspecific immunity. A sampling group of patients with schizophrenia as a whole, without division into groups, supplemented up to 90 people [105], was analyzed.

Thus, with the expansion of the perivascular spaces, the percentage of lymphocytes and the total number of neutrophils are significantly lower, with the expansion of the subarachnoid spaces in the frontal lobes—the level of IgM to EBV is lower, and in the parietal—the percentage of T-helpers is higher. With the expansion of the furrows of the cortex, IgG levels to HSV-2 are lower and above is the paranoid BPRS factor. The local expansion of the cortical furrows in the frontal lobes corresponds to significantly higher levels of the percentage of natural killers, and in the parietal—total IgG.

The presence of anomalies (change in size, deformation) in the ventricular system corresponds to higher levels of IgG to EBV, indicators of "acute psychotic factor," "mannerisms and posture," "unusual thoughts," and the total score of the BPR Scale, as well as with a higher frequency of cases of leading paranoid and catatonic-paranoid syndromes in mental status. The presence of expansion of the anterior horns of the lateral ventricles is associated with a higher score on the parameter "hallucinations," and posterior—with higher levels of IgA. In patients with cerebral circulation disorders, lower levels of IgA and the parameter "excitation," higher scores on the signs of "motor inhibition" and "somatic concern." The weakening of the signals of certain venous sinuses corresponds to lower values of the parameter "excitation." The weakening of the signal of the sagittal sinuses (mainly left) corresponds to a lower percentage of cytotoxic cells as well as higher values of the parameters "idea of greatness," "hostility" and lower—"hallucinations."

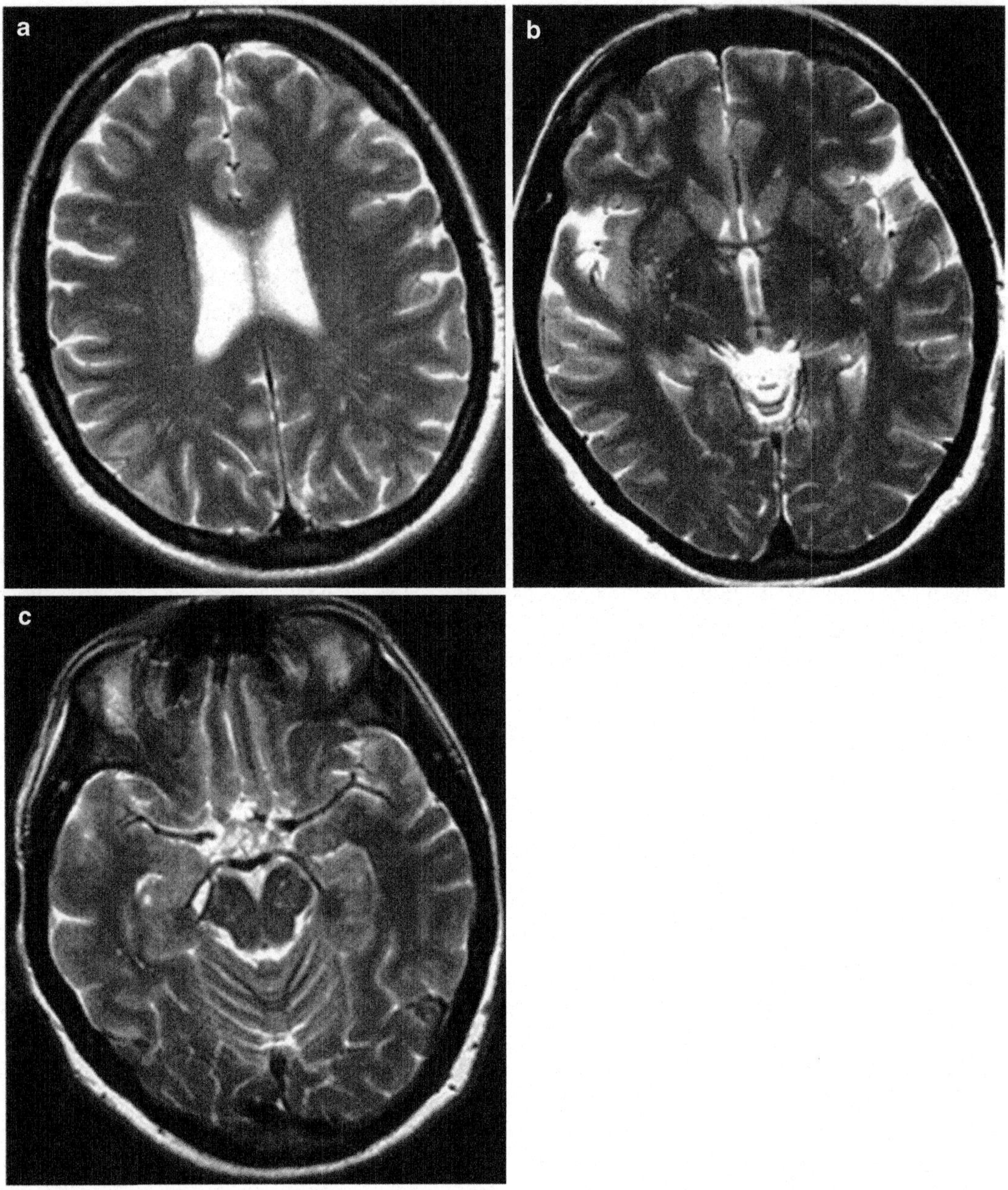

Fig. 20.1 MR tomograms of a patient with schizophrenia P., in T2 mode. Extended perivascular spaces (PVP) look like linear sections of a high MR signal and represent an accumulation of fluid along the walls of small vessels. (**a**) expansion of PVP in the white matter of the brain at the border of the temporal and occipital lobes, (**b**) expansion of PVP in the basal nuclei, (**c**) expansion of PVP in the brain stem. Courtesy of T.P. Berezovskaya

In a group of 48 patients with episodic paranoid schizophrenia (F20.01–03) (24 men and 24 women), anomalies of latent periods and amplitudes of auditory evoked potentials (EP) were identified [106].

The average values of latent periods and amplitudes of auditory EP in the studied patients revealed anomalies, differing from the normative indicators. Latency of early components of auditory cognitive EP (ACEP) was detected both shortening in an unfavorable form of the disease with a tendency to transition to a continuous course, and elongation (to a greater extent with a distinct episodic course). Previously, shortening of the latent period of EP in a neurological clinic was noted in inflammatory processes in the brain [107] which, as indicated earlier, are also discussed in schizophrenia [108, 109]. Latency of long-latent auditory EP (LAEP) P1 and N1 exceeded the norm by more than 2 times.

The revealed relationships between the characteristics of the studied EP and the level of antibodies to herpesviruses indicate the possibility of modifying the work of neural populations by them. In particular, in the increase in the latent period of ACEP, indicating a slowdown in the onset of the response process to the stimulus, antibodies to HSV-1, EBV and CMV contribute in different examined groups of patients. Elongation of LAEP latency is associated with the level of antibodies to HSV-2, EBV, and CMV.

The mechanisms of the noted antibody influences can be associated with the infectious process-induced restructuring of neuronal synapses, changes in cellular activity, a decrease in the number of neuronal populations, as well as the process of demyelination. The latter disrupts the work of ion channels and is described, as noted above, in herpesvirus infections and schizophrenia. Correlations of ACVP N1-P2 and P2-N2 with IgG levels to EBV and CMV may reflect changes in the functioning of the membrane of neurons in the auditory cortex under the influence of these viruses. The same characteristics of EP in patients correlate with such psychopathological parameters as "suspicion," "anxiety," "total BPRS score."

The relationship of pathological changes in the state of microstructures of the nervous system with herpetic infection was shown on the material of 56 patients (24 men, 32 women) with SHAP (F-25) in comparison with a control group of 100 mentally healthy subjects by identifying deviations in the indicators of the corresponding auto-Ab in peripheral blood and their correlations with antiherpes antibodies [110].

Anomalies of serum immunoreactivity profiles caused by the auto-Ab studied were found in the majority patients of the main group (94.6%) and only 3% of the examined control group. The prevailing increase in the amplitude of peaks (10.6% of the total number of indicators excluding boundary values), their abnormal decrease (1.5%) was less common, which differed significantly from the corresponding indicators of the control group (2.5% and 0.7%, respectively).

An increase in the amplitude of auto-Ab peaks to MBP (the main myelin protein) (27% of cases, and only in the main group of patients) in combination with an increase in auto-Ab levels to a specific axon protein NF-200 (15.7% in patients against 2% in control group individuals, $p = 0.003$) with a high degree of probability indicates degenerative changes in axons, including their demyelination [111].

An increase in the content of auto-Ab to GABA receptors (23.5% vs. 1% in control) reflects changes in the GABAergic system of neurons.

In 21.8% of patients of the main group and only 3% in the control group ($p = 0.000$), there was an increase in the content of auto-Ab to the proteins of the S100 group—calcium-dependent regulators of a number of cellular roles that provide functional homeostasis of brain cells by conjugating and integrating diverse metabolic processes [112]. The increase in the content of auto-Ab to such a representative of proteins of this group as S-100B, apparently reflects destructive changes in nervous tissue and its involvement in an inflammatory response, often associated with a viral infection (due to the similarity of the epitopes of S100 proteins with the epitopes of some viruses, for example, HPV).

In addition, since S100 proteins in the extracellular sector exhibit the properties of cytokines and interact with RAGE receptors [113], which are expressed in the nervous system not only by neurons, microglia, and astrocytes, but also by cells of the vascular wall, it is possible to assume involvement in the inflammatory response of the vascular network as well.

An increase in the levels of auto-Ab to S-100B may indicate the activation of pathological processes in the astrocytic glia [114]. This position is confirmed by the analysis of auto-Ab levels to the

GFAP protein (glial fibrillary acid protein) in the studied patients. In 14.3% of cases (against 3% in the control group), there was an increase in the level of auto-Ab to this protein, which may indicate the activation of astrocytic glia in response to damage to neurons of various, including infectious-inflammatory, genesis and may indicate a violation of the function of the blood-brain barrier (BBB) [115].

Other deviations in the levels of auto-Ab (to dopamine, serotonin, and H-cholinergic cells, to double-helix DNA and β-2-glycoprotein) were less common (10–11% vs. 2–3% in control) and reflected changes in the dopamine, serotonin, and cholinergic systems of neurons, violations of the water-electrolyte balance and energy metabolism of neurons, changes in the ratios between excitatory and inhibitory processes in the nervous system, as well as the likely association of the described changes with nonspecific immune activation (systemic inflammation, including inflammation in the vascular network, usually viral etiology) [111].

Indicators of specific antiherpes immunity were studied in 25 out of 56 patients. Their deviations were similar to those in the rest of the samples. Thus, elevated levels of certain antiherpes IgG were observed in all cases, most often to HSV-1 (84%), to capsid (87%) and nuclear (71%) EBV antigens, to CMV (54%).

As shown by the results of nonparametric correlation analysis, the content of auto-Ab to MBP correlates with the level of IgG to the capsid antigen EBV ($r = 0.55$) and the level of IgM к CMV (r = 0.34), auto-Ab to NF-200—with the content of IgM to EBV ($r = -0.68$). Auto-Ab levels to dopamine receptors correlated with IgG content for capsid ($r = -0.6$) and for nuclear EBV antigens ($r = -0.49$), auto-Ab for glutamate receptors with IgM content for EBV ($r = -0.5$) and IgG for HSV-6 ($r = -0.51$) ($p < 0.05$ for all correlations).

These data showed not only the cerebral localization of the inflammatory process, but also its activity at the time of examination, as well as the etiological role of the studied herpesviruses, especially EBV, in this process.

Additionally, in a group of 35 patients with SHAP (F25), which was part of the previous sample (14 men and 25 women), an analysis of the indicators of the erythrocyte link of peripheral blood was carried out in the context of the connection of an acute psychotic state with herpesvirus infection [116].

Any deviations from the norm in the clinical blood test were observed in 57% of cases. Deviation from the norm of leukocyte levels mainly upwards was noted in 28.2% of cases, decreases in 10% of cases, and the erythrocyte link (total erythrocyte content and hematocrit) in 41% of cases (of which upwards in 35.9% of patients, decreases in 13%). Hematocrit in all cases was close to the upper limit of the norm. An increase in the level of certain antiherpes antibodies was noted in all cases: IgG to HSV-1 in 70%, IgG to capsid hypertension EBV in 90%, and IgG to nuclear hypertension EBV in 73%. The number of cases of increase in IgG levels to CMV was 54.6%.

Methods of nonparametric statistics revealed positive correlations of the average hemoglobin content in the erythrocyte with the level of IgM to HSV 2 ($r = 0.47$ in 22 cases), the average volume of erythrocyte with IgM to HSV 1 ($r = 0.42$ in 27 cases), and the hemoglobin content with IgG to HSV-1 ($r = 0.48$ in 31 cases) (in all cases $p < 0.05$). The direct orientation of the correlations of herpes infection with the parameters of the erythrocyte link of peripheral blood may be associated with a decrease in the infectious load of specific antibodies. The revealed correlations reflect the destructive effect of herpes infection on red blood cells.

The facts obtained need additional study, being potentially significant for understanding additional aspects of the pathogenesis of SHAP (F25) and schizophrenia (F20). In particular, these conjugations may reflect the significance of violations of the transport and exchange function of the blood due to the change under the influence of viruses of negative charges on the surface of erythrocytes and the deformation of the "electrostatic space." The latter reduces the possibility of blood plasma passing between erythrocytes (A.L. Chizhevsky, citated by 118), which leads to a violation of metabolism as a whole. According to T.P. Teterina [117], due to neuro-regulatory mechanisms, the spatial-regulatory system of moving blood is capable of being able to comprise response to certain fluctuations in the electromagnetic radiation of the atmosphere. Thus, this system is an adaptive mechanism that provides a constant balance in the organism itself and between the organism and the external environment. Damage to the membranes of erythrocytes, a decrease in their charge should inevitably lead to a violation of this adaptive function.

In addition to the above, it should be noted that the interaction of herpesvirus infection with the erythrocyte link of the blood may include a violation of the regulation of the production of erythropoietin in infected cells [118]. Additional importance to this mechanism is given by the tropism of herpesviruses to the vascular endothelium, including in the kidneys, the cells of which are also attributed to the function of producing erythropoietin [119]. In addition, there are possible direct ways of violation of erythropoiesis by herpesviruses in the bone marrow. The tropism of herpesviruses to the hematopoietic system was noted in a number of works [120].

Of particular importance is the participation of erythropoietin in the infectious process in SHAP (F25) giving its diverse cerebroprotective effect. In particular, erythropoietin plays an important role in the brain's response to neuronal damage [121], enhances the antihypoxic reactions of the hippocampus, and increases neural plasticity [122]. The direct neuroprotective effect of erythropoietin may be to protect neurons from glutamate intoxication or to reduce the production of damaging molecules, such as active forms of oxygen [123]. These factors are likely to contribute to a decrease in apoptosis level [124, 125]. Some researchers tend to believe that erythropoietin may serve as a neurotransmitter by providing synaptic plasticity in the brain. A number of authors suggest the ability of erythropoietin to stimulate neoangiogenesis [126] and inhibit anti-inflammatory cytokines, increase the expression of brain neurotrophic factors [127]. Since cerebroprotection is carried out by small doses of erythropoietin [128], a violation of hormone production in SHAP (F25) can affect the mental state without leading to a change in the number of red blood cells.

In general, the considered data show links between psychopathology, cerebral neuropathology, and hemodynamic disturbances, disorders of immunity, erythrocyte links of the blood, deviations in the levels of autoantibodies to the nervous tissue, and levels of antibodies to herpesviruses, which allows us to conclude about the unified nature of the current psychosis in patients of the sampling group, an important role in which is played by the inflammatory-degenerative process of infectious genesis.

Below is our material showing the relationship of the studied indicators of different levels with the forms of schizophrenia.

On a sample consisting of 74 patients with schizophrenia with different types of courses, compared with a control group of mentally healthy individuals (10 people), associations of the severity of psychopathological symptoms with antiherpes antibodies characteristic of different types of schizophrenia [129] were revealed.

In 27 patients (first group) was diagnosed with episodic paranoid schizophrenia with a tendency to transition into a continuous course with the preservation of reduced paranoid symptoms in remissions, a stable or increasing defect (F20.00, F20.01 according to ICD-10), in 16 (second group)—episodic paranoid with remissions of higher quality with the preservation of rudimentary subpsychotic manifestations, a stable defect (F20.02), in 31 (3rd group)—remitting with complete remissions (F20.03).

Differences in serological indicators between groups of patients with different forms of schizophrenia were unreliable, but the levels of IgM to HSV-2 and EBV in all groups of patients with schizophrenia were significantly higher than in control (10 mentally healthy individuals) (Table 20.5)

Despite the small number of groups, this table shows clear differences in infectious processes in patients with different forms of schizophrenia.

Different types of schizophrenia are characterized by a different spectrum of viruses involved in the development of the disease, their different interactions (synergistic, antagonistic) and correlations between the content of specific antiherpes Ab in the blood serum, and the severity of clinical symptoms. The severity of the course of the disease, the tendency to reduce the quality of remissions correspond to an increase in the number of herpesviruses associated with the

Table 20.5 Correlations between serological, as well as serological and clinical parameters in groups of patients with schizophrenia

Group, *N*	Levels of antibodies to herpes viruses	Levels of antibodies to herpes viruses, BPRS parameters	*r**
1 (F20.00-01), *N* = 27	IgG HSV -1	IgM HSV - 1	0.52**
		IgG HSV -2	0.46*
		IgM CMV	0.42*
	IgM HSV - 1	IgM HSV - 2	0.47*
	IgG HSV -2	IgM HSV -2	–0.41*
		IgG CMV	0.49*
	IgM CMV		0.45*
	IgM HSV - 1	Feeling of guilt	0.48*
	IgG HSV -2	Excitement	0.42*
	IgM HSV -2		–0.5*
	IgG CMV	Excitement	0.51*
		Motor retardation	–0.5*
	IgG EBV	Tension	0.41*
	IgM EBV	Megalomania	–0.5*
		Depressive mood	0.57**
2 (F20.01-02), *N* = 16	IgG HSV -1	IgM HSV -1	0.68**
		IgG HSV -2	0.57*
		IgM HSV -2	0.53*
	IgM HSV - 1	IgM HSV - 2	0.87*
	IgM CMV	IgM EBV	–0.65*
	IgM CMV	Tension	0.56*
	IgM EBV		–0.68*
		Suspicious	–0.56
3 (F20.03), *N* = 31	IgM EBV	IgG EBV	–0.46*
	IgM HSV - 2	Somatic anxiety	0.48*
		Anxiety	0.54**
		Feeling of guilt	0.5**
		Tension	0.48*
		Noncooperation	0.47*
	IgM EBV	Suspicious	0.46*
		Extraordinary thoughts	0.47*

$*p \leq 0.05$, $**p \leq 0.005$

symptoms of the disease, their synergism, the severity of immunodeficiency. Different forms of schizophrenia correspond to the features of general and local immune reactivity.

Below we show the results of our studies of EP in samples of patients with the same forms of schizophrenia—16 patients in each [106, 130].

The parameters of the studied EP revealed a reliable intergroup difference in U-test for the parameters of latencies N2 of ACEP and P1 of LAEP when comparing groups of episodic paranoid schizophrenia with an increasing or stable defect (F20.01-02) and with remissions without any psychopathological symptoms (F20.03), for latency P2 ACEP when comparing groups with a tendency to a continuous course and without this trend. Amplitudes of ACEP were identified as a decrease (more often with the most severe form of the course in patients of the first group), and increase (in patients of the second group). The amplitudes of N1-P2 LAEP significantly differed in U-test in patients of the first and second groups.

The conjugation of EP parameters with the levels of antiherpes antibodies was revealed (Table 20.6).

Attention is drawn to the significantly higher frequency of detection of the studied correlations in groups with a more severe course of the dis-

Table 20.6 Correlations between the parameters of the studied EP (latent period —LP, amplitude—A) and the levels of antibodies to herpes viruses in groups of patients with schizophrenia with different types of course

Parameter of auditory EP	Episodic paranoid schizophrenia, a tendency to a continuous course (F20.01)		Episodic paranoid schizophrenia, stable defect (F20.02)		Episodic paranoid schizophrenia, remittent (F20.03)	
	AT	R	AT	R	AT	R
LP ACEP P1					IgG HSV -2	−0.7**
LP ACEP N2			IgG HSV -2	−0.6		
LP ACEP P3	IgG HSV -1	0.72*				
LP ACEP P2		0.65	IgM EBV	0.59		
LP ACEP N3			IgG CMV	0.56	IgM HSV -1	−0.53
A ACEP N1–P2			IgG EBV	0.63		
			IgG CMV	0.71		
A ACEP P2– N2	IgG CMV	−0.9**	IgG EBV	0.81**		
LP LAEP P1	IgG EBV	0.9	IgM HSV -2	0.73		
LP LAEP P2	IgM CMV	0.82			IgM HSV-1	−0.62
LP LAEP P3			IgG HSV -2	0.78		
			IgG CMV	−0.68		

$*p < 0.01$; $**p < 0.005$, in all other cases $p < 0.05$

ease compared to the group of recurrent schizophrenia. However, in a more favorable group of recurrent schizophrenia, IgM to herpesviruses were more often involved in correlations, reflecting an acute early reaction to the infect. In general, the multidirectional correlations can reflect different effects of the interaction of antiviral antibodies with the same or with different cell receptors and the possibility of changing different types of mediator metabolism, which leads to both excitation and inhibition of neurons.

A more detailed study was conducted on a sampling group of 62 patients with different variants of episodic paranoid schizophrenia (30 cases—F20.01-02 and 32 cases—F20.03), in age and sex composition, as well as mental status comparable to the first sample described. It did not include patients with a pronounced tendency to a continuous course of the disease (F20.00) [131].

The data from the immune screening and serological study on the sample were generally similar to those in the first sample described (Table 20.7).

This table at all levels reflect the great acuity of the infectious process in the remitting course of paranoid schizophrenia (F20.03) and the tendency to chronicity and immune deficiency in its episodic course with an increasing or stable defect (F20.01-02).

Table 20.7 The frequency of occurrence of abnormal immunological, serological, MR—parameters in groups of patients with different forms of episodic paranoid schizophrenia, significantly differing in groups

Abnormal immunological, serological, MR—parameters	F20.01-02 (%)	F20.03 (%)
Decrease in the level of T-helpers	47	21.7
Relative lymphocytosis	26	47.8
Slight increase in the CIC	40	8
Increase IgM HSV2	0	14
Increase IgM CMV	14	3.5
Focuses of dystrophy	10	32
Perivascular space dilation in basal ganglia	40	75
Native abnormality of structure of brain arteries	33	10

When calculating intralevel and interlevel relationships in each group of patients, complexes of indicators were identified that were significantly related to each other directly or indirectly (association with the same indicator of several unrelated indicators). Relationships that were significant according to the criteria of the Spearman rank correlation coefficient and the Mann-Whitney U-test were taken into account. The complexes were given names reflecting their clinical content.

Comparative analysis of the obtained complexes showed obvious intergroup differences in

Table 20.8 The structure of clinical and paraclinical complexes in the studied groups of patients with schizophrenia

Form of schizophrenia	Episodic paranoid schizophrenia, a course with an increasing or stable defect (F20.01-02) (main group)		Episodic paranoid schizophrenia, remitting course (F20.03)	
The name of complex	BPRS parameters	Immunological and morphological parameters	BPRS parameters	Immunological and morphological parameters
1. "Partial-depressive" complex	"Guilt"	HSV-1 IgM, B-lymphocytes (%), Natural killers (%), venous circulation disorder, ventriculi enlargement, pathology of sinuses	"Somatic concern"	HSV-2 IgM*, IgA (g/l), Cytotoxic cells(%), T-lymphocytes (%), T-helpers (%), B- lymphocytes (%), phagocytic coefficient(%), distention of perivascular spaces of subcortical area, asymmetry of the sigmoid sinuses signal
2. "Affective" complex	"Anxiety", "Hostility", "Tension", "Excitement", "Depression", "Motor retardation", Total BPRS value.	HSV-2 IgM*, HSV-2 IgG (IU/ml), EBV IgM*, EBV IgG*, CMV IgG*, IgA(g/l), T-lymphocytes %, Neutrophils (10 × 9/l), T-helpers(μl), cytotoxic cells(μl), cortex sulci enlargement, perivascular space dilation in basal ganglia and in the parietal lobes white matter	"Anxiety", "Tension", "Guilt", "Depression".	HSV-2 IgM*, CIC, phagocytic coefficient(%), T-lymphocytes %, T-helpers %, B-lymphocytes %, natural killers%, lateral ventricles asymmetry, subcortical perivascular space dilation
3. "Psychotic" complex	"Unusual thought content", "Hallucinations", "Suspiciousness", "Grandiosity".	HSV-1 IgM*, HSV-2 IgG(IU/ml), EBV IgM*, IgM(g/l), IgG(g/l), CIC, Natural killers %, B-lymph (μl), Ventricli enlargement, venous circulation disorder, asymmetry of the sigmoid sinuses signal.	"Unusual thought content", "Hallucinations", "Suspiciousness", "Grandiosity", "Hostility", "Uncooperativeness".	HSV-2 IgM*, EBV IgM*, EBV IgG*, phagocytic coefficient(%), ventriculi enlargement, perivascular space dilation, venous circulation disorder.
4. "Catatono-disorganized" complex	"Mannerisms and posturing", "Conceptual disorganization"	T-helpers(μl), cytotoxic cells(μl), T-lymphocytes(μl), diffuse perivascular cysts	–	

the identified complexes for paraclinical signs with a common clinical one. Thus, the parameters of the BPRS scale in both groups were combined into similar complexes: partial-depressive (with a predominance of the cognitive component of depressive affect), affective, psychotic, catatonic (for a group with a more severe course), but in each group of patients they were associated with different paraclinical parameters.

The data of Table 20.8 show the relationship of each psychopathological syndrome with a certain aspect of a single infectious process involving herpesviruses, manifested by inflammatory-degenerative processes in brain tissue, cerebral vessels, and the collector system. In different forms of schizophrenia, these processes have significant differences. In this case, they can be roughly designated as a polyetiological with significant role of CMV, immune deficiency, and a tendency to neurodegenerative processes in adverse forms of episodic paranoid schizophrenia (F 20.01-02) and the preservation of immunity in combination with the predominance of inflammatory manifestations in a milder form (F20.03).

The frequency of occurrence in the examined patients both of anomalies of the ventricular system (especially lateral) and MR signs of damage to the cerebral vascular system (hemodynamic disorders, including in the collector system, expansion of the perivascular spaces) and dynamics of liquor (signs of external and internal hydrocephalus), taking into account the central place of the choroid plexus, suggests its special role in the infectious process.

The presented material shows the presence of significant relationships between all the studied parameters at all levels, both within the current state and in the dynamics of the disease. This is highly likely to indicate the etiological and pathogenic unity of a mental disorder and a persistent infection.

The final analysis of the obtained data allows us to formulate following conclusions:

1. In the pathogenesis of schizophrenia, an important role is played by the chronic polyinfectious process, in which herpesviruses are a significant etiological factor. The latter is manifested by inflammatory and degenerative processes in brain tissues, cerebral vessels, and the collector system. Thus, it seems reasonable to raise the question of the definition of schizophrenia as atypical encephalitis.
2. Changes in the speed of information processing in schizophrenia, associated with disruption of neural networks and detected by the method of evoked potentials, can be largely associated with the molecular mimicry of herpesviruses and the cascade of autoimmune reactions in the brain that develop as part of the infectious process.
3. Inflammatory morphological and autoimmune changes have an infectious etiology and are associated with symptoms of schizophrenia and SHAP.
4. Three highlighted types of infectious process underlying schizophrenia may differ in the severity of immune compromise (indicators of lymphocytes and phagocytic index) and associations of herpesviruses, which is associated with different quality of remissions with the similarity of the clinical picture of seizures. This circumstance requires a differentiated therapeutic approach.
5. In patients with schizophrenia, CMV and EBV are of particular importance for the formation of the insolvency of the lymphocytic link of immunity, and the latter for morphological changes in the tissue and vessels of the brain, as well as the severity of psychotic manifestations of the disease.
6. The study of the probable special role of choroid plexus lesions in the formation of the type of course and prognosis of schizophrenia requires special attention.
7. Standard laboratory methods for diagnosing infections in patients with schizophrenia are unacceptable due to immune disorders. It is advisable to develop special criteria for laboratory diagnostics for this category of patients.

Some aspects of our study, as noted above, suggest the participation in the infectious process in schizophrenia not only of viral factors, but also of bacterial flora. It should be noted that at present a strategy for complex differentiation of herpesvirus infections [73, 120] has been developed, which involves the identification of viral-viral and viral-bacterial associations, including associations of herpesviruses and other pathogens (*Chlamydia, Ureaplasma*, etc.), herpesviruses and other conditionally pathogenic microorganisms (*Staphylococcus* spp.; *Streptococcus* spp., *Clostridium* spp., *Esherichia coli*, etc.). Some works show the effects of various microbial associations on the clinical picture and pathological disorders in diseases associated with brain pathology [132]. Taking into account the indicated strategy, as well as the available literature data on the possible involvement of other microorganisms in the pathogenesis of schizophrenia, in particular, toxoplasma [133, 134], a broad study of the microbial landscape of all biological fluids of the body of patients with schizophrenia, as well as intestinal contents, is necessary. Many pathogenic viruses, including herpes, influenza, etc., have tropism to the tissues of the gastrointestinal tract (GIT), where more than 70% of immune cells are located [135]. The microflora of the gastrointestinal tract is currently recognized as a central factor determining health or disease [46]. It largely determines the state of immunity, including immune response or immunological tolerance [136]. The introduction of pathogenic viral agents can introduce an imbalance in its microbiota and disrupt the intercellular networks that represent the system of trophic and energy interconnections within the intestinal microbiocenosis. The gastrointestinal tract, including the oropharynx, accounts for the largest number of microorganisms—75–78% (the total mass of the intestinal microflora is from 1 to 3 kg). On the other hand, primary dysbiosis of the gastrointestinal microflora, considered in the light of recent studies as a separate organ, can contribute to the introduction of viral agents into the tissues of the gastrointestinal tract, and through it into the blood and other tissues and organs. At the same time, if a person is considered as a "superorganism," the metabolism of which is provided by the well-organized work of enzymes encoded not only by the genome of *Homo sapiens* proper, but also by the genomes of all symbiotic microorganisms, we can expect manifestations of not only local, but also generalized metabolic, including mediator, disorders, manifestations of inflammatory processes. New evidence suggests that the gut microbiota may promote brain development, modulate its functions and behavior of the individual [137, 138], and prevent the development of demyelinating autoimmune diseases [139]. This circumstance stimulated the study of the microbiota-gut-brain (MGB) axis [140–142] in mental diseases, currently considered as one of the highest priorities.

Most of the work performed focused on the bacterial components of the human gut microbiome, including patients with endogenous mental illness, but the modern methods of whole-genome sequencing allow to study also virom. Studies have shown that the virom of most human mucous membranes includes a wide range of bacteriophages [143]. Bacteriophages are viruses that infect bacteria. It has been hypothesized that the pharyngeal bacteriophage community, characterized as a "phage," plays an important and as yet uncharacterized role in maintaining human health and developing diseases. Within this hypothesis, R.H. Yolken et al. [144], studying by metagenome sequencing of human oropharyngeal bactoriophagic virom, found an increased content of *Lactobacillus* bacteriophages in patients with schizophrenia compared with individuals from the control group. *Lactobacillus phage phiadh* is a phage that predominantly infects the bacteria *Lactobacillus gasseri*, which are a common component of the oral mucosa and gastrointestinal tract and are able to bind to the intestinal epithelium. The quantitative content of *Lactobacillu sphage phiadh* and the quantitative content of *Lactobacillus gasseri* in patients with schizophrenia were conjugated. *Lactobacillus gasseri* is known to modulate the immune system, mainly by altering the function of dendritic cells, enterocytes, and components of innate immunity. The introduction of *Lactobacillus gasseri* to humans has a number of beneficial effects on the immune system and the functioning of the gastrointestinal tract. *Lactobacillus phage phiadh* can change the number of relevant bacteria either by directly destroying them or by establishing a prolonged lysogenic state in the genome of the host bacterium (that is, a state in which a phage embeds its genome into the genome of a bacterium with doubling each division of the host cell with the subsequent weakening of its function). Thus, the altered quantitative level of *Lactobacillus phage phiadh* indirectly through changes in the number and function of lactobacilli can affect the human immune system and the ecology of its microbiota as a whole.

Works concerning the study of the representation of other viruses in the composition of the virom, which characterizes the microbial community of the gastrointestinal tract of patients with endogenous mental diseases, are also seldom. Meanwhile, the ability of herpesviruses, which make up 18% of human virom [145], to affect the gastrointestinal tract is well known, which dictates the need for research in this direction.

In our [146] small comprehensive study, which included a group of patients with schizophrenia and SHAP, the microbiota of the posterior wall of the oropharynx was studied by the method of chromato-mass spectrometry of microbial markers (MSMM), which allows simultaneous identification of markers of 57 microorganisms. Along with coccal microflora which is the characteristic of chronic tonsillitis and pharyngitis, fungi (Aspergillus, Candida, Actinomycetes) as well as microorganisms "traditionally" found in the intestine and not found in the throat (anaerobic Streptococci—*Peptostreptococci, Enterococci, Clostridia* of various species, gram-negative bacteria (*Kingella, Flavobacterium* etc.)) and a decrease in the content of beneficial microflora (lacto- and bifidobacteria), herpes viruses were found (including HSV-1 and HSV-2, CMV and EBV). An increased total number of microorganisms, a high level of toxins, the appearance of pathogenic microflora, which is not normally found in the throat, a decrease in normal microflora negatively affect the state of the central nervous system. Currently, it is proved that pathogenic, in particular, viral, microbiota not only through hematogenic but also neural pathways can reach the brain [73]. In the same patients, in addition to anomalies in the content of autoantibodies to the structures of nervous tissue, innovative methods of studying physiological autoimmunity found an increase in the titer of autoantibodies against antigens of stomach, small and large intestine, liver, as well as to insulin and its receptors [146]. Despite the fact that the studies of the gastrointestinal microbiome of patients with endogenous psychosis are at an initial stage, it can already be concluded that the intestinal microflora in patients with schizophrenia is more scarce in the number and diversity of microorganisms, is characterized by a disproportion in the content of representatives of some families of microbes compared to mentally healthy individuals [147–151], and also reveals translocation between the gastrointestinal tract (in particular, characteristic representatives of the intestinal microbiota—in the oropharynx [146]). A number of microbial taxa show conjugation with psychotic, depressive, and negative symptoms [150, 152], as well as somatic characteristics. The latter may include inflammatory changes in the intestine [146, 147, 149], oropharynx [146], diabetes mellitus [144], as well as the risk of developing coronary heart disease [152]. Also revealed the conjugation of disorders in the composition of the intestinal microflora with abnormalities of brain structures: the volume of the right middle frontal gyrus [153]. Transplantation of the intestinal microbiome from patients with schizophrenia to gnotobiont mice causes a decrease in the concentration of glutamate and an increase in glutamine and GABA in the hippocampus, as well as behavioral disorders similar to those in models of schizophrenia with glutamatergic hypofunction in mice [150]. Specific patterns of microbiome community structure, studied more in terms of bacterial composition, vary in patients with schizophrenia [154] and need further research, including with increased study of the viral aspect.

20.1.4 Will Final Evidence Be Obtained?

The final proof of the etiological and pathogenic relationship of schizophrenia with infection will be the identification of infectious agents in the brain tissue in postmortem studies. Some peculiarities of the neuropathological picture in schizophrenia allowed some pathologists to assume the viral nature of brain damage in patients with schizophrenia. This applies to the characteristic for the disease nesting discharges of cytoarchitectonics of the surface layers of the cerebral cortex (bald spots), which may be, according to a number of authors [53], a consequence of viral lesion. According to A.I. Oifa [53], in a situation where the virus is embedded in the genome and does not replicate, mass death of neurons may not occur and it can be judged only by areas with shadow cells. Latent viral infection of the human brain is not manifested by classical signs of inflammation. Pathological anatomy of encephalopathy is not studied at all.

When the nature of the "pathy" is revealed, it becomes obvious that, at least in some cases, we are talking about viruses. In this regard, the allocation of so-called functional psychoses, which include, among other things, schizophrenia, is nothing more than a "psychiatric myth" [53].

Currently, postmortem neuropathological studies [18, 155] demonstrate the defeat of the myelin sheaths of the nerves as characteristic of schizophrenia. It should be noted that it is also characteristic of a number of neuroinfections, in particular, due to herpes [156]. Although most modern studies have confirmed the absence of astrogliosis in schizophrenia, the question of its presence in the periventricular zones of the brain, in certain forms of the course of schizophrenia, as well as its relationship with regional specificity [157] has not been resolved. At the same time, there is evidence of changes in the ultrastructure of astrocytes in particular, a decrease in the numerical density and volume fraction of their mitochondria associated with the duration of the disease [158] and the expression of their markers, which indicates the active involvement of astrocytes in the pathological process in schizophrenia and their activation [157]. At the same time, the functional inferiority of astrocytes in this disease prevents the formation of classical signs of astrogliosis. Since astrocytes are resident immunocompetent brain cells, one of the possible reasons for their activation, which requires study, is involvement in immune reactions and neuroinflammation [157]. Nonspecific ultrastructural anomalies of capillaries in schizophrenia were found, including thickening, deformation of the basal plate, vacuolization of the cytoplasm of endothelial cells, basal plate and astrocytic terminal legs, swelling of the latter, a decrease in the number of perivascular oligodendrocytes with ultrastructural dystrophic and degenerative damage and signs of activation of microglia cells [159, 160]. The revealed ultrastructural anomalies of capillaries and the cellular environment of the pericapillaries indicate dysfunction of the BBB. Interpreting the identified changes, the authors suggest that the damaged BBB can cause the penetration of infectious agents, an increase in the diffusion of water, immunoglobulins, cytokines, autoantibodies, and other serum macromolecules in the parenchyma of the brain. As a consequence of these events, damage to cell and myelin membranes may occur, in particular, with the subsequent activation of phagocytosis using microglia.

The identified ultrastructural anomalies of capillaries in schizophrenia can explain the development of the very common spongiosis in the white matter of the marginal layer of the cortex and subependymal zones, considering it as a manifestation of cerebral edema due to impaired cerebral fluids dynamics [53].

It should be added that in cases of a rare hypertoxic form of schizophrenia (febrile catatonia, lethal catatonia), occurring with catatonic symptoms, confusion of consciousness and autonomic dysfunction in the form of hyperthermia along with acute changes in nerve cells in various parts of the brain in the form of swelling of their bodies and processes, chromatolysis, karyolysis, cytolysis, ischemic changes, vacuolization, perivascular hemorrhages, plasmorrhagia chronic changes (wrinkling, atrophy, lipoid sclerosis) are described as well. During macroscopic examination are noted edema and swelling of the brain, its sharp fullness with pronounced hyperemia of the soft meninges and substances, mainly petechial [53]. In microglia and oligodendroglia, proliferative-dystrophic processes prevail. Histopathology of internal organs in hypertoxic schizophrenia reveals parenchyma reversal alteration, stagnant fullness, and edema of organs; possible spotted and point hemorrhages in them, as well as in the skin [2]. To the line-turbulent, often lethal, process in the brain, some pathologists [53] justify the chain mutagenesis associated with the effects of viral factors (virogenic mutations—inserts). At the same time, the possibility of a congenital persistent infection (influenza, herpes, measles, viruses, etc) is allowed, which can be activated by various factors, including a new exogenous infection. Note that herpes labialis is almost constantly detected in patients with febrile schizophrenia [53].

Studies to identify microbial factors in the brains of deceased patients with schizophrenia are few and contradictory. A case of detection of viral inclusions in neuronal processes [161] in febrile schizophrenia was described; it was not possible to identify viruses. This circumstance again raised the question of a possible defective type of viruses that "elude" an adequate immune response.

In separate studies in the brains of patients, HSV-1 [162] and beta-herpesvirus 6A (HHV-6B) [163] and CMV [163] were found. The study is complicated by the widespread of herpesviruses in the population with the possibility of persistence in the brain in a latent state, as well as their involvement in the pathogenesis of a number of human diseases. Apparently, the results of the work [164] detected the viral RNA of EBV, CMV, HSV, and VZV both in brain samples of patients with schizophrenia and controls are connected with this circumstance. A difficult situation is also characteristic of studies related to the detection of retroviruses in the brain of patients in schizophrenia. In particular, it was found that the GAG protein encoded by the family of multicopy genes HERV-W is also expressed in the cells of the central nervous system in the norm [165]. However, a change in the expression of this protein in schizophrenia [165] has been shown, and a tendency to increase the expression of total HERV and the HERV-W family in brain samples of patients with schizophrenia has been demonstrated [166].

Research in this important direction should be continued and intensified, as well as using modern methods for diagnosing microbial flora.

20.1.5 Prospects of Anti-infectious Therapy in the Treatment and Prevention of Mental Illness

Taking into account the above data, an important component of the fight against mental pathology may be the inclusion of anti-infectious drugs in the treatment regimens for mental diseases, including antiviral drugs. Attempts to use such drugs in the treatment of schizophrenia have been repeatedly made and in some cases have given a positive result [167]. The tasks of anti-infective therapy in schizophrenia and SHAP are to suppress pathogens that cause inflammatory processes in the body of patients identified in numerous studies, which will contribute to the correction of immunological shifts observed in these patients. Another important therapeutic area may be the use of probiotic and prebiotic drugs [154]. Microbiologically oriented methods of treatment, aimed, among other things, at the correction of the intestinal microbiota, are currently one of the most promising areas in psychiatry [168]. Violations in the composition of the gastrointestinal microbiota, associated in patients with schizophrenia with a number of somatic problems (inflammatory manifestations in the gastrointestinal tract, oropharynx, etc.) dictate the need for careful sanitation of foci of infection in the body. These measures can be considered as elements of an integrative approach that considers the human body as an integral system in which various aspects of life, including the function of various parts of the nervous system, internal organs, immune system, etc. are interrelated and are in inseparable unity with the external environment [44].

Since anti-infective therapy is inextricably linked with the diagnosis of the presence of a microbial agent in the body, it is necessary to emphasize that due to the atypical manifestations of infection in schizophrenia, it is advisable to use various methods of microbial diagnosis with repeated repetitions of analyses. Among the promising diagnostic methods for everyday medical practice can be attributed to chromato-mass spectrometry of microbial markers (MSMM) [169], certified for clinical use and allowing simultaneous study of any biological material for 57 microorganisms. Unlike genetic methods, MSMM allows quickly, within 3 hours after the sample enters the laboratory, to determine the content of herpes viruses (CMV, herpes types 1 and 2, EBV); microbes—pathogenic and conditionally pathogenic, aerobic and anaerobic, gram-negative "sticks," actinomycetes; mushrooms; assess the content of toxins, the total level of microorganisms and the amount of normal flora (bifido- and lactobacilli). As we discussed earlier [44], the interaction of viral factors with the immune system, and some of them (in particular, herpes viruses) with all organs and tissues, dictates the need not only for a thorough immunological study, taking into account the characteristic features of immunity for endogenous mental diseases (including its anti-infectious characteristics), but also for a detailed somatic examination. To identify erased and clinically non-manifested lesions of the part of internal organs, it is promising to use a comprehensive assessment of physiological autoimmunity, which makes it possible to determine by the changed level of specific autoantibodies disorders both in the nervous system (neurons, axons, glia, the main myelin protein, neurotransmitter system) and in other systems (cardiovascular system, gastrointestinal tract, endocrine organs, urogenital system), as well as to assess the level of systemic inflammation. The method makes it possible to assess the effectiveness of therapy and the quality of remission achieved on therapy [170]. The fight against infectious, including viral, diseases (timely high-quality therapy of acute infections, sanitation of foci of chronic infections, specific immunoprophylaxis), along with increasing the body's defenses aimed at counteracting infections, may be one of the likely directions for reducing the level of mental morbidity among the population. It can be very relevant for working with persons from the high-risk group for schizophrenia.

20.1.6 Conclusion

The direction of research considered in this work is extremely important and promising from the point of view of obtaining new knowledge about the pathogenic features of the occurrence and development of psychoses on the example of schizophrenia. The infectious hypothesis of schizophrenia can be considered as integrating other known hypotheses, only stating individual pathogenetic links of the disease—changes in dopamine transmission, GABA and glutamate metabolism, serotonin metabolism, and others, including the hypothesis of neuroinflammation, since it can explain the causes of neurotransmitter metabolism disorders and the development of inflammation processes in the nervous tissue.

Every year the number of facts indicating the direct or indirect participation of a number of microbial agents, including viruses, in the occurrence and development of mental pathology, including such common psychoses as schizophrenia, is increasing. This made it possible to formulate a position that schizophrenia can be a disease in the etiology of which external factors of infectious or other nature play a major role, and genetic factors determine the degree of susceptibility to these factors [171]. Measures for timely immunoprophylaxis, diagnosis, and treatment of infections with a high degree of probability will help to significantly improve the prevention of the disease and the prognosis of its course. Based on the data presented, a very promising therapeutic direction in the fight against endogenous psychosis could be the inclusion in the schemes of their treatment of antiviral, and, if necessary, antibacterial drugs along with anti-inflammatory drugs (which have already shown effectiveness in a number of studies—[172, 173]) and means that correct disturbed metabolic processes, eliminate toxic products that restore the function of the vascular endothelium and the balance of the gastrointestinal microbiota.

20.2 Infectious Etiology in the Genesis of Alzheimer's Disease[3]

Progress in the development of medicine has led to an increase in the proportion of elderly people in the population, often with cognitive impairments and dementia. Four to seven million new cases of dementia are registered annually. It is assumed that by 2030 their number may double (up to 78 million), and by 2050 triple (up to 139 million), given the continuous increase in the number of such patients [174, 175]. Currently, more than 55 million people in the world suffer from dementia, of which 50–60% is diagnosed with Alzheimer's disease (AD) [174–178]. By

[3]With contribution of A.A. Garbuzov, D.A. Khavkina, P.V. Chukhliaev, T.A. Ruzhentsova.

2030, this figure is projected to increase to 66 million, and by 2050 to 115 million [176].

AD is a neurodegenerative disease that leads to the development of cognitive impairment and complete destruction of intelligence in general.

Most often, it is found in people over 65 years of age, rarely occurring early AD is distinguished as a separate form.

According to statistics, the incidence depends on the age of patients: among people 65–85 years old, it is 4–6%, and among people over 85 years old—up to 32% [177, 179–181].

According to WHO, AD and other forms of dementia were among the top ten causes of death worldwide in 2019, taking the third place in this list in the countries of America and Europe. Sixty-five percent are women among those who died from AD and other forms of dementia [182–184].

20.2.1 Theories of the Pathogenesis of Alzheimer's Disease

Various hypotheses for the development of AD during the period of studying this pathology have been formulated. The "cholinergic hypothesis" was proposed initially [185]. Its essence is to reduce the synthesis of the neurotransmitter acetylcholine, which causes the development of AD. However, treatment regimens show very low effectiveness based on this theory.

The "amyloid hypothesis" was formed with the development of molecular diagnostic methods in 1991–1995 [186, 187]. Intracerebral deposition of Aß-peptide (one of the forms of amyloid) plays a role in the pathogenesis of AD development according to this theory. However, scientists did not find a reliable correlation between amyloid accumulation and neuronal loss in the course of the following studies.

The next step was the "TAU hypothesis," according to which the hyperphosphorylation of tau protein—the main component of intracellular transport connecting microtubules of axoplasmic current should be considered the basis of the changes [188–190]. Deposition of Aß-peptide causes a number of pathological changes: disruption of synapses and cellular communication, ion homeostasis disorders, activation of glial cells, oxidative damage, mitochondrial dysfunction, formation of neurofibrillary tangles, and hyperphosphorylation of tau protein, which triggers a cascade of metabolic disorders with the formation of filaments from it, grouped into neurofibrillary conglomerates inside nerve cells. This process causes the disintegration of microtubules and blocks the transport of metabolites of almost all metabolic systems in neurons, which as a result leads to amyloidosis of the neuron and its death [189, 191–193]. A number of researchers have noted that cell death in AD is associated with the expression of apoptosis inducer genes (c–jun) due to the effects of both amyloid protein and its precursor (amyloid precursor protein, APP) [180, 194].

It was noted that the deposition of amyloid protein occurs more actively when exposed to pathological forms of apolipoprotein E. The probability of AD disease increases by 18 times in heterozygous or homozygous carriers of the apolipoprotein E e4 [180, 195–199]. In general, observations show that hyperlipidemia, which leads to changes in the walls of cerebral vessels, contributes to the accumulation of amyloid protein and is an important factor in the progression of the disease [200, 201].

Additional experimental studies have shown that a decrease in the level of estrogens also contributes to the deposition of amyloid [202, 203].

For the prevention and effective treatment of the disease, the identification of triggers and causes that stimulate the pathological process is of the greatest importance. The search for an infectious agent involved in the genesis of degenerative diseases, in particular AD is not popular, although degeneration and death of neurons are the main features of AD and there are signs of cellular inflammation in the area of neuronal death. Activation of microglial elements with accumulation of proinflammatory cytokines is noted around senile plaques [204].

Back in the 1990s, the first data were obtained indicating a high probability of AD being linked to a number of infectious agents. The results of studies was published by M. Sochocka et al. confirmed the hypothesis about the role of neurotropic viruses from the *Herpesviridae* family, primarily herpes simplex virus types 1 and 2, cytomegalovirus, and virus hepatitis C in the formation of AD [205]. Among the bacteria, the family of *Spirochaetes* and periodontal pathogens, such as *Porphyromonas gingivalis* or *Treponema denticola*, were shown as agents stimulating the development of dementia. *Spirochaetes* were detected during autopsies of deceased with a confirmed diagnosis of AD in the blood, cerebrospinal fluid, and brain tissues. Researchers found another pathogen in the areas of neurodegeneration in the autopsy material of the brain—*Chlamydia pneumoniae* while no pathogens were found in other parts of the brain without signs of degeneration. *Chlamydiae* were detected at the sites of amyloid accumulation in astroglial cells, microglia, perivascular macrophages, and neurons. In the course of the study was shown that *Chlamydia pneumoniae* can increase the risk of AD by 5 times. This was also confirmed by the presence of elevated levels of antibodies to *Chlamydia* in many patients with AD [205].

But despite the fact that different microorganisms were considered as an infectious trigger of the disease (with a common genetically nondeterministic form of AD with a so-called late onset), taking into account the biological characteristics of *Chlamydia pneumoniae*, its main contribution to the development of AD seems most likely [206].

Only a few studies have been published that showed this pathogen in the brains of patients with AD. The vast majority of them were held at different times by a group with the participation of B Balin [207] and only two by independent researchers, but the results are comparable. Other attempts to detect *Chlamydia pneumoniae* in the brain were unsuccessful.

Typical intracellular and atypical extracellular *Chlamydia pneumoniae*—antigens were identified in the frontal and temporal cortex of patients with AD and were not detected in the control group when examining the brains of other patients (5 with AD and 5 without AD) using specially developed clarifying methodological protocols [208].

Astrocytes, microglia, and neurons were host cells for *Chlamydia pneumoniae* in the brains of patients with AD according to immunohistochemical study. Infected cells were found in close proximity to senile plaques and neurofibrillary glomeruli [209]. Subsequently, similar results were obtained using cultural studies and in situ hybridization [210].

Chlamydia pneumoniae antigens were also detected inside the cells of neurons, neuroglia, endothelial and periendothelial cells and extracellularly on biological material from other patients with AD. *Chlamydia pneumoniae*, amyloid deposits, and neurofibrillary tangles were located near each other. The microorganism did not directly contact the amyloid plaque according to the results of the assessment using staining with theoflavin S [208].

Part of *Chlamydia pneumoniae* detected and visualized in patient with AD cells located near senile plaques and neurofibrillary tangles showed metabolic activity in frozen brain tissue samples (by specific RNA transcriptase during RT-PCR), and after isolation from the tissue, they multiplied on cell culture [211]. *Chlamydia pneumoniae* behaved not as a persistent, but as an active form in the culture of astrocytes and microglia. Obviously, this accompanies the destruction and lysis of some part of the host cells at the end of the life cycle.

Intranasal infection *Chlamydia pneumoniae* of non-transgenic young female mice balb/c promotes the production in the mouse brain of amyloid (AB1-42), similar to plaques and found in neurons, according to an experimental study. This suggests a model of the primary trigger for the development of the pathological process of AD in sporadic cases of the disease [212].

In addition, *Chlamydia pneumoniae* was found in olfactory bulbs by intranasal infection of mice ,which correlated with the results of autopsies in Alzheimer's disease [212]. It is assumed that the cells of the olfactory epithelium in the nasal passages serve as a target for *Chlamydia pneumoniae*, and after infection, potential cell damage or death can occur in the olfactory bulb and olfactory cortex, creating conditions for further retrograde damage to neurons.

Nonsteroidal anti-inflammatory drugs are included in the treatment regimens of AD taking into account the detection of inflammatory reactions. A randomized, placebo-controlled multicenter clinical trial was conducted to determine the effectiveness of antibacterial therapy against *Chlamydia pneumoniae* (doxycycline and rifampicin) in the clinical course of the disease presupposing the participation of *Chlamydia pneumoniae* in the development of AD. According to the results, the progression of cognitive decline in the group of patients receiving antibiotics was less intense than in the control group [213].

Also, experimental work has shown that *Borrelia burgdorferi*, which causes Lyme disease, in contact with mammalian glial cells cause the formation of Aß-immunoreactive amyloid plaques.

Professor R. Itzhaki has been studying the effects of the herpes virus type 1 (HSV-1) on the development of AD for more than 25 years in the University of Manchester. She claims that this infection is the cause of more 50% of cases of AD [30, 31]. Antiviral drugs reduced the risk of dementia in patients with severe herpes infection, according to the study [214]. The results, published by Cairns et al. in the journal *Science Advances* (2020), clearly showed the possibility of the presence of herpes infection in the nervous system, as shown in Figure 20.2 [215].

The results of another work showed that in elderly patients with confirmed herpes simplex virus-1 (HSV-1) infection, toxic amounts of amyloid (Aß) and phosphorylated (p) tau protein can be deposited in the brain [216–218]. At the same time, MR White et al, have shown that amyloid is able to inhibit the replication of seasonal and pandemic strains of influenza A H3N2 and H1N1 viruses in vitro [219]. Atherosclerosis can increase the degree of changes, which often develops in direct connection with infectious pathology, primarily the herpes simplex virus infection [220] (see also Sect. 20.3).

Cytomegalovirus (CMV) is another virus of this family considered as a significant factor for the development of AD. It was found on the postmortem material that in persons suffering from AD, there is a significant positive correlation between the presence of antibodies to CMV in the blood serum and the level of formation of the pathological protein β-amyloid (p = 0.27), as well as τ-protein (p = 0.11) [221]. It is shown that the presence of antibodies to CMV in the blood is accompanied by a more significant rate of cognitive decline, as well as an increase in the likelihood of dementia (risk ratio = 2.15). These data followed a 5-year follow-up of a cohort of 849 older adults who had AD formation in 93 cases [222]. Another study showed a possible effect of CMV on cognitive function [223]. The researchers found worse results on MMCE and telephone cognitive status interviews (telephone interview for cognitive status) in a group of individuals who had IgG antibodies to CMV compared to uninfected individuals when followed over 1625 patients. Relationship was found between the titer of antibodies and the rate of decrease in higher cortical functions. A 4-year follow-up determined that cognitive deficits form faster in patients with high levels of immunoglobulin G to CMV among more than 1000 elderly individuals aged 60 to 100 years. [224]. Also, it was determined that the formation of the clinical picture of AD is accompanied by a significant increase in IgG titer to CMV, compared with persons without dementia [225].

To date, a number of data have been received on the impact on the development of AD and other representatives of *Herpesviridae*. In particular, some studies indicate the possible role of the Epstein-Barr virus (EBV). It was found that 45% of patients with AD have EBV DNA in their blood. At the same time, only 31% of persons without neurodegeneration have EBV DNA. The differences obtained were statistically reliable. The virus was found in 6% of patients with postmortem study in brain tissue samples. Interesting is the fact that they were all carriers of the APOE gene-ε4 [226].

Some researchers have also pointed to the possible involvement of herpes virus type 6 (HHV-6) in the development of AD. HHV-6 is found in the brain in 70% of patients who suffered from Alzheimer's type dementia during their lifetime, while the virus is found only in 40% in samples obtained from persons of the appropriate age, but did not have AD (p = 0.003)

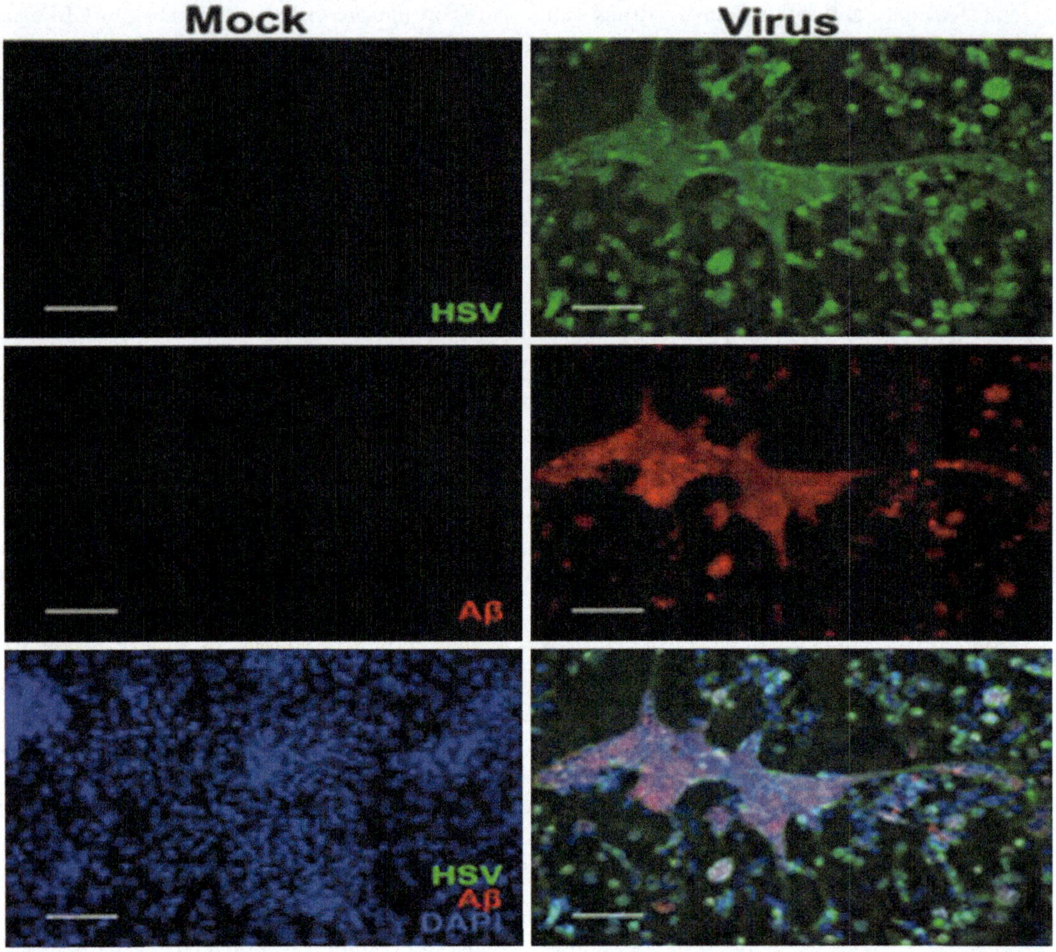

Fig. 20.2 A culture of neurons infected with herpes simplex virus type 1. The control culture is on the left, the infected culture is on the right. Green staining—herpes virus, blue—cell nuclei, red—beta-amyloid. A large "cell" with appendages in an infected culture is the result of the fusion of several neurons [31]. https://www.ncbi.nlm.nih.gov/pmc/articles/PMC7202879/figure/F5/

[226]. However, other scientists have not established differences in titers of IgG antibodies to HHV-6 when compared in groups of patients with AD, mild cognitive impairment syndrome (MCI), and in patients who do not suffer from disorders of higher cortical functions [227].

The results of another study indicate a possible role of *Helicobacter pylori*. Subjects aged 60–90 years who were diagnosed with *Helicobacter pylori* showed lower results when performing tests for verbal memory, compared with persons in whom *Helicobacter pylori* was not detected [228].

The researchers noted elevated serum levels of Aß40, Aß42, and total Aß in the AD group of patients who were found to have *Helicobacter pylori* against the background of an increase in the content of TNF-alpha, IL-1B, and IL-6 [229]. Another study found that the presence of *Helicobacter pylori* was accompanied by worse MMSE testing values in patients with Alzheimer's dementia ($p = 0.017$) [230]. It is shown that there is a positive correlation between the presence of *Helicobacter pylori* and the level of hyperphosphorylation of the protein τ, which opens up new ways of studying AD [231]. Also, based on a number of studies, it has been suggested that *Helicobacter pylori* can influence AD through involvement in several pathophysiological processes, such as intracellular signaling, prolifera-

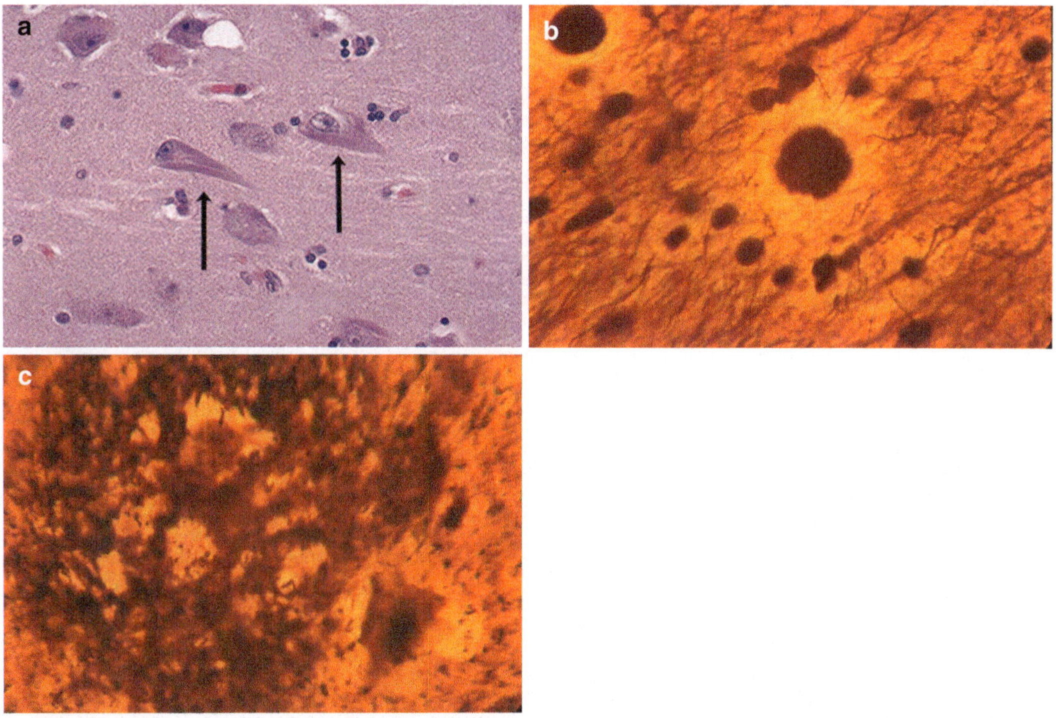

Fig 20.3 Histopathological picture of Alzheimer disease. (**a**) Intracellular tangles in neurons. H-E ×400; (**b**) "Young" Alzheimer (senile) plaque. Silver impregnation; ×200, (**c**) Destructed plaque. Silver impregnation. ×600

tion, as well as the organization of the immune response [232].

The basis of the pathological picture of AD is cerebral amyloidosis of intra- and extracellular (mainly circulatory) localization, intracellular neurofibrillary tangles, and neuronal death (Fig. 20.3). Morphological changes occur in a certain sequence, starting with the mediobasal parts of the frontal lobes, which carry out cholinergic mediation of the posterior parts of the brain [193, 233]. Further, these morphological changes extend to the area of the hippocampus, the amygdala nucleus, and the medial parts of the temporal lobes. This stage is characterized by a significant decrease in the number and density of neuronal synapses in the hippocampus [193, 234].

20.2.2 Clinical Manifestations and Diagnosis of AD

The most common early signs of AD are emotional and affective disorders, which makes it difficult for early diagnosis. In this regard, in patients with depression, the possibility of developing an early stage of AD should be excluded [180, 235–237]. The severity of symptoms increases, the pathological process causes neuronal death and reactive astrogliosis of the associative zone of the temporoparietal and frontal parts of the brain, increasing the progression of dementia with the progression of the disease. Memory starts deteriorating, both long-term and short-term memorization of things and events suffers. The symptoms are joined by amnestic and sensory aphasia, apracto-agnostic disorders in the form of spatial and somatotopic apraxia and agnosia. The progressive neurodegenerative process reaches the anterior parts of the brain, causing disorientation in the patient, difficulty in self-service. Pelvic disorders may join with severe brain damage [180, 238].

Modern methods make it possible to detect the development of the disease in the early stages, before the appearance of clinical symptoms. Thus, with the help of MRI diagnostics, it is possible to detect a decrease in the volume of the hippocampus, amygdala, medial temporal lobe, posterior cingulate gyrus [239–242]. The use of a positron emission tomograph with a Pittsburgh substance makes it possible to detect the accumulation of amyloid protein in cerebral structures before the development of anamnestic symptoms [243]. Early diagnosis of AD is possible by determining biomarkers: beta-amyloid and hyperphosphorylated forms of tau protein in cerebrospinal fluid [238, 242]. At the same time, it has to be stated that in many cases reliable diagnosis of AD is not carried out either in vivo or posthumously.

20.2.3 Treatment and Prevention of AD

The approach to the treatment of AD should be comprehensive, the complex etiology and involvement of mental disorders involves the use of drugs of different groups, as well as nonmedicinal methods of treatment [244–249]. Unfortunately, in most cases, the currently recommended treatment for AD is ineffective.

These data show that there are no generally accepted views on the role of infectious factors in the etiology and pathogenesis of AD. At the same time, many studies provide significant evidence of the role of viruses, bacteria, and other pathogens, which allows us to take a fresh look at the pathogenesis and prospects of AD therapy. It can be assumed that various pathogens are associated with AD, among which *Chlamydia* and viruses of the *Herpesviridae* family play a leading role. Many issues are subject to comprehensive study.

20.3 Infection as an Etiological Factor in the Genesis of Atherosclerotic Lesions of Cerebral Vessels[4]

Atherosclerosis being the basis for the formation of coronary heart disease, strokes, and many other pathological processes, currently occupies a leading place among diseases of the circulatory system [250]. These diseases are the leading cause of death worldwide. The main morphological substrate of atherosclerosis is traditionally considered to be the formation of atherosclerotic plaques associated with a disturbance of cholesterol metabolism characterized by predominance of low and very low density lipoproteins. The causes of atherosclerosis are currently associated not only with the nature of nutrition and genetic predisposition, but also with the influence of other endogenous and exogenous factors. Numerous studies of recent decades have shown a significant influence on the onset and progression of the atherosclerotic process of various infectious agents [251].

To date, the most convincing data are presented for *Chlamydia pneumoniae, Chlamydia trachomatis*, cytomegalovirus, herpes simplex virus types 1 and 2 (HSV-1 and HSV-2) and a number of representatives of the intestinal microbiota on the participation of microorganisms in the mechanism of atherosclerosis development [250–253].

Currently, it is generally accepted that primary vascular changes occur with atherosclerosis in childhood, and then progress in waves, which does not exclude infection in the perinatal period with the subsequent development of a chronic inflammatory process [254, 255]. Traditionally, the main pathogenetic factor for the development of acute cerebral circulatory disorders is considered to be atherosclerosis of intra- and extracranial vessels, especially of the ischemic type [256]. However, in many patients, especially young ones, such a connection cannot be traced [257].

American scientist C. Gross presented the role of infectious agents in the pathogenesis of acute disorders of cerebral blood supply in 2016. According to his data, herpes simplex viruses of types 1 and 2 (HSV-1 and HSV-2) have been present and persist in the ganglia for a long time, but in certain periods of time they can migrate along efferent fibers directly to the adventitia of the cerebral arteries, where they replicate, thereby damaging the vascular wall [252]. This conclusion is based on the results of morpho-

[4]With contribution of D.A. Khavkina, P.V. Chukhliaev, T.A. Ruzhentsova.

logical studies of the temporal arteries in stroke patients. The study included 70 children aged 5 to 14 years. Acute cerebrovascular accident was diagnosed after an episode of chickenpox in 90% or herpes zoster in 10%. Two children had a stroke after vaccination against chickenpox. The average interval between an episode of chickenpox or shingles and a subsequent stroke was 18 weeks. Clinical symptoms of stroke in children were, as a rule, expressed and typical of this pathology. Hemiparesis, speech disorders, facial asymmetry, and headache were most frequently recorded [252].

Similar conclusions were made by Russian scientists in 2014, who conducted a postmortem study of 30 patients who died from acute heart attack and its complications [258]. The DNA of eight types of herpes virus was determined using polymerase chain reaction (PCR). Areas of intact coronary arteries were studied in comparison with those that had signs of atherosclerosis of varying severity. HSV-1,2 types and/or varicella zoster virus were detected in more than 80% of vascular lesions (p=0.05).

Later, in 2018, M.E. Evseyeva et al. presented the results of a survey of young individuals for the presence of foci of chronic infection and its association with the development of atherosclerosis. Sixty-six (35.1%) of the 232 examined conscripts, had foci of chronic infection, the most common being chronic tonsillitis. These patients showed signs of rigidity of the vascular wall of the aorta and large arteries, which indicates the preclinical stage of atherosclerosis. There was also a tendency to develop left ventricular dysfunction, expressed in a decrease in the maximum rate of pressure buildup and an increase in the period of expulsion of the left ventricle. In the group of healthy individuals, these indicators corresponded to the norm [259]. Ya.V. Alekseeva et al. confirmed the presence of viruses in the plaques of coronary vessels of patients who died in the stage of acute infarction in 2019 [260]. Antigens were found in all samples, HSV-6 and enteroviruses were the most common.

American scientists conducted an experiment in 2019. Mice receiving apolipoprotein were intraperitoneally injected with *Chlamydia muridarum*. Lesions of the aorta sinuses and its descending part were evaluated after 8 weeks. Compared with the uninfected group, infected mice developed significantly more atherosclerotic lesions, which was accompanied by higher levels of serum amyloid A-1, IL-1ß [261].

A large study was conducted in 2019 to detect the intestinal microbiota among 119 patients with coronary heart disease and acquired heart defects. The 16S rRNA gene was sequenced. It was found that the intestinal microbiota of patients in the main group significantly differed in the level of beta diversity from the comparison group. A large number of *Veillonella dispar, Bacteroides plebeius,* and *Fusobacterium* were detected, while the number of *Collinsella aerofaciens, Megamonas, Enterococcus, Megasphaera, Dorea,* and *Blautia* was reduced in the group with heart defects [262]. Seven main representatives were identified among the main pathogens associated with dyslipidemia: *Bacteroides* spp., *Bacteroides plebeius, Fusobacterium, Lactobacillus, Megamonas, Parabacteroides distasonis,* and *Prevotella copri*. It was proved that the constituent of the intestinal microbiome is associated with the clinical characteristics of diseases, as a result of the study, which can be used as a new direction in therapy [262].

Finnish scientists assessed the frequency of the main representatives of the intestinal microflora in different age groups as causes of sudden death. It was noted that the number of *Clostridium leptum, Enterobacteriaceae,* and *Streptococcus* spp. increases with age. At the same time, the number of *Enterobacteria* is directly related to the area of coronary vascular fibrosis ($p = 0.001$), and the number of *Clostridium leptum* is directly related to the area of calcification ($p = 0.015$). Intestinal bacterial DNA was detected in 67.6% of coronary plaques. Most frequently were detected *Streptococcus* spp. (41.0%), *Enterobacteriaceae* (12.1%), *Clostridium septicum* (2.4%), and *Lactobacillus* spp. (2.4%), as shown in Figure 20.3. By strains of *Lactobacillus* spp., *Bifidobacterium* spp., *Clostridium coccoides,* and *Bacteroides* spp., there were no differences among the deceased of different ages [263] (Fig. 20.4).

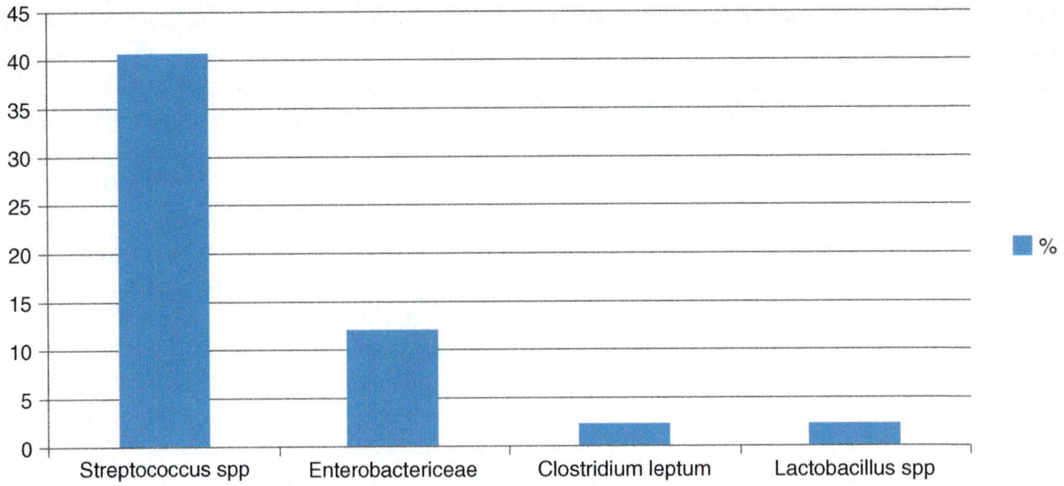

Fig. 20.4 Distribution of the intestinal microbiome by association with the development of atherosclerosis, % [254, 263]

It can be assumed that damage to the vascular wall occurs under the action of an infectious agent, and low and very low density lipoproteins play a leading role in the progression of the disease. Studies have shown that cytomegalovirus (CMV), HSV-1, and HSV-2 can synthesize specific Toll receptors (FC and C3) on the surface of endothelial cells involved in atherogenesis with the formation of immune circulating complexes.

We (V.A. Zinserling together with A.L. Lozovator) previously performed a study of 30 people who died from ischemic stroke from 48 to 89 years old with a disease duration of 1–4 days (6 people), 5–10 days (6 people), 11–15 days (18 people) within a random sampling. The detection of herpes simplex viruses of types 1 and 2 was carried out by dot hybridization on disks and in situ hybridization in paraffin sections using dioxygenin of the Dianova diagnostic kit (Germany).

A typical picture of acute cerebral circulation disorders was observed clinically in all observations in the right or left hemisphere, 24 people developed bilateral focal pneumonia. A typical picture of ischemic stroke corresponding to the terms of the disease was noted at the autopsy and at the standard histological examination. In addition, muff–like perivascular infiltrates were found in some of the deceased (9 on 11–15 days, 6 – in the first three days and 6 – during 5–10 days, Fig. 20.5). There were also cellular changes similar to those observed in herpetic encephalitis (see Chap. 5).

We detected HSV1 (in 4), HSV2 (in 1), HSV1+2 (in 1) by method of dot hybridization in all six specimens in the deceased in first 3 days of the disease. HSV1+ was positive in two cases by in situ hybridization (done in three cases), and HSV2– in one case (Fig. 20.6).

The dot hybridization method detected nucleic acids of the HSV 1 virus in three deceased (out of six) during 5–10 days from the onset of the disease. By in situ hybridization (done in three cases)—HSV 1+ was positive in one case.

By the dot hybridization method, nucleic acids of HSV1-2 and HSV2-1 viruses were detected in 3 out of 18 deceased on 10–15 days from the onset of the disease. By in situ hybridization (done in 3 cases)—the results were same.

Thus, the study independently conducted using two sensitive modern methods reliably showed the presence of the herpes virus in the foci of ischemic stroke. At the same time, the virus was present initially in all observations, later the frequency of its detection decreased. Presumably, this can be attributed either to the gradual elimination of the virus, or to its deeper integration. Of course, a larger comprehensive study is required to verify the facts obtained.

Important data were obtained during the study of autopsy material of brain tissue in 15 patients

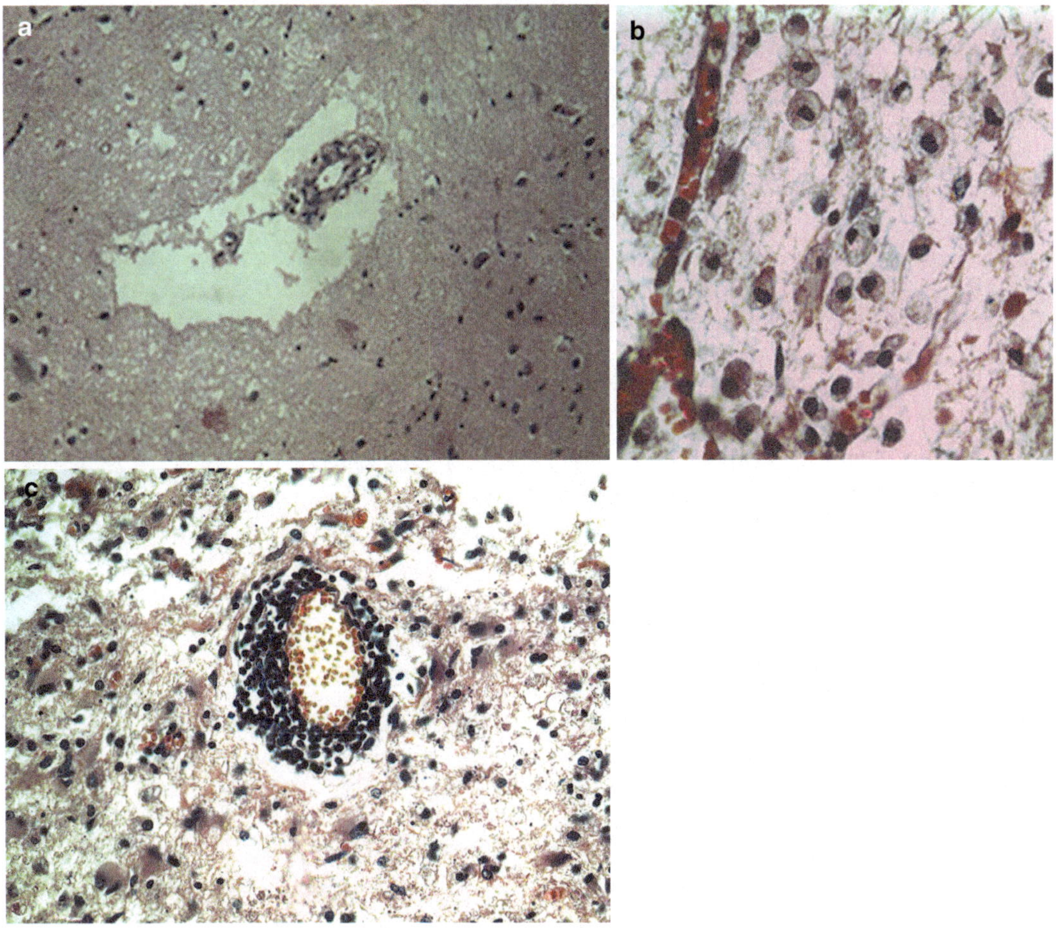

Fig. 20.5 Histopathological picture of ischemic stroke. H-E. (**a**) Perivascular edema and degenerative changes in surrounding tissue at the early stage. ×100; (**b**) Accumulation of macrophages (foamy cells) in the necrotic focus. ×400; (**c**) Dense perivascular lymphoid infiltration. ×200

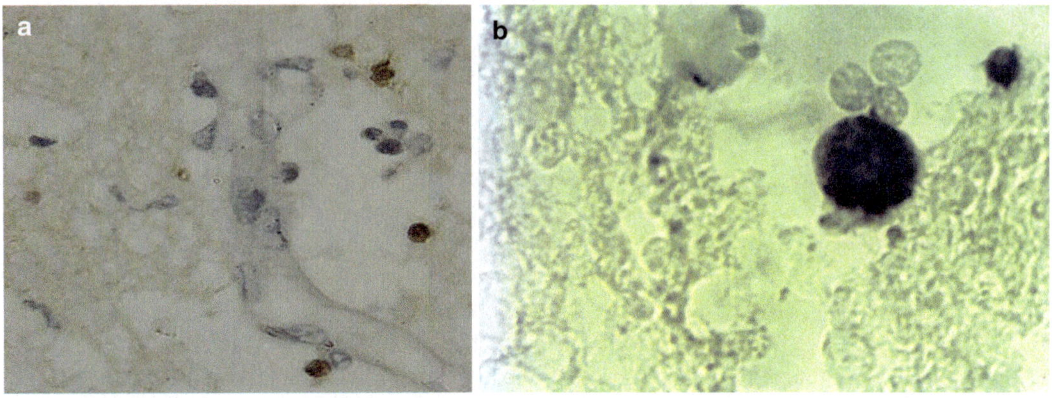

Fig. 20.6. DNA of HSV1 in perivascular space in the patient with stroke. In situ hybridization. (**a**) ×400, (**b**) ×1000

who died of natural causes (Khavkina D.A., Chukhliaev P.V., Ruzhentsova T.A.). The main group included those who died with pronounced signs of cerebrovascular disease, both according to clinical data from medical documentation and structural changes. Pronounced cognitive impairments were noted: in six cases with predominance of atherosclerotic changes, in three cases—in the presence of a malignant neoplasm of the brain (1 patient) and lungs with metastases (2 patients), in 1 case—in the presence of diabetic angiopathy. The comparison group included 6 patients who died without clinical and pathological signs of significant damage to the central nervous system. The causes of death were pulmonary embolism (PE) in three cases, cardiomyopathy, bronchial cancer, laryngeal cancer (in one case accordingly).

The authors investigated areas of the cerebral cortex and medulla oblongata with corresponding vessels. Specimen were collected at the autopsy under sterile conditions using disposable instruments and placed in sterile containers with 50 ml of 0.9% sodium chloride solution. The material was transported in a thermal container using refrigerants at a temperature of $0^0/+5^0$C. The specimen were stored at a temperature of - 30^0C and then examined by PCR in order to detect microorganisms in the tissues.

We detected the DNA of *Acinetobacter baumannii, Enterovirus* spp., *Escherichia coli, Enterococcus* spp., Human alphaherpesvirus 1 (HSV-1), Human alphaherpesvirus 2 (HSV-2), Human gammaherpesvirus 4 (CMV), Human betaherpesvirus 5 (EBV), Human betaherpesvirus 6A/B (HHV6), *Klebsiella pneumoniae, Neisseria meningitidis, Pseudomonas aeruginosa, Staphylococcus* spp., *Staphylococcus MRSA, Streptococcus* spp., *Streptococcus agalactiae, Streptococcus pneumoniae, Streptococcus pyogenes* by PCR with hybridization-fluorescence detection of amplification products in "real time" mode (PCR-RT) in qualitative or quantitative format using reagent kits manufactured by the Federal Research Institute of Epidemiology (RF). DNA extraction was carried from the analyzed samples of biological material out using a set of reagents "RIBOT-prep" (RU No. FSR 2008/03147, FBUN Central Research Institute of Epidemiology, RF). The formulation and analysis of the amplification results were carried out on a device with a "real-time" fluorescence signal detection system "Rotor-Gene Q" ("Qiagen", Germany).

The material was taken from deceased patients, men and women aged 52–90 years, the average age was 74.3±14.5.

Table 20.9 presents data on the frequency of detection of certain viruses and bacteria in the brain tissue of the deceased. As it can be seen

Table 20.9 Frequency of pathogens in brain tissue in the compared groups (*n*, %)

Infectious agent	Main group, *n* = 9 (100%)	Comparison group, *n* = 6 (100%)
HSV1	1 (11%)	0
CMV	0	0
EBV	3 (33%)	0
HHV6	5 (56%)	1 (17%)
Enterovirus	0	0
Frequency of virus detection	5 (56%)	1 (17%)
Enterococcus	3 (33%)	0
Escherichia coli	3 (33%)	0
Klebsiella pneumoniae	0	0
Neisseria meningitidis,	0	0
Pseudomonas aeruginosa	1 (11%)	0
Staphylococcus spp.	6 (67%)	2 (33%)
Staphylococcus MRSA	1 (11%)	0
Streptococcus spp.	5 (56%)	2 (33%)
Streptococcus agalactiae	0	0
Streptococcus pyogenes	0	0
Streptococcus pneumoniae	3 (33%)	0
Acinetobacter baumannii	0	0
Frequency of detection of bacteria	8 (89%)*	2 (33%)
Frequency of detection of a combination of pathogenic bacteria	4 (44%)*	0
Frequency of detection of various microorganisms	9 (100%)*	2 (33%)
Frequency of detection of 4 or more different microorganisms	6 (67%)*	0

*The differences are significant, one-sided Z-criterion, $p < 0.05$

from it, infectious agents were found in all those who died with cerebrovascular disease, most often bacteria. Attention is drawn to the detection of *Pneumococcus, Staphylococcus MRSA, and Pseudomonas aeruginosa* in the main group, which was not detected in any case in the comparison group. Four or more pathogens were detected in various combinations at once significantly more often against the background of cerebrovascular disease.

Infectious agents were detected in the comparison group in those who died from oncological pathology, which can be explained by a decrease in the immune response in this category of patients.

Thus, the hypothesis is quite of a close relationship between infectious processes of various etiologies and vascular atherosclerosis convincing today, the prospects for modernizing approaches to therapy are obvious. However, of course, further research is required to form practical recommendations.

20.4 New Approaches to the Study of the Etiology and Pathogenesis of Migraine and Patient Management. The Importance of the Throat Microbiota[5]

According to a WHO study, migraine ranks fourth in terms of the number of years of life lost due to persistent deterioration of health in people aged 15–49 years [264].

Migraine remains the second among the causes of disability in the world and the first among young women according to [265].

The prevalence in Europe and USA is 11–25% for women, 4–10% for men; in Russia, this indicator is significantly higher (about 21%). Migraine significantly reduces the quality of life, working capacity, and daily activity: 92% of women and 89% of men suffering from migraines experience difficulties in everyday life, and half of them are forced to stay in bed due to severe headache attacks [266]. The applied methods of treatment are not always effective enough, so the search for new approaches is relevant.

The relationship between migraine and gastrointestinal (GI) disorders has been shown [267]. The frequency of migraines in gastrointestinal disorders: *Helicobacter pylori (HP) infections*—45% (according to the results of a meta-analysis of five case-control studies); irritable bowel syndrome (IBS)—from 4% to 40%; celiac disease (C) 21–28%; inflammatory bowel diseases (IBD)—46%; Crohn's disease—36%; ulcerative colitis—14.8%; gastroparesis—47%; children's colic—5 to 19%.

Traditional migraine therapy includes relief of an already developed attack with nonsteroidal anti-inflammatory drugs and triptans and preventive treatment. Recently, it has been shown that the key to successful treatment of migraines is also the prevention and treatment of comorbid disorders, which allows preventing the progression (chronization) of migraines and improving the quality of life of patients.

There is data in the literature on the significance of chronic infection of the gastrointestinal organs in migraines. Up to 70% of the examined patients have comorbid diseases—chronic tonsillitis, rhinitis, sinusitis, etc. belonging to the group of "often and long-term ill people" [268].

In patients suffering from chronic subclinical sinusitis, migraine is subsequently detected [269]. In this study, 63 patients with migraine had a history of allergic rhinitis (54%), previously suffered acute (76%) and chronic (14%) rhinosinusitis.

However, despite these data, revealing the significance of infections and inflammatory processes in the nasopharynx and gastrointestinal tract, the analysis of the microbiota in these biotopes in patients with migraine was not carried out [270].

Our aim was to study the characteristics of the microbiota in the throat and their correlation with the clinical manifestations of the disease in patients with migraine. An additional task of this

[5]With contribution of I. L. Naidenova, A. B. Danilov, A.V. Simonova, E. G. Filatova, I. A. Pavlovsky, O. V. Bystrova.

Table 20.10 Clinical characteristics of patients with migraine (*N* = 58)

Migraine indicator	Migraine (*N* = 58)	Control group (*N* = 15)
Age, years, Average value ±σ (min.–max.)	39.2 ± 8.08 (21-56)	34 ± 5.0
Gender of the person (m/w)	8/50	5/10
The number of days of migraine, days Average value ±σ	8.60 ± 5.1	–
The number of days of taking the drug, the dose Average value ±σ	9.52 ± 7.3	–
MIDAS Average value ±σ	47.44 ± 49.8	–

work was to evaluate the clinical and diagnostic value of the method of chromatography-mass spectrometry of microbial markers (MSMM) in patients with migraine.

20.4.1 Materials and Methods

A survey of 58 patients with migraine (with unilateral debilitating headache with light and sound phobia, nausea and vomiting—from 4 to 8 days a month) was conducted. Among the examined individuals, there were 8 men and 50 women. The age of patients ranged from 21 to 56 years, average—35 years. The duration of the disease varied from 15 to 25 years. The control group was formed by 15 healthy individuals aged 18 to 55 years (average 34) (Table 20.10).

20.4.1.1 Clinical and Neurological Examination

A traditional neurological examination was conducted; a study of the characteristics of headache and its impact on vital activity was conducted:

- Headache diary—MIDAS (Migraine Disability Assessment) scale [271], assessing the impact of migraine on daily activity and working capacity (Table 20.10).

The patients were repeatedly treated by neurologists using combinations of nonsteroidal anti-inflammatory drugs and triptans, which was ineffective. All patients with migraine during the examination had complaints of a throbbing headache with light and sound phobia, nausea, and vomiting. Some patients had a visual or sensory aura at the beginning of an attack lasting from 5 to 60 min. The seizures were assessed as severe, debilitating. On average, patients were disabled for 8 days in a month. The examination was carried out at the stage of migraine exacerbation.

People with migraine had concomitant diseases. Among them were chronic diseases of the nasopharynx (chronic tonsillitis, chronic pharyngitis, chronic sinusitis) and diseases of the upper respiratory tract.

Exclusion criteria: chronic gastrointestinal diseases (Crohn's disease, gastritis, gastric and duodenum ulcer, enterocolitis), chronic diseases of the upper respiratory tract (tonsillitis, sinusitis), diseases of the teeth and oral cavity, mental diseases (including disorders of schizophrenic spectrum, depressive states), pregnant and lactating women, persons under 18 years and over 65 years of age.

The control group had no complaints of migraine headache, there were no diseases of the gastrointestinal tract and nasopharyngeal organs.

20.4.1.2 Microbiological Examination

The level of 57 microorganisms, including viruses and fungi, as well as the level of endotoxin in the throat were determined. Microorganisms were estimated by mass spectrometry of microbial markers (MSMM).

The sampling of biological material (throat swab) was carried out under the supervision of a doctor. The delivery time of the clinical material to the laboratory for analysis did not exceed 2 h from the moment of sampling.

20.4.1.3 Evaluation of Microbiota in Throat Swabs in Patients with Migraine

The modern MSMM method was used to detect 57 microorganisms, including fungi and viruses. The analysis allows us to determine the qualitative and quantitative composition of microorganisms by their biochemical markers (molecules of higher fatty acids (HFA), aldehydes, alcohols) in the biomaterial of patients. MSMM analysis makes it possible to quickly obtain expanded information about anaerobes and difficult-to-cultivate aerobes, as well as *actinobacteria,* viruses, and different *fungi* of the genus *Candida, Aspergillus,* etc. from the same sample. This possibility is sufficient to learn the microbial landscape of the studied area and understand its role in the pathogenesis of the disease. Since the content of HFA in the cells of microorganisms of a certain type is the same and specific, their concentration in the clinical material is proportional to the number of this type of microorganisms. According to the content of microbial markers, their level is recalculated by the number of microbial cells per gram of biomaterial using mathematical methods [276]. The concentration of 57 microorganisms (10 × 5 cells/gram of the sample) in the biological material is known already 3 h after its receipt in the laboratory (Table 20.10). The technology was developed by Professor of Microbiology G. A. Osipov and others [272–275] ("Institute of Analytical Toxicology").

As follows from Table 20.11, in the throat of patients with migraine, using the MSMM method:

- An increase in the microflora often sown in chronic diseases of the nasopharynx: *Staphylococcus aureus, Staphylococcus epidermidis, Streptococci*
- An increase in the content of microbial markers that are not characteristic of the mycobiota of the upper respiratory tract: anaerobic microorganisms—*Peptostreptococcus anaerobius, Fusobacterium* spp./*Haemophilus* spp.
- Appearance of transient microorganisms that are absent in the norm: *Clostridium,* gram-negative microorganisms 12 *(Porphyromonas* spp.*), Kingella* spp., *Porphyromonas* spp.

Revealed the following relationship between level of microorganisms in the throat of migraine patients and their clinical status:

1. From 30% to 50% of persons with migraine have high levels of *Helicobacter pylori*, one or more microorganisms that characterize of the intestinal microflora; for these patients, typical comorbidities and concomitant diseases of the gastrointestinal tract (GIT) : functional gastrointestinal disorders (violation of a chair, meteorism), chronic gastritis, gastroesophageal reflux disease, irritable bowel syndrome.
2. A decrease in bifidobacteria (by 2.1 or more times compared to the norm) was found in 43% of patients with migraine; they have more frequent migraine episodes.
3. Herpes viruses were detected in 16-43% of people with migraine; it was noted that a high level of viral markers correlates with a more severe course of migraine, a simultaneous increase in the content of several viruses in a particular patient exacerbates the severity of the migraine.
4. Patients with migraine who have an increased level of one or more microorganisms in the throat have a history of chronic nasopharyngeal diseases—chronic pharyngitis , chronic tonsillitis, chronic sinusitis.

Complex therapy of patients with migraine (*n* = 38) was performed, which showed high clinical efficacy. It included: "basic" therapy-treatment and observation by a neurologist, rehabilitation of chronic foci of infection in the nasopharynx under the control of otolaryngologists, correction of dysbiosis of the throat microbiota with the help of local and systemic probiotics (Bifidumbacterin forte® , Hepafor®, Probifor®, Florin ® Forte, Avan company, Russia), treatment of diseases of the gastrointestinal tract with the involvement of consultations of a gastroenterologist, compliance with diet therapy.

As a result of the treatment, for the first time in the entire history of their disease, a reduction or complete disappearance of migraine attacks was achieved in patients. Along with this, it became possible to reduce the dosages of painkillers and triptans, or completely cancel them. In patients whose seizures became more rare, but persisted,

Table 20.11 Significantly different mean values of microorganisms (M) and their standard deviations (σ) in patients with migraine and in the control group, % of individuals with an increase in the level of microorganisms by 2.1 or more times

Types of microorganisms	Name of the microorganism	% of people with migraine who have an Increase/decrease microorganisms in the level of the microorganism by 2.1. or more times compared to the norm	M ± σ Control group, (n = 15) Units of measurement	Patients with migraine, (n = 58) Units of measurement	Reliability (p)
Cocci	*Enterococcus* spp.	86%	0	31.33 ± 39.89	<0.05
	Streptococcus spp.	55%	45.4 ± 38.2	272.71 ± 409.82	<0.05
	Streptococcus mutans	47%	114.4 ± 92.1	297.74 ± 314.17	<0.05
	Staphylococcus aureus	90%	30.5 ± 23.3	301.28 ± 267.22	<0.05
Anaerobes	*Bacteroides fragilis*	47%	10.3 ± 21.4	52.74 ± 99.09	<0.05
	Bifidobacterium spp.**	43%	225.3 ± 132.1	308.31 ± 399.16	<0.05
	Blautia coccoides	38%	0	58.67 ± 84.52	<0.05
	Clostridium spp. *(rpynna C. tetani)*	71%	350.4 ± 243.2	566.19 ± 505.92	<0.05
	Clostridium difficile	60%	0	26.5 ± 41.75	<0.05
	Cl. Hystolyticum/Str. pneumonia	29%	50.4 ± 41.5	184.4 ± 443.82	<0.05
	Clostridium perfringens	29%	84.5 ± 74.1	392.76 ± 832.48	<0.05
	Clostridium propionicum	28%	94.4 ± 81.3	196.17 ± 311.95	<0.05
	Fusobacterium spp./*Haemophilus* spp.	34%	18.4 ± 43.2	38.28 ± 61.03	<0.05
	Lactobacillus spp.**	10%	659 ± 541.3	1450.41 ± 1067.21	<0.05
	Peptostreptococcus anaerobius 18623	36%	378.3 ± 660.8	843 ± 1124.01	<0.05
	Propionibacterium acnes	31%	44.2 ± 63.4	118.76 ± 259.8	<0.05
Enterobacteria	*Helicobacter pylori*	31%	15 ± 19.1	38.52 ± 75.16	<0.05
Gram-negative sticks	*Kingella* spp.	40%	0	58.62 ± 176.94	<0.05
	Porphyromonas spp.	33%	0	4.41 ± 9	<0.05
Viruses	*Herpes* spp.	40%	0	5.45 ± 11.76	<0.05
	Cytomegalovirus	43%	0	17.57 ± 82.17	<0.05
	Epstein-Barr virus	16%		7.95 ± 13.91	<0.05

** a significant decrease in the content of normal flora by more than two times their severity changed: the seizures became much milder. The patients ability to work has been restored.

Thus, based on the study that revealed the features of the microbial landscape of the pharynx of patients with migraine, its correlation with the severity of the clinical picture of the disease, as well as the effectiveness of antimicrobial therapy aimed at the identified infections, it can be stated that the association of pathogenic microorganisms (herpes viruses, cocci) in the presence of dysbiosis in the throat (a decrease in the content of normal microflora characteristic of the oropharynx and the appearance of intestinal microflora, normally not characteristic of it) can be considered as etiologic and pathogenetic factor in the development of migraine. This occasion should be taken into account when examining patients and developing therapeutic approaches. The mechanisms of influence of the pharyngeal microbiota on migraine need further study.

20.5 Role of Infectious Agents and Microbiomes in the Development of Autism Spectrum Disorders (ASD)[6]

ASD, according to ICD-10—diseases that are included in the large block of "disorders of psychological (mental) development" (F80-89). This means that, manifesting in childhood, these disorders then accompany a person throughout his life, they can change, but are never cured. Within this block, spectrum disorders are referred to as F84 ("general developmental disorders"), and include: childhood autism, atypical autism, Rett syndrome, other childhood disintegrative disorder, hyperactive disorder associated with mental retardation and stereotypical movements, Asperger's syndrome, other common developmental disorders and general developmental disorder, unspecified.

In the DSM-V, ASD is classified differently: here four disorders (autism, Asperger's syndrome, childhood disintegrative disorder, and pervasive developmental disorder without further specification) are combined into one—autism spectrum disorder (299.00), which corresponds to heading 84.00 of ICD-10.

Autism is a central symptom of ASD. The concept of "autism" was introduced by E. Bleuler to designate such an important symptom of schizophrenia as a disconnection from reality and focus on inner experiences that arise during the course of the disease. Subsequently, the question was raised about the possibility of developing schizoid personality disorders in childhood, and in 1943, Kanner described children who were incapable of verbal and affective contact with others. At that time, there were already ideas about the possibility of developing schizophrenia in children, in connection with which Kanner admitted that he belonged to the disorders of the schizophrenic spectrum, but distinguished it from schizophrenia and schizoidia. The more mildly symptomatic autistic disorder, referred to as Asperger's syndrome, has since been described as a manifestation of autistic (schizoid) personality disorder. [1].

Other common features of diseases related to ASD are cognitive, behavioral, and social dysfunctions [277], as well as stereotypes and mannerisms that manifest themselves not only in motor skills, but also in thought processes. The manifestation of "additional" symptoms in the form of phobias, irritability, sleep disorders, eating disorders, aggressiveness, etc. is possible.

The etiology of ASD is poorly understood. They belong to multifactorial diseases, the development of which is associated with both genetic factors and environmental factors [277–280].

Currently, the probable role of microorganisms is considered within the framework of two pathogenetic concepts: (1) disruption of the intestinal microbiome (and, possibly, other localizations), affecting both the central and enteric nervous systems; (2) the latent course of the infectious process directly in the central nervous system during perinatal infection.

The enteric nervous system has been studied in medicine and physiology for over 150 years.

[6]With contribution of Zatevalov A.M., Bezrodny S.L., Sadekov T.Sh., Ruzhentsova T.A.

The first publication "The Abdominal and Pelvic Brain" by the American physician Byron Robinson, devoted to the study of the enteric nervous system, was published in 1907. The term "gastrointestinal nervous system" was coined by Newport Langley, a physiologist who noted that the villi of the intestinal wall contain more than 100 millions of nerve cells [281]. Nerve cells are located throughout the entire digestive tract and make up the enteric nervous system (ENS), which controls gastroenterological processes almost autonomously, for which in the literature it is called neurogastroenterological, or viscerotonic, or simply the second brain [282]. It is known that the second brain affects the central nervous system and mental processes, since the ENS releases more than 70 neurotransmitters, similar to those involved in the work of the brain [283]. The neurons of the ENS provide 70% of the functioning of the body's immune system, are responsible for mobility and secretion, and are involved in the regulation of the inflammatory process [284].

The relationship between the ENS and the brain is carried out through the nervous, endocrine, immune systems and nonspecific natural immunity. The nervous system includes the vagus, sympathetic and spinal nerves; humoral signaling pathways include cytokines, hormones, and neuropeptides. More than 90% of information is directed from the ENS to the brain, that is, the intestine informs the brain and contributes to the formation of our well-being [285].

As discussed above (see Sect. 20.1), the intestinal microflora not only has a significant effect on intestinal functions, but can also interact with higher nerve centers. The interaction of the gut microbiota with these centers can cause anxiety, depression, and cognitive impairment. Thus, M. Lyte et al. showed that in acute infection with *Campylobacter jejuni*, mice exhibit anxious behavior, which is noted several hours after the introduction of the pathogen into the stomach, before an immune response has been formed. Thus, it can be assumed that the response to the introduction of a pathogen is cytokine-induced behavior during the development of the disease. Further studies have shown that administration of *Campylobacter jejuni* triggers the activity of the vagus-associated ascending pathway. As a result, a specific pattern of activation of many areas of the brain responsible for anxious behavior is observed. This mechanism is provided by evolution for the detection of acute changes in the intestine by the nervous system with the ability to selectively identify the pathogen [285–287].

In another study, P Bercík. et al. showed that *Helicobacter pylori* also affects the behavior of mice. During the experiment, it was noted that a slowdown in gastrointestinal emptying during infection with *H. pylori* is accompanied by a decrease in visceral sensitivity through the regulatory mechanisms of the nervous system of the stomach and spinal cord. Chronic *H. pylori* infection is characterized by frequent bouts of hunger, characteristic of patients with functional dyspepsia. Further in-depth studies showed that abnormal eating behavior was accompanied by a decrease in the level of the regulatory peptide proopiomelanocortin in the arcuate nucleus and an increase in the proinflammatory cytokine TNF-α in the median eminence of the hypothalamus, where the blood-brain barrier is more permeable than its other regions. Violation of the blood-brain barrier allows metabolites and small molecules from the systemic circulation to enter the central nervous system. The alarming behavior caused by this and biochemical abnormalities in animals persisted for 2 months after the eradication of the pathogen, which allows us to regard the infectious agent as a trigger factor provoking long-term or even permanent changes in the central nervous system that develop as a result of infection [288, 289].

Comparison of gnotobiont and infected mice by R.D Heijtz. et al showed that gnotobiont mice have a higher level of exploratory behavior and a lower level of anxiety behavior than infected animals. To confirm these conclusions, standard behavioral tests were used—open field and preference for light or dark. As a result of biochemical studies, it was found that the infected animals had a higher expression of neutrophilic nerve growth factors (NGF) and brain neutrophilic factor (BDNF). Differential expression of multiple genes involved in secondary pathways of information transmission, synaptic long-term potentiation in the hippocampus, frontal lobes of the cortex, and striatum was observed [290]. Neufeld K.M. et al showed that in infected mice, compared to gnotobionts, there is an increased expression of the nr2b subunit of the NMDA receptor in the central amygdala and an increased expression of the serotonin 1A receptor (5-HT 1A) in the hippocampus [291].

In addition to infectious agents, commensal bacteria also have an effect on the central nervous system. Thus, in the works of N. Sudo et al., It was shown that gnotobiont mice exhibit abnormal activity of the hypothalamic-pituitary-adrenal (HPA) axis with increased levels of ACTH and corticosterone in response to stress. Normalization of HPA axis activity is observed after colonization of animals with commensal bacteria. Also, gnotobiont animals had lower levels of the brain neutrophilic factor in the cortex and hippocampus [292]. Thus, in mice whose intestines are colonized by a complex microbiota, it has been shown that bacteria can influence various aspects of immunity, physiology, and metabolism. In the works of L.V. Hooper et al. is noted that colonization of a single commensal bacterium *Bacteroides thetaiotaomicron* alters the expression of a wide range of genes responsible for metabolism, intestinal permeability and angiogenesis, as well as glutamate uptake, GABA production, and neurotransmitter release [293]. Currently, the microbiome features of patients with autism spectrum disorders (ASD) are being actively studied.

It is known that a significant number, and, according to some authors [277], all patients with ASD have certain diseases of the gastrointestinal tract. They are characterized by a special composition of the intestinal microbiocenosis, which differs from the healthy microbiocenosis. Changes in the composition of the intestinal microbiocenosis of patients with ASD lead to increased production of toxins that negatively affect the immune system and the brain, as well as provoke an immune system response and intensify the inflammatory process.

The composition of the intestinal microbiota in patients with ASD plays a significant role in the development of chronic endotoxemia due to the production of neurotoxins, an increase in the permeability of the intestinal wall, and/or disruption of the blood-brain barrier. In the review by A.S. Blagonravova et al. are provided descriptions of intestinal dysbiosis in children with ASD, established by studies of the last decade [280]. Despite the inconsistency of the data, the main characteristic features related to the imbalance of the bacterial and fungal flora were highlighted. By the method of sequencing of the intestinal microbiota genome, as well as PCR, in patients with ASD, in almost all studies, a statistically significant increase in the number of *Clostridium* spp. was found in comparison with the control groups. A specific species of *Clostridium bolteae* was found, which was detected only in patients with ASD. The ability of *Clostridium* spp. to the production of phenols, derivatives of p-cresol and indole, which are toxins for humans. Studies have shown that these substances are present in the feces of patients with ASD. The importance of clostridial titer-dominated dysbiosis has been confirmed by the efficacy of vancomycin in improving both behavioral and gastrointestinal disturbances. The review also highlights the possible role of other microorganisms present in more patients with ASD than in healthy people. There is a strong correlation between the abundance of *Desulfovibrio* spp. with the severity of autism. This type of microorganism is a producer of propionic acid, which affects the permeability of the intestinal wall, can disrupt the blood-brain barrier, which contributes to the development of chronic endotoxemia and can provoke exacerbation of symptoms in patients with ASD. There is a high probability of the significance of the predominance of representatives of the *Bacteroidetes* type in the intestinal microbiocenosis and the violation of the *Bacteroidetes / Firmicutes* ratio. In some studies, increased levels of *Lactobacillus* spp. as well as *Bifidobacterium* spp. were noted in children with ASD compared with healthy children. At the same time, when studying these bacteria, it is necessary to take into account whether probiotic therapy was carried out, but this issue was not specified in the relevant publications. At the same time, data on a decrease in the number of bifidobacteria in patients with ASD are more numerous. The use of probiotic preparations based on strains of *Bifidobacterium* spp. has a positive effect in such cases due to their anti-inflammatory properties. Among other microorganisms, the level of which correlates with the severity of autism manifestations, *Candida albicans* has been isolated. It is important that aggressive forms of this fungus with pseudohyphae are found, which indicates the possibility of their facilitated adhesion to the intestinal mucosa. Fungi of the genus *Candida* can release ammonia, D-arabinitol and other toxins, which can be easily absorbed into the blood when the intestinal wall is permeable and can be associated with changes in behavior.

As shown by the results of studies by A.A. Maksimova [294], there are clear correlations between the severity of the manifestations of autism, the growth of certain microorganisms in the intestines of patients and the content of fecal calprotectin and zonulin in the feces. Elimination of bacterial and fungal infections leads to the normalization of the content of the latter and a decrease or disappearance of the negative behavior of children. Dysbiosis associated with excessive growth of *hemolytic enterococci* (*Enterococcus*), *hemolytic E. coli* (*Escherichia coli*), *Pseudomonas aeruginosa* in the large intestine was accompanied by sleep disorders, low concentration, and aggression. Antimicrobial therapy based on the sensitivity of the above pathogens to antibiotics, as well as the elimination of fast carbohydrates, sweets, and starch from the diet, reduced the severity of autism manifestations. In intestinal dysbiosis associated with the overgrowth of *Candida albicans* in the large and small intestines, there were manifestations in the form of attacks of sudden hysterical laughter, which often ended in outbursts of aggression or self-aggression. Excessive anxiety during sleep was noted, which was accompanied by frequent awakenings with crying and/or severe aggression. A decrease in the severity of these manifestations was achieved after a course of antifungal therapy, exclusion of sweets from the diet, including sweet fruits, sugary carbonated drinks, and bakery products. Infection with *Helicobacter pylori* was associated with hyperactivity or "shutdown" of the child from cognitive processes, as well as with sleep disorders. A decrease in autistic manifestations occurred after the eradication of the pathogen, the use of a special low-carbohydrate diet, and the appointment of probiotics. With excessive colonization of *Streptococcus mutans* in the small intestine, a high level of anxiety and periodic outbursts of aggression and self-aggression were noted, but without disturbances in sleep function. A positive effect was achieved by therapy with bacteriophages with the additional appointment of probiotics, prebiotics, and detoxification therapy using silicon-containing enterosorbents. Intestinal dysbiosis associated with a high intensity of small intestine colonization by *Clostridium perfringens* led to sleep disturbances, high levels of anxiety and emotional lability, severity of phobic manifestations and stereotypes. Long-term treatment, including antibiotic therapy and an anti-inflammatory nutritional protocol, was required to normalize *Clostridium perfringens*-associated disorders. However, the improvements were unstable and reversible due to the difficulties in suppressing this pathogen.

The author rightly draws attention to the fact that parents and medical professionals should not attribute all manifestations of negative behavior of children to the features of autism. It should be remembered that these manifestations may be the result of pathological changes in the child's gastrointestinal tract, which need to be diagnosed and corrected. Accordingly, it is necessary to connect a gastroenterologist to the patient's management. It is significant that none of the parents of all the children involved in the study (41 people) were ever told about such a need. This situation is widespread in all countries. These recommendations directly apply to psychiatrists, psychologists, behavioral analysts, defectologists, tutors, and other professionals who constantly work with children diagnosed with ASD. If there is a suspicion of the existence of medical reasons for negative behavior, children should be sent for a specialized consultation, and not increase the corrective and cognitive load on them. Moreover, with the disappearance of negative behavior, the effectiveness of any behavioral and corrective therapy increases many times over. Disorders of the gastrointestinal tract can be associated with pathological changes in other body systems. This dictates the need for an interdisciplinary medical approach in the diagnosis of pathological conditions in children with ASD. Psychiatrists need to take into account the possible connection between the negative behavior of patients with pathological conditions of the gastrointestinal tract and other organs. Only after the mentioned pathological conditions are confidently excluded from the list of causes of negative behavior, the doctor can consider the possibility of connecting psychotropic drugs to therapy.

Thus, deformation of the intestinal microbiocenosis and changes in the structure of its functional activity play a significant role in the development of autism (as well as other neuropsychiatric diseases (see 20.1.3)). As you know, normally the intestinal microflora synthesizes vitamins of the B and K groups, participates in the synthesis of essential amino acids, in the metabolism of fats, fatty acids, bilirubin, bile acids, water-salt metabolism and heat exchange. The intestinal microflora is responsible for the elimination of toxins, regulation of cellular and humoral immunity, and stimulation of peristalsis [295].

An important role in maintaining homeostasis is played by the production of metabolites by the intestinal microflora, among which short-chain fatty acids should be especially noted. Short-chain fatty acids are saturated monocarboxylic acids in the homologous range from acetic to nylon, including isoforms. Of the total pool produced by the microflora, 90% are acetic, propionic, and butyric acids. Butyric acid is not absorbed into the blood, but is involved in the energy supply of the absorption of other metabolites and nutrients from the intestine into the blood through colonocytes [296]. Acetic and propionic acids are absorbed into the bloodstream and participate in further biochemical processes. Acetic acid circulates through the systemic circulation and provides energy to the peripheral cells of the body [297]. Excessive concentration of propionic acid leads to stimulation of intestinal smooth muscles and, accordingly, to accelerated evacuation of feces, increases intestinal permeability due to the weakening of tight contacts between the cells of its wall, followed by the penetration of undissolved molecules into the systemic circulation [297]. Propionic acid from the portal vein enters the liver, where it is burned in the liver peroxisomes. An increase in the concentration of propionic acid in the systemic circulation promotes the launch of inflammatory processes and the activation of the immune system response. Further impairment of mitochondrial function is noted, which affects the distribution of energy in the brain. Oxidative stress is provoked and the content of antioxidant molecules, neurotransmitters, omega-3 fatty acids decreases [298].

The result of dysfunction of the intestinal barrier, as already mentioned, is the formation of chronic endotoxemia. A high level of toxins in the blood forms a stable inflammatory state in the periventricular areas of the brain, followed by destabilization of the blood-brain barrier and the spread of inflammation to other parts of the brain, which can subsequently contribute to the development of neurodegeneration [299].

It should be noted that studies devoted to the study of the microbiota of patients with ASD in other biotopes, in particular, the oral cavity and oropharynx, are few in number. However, as discussed above (Sects. 20.1 and 20.4), the disturbance of microflora in the oropharynx associated with the presence of pathogens and their toxins reaching the brain through the neural and hematogenous pathways can negatively affect the state of its structures. According to several studies, the oral microflora of children with autism is characterized by a general decrease in the number of bacteria and an increase in the number of pathogens such as *Haemophilus* in saliva and *Streptococcus* in plaque, as well as a decrease in the number of some commensal bacteria (*Prevotella, Selenomonas, Actinomyces, Porphyromonas and Fusobacterium*). Plaque also showed a significant decrease in all *Prevotellaceae*, a family that can interact with the immune system, and a high concentration of *Rothia*, a bacterium often associated with dental disease [300, 301]. The data for *Rothia* are consistent with those for saliva [302].

In the literature, we were unable to find works analyzing the microbiome of the posterior pharyngeal wall in patients with ASD; however, this is an important anatomical region containing elements of lymphoid tissue that can be a reservoir of infection. In this regard, we have begun to study the microbiota of the posterior pharyngeal wall in patients with ASD. Preliminary data were obtained on a general group of children with speech disorders, of which eight people was diagnosed with ASD [303]. The study of scraping of the posterior pharyngeal wall was carried out by the method of chromatography-mass spectrometry of microbial markers (MSMM) [272], which, as noted, makes it possible to identify 57 markers of bacterial, fungal, and viral flora. All patients underwent a comprehensive assessment of the state of the main organs according to the previously mentioned (Sects. 20.1 and 20.4) method of comprehensive assessment of autoimmunity, including the assessment of autoantibodies to antigens of 16 major organs (including the microstructures of the brain—neurons, glia, myelin sheaths of nerves) and markers of systemic inflammation (8) (ELI-viscerotest-24) [170]. All children had an increased content of coccal microflora in the throat, characteristic of chronic tonsillitis (CT) and chronic pharyngitis (CP) (*epidermal Staphylococcus aureus* and *S. epidermidis*, *pyogenic Streptococcus*) with an increase in the level of anaerobic streptococci (peptostreptococci, characteristic of the intestinal flora). There was also a high level of other microflora characteristic of the intestine - enterococci, clostridia of various species, gram-negative bacteria (*kingella, flavo*, etc.). In some patients, viruses of the herpes group were detected—more often HSV-2, less often CMV and EBV, as well as an increase in fungal microflora (*Aspergillus, Candida*, as well as actinomycetes of various types). Clinically, all patients had chronic diseases of the upper respiratory tract: CP and CT, sinusitis, vasomotor rhinitis. Lymphadenopathies of the cervical lymph nodes, labial herpes, frequent ARVI were also noted. The treatment-resistant variant of CP and CT in the examined children was combined with an increase in the content in the pharynx of bacteria characteristic of stomach diseases—*Helicobacter* and *Campylobacter*, which indicated the presence of reflux—esophagitis.

The study of autoimmunity revealed an increase in titers of autoantibodies to antigens of the gastrointestinal tract in 100% of cases: stomach, small intestine, liver, insulin, insulin receptors. All examined children had increased antibodies to one of the markers of the uneven system (S-100 proteins, glia, myelin basic protein). Most often, an increase in antibodies to glia (glial acidic fibrillar protein) was detected, which raises the question of the presence of an inflammatory process in the brain. Normalization of the microbiota in the pharynx, treatment of CP and CT, correction of changes in the main organs and systems (treatment of gastrointestinal diseases, restoration of the hepato-biliary system, etc.) made it possible to significantly improve the condition of patients. Additionally, the study showed the feasibility of using the considered autoimmunity research method to monitor the effectiveness of the treatment.

As can be seen from the above study, the characteristics of the autoimmunity of patients with ASD indicate that such children are predisposed to infectious diseases. The little person is gradually moving towards adulthood, and along the way, he can meet with a wide variety of infections. New infections can contribute to both the aggravation of the imbalance of its microbiota and the aggravation of autoimmunity disorders. On the other hand, the addition of new infections in children with ASD can be more severe. In particular, this applies to coronavirus infection. French scientists have published the results of a study in which 16 autistic patients aged 12 to 43 years old (average age—20.8 years) took part [304]. The manifestations of the main diagnosis were: limited social interaction ($N = 16$; 100%), stereotypical limited behavior ($N = 15$; 93.8%), other complex behavior ($N = 11$; 68.8%). Eleven of them were diagnosed with COVID-19 with corresponding symptoms: signs of upper respiratory tract infection (rhinitis, $N = 9$; 81.8%), diarrhea ($N = 7$; 63.6%), fatigue (N = 7; 63, 6%), fever (N = 4; 36.4%), and various respiratory manifestations (N = 5; 45.5%).

As the study showed, autistic children, when infected with the SARS-CoV-2 virus, were observed both common signs of the disease of the new coronavirus infection COVID-19, such as fever, fatigue, shortness of breath and diarrhea, and uncharacteristic for this viral infection. Since people with autism are more susceptible to diseases and disorders of the gastrointestinal tract, the prevalence of diarrhea among them is higher than the average for coronavirus infection, which can aggravate the symptoms of COVID-19 [305, 306]. There is no evidence to support the ability of the new coronavirus infection to contribute to the development of autism, but there is no doubt that this infection aggravates the symptoms of autistic disorder.

Studies of the influence of genetic and environmental factors show that the pathophysiological changes characteristic of autism originate during intrauterine development [307, 308].

Infections during pregnancy, including coronavirus infection, are accompanied by an increase in proinflammatory cytokines in a woman's body [309, 310], which contributes to an increase in type 6 interleukin (IL-6) and changes in gene expression in the placental environment. This activates the signaling pathway of Janus kinase (JAK)—signal transducer and activator of transcription proteins (STAT)—JAK / STAT-3, which contributes to a decrease in placental synthesis of growth hormone and insulin-like growth factor (IGF-1) [311]. This, in turn, leads to a decrease in the ability of the fetus to myelination of the developing nervous system, and, accordingly, to disruption of neural connections in the brain, and may be associated with the development of a number of pathologies of the nervous system, including autism [312, 313]. It is assumed that autoreactive T-lymphocytes can migrate across the blood-brain barrier and cause the activation of local antigen-presenting cells, such as microglia and astrocytes [314, 315]. The production of interleukins (IL) -2, -6 types, interferon (IFN) -γ and tumor necrosis factor (TNF) -α at an early prenatal stage can lead to damage to oligodendrocytes and demyelination, which can also contribute to the development of autism [316]. Thus, the mother's immune response to infection includes the formation / release of antibodies and cytokines that can cross the immature blood-brain barrier of the fetus, which subsequently increases the risk of developing autism [317].

To the above, it should be added that during pregnancy there is a powerful restructuring of all systems, including immunity. Pregnancy itself is a physiological immunosuppressive factor, since there is a natural decrease in the protective properties of the body in order to prevent miscarriage. The flip side of this phenomenon is the manifestation, and possibly subclinical activation, of previously "dormant" infections, for example, genital herpes. The question is raised about the possibility of vertical transmission of the SARS-CoV-2 virus from mother to fetus during pregnancy associated with COVID-19; however, there is little reliable data confirming this possibility [318]. It is possible that lactoferrin existing in the placenta, amniotic fluid and milk secretions may have a protective effect in these cases [316].

Probably, transplacental infection can occur not only with active forms of infections, but also with their erased course (see Chap. 17). In cases of the latter option, malformations of various organs of the fetus may be absent, including pronounced pathology of brain structures. Not only infectious agents themselves, but also antimicrobial antibodies that penetrate through the placenta, negatively interacting with the noted microstructures by the mechanism of molecular mimicry, can have a damaging effect on the microstructures of the brain. The situation can be aggravated if, in connection with the infectious disease in question, in the body of a pregnant woman there are autoimmune processes with excessive production of autoantibodies to the brain tissue, which are able to penetrate the placental and blood-brain barriers. As a result, hypothetically, by the time a child is born, an autoimmune process can take place in his nerve tissue. Any adverse effects of the external environment after birth can lead to its aggravation and manifestations of autistic disorder, or aggravate symptoms that are already present from birth. Probably, in parallel, the disturbances of the microbiota are becoming more severe due to a decrease in immunity under these conditions, the activation of the existing pathogenic microflora, and/or the introduction of new pathogens.

Thus, to assess the state of the organism in patients with ASD, not only psychiatric and psychological examinations are required, but also the study of the characteristics of the microbiome, preferably in various biotopes. It is also necessary to determine the functional activity of the intestinal microbiocenosis, including the concentration of metabolites, especially the concentration of propionic and butyric acids. An interdisciplinary approach to the examination and management of patients, as well as the identification of preclinical forms of pathology, is important.

In addition to using the possibilities of antimicrobial therapy individualized in each specific case, the use of neurodietology in combination with personalized probiotic therapy is an important direction in the treatment of ASD. The main tool of neurodietology is the application of the ketogenic, gluten-free, gluten-free Atkinson diet and the low glycemic index diet, which promotes neuroprotection in a wide range of brain diseases. Studies have shown that after its use, 51.5% of patients experience a positive change in attention indicators, an improvement in cognitive function and an improvement in adaptive abilities [319]. It is especially important to reduce the amount of carbohydrates consumed in patients with dysbiosis, characterized by a large number of *Clostridium* spp. It has been shown that with such a composition of the intestinal microbiocenosis, patients consume excessively foods with a high content of carbohydrates, which contribute to the growth of *Clostridia*.

The inclusion of probiotics in the general treatment regimen for patients with ASD, as already mentioned, had a positive role, in particular, in conditions characterized by anxiety and aggression [294]. The feasibility of using probiotics was also justified in cases of anxiety and depressive disorders caused by chronic bowel diseases (irritable bowel syndrome, inflammatory bowel diseases). In experiments *in vivo* on mice, it was shown that a probiotic based on bifidobacteria *Bifidobacterium longum* NC3001 relieved anxiety. In *ex vivo* experiments, it was found that the action of the probiotic is neurally mediated. The essence of the experiment was to record the electrical response of enteric neurons, which was assessed after perfusion over *B. longum* sedimentary fluid. Neurons treated with the probiotic generated fewer action potentials in response to a suprathreshold depolarizing current compared to intact neurons. At the same time, in the experiment *in vivo*, there was no improvement in the state of the inflamed intestine or cytokine circulation [320, 321].

In another study by Desbonnet L. et al, it was shown that administration of *Bifidobacterium infantis* to healthy rats reduced the concentration of serotonin and dopamine metabolites in the corresponding lobes of the cerebral cortex [322, 323].

Research on a probiotic based on *L. rhamnosus* JB1 strain by Bravo J.A. and colleagues showed that administering this probiotic to healthy mice stimulated their exploratory behavior in the maze test and reduced feelings of despair in the forced swim test. This was accompanied by some changes in the levels of GABA mRNA in the brain, which were obviously vago-dependent, since no changes in brain biochemistry and in the behavior of subjects were observed during subdiaphragmatic vagotomy [324].

Thus, studies have confirmed the assumptions that commensal bacteria and specific probiotics may affect brain chemistry and alter the function of the central nervous system. Taking into account the data obtained, including the practical experience of using probiotic drugs for the treatment of ASD [294], it is obvious that these drugs are widely used in correction schemes for children with ASD.

Summarizing the above data, it should be concluded that the studies have demonstrated the presence of pronounced microbiota disorders in patients with ASD, their association with the severity of autistic disorders and reduction after specific antimicrobial therapy in combination with the use of pre- and probiotics and diet therapy. The foregoing provides a basis for considering the role of microbial agents and microbiome disorders as probable etiopathogenetic factors of ASD. Further research should be focused on studying the microbiota of patients with ASD in other biotopes, in particular, the upper respiratory tract, including taking into account the viral component of the microbiome and its possible disorders in this contingent of patients. A wide diagnostic range of methods for detecting pathogens should be used, including metagenomic analysis of the microbiome by molecular genetic methods and determination of the content of metabolites of the microbial flora. It is also necessary to study the interaction of the microbiota in patients with ASD and environmental factors affecting the individual development of the organism.

Regardless of whether infections are considered as the etiological factor of ASD or as a factor aggravating the course of the disease, each patient with this diagnosis should be investigated interdisciplinary, taking into account the possible pathology of the gastrointestinal tract and respiratory tract, and the most complete definition of microbiota as an indicator of the state of factors of natural resistance and adaptive immunity. It is important to identify undetected forms of pathology, including by methods of autoimmunity research.

In the programs for the prevention of ASD, it is advisable to include screening of the microbiota of the gastrointestinal tract of newborns during the period of transformation of the microbial landscape (4–5 days after birth) (with special attention to the data of the study of children from risk groups—with a complicated course of pregnancy and childbirth, bacterial vaginosis, herpes infection, and others diseases of the mother, low assessment of the newborn on the Apgar scale, etc.), as well as a comprehensive immunochemical study of autoimmunity. The same studies should be included in the protocols for examining children before vaccination.

References

1. Tiganov AS. A Guide to Psychiatry. Ch. 1, 2. M: Medicine, 1999. (In Russian).
2. Orlovskaya DD. Pathological anatomy of psychosis. In: Snezhnevsky AV, editor. A guide to psychiatry, Part 1. M.: Medicine; 1983. p. 158–86. (In Russian).
3. Tiganov AS. Pathological anatomy of schizophrenia. In: Tiganov AS, editor. A guide to psychiatry, Ch.1. M.: Medicine; 1999. p. 506–10. (In Russian).
4. Orlova VA, Savina TD, Trubnikov V and., Yu SN. etc. Structural features of the brain (according to magnetic resonance imaging) and their functional connections in the families of patients with schizophrenia. Russian Psychiatr J. 6: 48-56. 199 (In Russian).
5. Gur RE, Pearlson GD. Neuroimaging in schizophrenia research. Schizophr Bull. 1993;19(2):337–53.
6. Pearlson GD. Marsh L Structural brain imaging in schizophrenia: a selective review. Biol Psychiatry. 1999;46(5):627–49.
7. Sigmundsson T, Suckling J, Maier M, et al. Structural abnormalities in frontal, temporal and limbic regions and interconnecting white matter tracts in schizophrenic patients with prominent negative symptoms. Am J Psychiatry. 2001;158:234–43.
8. Mc Donald C, Grech A, Toulopoulou T, et al. Brain volumes in familial and non-familial schizophrenic probands and their unaffected relatives. Am J Med Genet. 2002;114:616–25.
9. Bogerts B. Recent advances in the neuropathology of schizophrenia. Schizophr Bull. 1993;19(2):431–45. https://doi.org/10.1093/schbul/19.2.431.
10. Chua SE, Murray RM. The neurodevelopment theory of schizophrenia: evidence concerning structure and neuropsychology. Acta Neuropsychiatry. 1996;8:25–34.
11. Jones P, Murray RM. The genetics of schizophrenia is the genetics of neurodevelopment. Br J Psychiatry. 1991;158:615–23.
12. Jakob H, Beckmann H. Prenatal developmental disturbances in the limbic allocortex in schizophrenics. J Neural Transm. 1986;65:303–26.
13. Jaskiw GE, Juliano DM, GoldbergT E, et al. Cerebral ventricular enlargement in schizophreniform disorder does not progress. A seven year follow-up study. Schizophr Res. 1994;14:23–8.
14. Lim KO, Harris D, Beal M, J. G., et al. Gray matter deficits in young onset schizophrenia are independent of age of onset. Biol Psychiatry. 1996;40:4–13.
15. Vita A, Dieci M, Giobbio GM, et al. CT scan abnormalities and outcome of chronic schizophrenia. Am J Psychiatry. 1991;148:1577–9.
16. Mathalon DH, Sullivan EV, Lim KO, et al. Progressive Brain Volume Changes and the Clinical Course of Schizophrenia in Men. A Longitudinal

Magnetic Resonance Imaging Study. Arch Genet Psychiatry. 2001;58(2):148–57. https://doi.org/10.1001/archpsyc.58.2.148.
17. Perez-Neri I, Ramirez-Bermudez J, Montes S, Rios C. Possible mechanisms of neurodegeneration in schizophrenia. Neurochem Res. 2006;31:1279–94.
18. Uranova N, Orlovskaya D, Vikhreva O, et al. Electron microscopy of oligodendroglia in severe mental illness. Brain Research Bulletin. 2001;55(5):597–610.
19. Keshavan MS. Development, disease and degeneration in schizophrenia: a unitary pathophysiological model. J Psych Research. 1999;33:513–21.
20. Orlova VA, Trubnikov VI, Odintsova SA, et al. Genetic analysis of the anatomical and morphological signs of the brain detected by magnetic resonance imaging in families of patients with schizophrenia. Genetics. 1999;35(7):998–1004. (In Russian)
21. Orlova VA. Clinical and genetic studies of schizophrenia (current state and development prospects). Russian Psychiatric J. 2003;1:31–5. (In Russian)
22. Miloserdov EA, Gubsky LV, Orlova VA, et al. Structural peculiarities of the brain in patients with schizophrenia and their relatives according to morphometric analysis of MRI images of the brain. Soc Clin Psychiatry. 2005;15(1):5–12. (In Russian)
23. Karlsson JL. Partly dominant transmission of schizophrenia in Iceland. Br J Psychiatry. 1988;152:324–9. https://doi.org/10.1192/bjp.152.3.324.
24. Kendler KS, Karkowski-Shuman L, Walsh D. The risk for psychiatric illness in siblings of schizophrenics: the impact of psychotic and non-psychotic affective illness and alcoholism in parents. Acta Psychiatr Scand. 1996;94(1):49–55. https://doi.org/10.1111/j.1600-0447.1996.tb09824.x.
25. Gottesman I. Schizophrenia genesis: the origins of madness. New York: NY: Freeman; 1991. p. 296. https://doi.org/10.1192/S0007125000030919.
26. Torrey EF. Are we overestimating the genetic contribution to schizophrenia? Schizophr Bull. 1992;18: 159–70. https://doi.org/10.1093/schbul/18.2.159.
27. Boyd JH, Pulver AE, Stewart W. Season of birth: schizophrenia and bipolar disorder. Schizophr Bull. 1986;12:173–85. https://doi.org/10.1093/schbul/12.2.173.
28. Bradbury TN, Miller GA. Season of birth in schizophrenia a review of evidence, methodology, and etiology. Psychol Bull. 1985;98(3):569–94. https://doi.org/10.1037/0033-2909.98.3.569.
29. Susser E, Lin SP. Schizophrenia after prenatal exposure to the Dutch hunger winter of 1944–1945. Arch Gen Psychiatry. 1994;51(333–334) https://doi.org/10.1001/archpsyc.1992.01820120071010.
30. Torrey EF, Bowler AE, Taylor EH, et al. Schizophrenia and manic depressive disorder: the biological roots of mental illness as revealed by a landmark study of identical twins. New York: Basic Books; 1994. p. 274. https://doi.org/10.1176/ajp.152.9.1395.
31. Adams W, Kendell RE, Hare EH, et al. Epidemiological evidence that maternal influenza contributes to the etiology of schizophrenia. An analysis of Scottish, English, and Danish data. Br J Psychiatry. 1993;163:522–34. https://doi.org/10.1192/bjp.163.4.522.
32. Buka SL, Cannon TD, Torrey EF, et al. Maternal exposure to herpes simplex virus and risk of psychosis among adult offspring. Biol Psychiatry. 2007;63:809–15. https://doi.org/10.1016/j.biopsych.2007.09.022.
33. Brown AS. Prenatal infection as a risk factor for schizophrenia. Schizophr Bull. 2006;32:200–2. https://doi.org/10.1093/schbul/sbj052.
34. Dalman C, Allebeck P, Gunnell D, et al. Infections in the CNS during childhood and the risk of subsequent psychotic illness: a cohort study of more than one million Swedish subjects. Am J Psychiatry. 2008;165:59–65. https://doi.org/10.1176/appi.ajp.2007.07050740.
35. Sham PC, MacLean CJ, Kendler KS. Risk of schizophrenia and age difference with older siblings: evidence for a maternal viral infection hypothesis? Br J Psychiatry. 1993;163:627–33. https://doi.org/10.1192/bjp.163.5.627.
36. Lewis GA, Andreasson DS, Allebeck P. Schizophrenia and city life. Lancet. 1992;340:137–40. https://doi.org/10.1016/0140-6736(92)93213-7.
37. Torrey EF. Schizophrenia and civilization. New York: Jason Aronson; 1980. p. 230.
38. Book JA, Wetterberg L, Modrzewska K. Schizophrenia in a North Swedish geographical isolate 1900–1977: epidemiology, genetics andbiochemistry. Clin Genet. 1978;14:373–94. https://doi.org/10.1111/j.1399-0004.1978.tb02105.x.
39. Kohn ML. Social class and schizophrenia: a review. J Psychiatr Res. 1968;6:155–73. https://doi.org/10.1016/0022-3956(68)90014-9.
40. Schweitzer L, Su W-H. Population density and the rate of mental illness. Am J Public Health. 1977;67:1165–72. https://doi.org/10.2105/AJPH.67.12.1165.
41. Eskirol J-E. 1845. Cit. by Oifa A.I. The brain and viruses. Moscow: Russkiy Mir Publishing House; 1999. p. 191. (In Russian)
42. Drecke T. On the germ-theory of disease. Am J Insanity. 1874;30:443–68.
43. Morozov VM. On the viral nature of schizophrenia. J Neuropathol Psychiatry named S. S. Korsakov. 1954;54:732–4. (In Russian)
44. Orlova VA, Mikhailova II, Lavrov VF, et al. The role of viral factors in the development of endogenous mental pathology (schizophrenia, schizoaffective psychosis): clinical-biological aspects. Mental Health. 2021;12:65–78.
45. Turnbaugh PJ, Ley RE, Hamady M, et al. The human microbiome project: exploring the microbial part of ourselves in a changing world. Nature. 2007;449(7164):804–10. https://doi.org/10.1038/nature06244.
46. Agorastos A, Bozikas VP. Gut microbiome and adaptive immunity in schizophrenia. Psychiatriki.

2019;30(3):189–92. https://doi.org/10.22365/jpsych.2019.303.189.
47. Global virome project. http://www.globalviromeproject.org/.
48. Carter CJ. Schizophrenia susceptibility genes directly implicated in the life cycle of pathogens: cytomegalovirus, influenza, herpes simplex, rubella, and toxoplasma gondii. Schizophr Bull. 2009;35(6):1163–82. https://doi.org/10.1093/schbul/sbn054.
49. Barinskij IF, Mahmudov FR. Gerpes. Baku: Victory, 2013; 352p. (In Russian).
50. Prokofieva-Belgovskaya A. A. Action of genes. Mutations. Population genetics. M.: Meditsina, 1969. 544 p. (In Russian)
51. Khesin R. B. Impermanence of the genome. M.: Nauka; 1985. 472 p. (In Russian)
52. Crow TJ. Psychosis as a continuum and the virogene concept. Br Med Bull. 1987;43:754–67.
53. Oifa A Brain and viruses (virus-genetic hypothesis of the origin of mental diseases). M: Russkii mir 1999. 190 p. (In Russian)
54. Perry VH, Cunningham C, Holmes C. Systemic infections and inflammation affect chronic neurodegeneration. Nat Rev Immunol. 2007;7(2):161–7. https://doi.org/10.1038/nri2015.
55. Cunningham C, Wilcockson DC, Campion S, Lunnon K, Perry VH. Central and systemic endotoxin challenges exacerbate the local inflammatory response and increase neuronal death during chronic neurodegeneration. J Neurosci. 2005;25(40):9275–84. https://doi.org/10.1523/JNEUROSCI.2614-05.2005.
56. Frank MG, Baratta MV, Sprunger DB, Watkins LR, Maier SF. Microglia serve as a neuroimmune substrate for stress-induced potentiation of CNS pro-inflammatory cytokine responses. Brain Behav Immun. 2007;21(1):47–59. https://doi.org/10.1016/j.bbi.2006.03.005.
57. Brown AS, Derkits EJ. Prenatal infection and schizophrenia: a review of epidemiologic and translational studies. Am J Psychiatry. 2010;167(3):261–80. https://doi.org/10.1176/appi.ajp.2009.09030361.
58. Khandaker GM, Zimbron J, Lewis G, Jones PB. Prenatal maternal infection, neurodevelopment and adult schizophrenia: a systematic review of population-based studies. Psychol Med. 2013;43(2):239–57. https://doi.org/10.1017/S0033291712000736.
59. Bramham CR, Wells DG. Dendritic mRNA: transport, translation and function. Nat Rev Neurosci. 2007;8:776–89.
60. Grohmann U, Fallarino F, Puccetti P. Tolerance, DCs and tryptophan: much ado about IDO. Trends Immunol. 2003;24:242–8.
61. Schwarcz R, Rassoulpour A, Wu HQ, Medoff D, Tamminga CA, Roberts RC. Increased cortical kynurenate content in schizophrenia. Biol Psychiatry. 2001;50(7):521–30.
62. Muller N, Schwarz MJ. The immunological basis of glutamatergic disturbance in schizophrenia: towards an integrated view. J Neural Transm Suppl. 2007;72:269–80.
63. Grayson DR, Jia X, Chen Y, Sharma RP, Mitchell CP, Guidotti A, et al. Reelin promoter hypermethylation in schizophrenia. Proc Natl Acad Sci USA. 2005;102:9341–6.
64. Domegan LM, Atkins GJ. Apoptosis induction by the Therien and vaccine RA27/3 strains of rubella virus causes depletion of oligodendrocytes from rat neural cell cultures. J Gen Virol. 2002;83:2135–43.
65. Bello-Morales R, Fedetz M, Alcina A, Tabares E, Lopez-Guerrero JA. High susceptibility of a human oligodendroglial cell line to herpes simplex type 1 infection. J Neurovirol. 2005;11:190–8.
66. Casanova AS, Lavrov VF, Zverev VV. Varicella Zoster virus and vascular diseases of the central nervous system. J Microbiol. 2015;3:106–16. (In Russian)
67. Lavrov VF, Svitich OA, Casanova AS, Kinkulkina AR, Zverev VV. Varicella zoster-viral infection: immunity, diagnosis and modeling in vivo. J Microbiol. 2019;4:82–9. (In Russian). https://doi.org/10.36233/0372-9311-2019-4-82-89.
68. Fatemi SH, Emamian ES, Kist D, Sidwell RW, Nakajima K, Akhter P, et al. Defective corticogenesis and reduction in reelin immunoreactivity in cortex and hippocampus of prenatally infected neonatal mice. Mol Psychiatry. 1999;4:145–54.
69. Zuev VA The many faces of the virus: the secrets of latent infections. M.; 2020. 370 p. (in Russian)
70. Brok HP, Boven L, van Meurs M, Kerlero de Rosbo N. The human CMV-UL86 peptide 981-1003 shares a crossreactive T-cell epitope with the encephalitogenic MOG peptide 34-56, but lacks the capacity to induce EAE in rhesus monkeys. J Neuroimmunol. 2007;182(1–2):135–52.
71. Sugita S, Takase H, Kawaguchi T, Taguchi C, Mochizuki M. Cross-reaction between tyrosinase peptides and cytomegalovirus antigen by T cells from patients with Vogt-Koyanagi-Harada disease. Int Ophthalmol. 2007;27(2-3):87–95.
72. Ou D, Mitchell LA, Metzger DL, Gillam S, Tingle AJ. Cross-reactive rubella virus and glutamic acid decarboxylase (65 and 67) protein determinants recognised by T cells of patients with type I diabetes mellitus. Diabetologia. 2000;43(6):750–62.
73. Lvov ND. Human herpesviruses—systemic, integrative, lymphoproliferative immuno-ocopatology. ILR (Russian Medical Journal). 2012;22:1133. (In Russian)
74. Witte L, Mierlo H, Litjens M, Klein H, Bahn S & Osterhaus AB. The association between antibodies to neurotropic pathogens and schizophrenia: a case-control study. npj Schizophrenia 1, Article number: 15041 (2015). http://www.nature.com/articles/npjschz201541
75. Mañanes-González S, Carrillo-Ávila JA, Gutiérrez B, Cervilla J, Sorlózano-Puerto A. Different presence of Chlamydia pneumoniae, herpes simplex virus type 1, human herpes virus 6, and Toxoplasma

gondii in schizophrenia: meta-analysis and analytical study. Neuropsychiatric Disease and Treatment. 2015;11:843–52.
76. Fukuda R, Sasaki T, Kunugi H, Nanko S. No changes in paired viral antibody titers during the course of acute schizophrenia. Neuropsychobiology. 1999;40(2):57–62.
77. Maltsev DV. Modern methods of diagnosis of human herpesvirus infections and principles of interpretation of their results. Clin Immunol Allergol Infectol. 2010;1(30):23–33. (In Russian)
78. Pokrovsky VI. Laboratory diagnostics of infectious diseases. Directory. M: Binom. 2016; 648 p. (In Russian).
79. Leweke FM, Gerth CW, Koethe D, Klosterkötter J, Ruslanova I, Krivogorsky B, Torrey EF, Yolken RH. Antibodies to infectious agents in individuals with recent onset schizophrenia. Eur Arch Psychiatry Neurosci. 2004;254(1):4–8. https://doi.org/10.1007/s00406-004-0481-6.
80. Krause D, Matz J, Weidinger E, Wagner J, Wildenauer A, Obermeier M, Riedel M, Müller N. The association of infectious agents and schizophrenia. World J Biol Psychiatry. 2010;11(5):739–43. https://doi.org/10.3109/15622971003653246.
81. Tedla Y, Shibre T, Ali O, Tadele G, Woldeamanuel Y, Asrat D, et al. Serum antibodies to Toxoplasma gondii and Herpesvidae family viruses in individuals with schizophrenia and bipolar disorder: a case-control study. Ethiop Med J. 2011;49(3):211–20.
82. Mohagheghia M, Alikhanib MY, Taheri M, Eftekhariane MM. Determining the IgM and IgG antibodies titer against HSV1, HSV2 and CMV in the serum of schizophrenia patients. Human Antibodies. 2017;26(2):1–6. https://doi.org/10.3233/HAB-170325.
83. Tanaka T, Matsuda T, Hayes LN, Yan S, Rodriguez KM, et al. Infection and inflammation in schizophrenia and bipolar disorder. Neurosci Res. 2017;115:59–63. https://doi.org/10.1016/j.neures.2016.11.002.
84. Dickerson F, Jones-Brando L, Ford G, Genovese G. Schizophrenia is associated with an aberrant immune response to Epstein–Barr Virus. Schizophr Bull. 2019;45(5):1112–9. https://doi.org/10.1093/schbul/sby164.
85. Torrey EF, Leweke MF, Schwarz MJ, Mueller N, Bachmann S, Schroeder J, et al. Cytomegalovirus and schizophrenia. CNS Drugs. 2006;20:879–85. https://doi.org/10.2165/00023210-200620110-00001.
86. Brusov OS, Kaleda VG, Kolyaskina GI, Lavrov VF, Ebralidze LK, et al. Cytomegalovirus infection as a factor in the formation of resistance to treatment with neuroleptics in adolescent patients with the first attack of endogenous psychosis. Psychiatry. 2007;4(28):62–71. (In Russian)
87. Arias I, Sorlozano A, Villegas E, et al. Infectious agents associated with schizophrenia: a meta-analysis. Schizophr. Res. 2012;136(1–3):128–36. https://doi.org/10.1016/j.schres.2011.10.026.
88. Niebuhr DW, Millikan AM, Yolken R, Li Y, Weber NS. Results from a hypothesis generating case-control study: Herpes family viruses and schizophrenia among military personnel. Schizophr Bull. 2008;34(6):1182–8. https://doi.org/10.1093/schbul/sbm139.
89. Wang H, Yolken RH, Hoekstra PJ, et al. Antibodies to infectious agents and the positive symptom dimension of subclinical psychosis: The TRAILS study. Schizophr Res. 2011;129(1):47–51. https://doi.org/10.1016/j.schres.2011.03.013.
90. Hannachi N, El Kissi Y, Samoud S, Jaafar NJ, Letaief L, Gaabout S, Ben Hadj Ali B, Boukadida J. High prevalence of Human Herpesvirus 8 in schizophrenic patients. Psychiatry Res. 2014;216(2):192–7. https://doi.org/10.1016/j.psychres.2013.12.035.
91. Yolken RH, Torrey EF, Lieberman JA, et al. Serological evidence of exposure to Herpes Simplex Virus type 1 is associated with cognitive deficits in the CATIE schizophrenia sample. Schizophr Res. 2011;128(1-3):61–5. https://doi.org/10.1016/j.schres.2011.01.020.
92. Schretlen DJ, Vannorsdall TD, Winicki JM, et al. Neuroanatomic and cognitive abnormalities related to herpes simplex virus type 1 in schizophrenia. Schizophr Res. 2010;118(1–3):224–31. https://doi.org/10.1016/j.schres.2010.01.008.
93. Prasad KM, Watson AM, Dickerson FB, et al. Exposure to herpes simplex virus type 1 and cognitive impairments in individuals with schizophrenia. Schizophr. Bull. 2012;38(6):1137–48. https://doi.org/10.1093/schbul/sbs046.
94. Zakharova MN, Logunov DY, Kochergin DA, Bakulin IS. Endogenous retroviruses: from basic research to etiotropic therapy of multiple sclerosis. Ann Clin Exp Neurol. 2015;1(5):49–51. (In Russian)
95. Yolken R. Viruses and schizophrenia: a focus on herpes simplex virus. Herpes. 2004;11(2):83A–8A.
96. Aftab A, Shah AA, Hashmi AM. Pathophysiological role of HERV-W in Schizophrenia. J Neuropsychiatry Clin Neurosci. 2016;28(1):17–25. https://doi.org/10.1176/appi.neuropsych.15030059.
97. Da R, Ren JK. Pathogenic significance and possible pathogenic mechanism of human endogenous viruses in development of schizophrenia. Bing Du Xue Bao. 2014;30(1):98–102.
98. Ellul P, Groc L, Leboyer M. Implication of human endogenous retroviruses in schizophrenia and bipolar disorder. Med Sci (Paris). 2017;33(4):404–9. (In French). https://doi.org/10.1051/medsci/20173304010.
99. Ermakov EA, Smirnova LP, Parkhomenko TA, et al. DNA-hydrolysing activity of IgG antibodies from the sera of patients with schizophrenia. Open. Biology. 2015;5:150064.
100. Khandaker GM, Cousins L, Deakin J, et al. Inflammation and immunity in schizophrenia: implications for pathophysiology and treatment. The Lancet. 2015;2(3):258–27.

101. Kolyaskina GI, Brusov OS, Sekirina TP, Androsova LV, Kushner SG, Vasilyeva EF, Lavrov VF, Ebralidze LK, Burbayeva OA, Ya M, Tsutsulkovskaya, Kaleda VG, Barkhatova AN. (Moscow). Immune system in juvenile schizophrenia at the moment of the first disease manifestation. Siberian Bulletin of Psychiatry and Narcology. 2008;1:22–6. (In Russian.)
102. Vetlugina TP, Lobacheva AO, Naidenova NN, et al. Psychoneuroimmunomodulation in schizophrenia. Pathogenesis. 2006;4(1):42–3. (In Russian)
103. Mikhailova II, Orlova VA, Berezovskaya TP, Shavladze NZ, Minutko VL. MRI- parameters of brain abnormality in attack-like schizophrenia: new data with angiography using. http://vestnik.rncrr.ru/vestnik/v13/papers/michail_v13.htm) (In Russian.)
104. Mikhailova II, Orlova VA, Minutko MIN, Eliseeva NA. Relationship between clinical symptomatology and the level of serum antibodies to human herpesvirus in patients with different types of schizophrenia. Russian Psychiatric Journal. 2014;3:61–6. (In Russian)
105. Mikhailova II, Orlova VA, Minutko VL, Simonova AV, Pogodina EA. The relationship between the features of immunity and the clinical parameters of episodic paranoid schizophrenia. Norwegian J Dev Int Sci. 2019;34:19–27. (In Russian)
106. Mikhailova II, Orlova VA, Minutko VL, Simonova AV, Pogodina EA. Episodic paranoid schizophrenia as an infectious process (multidisciplinary study). Norwegian J Dev Int Sci. 2019;37:31–5. (In Russian).
107. Orlova VA, Gerasimova OV, Mikhailova II, Minutko VL, Gnezdickij VV. Correlation between the functional state of the central link of the auditory analyzer (according to cognitive EP data) and the level of serum antibodies to herpes viruses in schizophrenia. Social and Clinical Psychiatry. 2017;1:13–9. (In Russian)
108. Kolker IA. Auditory evoked potentials in neurology. Int Neurol J. 2006;6:10. http://www.mif-ua.com/archive/article_print/2343 (In Russian).
109. Bechter K, Reiber H, Herzog S, et al. Cerebrospinal fl uid analysis in affective and schizophrenic spectrum disorders: identification of subgroups with immune responses and blood-CSF barrier dysfunction. J Psychiatry Res. 2010;44:321–30.
110. Lee EE, Hong S, Martin AS, Eyler LT, Jeste DV. Inflammation in schizophrenia: cytokine levels and their relationships to demographic and clinical variables. Am J Geriatr Psychiatry. 2017;25(1):50–61. https://doi.org/10.1016/j.jagp.2016.09.009.
111. Orlova VA, Mikhaylova II, Minutko VL, Simonova AV, Pogodina EA. Anomalies in the levels of serum autoantibodies to antigens of nervous tissue in patients with schizoaffective psychosis: association with herpes viruses. Doctor RU Neurol Psychiatry. 2020;19(4):43–9. (in Russian)
112. Poletaev AB. Immunology and immunopathology. M.: MIA; 2008: 207 p. (in Russian).
113. Poletaev AB, Sherstnev VV. S100 proteins: overview of functional properties. Advances in Contemporary Biology. 1987;10(1):124–32. (in Russian)
114. Arumugam T, Simeone DM, Schmidt AM, Logsdon CD. S100P stimulates cell proliferation and survival via receptor for activated glycation end products (RAGE). J Biol Chem. 2004;279(7):5059–65. https://doi.org/10.1074/jbc.M310124200.
115. Sheng JG, Mrak RE, Griffin WST. Glial-neuronal interactions in Alzheimer disease: progressive association of IL-1α+ microglia and S100β+ astrocytes with neurofibrillary tangle stage. J Neuropath Exp Neurol. 1997;56(3):285–90.
116. Rasulova KA, Azizova RB. Natural neurotropic autoantibodies in blood serum of epilepsy patients. Ann Russian Acad Med Sci. 2014;5–6:111–5. (in Russian.)
117. Mikhaylova II, Orlova VA, Minutko VL, Simonova AV, Pogodina EA. Clinical significance of laboratory parameters of the erythrocyte level of peripheral blood in the acute period of schizoaffective psychosis. Soc Clin Psychiatry. 2018;2:39–44. (in Russian)
118. Teterina TP, Light, eye, brain. Principles of color therapy. Kaluga: "Oblizdat". 1998;1:216c. (in Russian). http://www.medsecret.net/ginekologiya/mochepolovye-infekcii/538-citomegalovirusnaja-infekcija.
119. Miskowiak K, Inkster B, Selvaraj S, Wise R, Goodwin GM, Harmer CJ. Erythropoietin improves mood and modulates the cognitive and neural processing of emotion 3 days post administration. Neuropsychopharmacology. 2007;33:611–8.
120. Lvov ND. Development of therapeutic antiherpetic drugs and diagnostic test systems: Author's abstract. diss. ... doct. honey. sciences. 1992. The original article was published on the RMJ website (Russian medical journal): https://www.rmj.ru/articles/dermatologiya/Gerpesvirusy_cheloveka__sistemnaya_integrativnayalimfoproliferativnaya_immunoonkopatologiya/#ixzz5BRm0gS5m. (in Russian).
121. Uranova N, Vikhreva O, Rachmanova V, Orlovskaya D. Ultrastructural alterations of myelinated fibers and oligodendrocytes in the prefrontal cortex in schizophrenia: a postmortem morphometric study. Schizophr Res Treat. 2011., Article ID;325789:13. https://doi.org/10.1155/2011/325789.
122. Porcellini E, Carbone I, et al. Alzheimer's disease gene signature says: beware of brain viral infections. Immun Ageing. 2010;14(7):16.
123. Konry S, Bondurant M, Konry M. Localization of erythropoietin synthesising cells in murine kidneys by in situ hybridization. Blood. 1988;71:524–7.
124. Tomilina NA, Bikbov BT. Chronic renal epidemiology insufficiency and new approaches to the classification and assessment of the severity of chronic progressive kidney disease. Therapeutic Archive. 2005;77(6):87–91. (In Russian)
125. Shilo VY, Khasabov NN. Anemia in chronic kidney disease. Therapist. 2008;1:25–31. (In Russian)

126. Maslov LN, Sazonova SI. Use of cytokines to stimulate neoangiogenesis and heart regeneration. Exp Clin Pharmacol. 2006;69(5):70–6. (In Russian)
127. Joyeux-Faure M. Cellular protection by erythropoietin: new therapeutic implications? J Pharmacol Exp Ther. 2007;323:759–62.
128. Kolesnik IM, Pokrovsky MV, Pokrovskaya TG, et al. Pharmacological preconditioning with erythropoietin in limb ischemia. Biomedicine. 2011;4:90–2. (In Russian)
129. Mikhailova II, Orlova VA, Minutko VL, Malysheva IN, Eliseeva NA. Relationships between clinical symptoms and the level of serum antibodies to herpes viruses in patients with different forms of schizophrenia. Russian Psychiatric J. 2014;3:61–6. (In Russian)
130. Orlova VA, Gerasimova OV, Mikhailova II, Minutko VL, Gnezditskiy VV. Correlations of the parameters of auditory EPs (long-latency, cognitive) with the level of serum antibodies to herpes viruses in schizophrenia. Magazine Evol Nat Sci. 2016;6:27–32. (In Russian)
131. Mikhailova II, Orlova VA, Minutko VL, Malisheva IN, Berezovskaya TP. The role of Herpes family viruses in the pathogenesis of paranoid schizophrenia: the data of multidimensional correlations of immunological, morphological and clinical characteristics. Int Neuropsychiatr Dis J. 2015;3(3):74–83.
132. Vainshaker YI, Ivchenko IM, Tsinzerling VA, Nuralova IV, Khlopunova OV, Berezina LA, Kulyashova LB, Vyazovaya AA, Kalinina OVV, Korotkov AD, Kataeva GV, Medvedev SV. Low-manifest infections with lesions of the central nervous system in patients with prolonged unconsciousness of non-inflammatory etiology. J Microbiol Epidemiol Immunobiol (ZhMEI). 2011;6:85–9.
133. Yolken RH, Bachmann S, Ruslanova I, Lillehoj E, Ford G, Torrey EF, Schroeder J, Rouslanova I. Antibodies to Toxoplasma gondii in individuals with first-episode schizophrenia. Clin Infect Dis. 2001;32:842–4.
134. Chaudhury A, Ramana BV. Schizophrenia and bipolar disorders: The Toxoplasma connection. Trop Parasitol. 2019;9(2):71–6. https://doi.org/10.4103/tp.TP_28_19.
135. Diagnostics by the GLC method (in Russian) http://www.labtechperm.ru/articles/636.
136. Severance EG, Yolken RH. From infection to the microbiome: an evolving role of microbes in schizophrenia. Version 2. Curr Top Behav Neurosci. 2020;44:67–84. https://doi.org/10.1007/7854_2018_84.
137. Cryan JF, Dinan TG. Talking about a microbiome revolution. Nat Microbiol. 2019;4(4):552. https://doi.org/10.1038/s41564-019-0422-9.
138. Valles-Colomer M, Falony G, Darzi Y, Tigchelaar EF, Wang J, Tito RY, Schiweck C, Kurilshikov A, Joossens M, Wijmenga C, Claes S, Van Oudenhove L, Zhernakova A, Vieira-Silva S, Raes J. The neuroactive potential of the human gut microbiota in quality of life and depression. Nat Microbiol. 2019;4(4):623–32. https://doi.org/10.1038/s41564-018-0337-x.
139. Mangalam A, Shahi SK, Luckey D, Ma K, Marietta E, et al. Human gut-derived commensal bacteria suppress CNS inflammatory and demyelinating disease. Cell Rep. 2017;20:1269–77. https://doi.org/10.1016/j.celrep.2017.07.031.
140. Cryan JF, Dinan TG. Mind-altering microorganisms: The impact of the gut microbiota on brain and behaviour. Nat Rev Neurosci. 2012;13:701–12. https://doi.org/10.1038/nrn3346.
141. Hsiao EY, McBride SW, Hsien S, Sharon G, Hyde ER, et al. Microbiota modulate behavioral and physiological abnormalities associated with neurodevelopmental disorders. Cell. 2013;155:1451–63. https://doi.org/10.1016/j.cell.2013.11.024.
142. Kanji S, Fonseka TM, Marshe VS, Sriretnakumar V, Hahn MK, Müller DJ. The microbiome-gut-brain axis: implications for schizophrenia and antipsychotic induced weight gain.Eur Arch Psychiatry. Clin Neurosci. 2018;268(1):3–15. https://doi.org/10.1007/s00406-017-0820-z.
143. De Paepe M, Leclerc M, Tinsley CR, Petit MA. Bacteriophages: an underestimated role in human and animal health? Front Cell Infect Microbiol. 2014;4:39. https://doi.org/10.3389/fcimb.2014.00039.
144. Yolken RH, Severance EG, Sabunciyan S, Gressitt KL, Chen O, Stallings C, Origoni A, Katsafanas E, Schweinfurth LA, Savage CL, Banis M, Khushalani S, Dickerson FB. Metagenomic sequencing indicates that the oropharyngeal phageome of individuals with schizophrenia differs from that of controls. Schizophr Bull. 2015;41(5):1153–61. https://doi.org/10.1093/schbul/sbu197.
145. Beketova GV, Savichuk NO. Virom of man and its role in the formation of diseases. Herpetic infection in children: modern approaches to therapy. Pediatr Eastern Europe. 2016;1:47–62. (In Russian)
146. Simonova AV, Mikhailova II, Orlova VA. An innovative interdisciplinary approach to the management of patients with psychoemotional disorders. Norwegian J development of the International Science. 2020;49:15–8. (In Russian)
147. Dickerson F, Severance E, Yolken R. The microbiome, immunity, and schizophrenia and bipolar disorder. Brain Behav Immun. 2017;62:46–52. https://doi.org/10.1016/j.bbi.2016.12.010.
148. Shen Y, Xu J, Li Z, Huang Y, Yuan Y, Wang J, Zhang M, Hu S, Liang Y. Analysis of gut microbiota diversity and auxiliary diagnosis as a biomarker in patients with schizophrenia: A cross-sectional study. Schizophr Res. 2018;197:470–7. https://doi.org/10.1016/j.schres.2018.01.002.
149. Nguyen TT, Kosciolek T, Eyler LT, Knight R, Jeste DV. Overview and Systematic Review of Studies of Microbiome in Schizophrenia and Bipolar Disorder. J Psychiatr Res. 2018;99:50–61. https://doi.org/10.1016/j.jpsychires.2018.01.013.

150. Zheng P, Zeng B, Liu M, Chen J, Pan J, et al. The gut microbiome from patients with schizophrenia modulates the glutamate-glutamine-GABA cycle and schizophrenia-relevant behaviors in mice. Science Advances. 2019;5(2):8317. https://doi.org/10.1126/sciadv.aau8317.
151. Zhu F, Ju Y, Wang W, Wang Q, Guo R, et al. Metagenome-wide association of gut microbiome features for schizophrenia. Nat Commun. 2020;11(1):1612. https://doi.org/10.1038/s41467-020-15457-9.
152. Nguyen TT, Kosciolek T, Maldonado Y, Daly RE, Martin AS, Mc Donald D, Knight R, Jeste DV. Differences in gut microbiome composition between persons with chronic schizophrenia and healthy comparison subjects. Schizophr Res. 2019;204:23–9. https://doi.org/10.1016/j.schres.2018.09.014.
153. Ma X, Asif H, Dai L, He Y, Zheng W, Wang D, Ren H, Tang J, Li C, Jin K, Li Z, Chen X. Alteration of the gut microbiome in first-episode drug-naïve and chronic medicated schizophrenia correlate with regional brain volumes. J Psychiatr Res. 2020;123:136–44. https://doi.org/10.1016/j.jpsychires.2020.02.005.
154. Macedo E, Cordeiro T, Zhang X, Graubics K, Colwell R, Teixeira AL. Microbiome and Schizophrenia: current evidence and future challenges. Curr Behav Neurosci Rep. 2020;7:51–61. https://doi.org/10.1007/s40473-020-00206-5.
155. Uranova NA, Kolomeets NS, Vikhreva OV, Zimina IS, Rakhmanova VI, Orlovskaya DD. Ultrastructural changes in myelin fibers in the brain with continuous and paroxysmal paranoid schizophrenia. J Neurol Psychiat S.S. Korsakov. 2017;117(2):104–9. https://doi.org/10.17116/jnevro201711721104-109. (In Russian)
156. Yushchuk N. D., Dekonenko E. P., Fedoseenko G. I., Klimova E. A. Herpetic neuroinfections. Ministry of Health of the Russian Federation, State Educational Institution All-Russian Educational-Scientific-Mertodic Center for Continuing Medical and Pharmaceutical Education. M., 2003; 31 p. (In Russian).
157. Kolomeets NS, Uranova NA. Modern ideas about the reactivity of astrocytes in schizophrenia. J. Neuropathol Psychiatr. 2014;114(5):92–9. (In Russian)
158. Kolomeets NS, Uranova NA. Ultrastructural abnormalities of astrocytes in the hippocampus in schizophrenia and duration of illness: a postmortem morphometric study. World J Biol Psychiatry. 2010;11:282–92.
159. Vostrikov V, Orlovskaya D, Uranova N. Deficit of pericapillary oligodendrocytes in the prefrontal cortex in schizophrenia. The World Journal of Biological Psychiatry. 2008;9(1):34–42. https://doi.org/10.3109/15622970903414188.
160. Uranova NA, Zimina IS, Vikhreva OV, Krukov NO, Rachmanova VI, Orlovskaya DD. Ultrastructural damage of capillaries in the neocortex in schizophrenia. World J Biol Psychiatry. 2010;11:567–78.
161. Vostrikov VM., Oifa A. I. Paramyxoviruses in the brain in febrile schizophrenia viruses, immunity, and mental disorders: 157–160.
162. Gordon L, McQuaid S, Cosby SL. Detection of herpes simplex virus (types 1 and 2) and human herpesvirus 6 DNA in human brain tissue by polymerase chain reaction. Clin Diagn Virol. 1996;6:33–40.
163. Moises HW, Ruger R, Reynolds GP, Fleckenstein B. Human cytomegalovirus DNA in the temporal cortex of a schizophrenic patient. Eur Arch Psychiatry Neurol Sci. 1988;238:110–3.
164. Tomasik J, Smits SL, Leweke FV, Eljasz PE, Pas S, Kahn RS, Osterhaus ADME, Sabine BS, Witte LD. Virus discovery analyses on post-mortem brain tissue and cerebrospinal fluid of schizophrenia patients. Schizophr Res. 2018;197:605–6. https://doi.org/10.1016/j.schres.2018.02.012.
165. Weis S, Llenos IC, Sabunciyan S, Dulay JR, Isler L, Yolken R, Perron H. Reduced expression of human endogenous retrovirus (HERV)-W GAG protein in the cingulate gyrus and hippocampus in schizophrenia, bipolar disorder, and depression. J Neural Transm (Vienna). 2007;114(5):645–55. https://doi.org/10.1007/s00702-006-0599-y.
166. Li F, Sarven S, Robert HY, Doheon L, Kim S, Hakan K. Transcription of human endogenous retroviruses in human brain by RNA-seq analysis. 2019;3, 14(1):e0207353. https://doi.org/10.1371/journal.pone.0207353. eCollection 2019
167. Dickerson FB, Boronow JJ, Stallings CR, Origoni AE, Yolken RH. Reduction of symptoms by valacyclovir in cytomegalovirus-seropositive individuals with schizophrenia. Am J Psychiatry. 2003;160:2234–6. https://doi.org/10.1176/appi.ajp.160.12.2234.
168. Fond GB, Lagier JC, Honore S, Lancon C, Korchia T, Verville PS, Llorca PM, Auquier P, Guedj E, Boyer L. Microbiota-orientated treatments for major depression and schizophrenia. Nutrients. 2020;12(4):1024. https://doi.org/10.3390/nu12041024.
169. Osipov G. Invisible organ—human microflora. Russian medical server. (In Russian). http://www.rusmedserv.com/microbdiag/invisibleorgan.htm
170. Poletaev A. Autoantibodies: serum content or profiles? In: Poletaev AB, editor. Physiologic autoimmunity and preventive medicine. Sharjah, Oak Park, Bussum: Bentham Science Publishers; 2013. p. 199–207.
171. Torrey EF, Yolken RH. Schizophrenia as a pseudogenetic disease: a call for more gene-тenvironmental studies. Psychiatry Res. 2019;278:146–50. https://doi.org/10.1016/j.psychres.2019.06.006.
172. Levkovitz Y, Mendlovich S, Riwkes S, et al. A double-blind, randomized study of minocycline for the treatment of negative and cognitive symptoms in ealy-phase schizophrenia. Journal of Clinical Psychiatry. 2010;71:138–49.

173. Miyaoka T, Yasukawa R, Yasuda H, et al. Minocycline as adjunctive therapy for schizophrenia: an open-label study. Clinical Neuropharmacology. 2008;31:287–92.
174. World failing to address dementia challenge. https://www.who.int/news/item/02-09-2021-world-failing--to-address-dementia-challenge.
175. Gauthier S., Rosa-Neto P., Morais J. A., Webster C. World Alzheimer Report 2021 Journey through the diagnosis of dementia. London: Alzheimer's Disease International, 2021. 314. https://www.alzint.org/u/World-Alzheimer-Report-2021.pdf
176. Livingston G, Sommerlad A, Orgeta V, et al. Dementia prevention, intervention and care. The Lancet. 2017;390(10113):2673–734.
177. Prince M, Bryce R, Albanese E, et al. The global prevalence of dementia: a systematic review and meta-analysis. Alzheimers Dement. 2013;9:63–75.
178. Danysz W, Parsons CG, Quack G. NMDA channel blockers: memantine and amino–alkylcyclohexanes—in vitro characterisation. Amino Acids. 2000;19:167–72. https://pubmed.ncbi.nlm.nih.gov/11026485/
179. Preobrazhenskaya IS. Diagnosis and treatment of Alzheimer's disease. Neurology, neuropsychiatry, psychosomatics. 2012;4(2S):5–10. https://doi.org/10.14412/2074-2711-2012-2502. (In Russian)
180. Akshulakov SK, Takenov ZT, Karibai SD. Alzheimer's disease, pathomorphology, clinical manifestations and modern treatment. J Neurosurg Neurol Kazakhstan. 2015;2(39):26–33. (In Russian)
181. Brookmeyer R, Johnson E, Ziegler-Graham K, Arrighi HM. Forecasting the global burden of Alzheimer's disease. Alzheimers Dement. 2007;3(3):186–91. https://doi.org/10.1016/j.jalz.2007.04.381.
182. WHO reveals leading causes of death and disability worldwide: 2000-2019. https://www.who.int/ru/news/item/09-12-2020-who-reveals-leading-causes-of-death-and-disability-worldwide-2000-2019
183. The top 10 causes of death. https://www.who.int/ru/news-room/fact-sheets/detail/the-top-10-causes-of-death.
184. Zhang XX, Tian Y, Wang ZT, et al. The epidemiology of Alzheimer's disease modifiable risk factors and prevention. J Prev Alzheimers Dis. 2021;8:313–21. https://doi.org/10.14283/jpad.2021.15.
185. Geula C, Mesulam MM. Cholinesterases and the pathology of Alzheimer disease. Alzheimer Dis Assoc Disord. 1995;2:23–8. https://doi.org/10.1097/00002093-199501002-00005.
186. Braak H, Braak E. Evolution of the neuropathology of Alzheimer's disease. Acta Neurol Scand. 1996;S165:3–12. https://doi.org/10.1111/j.1600-0404.1996.tb05866.x.
187. Yanagisawa K, Ihara Y, Miyatake T. Secretory pathway of beta/A4 amyloid protein precursor in familial Alzheimer's disease with Val717 to Ile mutation. Neurosci Lett. 1992;144(1-2):43–5. https://doi.org/10.1016/0304-3940(92)90711-f.
188. Morley JE, Armbrecht HJ, Farr SA, Kumar VB. The senescence accelerated mouse (SAMP8) as a model for oxidative stress and Alzheimer's disease. Biochim Biophys Acta. 2012;1822(5):650–6. https://doi.org/10.1016/j.bbadis.2011.11.015.
189. Iqbal K, Alonso-Adel C, Chen S, et al. Tau pathology in Alzheimer disease and other tauopathies. Biochim Biophys Acta. 2005;1739(2-3):198–210. https://doi.org/10.1016/j.bbadis.2004.09.008.
190. Johnson GV, Bailey CD. Tau, where are we now? J Alzheimers Dis. 2002;4:375–98.
191. Alvarez XA, Ruether E, Moessler H. Efficacy of cerebrolysin in moderate to moderately severe Alzheimer's disease. In: Research and practice in Alzheimer's disease, vol. 5. Paris: Serdi Publishing; 2009. p. 179–86. Springer Publishing Company (NY); https://pubmed.ncbi.nlm.nih.gov/20500802/.
192. Chun W, Johnson GV. The role of tau phosphorylation and cleavage in neuronal cell death. Front Biosci. 2007;12:733–56.
193. Maltsev AV, Dovidchenko NV, Uteshev VK, et al. Intensive protein synthesis in neurons and phosphorylation of beta-amyloid precursor protein and tau protein are triggering factors of neuronal amyloidosis and Alzheimer's disease. Biomed Chem. 2013;59(2):144–70. (In Russian)
194. Dolev I, Michaelson DM. A nontransgenic mouse model shows inducible amyloid–b (Ab) peptide deposition and elucidates the role of apolipoprotein E in the amyloid cascade. Neuroscience. 2004;10(38):13909–14. https://pubmed.ncbi.nlm.nih.gov/15365176/.
195. Lyketsos CG, Breitner JC. Mental and behavioral disturbances in dementia: findeigs from the cache county study on memory in aging. In: Research and practice in Alzheimer's disease, vol. 5. Paris: Serdi Publishing. Springer Publishing Company (NY); 2001. p. 144–50. https://pubmed.ncbi.nlm.nih.gov/10784462/.
196. Lannfelt L, Basun H, Vigo-Pelfrey C, et al. Amyloid β-peptide in cerebrospinal fluid in individuals with the Swedish Alzheimer amyloid precursor protein mutation. Neurosci Lett. 1999;199(3):203–6. https://doi.org/10.1016/0304-3940(95)12059-D.
197. Lannfelt L, Basun H, Wahlund LO, et al. Decreased alpha-secretase-cleaved amyloid precursor protein as a diagnostic marker for Alzheimer's disease. Nat Med. 1995;1(8):829–32.
198. Lehtimaki T, Pirttila T, Mehta PD, et al. Apolipoprotein E (apoE) polymorphism and its influence on ApoE concentrations in the cerebrospinal fluid in Finnish patients with Alzheimer's disease. Hum Genet. 1995;5(1):39–42.
199. Williams KR, Pye V, Saunders AM, et al. Apolipoprotein E uptake and low–density lipoprotein receptor–related protein expression by the NTera2/ D1 cell line: a cell culture model of relevance for late–onset Alzheimer's disease. Neurobiol Dis. 1997;4(1):58–67.

200. Masse I, Bordet R, Deplanque D, et al. Lipid lowering agents are associated with a slower cognitive decline in Alzheimer's disease. J Neurol Neurosurg Psychiatry. 2005;76:1624–9. https://pubmed.ncbi.nlm.nih.gov/16291883/
201. Southwick PC, Yamagata SK, Echols CL, et al. Assessment of amyloid β-protein in cerebrospinal fluid as an aid in the diagnosis of Alzheimer's disease. J Neurochem. 1996;66(1):259–65. https://doi.org/10.1046/j.1471-4159.1996.66010259.x.
202. Yamada M, Sodeyama N, Itoh Y, et al. Association of neprilysin polymorphism with cerebral amyloid angiopathy. J Neurol Neurosurg Psychiatry. 2003;74:749–51. https://jnnp.bmj.com/content/74/6/749.
203. Yue X, Lu M, Lancaster T, et al. Brain estrogen deficiency accelerates A plaque formation in an Alzheimer's disease animal model. Neuroscience. 2005;102(52):19198–203. https://pubmed.ncbi.nlm.nih.gov/16365303/
204. Akiyama H, Barger S, Barnum S, et al. Inflammation and Alzheimerrs Disease. Neurobiol Aging. 2000;21(3):383–421.
205. Sochocka M, Zwolińska K, Leszek J. The infectious etiology of Alzheimer's disease. Curr Neuropharmacol. 2017;15:996–1009. https://pubmed.ncbi.nlm.nih.gov/28294067/
206. Vainshenker YI, Nuralova IV, Onishchenko LS. Chlamydia of the central nervous system. Laboratory diagnostics and clinical and morphological features. Pathol Archive. 2014;76(1):57–62.
207. Balin BJ, Appelt DM. The role of infection in Alzheimer's disease. J Am Osteopathic Assoc. 2001;101(12, S1):S1–6.
208. Hammond CJ, Hallock LR, Howanski RJ, et al. Immunohistological detection of Chlamydia pneumoniae in the Alzheimer's disease brain. BMC Neurosci. 2010;11:121.
209. Balin BJ, Gérard HC, Arking EJ, et al. Identification and localization of Chlamydia pneumoniae in the Alzheimer's brain. Med Microbiol Immunol. 1998;187(1):23–42.
210. Gérard HC, Dreses-Werringloer U, Wildt KS, et al. Chlamydophila (Chlamydia) pneumoniae in the Alzheimer's brain. FEMS Immunol Med Microbiol. 2006;48(3):355–66.
211. Dreses-Werringloer U, Bhuiyan M, Zhao Y, et al. Initial characterization of Chlamydophila (Chlamydia) pneumoniae cultured from the late-onset Alzheimer brain. Int J Med Microbiol. 2009;299(3):187–201.
212. Little CS, Hammond CJ, MacIntyre A, et al. Chlamydia pneumoniae induces Alzheimer-like amyloid plaques in brains of BALB/c mice. Neurobiol Aging. 2004;25(4):419–29.
213. Loeb MB, Molloy DW, Smieja M, et al. A randomized, controlled trial of doxycycline and rifampin for patients with Alzheimer's disease. J Am Geriatr Soc. 2004;52(3):381–7.
214. Itzhaki RF. Corroboration of a major role for herpes simplex virus type 1 in Alzheimer's Disease. Front Aging Neurosci. 2018;10:324. https://doi.org/10.3389/fnagi.2018.00324.
215. Cairns DM, Rouleau N, Parker RN, et al. A 3D human brain-like tissue model of herpes-induced Alzheimer's disease. Sci Adv. 2020;6(19):8828. https://doi.org/10.1126/sciadv.aay8828.
216. Belodurina AD, Muginova RF. The infectious and inflammatory nature of Alzheimer's Disease. Bulletin of the Council of Young Scientists and Specialists of the Chelyabinsk region. 2019;3(26):70–4. (In Russian)
217. Al-Obaidi M, Desa M. Mechanisms of blood brain barrier disruption by different types of bacteria, and bacterial-host interactions facilitate the bacterial pathogen invading the brain. Cell Mol Neurobiol. 2018;38:1349–68. https://pubmed.ncbi.nlm.nih.gov/30117097/
218. Cao W, Zheng H. Peripheral immune system in aging and Alzheimer's disease. Mol Neurodegener. 2018;13:51. https://pubmed.ncbi.nlm.nih.gov/30285785/
219. White MR, Kandel R, Tripathi S, et al. Alzheimer's associated β-amyloid protein inhibits influenza A virus and modulates viral interactions with phagocytes. PLoS One. 2014;9(7):e101364. https://doi.org/10.1371/journal.pone.0101364.
220. Khavkina DA, Ruzhentsova TA, Chukhliaev PV. The role of infectious agents in the genesis of atherosclerosis. Academy of Medicine and Sports. 2020;1(1):22–6. https://doi.org/10.15829/2712-7567-2020-1-22-26.
221. Lurain NS, Hanson BA, Martinson J, et al. Virological and immunological characteristics of human cytomegalovirus infection associated with Alzheimer disease. J Infect Dis. 2013;208(4):564–72. https://doi.org/10.1093/infdis/jit210.
222. Barnes LL, Capuano AW, Aiello AE, et al. Cytomegalovirus infection and risk of Alzheimer disease in older black and white individuals. J Infect Dis. 2015;211:230–7.
223. Katan M, Moon YP, Paik MC, et al. Infectious burden and cognitive function: The Northern Manhattan Study. Neurology. 2013;80:1209–15.
224. Aiello AE, Haan M, Blythe L, et al. The influence of latent viral infection on rate of cognitive decline over 4 years. J Am Geriatr Soc. 2006;54:1046–54.
225. Carbone I, Lazzarotto T, Ianni M, et al. Herpes virus in Alzheimer's disease: relation to progression of the disease. Neurobiol Aging. 2014;35:122–9.
226. Lin WR, Wozniak MA, Cooper RJ, et al. Herpesviruses in brain and Alzheimer's disease. J Pathol. 2002;197:395–402.
227. Agostini S, Mancuso R, Baglio F, et al. Lack of evidence for a role of HHV-6 in the pathogenesis of Alzheimer's disease. J Alzheimers Dis. 2015;49:229–35.
228. Beydoun MA, Beydoun HA, Shroff MR, et al. Helicobacter pylori seropositivity and cognitive performance among US adults: evidence from a large national survey. Psychosom Med. 2013;75:486–96.

229. Bu XL, Yao XQ, Jiao SS, et al. A study on the association between infectious burden and Alzheimer's disease. Eur J Neurol. 2015;22:1519–22.
230. Roubaud-Baudron C, Krolak-Salmon P, Quadrio I, et al. Impact of chronic Helicobacter pylori infection on Alzheimer's disease: preliminary results. Neurobiol Aging. 2012;33(1009):11–9.
231. Wang XL, Zeng J, Yang Y, et al. Helicobacter pylori filtrate induces Alzheimer-like tau hyperphosphorylation by activating glycogen synthase kinase-3β. J Alzheimers Dis. 2015;43:153–65.
232. Boziki M, Polyzos SA, Deretzi G, et al. A potential impact of Helicobacter pylori-related galectin-3 in neurodegeneration. Neurochem Int. 2017;113:137–51.
233. Deller T, Frotscher M, Nitsch R. Sprouting of crossed entorhinodentate fibers after a unilateral entorhinal lesion: anterograde tracing of fiber reorganization with phaseolus vulgaris-leucoagglutinin (PHAL). J Comp Neurol. 1996;365(1):42–55. https://doi.org/10.1002/(SICI)1096-9861(19960129)365:1<42::AID-CNE4>3.0.CO;2-J.
234. Bertoni-Freddari C, Fattoretti P, Paoloni R, et al. Cerebrovascular pathology in Alzheimer's disease. Ann NY Acad Sci. 1997;826:479–82.
235. Jorm AF. Depression as a risk factor for dementia. In: Research and practice in Alzheimer's disease, vol. 5. Paris: Serdi Publishing. Springer Publishing Company (NY); 2001. p. 139–43. https://pubmed.ncbi.nlm.nih.gov/23906002/.
236. Koberskaya NN, Kovalchuk NA. Alzheimer's disease with early onset. Medical Advice. 2019;1:10–6. https://doi.org/10.21518/2079-701X-2019-1-10-16. (In Russian)
237. Maat-Schieman ML, Rozemuller AJ, van Duinen SG, et al. Microglia in diffuse plaques in hereditary cerebral hemorrhage with amyloidosis. An immunohistochemical study. J Neuropathol Exp Neurol. 1994;53(5):483–91. https://pubmed.ncbi.nlm.nih.gov/7521904/ (In Dutch)
238. Naumenko AA, Gromova DO, Trofimova NV, Preobrazhenskaya IS. Diagnosis and treatment of Alzheimer's disease. Neurol Neuropsychiatry Psychosom. 2016;8(4):91–7. (In Russian)
239. Scahill RI, Schott JM, Stevens JM, et al. Mapping the evolution of regional atrophy in Alzheimer's disease: Unbiased analysis of fluidregistered serial MRI. Proc Natl Acad Sci USA. 2002;99(7):4703–7. https://pubmed.ncbi.nlm.nih.gov/11930016/
240. Chan D, Fox NC, Scahill RI, et al. Patterns of temporal lobe atrophy in semantic dementia and Alzheimer's disease. Ann Neurol. 2001;49(4):433–42. https://pubmed.ncbi.nlm.nih.gov/11310620/
241. Dickerson BC, Goncharova II, Sullivan MP, et al. MRI-derived entorhinal and hippocampal atrophy in incipient and very mild Alzheimer's disease. Neurobiol Aging. 2001;22(5):747–54. https://pubmed.ncbi.nlm.nih.gov/11705634/
242. Jack CR, Knopman DS, Jagust WJ, et al. Hypothetical model of dynamic biomarkers of the Alzheimer's pathological cascade. Lancet Neurol. 2010;9(1):119–28. https://pubmed.ncbi.nlm.nih.gov/20083042/
243. Ksiezak-Reding H, Tracz E, Yang LS, et al. Ultrastructural instability of paired helical filaments from corticobasal degeneration as examined by scanning transmission electron microscopy. Am J Pathol. 2001;149(2):639–51. https://pubmed.ncbi.nlm.nih.gov/8702002/
244. Wilkinson D. Drugs for treatment of Alzheimer's disease. Int J Clin Pract. 2008;55(2):129–34.
245. Jones MW, McClean M, Parsons CG, et al. The in vivo relevance of the varied channel–blocking properties of uncompetitive NMDA antagonists: tests on spinal neurones. Neuropharmacology. 2008;41(1):50–61. https://www.semanticscholar.org/paper/The-in-vivo-relevance-of-the-varied-properties-of-Jones-McClean/7639d0c060d136ca6dc53d760b11e4dfeda5a8f5
246. Love S. Contribution of cerebral amyloid angiopathy to Alzheimer's disease. J Neurol Neurosurg Psychiatry. 2004;75:1–4. https://jnnp.bmj.com/content/75/1/1.2
247. Grossberg GT, Manes F, Allegri RF, et al. The safety, tolerability, and efficacy of once-daily memantine (28 mg): a multinational, randomized, double-blind, placebo-controlled trial in patients with moderate-to-severe Alzheimer's disease taking cholinesterase inhibitors. CNS Drugs. 2013;27(6):469–78. https://doi.org/10.1007/s40263-013-0077-7. https://pubmed.ncbi.nlm.nih.gov/23733403/
248. Bassil N, Thaipisuttikul P, Grossberg GT, Memantine ER. A once-daily formulation for the treatment of Alzheimer's disease. Expert Opin Pharmacother. 2010;11(10):1765–71. https://doi.org/10.1517/14656566.2010.493874. https://pubmed.ncbi.nlm.nih.gov/23733403/
249. Shao ZQ. Comparison of the efficacy of four cholinesterase inhibitors in combination with memantine for the treatment of Alzheimer's disease. Int J Clin Exp Med. 2015;8(2):2944–8. https://pubmed.ncbi.nlm.nih.gov/25932260/
250. Eckel RH, Jakicic JM, Ard JD, et al. 2013 AHA/ACC guideline on lifestyle management to reduce cardiovascular risk: a report of the American College of Cardiology. American Heart Association Task Force on Practice Guidelines. J Am Coll Cardiol. 2014;63:2960–84.
251. Jie Z, Xia H, Zhong SL, et al. The gut microbiome in atherosclerotic cardiovascular disease. Nat Commun. 2017;8:845.
252. Grose C. Biological plausibility of a link between arterial ischemic stroke and infection with Varicella-Zoster virus or Herpes Simplex virus. Circulation. 2016;133(8):695–7. https://doi.org/10.1161/circulationaha.116.021459.
253. Gozd-Barszczewska A, Koziol-Montewka M, Barszczewski P, et al. Gut microbiome as a biomarker of cardiometabolic disorders. Ann Agric Environ Med. 2017;24:416–22.

254. Zinserling WD. Untersuchungen über Atherosklerose. Über die Aorta Verfettung bei Kindern Virchow's Archiv. 1924. S: 678–705.
255. Alieva SZ, Maksudova MH. Modern ideas about etiopathogenetic mechanisms of myocardial infarction in young people. Avicenna. 2019;40:19–24. (In Russian)
256. Sacco RL, Kasner SE, Broderick JP, et al. An updated definition of stroke for the 21st century: a statement for healthcare professionals from the American Heart Association/American Stroke Association. Stroke. 2013;44:2064–89.
257. Montanaro VV, Freitas DD, Ruiz MC, et al. Ischemic stroke in young adults: Profile of SARAH Hospital Brasília from 2008 to 2012. Neurologist. 2017;22(2):61–3. https://doi.org/10.1097/NRL.0000000000000110.
258. Nikitskaya EA, Maryukhnich EV, Savvinova PP, et al. Human herpes viruses and atherosclerosis. A modern look. Creat Cardiol. 2015;2:54–61. (In Russian)
259. Evsevyeva ME, Eremin MV, Italiceva EV, et al. Foci of chronic infection and vascular rigidity in persons of military age. Bull Russian Military Med Acad. 2018;1(61):149–53. (In Russian)
260. Alekseeva Ya V, Rebenkova MS, Gombozhapova AE, et al. Detection of cardiotropic viral antigens in atherosclerotic plaques of coronary arteries in patients with fatal myocardial infarction. Cardiology. 2019;59(7):38–43. (In Russian)
261. Nagarajan UM, Sikes JD, Burris RL, et al. Genital Chlamydia infection in hyperlipidemic mouse models exacerbates atherosclerosis. Atherosclerosis. 2019;290:103–10. https://doi.org/10.1016/j.atherosclerosis.2019.09.021.
262. Liu Z, Li J, Liu H, et al. The intestinal microbiota associated with cardiac valve calcification differs from that of coronary artery disease. Atherosclerosis. 2019;284:121–8. https://doi.org/10.1016/j.atherosclerosis.2018.11.038.
263. Tuomisto S, Huhtala H, Martiskainen M, et al. Age-dependent association of gut bacteria with coronary atherosclerosis: Tampere Sudden Death Study. PLoS One. 2019;14(8):e0221345. https://doi.org/10.1371/journal.pone.0221345.
264. Vos T, Lim SS, Abbafati C, Abbas KM, Abbasi M. Global burden of 369 diseases and injuries in 204 countries and territories, 1990–2019: a systematic analysis for the Global Burden of Disease Study 2019. The Lancet. 2020;396(10258):1204–22. https://doi.org/10.1016/S0140-6736(20)30925-9.
265. Steiner TJ, Stovner LJ, Jensen R, Uluduz D, Katsarava Z. Migraine remains second among the world's causes of disability, and first among young women: findings from GBD 2019. The Journal of Headache and Pain. 2020. Published online 2020 Dec 2;21:137. https://doi.org/10.1186/s10194-020-01208-0.
266. Ryvlin P, Skorobogatykh K, Negro A, Sanchez-De La Rosa R, Israel-Willner H, Sundal C, Mac Gregor EA, Guerrero AL. Current clinical practice in disabling and chronic migraine in the primary care setting: results from the European My-LIFE anamnesis. BMC Neurol. 2021;21(1):1. https://doi.org/10.1186/s12883-020-02014-6.
267. Hemert S, Breedveld AC, Rovers JMP, Vermeiden JPV, Witteman BJM, Marcel GS, Nicole M. Migraine associated with gastrointestinal disorders: review of the literature and clinical implications. Front Neurol. 2014; https://doi.org/10.3389/fneur.2014.00241.
268. Mehle ME. Sinus headache, migraine, and the otolaryngologist a comprehensive clinical guide; 2017. Chapter 1, pages 3-5. Springer International Publishing AG 2017. Doi https://doi.org/10.1007/978-3-319-50376-9_1
269. Patel ZM, Kennedy DW, Setzen M, Poetker DM, John MDG. "Sinus headache": rhinogenic headache or migraine? An evidence-based guide to diagnosis and treatment 05 November; 2012
270. Proctor DM, Relman DA. The landscape ecology and microbiota of the human nose, mouth, and throat. Cell Host Microbe. 2017;21(4):421–32. https://doi.org/10.1016/j.chom.2017.03.011.
271. Oiconomidi T, Vikelis M, Artemiadis A, Chrousos GP, Darviri C. Reliability and validity of the Greek Migraine Disability Assessment (MIDAS). Questionnaire PharmacoEconomics. 2018;2: 77–85.
272. Osipov GA. Determination of the composition and number of microorganisms of the intestinal wall by chromatography-mass spectrometry of cellular fatty acids. Bull Russian Acad Med Sci. 1999;16(7):25–31. Exp and klin gastroenterology No. 4 pp. 59-67; 2003. (In Russian)
273. Osipov GA. Method for determining the generic (species) composition of the association of microorganisms. //Russian Patent No. 2086642. C12N 1/00, 1/20, C12Q 1/4. Priority from 24 Dec. 1993. (In Russian).
274. Osipov GA, Shabanova EA, Nedorezova TP, Istratov VG, Sergeeva TI. Method of diagnosis of clostridial anaerobic gas infection. Patent of the Russian Federation No. 2021608 cl. G01N 33/50. - Registered in the state register on 15.10.94. - Byul. No19. (In Russian).
275. Osipov G.A., Beloborodova N. V. Patent for invention No. 2146368 "Method for detecting the causative agent of an infectious process in sterile biological environments of a macroorganism", The patent was registered in the State Register of Inventions of the Russian Federation on 10.03.2000. (In Russian).
276. R: The main R command: a language and environment for statistical computing. R Foundation for Statistical Computing, Vienna, Austria. URL Address https://www.R-project.org/); 2021.
277. Arberas C, Ruggieri V. Autism. Genetic and biological aspects. Medicina (B Aires). 2019;79(S1):16–21.
278. Bhandari R, Paliwal JK, Kuhad A. Neuropsychopathology of Autism spectrum disorder: complex interplay of genetic, epigen-

etic, and environmental factors. Adv Neurobiol. 2020;24:97–141.
279. Sealey LA, Hughes BW, Sriskanda AN, et al. Environmental factors in the development of autism spectrum disorders. Review. Environ Int. 2016;88:288–98.
280. Blagonravova AS, Zhilyaeva TV, Kvashnina DV. Gut microbiota disorders in autism spectrum disorders: new horizons in the search for pathogenetic approaches to therapy. Part 1. Features of the gut microbiota in autism spectrum disorders. J Microbiol Epidemiol Immunobiol. 2021;98:1. https://doi.org/10.36233/0372-9311-62. (In Russian)
281. Langley JN. Connessions of the enteric nerve cells. J Physiol (London). 1922;56:39.
282. Gershon M. The enteric nervous system: a second brain. Hosp Pract (Minneap). 1999;34(7):31–2. 35–38, 41–42
283. Damasio A. The feeling of what happens: body and emotion in the making of consciousness. New York: Harcourt Brace; 1999. p. 365. https://doi.org/10.5860/choice.37-6553.
284. Niesler B, Kuerten S, Demir IE, et al. Disorders of the enteric nervous system—a holistic view. Nat Rev Gastroenterol Hepatol. 2021;18:393–410. https://doi.org/10.1038/s41575-020-00385-2.
285. Lyte M, Varcoe JJ, Bailey MT. Anxiogenic effect of subclinical bacterial infection in mice in the absence of overt immune activation. Physiol Behav. 1998;65(1):63–8.
286. Gaykema RP, Goehler LE, Lyte M. Brain response to cecal infection with Campylobacter jejuni: analysis with fos immunohistochemistry. Brain Behav Immun. 2004;18(3):238–45.
287. Goehler LE, Gaykema RP, Opitz N, et al. Activation in vagal afferents and central autonomic pathways: early responses to intestinal infection with Campylobacter jejuni. Brain Behav Immun. 2005;19(4):334–44.
288. Bercík P, De Giorgio R, Blennerhassett P, et al. Immunemediated neural dysfunction in a murine model of chronic Helico—bacter pylori infection. Gastroenterology. 2002;123(4):1. 205–15.
289. Bercik P, Verdú EF, Foster JA, et al. Role of gut-brain axis in persistent abnormal feeding behavior in mice following eradication of Helicobacter pylori infection. Am J Physiol Regul Integr Comp Physiol. 2009;296(3):R587–94.
290. Heijtz RD, Wang S, Anuar F, et al. Normal gut microbiota modulates brain development and behavior. Proc Natl Acad Sci USA. 2011;108(7):3.047-3.052.
291. Neufeld KM, Kang N, Bienenstock J, Foster JA. Reduced anxiety-like behavior and central neurochemical change in germ-free mice. Neurogastroenterol Motil. 2011;23(3):255–64.
292. Sudo N, Chida Y, Aiba Y, et al. Postnatal microbial colonization programs the hypothalamic-pituitary-adrenal system for stress response in mice. J Physiol. 2004;558(Pt 1):263–75.
293. Hooper LV, Wong MH, Thelin A, et al. Molecular analysis of commensal host-microbial relationships in the intestine. Science. 2001;291(5505):881–4.
294. Maksimova AA. Influence of pathological changes in intestinal microbiocenosis on the appearance or intensification of negative behavior in children with ASD. Int Res J. 2020;9(99):114–25. Part 1. - P. (In Russian)
295. Zatevalov AM, Selkova EP, Afanasyev SS, Aleshkin AV, Mironov AY, Gusarova MP, Gudova NV. Assessment of the degree of microbiological disorders of the microflora of the oropharynx and intestines using mathematical modeling methods. Clin Lab Diagn. 2016;61(2):117–21. (In Russian)
296. Zatevalov AM, Alyoshkin VA, Selkova EP, Grenkova TA. Determination of the concentration of butyric acid in feces, critical for the functional activity of normal intestinal and oropharyngeal microflora, of the concentration of butyric acid in the feces of patients of the intensive care unit and intensive care who are on tube feeding. Fundam Clin Med. 2017;2(1):14–22. (In Russian)
297. Kondrakova OA, Mazankova LN, Zatevalov AM, Begiashvili LV, Babin VN, Dubinin AV. Disorders of intestinal microbiocenosis in young children with secondary lactase deficiency. Russian Bull Perinatol Pediatr. 2008;53(2):74–81.
298. Kondrakova OA, Novikova TA, Eroshkina TD, Khachaturova EA, Zatevalov AM, Blinova OV, Musin II, Veresov KV, Balabashin AN. Correction of metabolic disorders in the early postoperative period in severe forms of ulcerative colitis and Crohn's disease. Russian J Gastroenterol Hepatol Coloproctol. 2003;4:63. (In Russian)
299. Chistyakova NV, Savostyanov KV. The hypothalamic-pituitary-adrenal axis and genetic variants affecting its activity. Genetics. 2011;47(8):1–13. (In Russian)
300. Strati F, Cavalieri D, Albanese D, De Felice C, Donati C, Hayek J, Jousson O, Leoncini S, Renzi D, Calabrò A, De Filippo C. New evidences on the altered gut microbiota in autism spectrum disorders. Microbiome. 2017;5(1):24. https://doi.org/10.1186/s40168-017-0242-1. PMID: 28222761; PMCID: PMC5320696
301. Qiao Y, Wu M, Feng Y, Zhou Z, Chen L, Chen F. Alterations of oral microbiota distinguish children with autism spectrum disorders from healthy controls. Sci Rep. 2018;8(1):1597. https://doi.org/10.1038/s41598-018-19982-y. PMID: 29371629; PMCID: PMC5785483
302. Ragusa M, Santagati M, Mirabella F, Lauretta G, Cirnigliaro M, Brex D, Barbagallo C, Domini CN, Gulisano M, Barone R, Trovato L. Potential Associations Among Alteration of Salivary miRNAs, saliva microbiome structure, and cognitive impairments in autistic children. Int J Mol Sci. 2020. 27 августа;21(17):6203. https://doi.org/10.3390/ijms21176203.

303. Simonova AV, Antonova IA, Pchelyakova VV. An interdisciplinary approach to the management of children with speech disorders. In the book: Innovative methods of prevention and correction of developmental disorders in children and adolescents. Collection of materials of the I international interdisciplinary scientific conference on April 17-18, 2019. Ed. HE. Usanova. M: Cogito-center, 2019. S: 240–242.
304. Nollace L, Cravero C, Abbou A, et al. Autism and COVID-19: a case series in a neurodevelopmental unit. J Clin Med. 2020;9(9):2937.
305. Xie M, Chen Q. Review Insight into 2019 novel coronavirus—An updated interim review and lessons from SARS-CoV and MERS-CoV. Int J Infect Dis. 2020;94:119–24.
306. Choi SH, Kim HW, Kang JM. Epidemiology and clinical features of coronavirus disease 2019 in children. Clin Exp Pediatr. 2020;63(4):125–32.
307. Christensen J, Grønborg TK, Sorensen MJ, et al. Prenatal valproate exposure and risk of autism spectrum disorders and childhood autism. JAMA. 2013;309(16):1696–703.
308. Parikshak NN, Luo R, Zhang A, et al. Integrative functional genomic analyzes implicate specific molecular pathways and circuits in autism. Cell. 2013;155(5):1008–21.
309. Tang Y, Liu J, Zhang D, Xu Z, Ji J, Wen C. Cytokine storm in COVID-19: the current evidence and treatment strategies. Front Immunol. 2020;11: 1708.
310. Edlow AG, Li JZ, Collier AY, et al. Assessment of maternal and neonatal SARS-CoV-2 viral load, transplacental antibody transfer, and placental pathology in pregnancies during the COVID-19 pandemic. JAMA Netw Open. 2020;3(12):e2030455.
311. Obregon D, Parker-Athill EC, Tan J, Murphy T. Psychotropic effects of antimicrobials and immune modulation by psychotropics: implications for neuroimmune disorders. Neuropsychiatry (London). 2012;2(4):331–43. https://doi.org/10.2217/npy.12.41.
312. Patterson PH. Maternal infection and immune involvement in autism. Trends Mol Med. 2011;17(7):389–94.
313. Brown AS, Derkits EJ. Review Prenatal infection and schizophrenia: a review of epidemiologic and translational studies. Am J Psychiatry. 2010;167(3):261–80.
314. Sciara AN, Beasley B, Crawford JD, et al. Neuroinflammatory gene expression alterations in anterior cingulate cortical white and gray matter of males with autism spectrum disorder. Autism Res. 2020;13(6):870–84.
315. Almehmadi KA, Tsilioni I, Theoharides TC. Increased expression of miR-155p5 in Amygdala of children with autism spectrum disorder. Autism Res. 2020;13(1):18–23.
316. Gumusoglu SB, Fine RS, Murray SJ, Bittle JL, Stevens HE. The role of IL-6 in neurodevelopment after prenatal stress. Brain Behav Immun. 2017;65:274–83.
317. Atladóttir HO, Thorsen P, Ostergaard L, et al. Maternal infection requiring hospitalization during pregnancy and autism spectrum disorders. J Autism Dev Disord. 2010;40:1423–30.
318. Musa SS, Bello UM, Zhao S, Abdullahi ZU, Lawan MA, He D. Vertical transmission of SARS-CoV-2: a systematic review of systematic reviews. Viruses. 2021;13(9):1877. Published 2021 Sep 20. https://doi.org/10.3390/v13091877.
319. Gasior M, Rogawski MA, Hartman AL. Neuroprotective and disease-modifying effects of the ketogenic diet. Behav Pharmacol. 2006;17(5-6):431–9. https://doi.org/10.1097/00008877-200609000-00009.
320. Bercik P, Verdu EF, Foster JA, et al. Chronic gastrointestinal inflammation induces anxiety-like behavior and alters central nervous system biochemistry in mice. Gastroenterology. 2010;139(6):2102–12.
321. Bercik P, Park AJ, Sinclair D, et al. The anxiolytic effect of Bifidobacterium longum NCC3001 involves vagal pathways for gut-brain communication. Neurogastroenterol Motil. 2011;23(12):1132–9.
322. Desbonnet L, Garrett L, Clarke G, et al. The probiotic Bifido - bacteria infantis: An assessment of potential antidepressant properties in the rat. J Psychiatr Res. 2008;43(2):164–74.
323. Desbonnet L, Garrett L, Clarke G, et al. Effects of the probiotic Bifidobacterium infantis in the maternal separation model of depression. Neuroscience. 2010;170(4):1179–88.
324. Bravo JA, Forsythe P, Chew MV, et al. Ingestion of Lactobacillus strain regulates emotional behavior and central GABA receptor expression in a mouse via the vagus nerve. Proc Natl Acad Sci USA. 2011;108(38):16050–5.

Conclusion. Questions Stay to be Investigated

This manual presents a variety of materials concerning many infectious lesions of the nervous system, especially those that are currently relevant for Russia. It is obvious that, despite the long history of studying neuroinfections and a significant number of works devoted to them, there are still a significant number of little or practically unexplored questions, which are of great theoretical and practical importance. In this regard, based on our many years of experience, we offer some provisions that should be taken into account when studying any infectious pathology of the nervous system: (1) The central nervous system is affected by all general laws of the infectious process, which involves a pathogen that is tropic to the affected tissue, characterized by an individual, sometimes changing properties during the disease and causing characteristic damage and response (inflammatory, immune, neuroendocrine, etc.) reactions of the body, the qualitative and quantitative characteristics of which depend on the general state of the host organism, the localization of the process, and the characteristics of the pathogen. (2) All infectious processes in the central nervous system can be classified according to: 1) ways of infection: neurogenic, hematogenic, contact, mixed; (2) features of course: acute, chronic, latent, slow infection, and carrier; (3) prevalence of the process: diffuse and focal (with damage to certain specific structures); (4) the nature of cellular reactions; and (5) etiology. (3) Infectious processes in the central nervous system are characterized by a number of significant features associated with the existence of the blood-brain barrier, which has a different structure in different zones and changes its properties during the disease, the ability to locally synthesize antibodies, interferons, and peptides with protective properties, the rapid loss of bactericidal properties by neutrophil granulocytes behind the BBB, while immune complexes lose their cytolytic properties. This creates the prerequisites for the formation of chronic, latent, and slow infections. The ineffectiveness of the functioning of neutrophils in the central nervous system leads to relatively more frequent adverse outcomes, including in the catamnesis. (4) Etiological diagnosis of infectious processes in the central nervous system must necessarily include the study of locally taken materials (CSF, brain tissue); the data obtained from the study of blood, nasopharyngeal flushes, etc. are not always informative. (5) In morphological studies, it is important to distinguish typical pathological processes: "ischemic" and "severe" changes in nerve cells, satellite disease, neuronophagy, replacement proliferation of astrocytic glia, vasculitis, pericellular and perivascular edema, demyelination, and changes characteristic of a certain etiology of the process, among which, along with the features of the inflammatory reaction, the most important role is played by cellular transformation, including the appearance of various variants of inclusions. Among the problems that, according to our view, need a comprehensive study, I would like to name, first of all, the study of the immune response in the brain cells. At the same time,

V. Zinserling, *Infectious Lesions of the Central Nervous System*,
https://doi.org/10.1007/978-3-030-96260-9

along with the study of complex cytokine interactions, it is very important to accurately topographically localize the phenomena that occur. The complement system in the central nervous system also needs a more precise characterization, since its features are presumably associated with the absence of both the cytolytic action of antibodies and the bactericidal action of neutrophils. The mechanisms of various cellular reactions, including the death of nerve cells, also need to be described in detail. The mechanisms of demyelination are not fully understood.

The nature of the interaction of many pathogens with CNS cells is also subject to clarification. The issue of long-term outcomes of perinatal infection of the central nervous system, which is almost not covered in the literature, is extremely important, both practically and theoretically. This list, of course, can be continued, including at the expense of questions concerning almost all individual nosological forms.

Currently, it is generally recognized that along with diseases belonging to the I class of ICD (infectious diseases), many other human diseases are associated with direct or indirect effects of biological pathogens. Nowadays, the "infectious component" is intensively studied in the pathogenesis of not only diseases such as pneumonia, cirrhosis of the liver, and pyelonephritis, but also many tumors, atherosclerosis, diabetes, bronchial asthma, glomerulonephritis, and other less common diseases. Neurology/neuropathology is no exception to the general trend—attempts continue to discuss the possible infectious nature of many diseases. It is obvious that the exact identification of pathogens that are in persistent and latent states and the proof of their significance in the most complex pathogenetic chains in many cases are significantly complicated by the methodological capabilities of modern science.

Significant progress in solving many of the issues raised in this chapter can only be achieved by using, along with a full-fledged classical morphological study, the entire arsenal of modern methods, primarily immunohistochemistry (including immunofluorescence microscopy), hybridization and PCR in situ, and confocal and electron microscopy. It should also be noted that in many cases we have to deal with combined pathology; in particular, lesions caused by biological pathogens can be combined with tumors, ischemic injuries, injuries, and malformations. In many cases, such combinations may have pathogenetic significance. Thus, it was shown that glioblastoma contamination with the herpes simplex virus is combined with increased endothelial cell proliferation and activation of angiogenesis and correlates with early tumor recurrence.

One of the most important questions in the modern neurosciences is neuroplasticity involved in development and aging of the brain and outcomes of different diseases. The linkage between neuroplasticity and biological pathogens has been discussed rarely, but we have to accept the possibility of direct lesions of different populations of progenitor cells by certain viruses, chlamydia, and mycoplasma and indirect mechanisms as well. Among the latter, very promising seems to be the study of toll-like receptors, which according to the modern data are involved in both innate immune response in the brain and proliferation and differentiation of neural progenitor cells.

It is obvious that the solution of these and other issues, which may not yet be formulated by anyone, is possible only with the use of the entire arsenal of modern molecular biological and radiological research methods. At the same time, sufficiently complete information can be obtained only by projecting the studied processes onto certain structures, i.e., by using modern morphological methods to study experimental and autopsy material. Pathomorphological tests designed to assess the neurovirulence of vaccine virus strains are also important in the development of vaccination methods.

In recent years, significant advances have been made in the diagnosis and treatment of infectious lesions of the central nervous system. All this led to a significant reduction in mortality in this pathology. However, further progress in the treatment of neuroinfections is possible only with a more complete account of the features of the course of infectious processes in the central nervous system.

Printed in Great Britain
by Amazon

44119581R00209